FIFTH CANADIAN EDITION

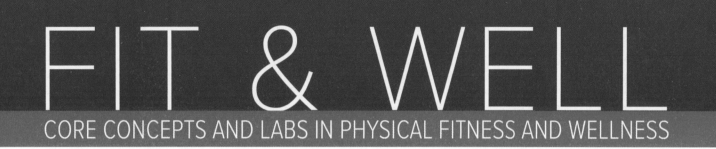

FIT & WELL

CORE CONCEPTS AND LABS IN PHYSICAL FITNESS AND WELLNESS

Thomas D. Fahey
California State University, Chico

Paul M. Insel
Stanford University

Walton T. Roth
Stanford University

Ilsa E. Wong
University of Lethbridge

Mc
Graw
Hill
Education

Fit & Well: Core Concepts and Labs in Physical Fitness and Wellness
Fifth Canadian Edition

The Internet addresses listed in the text were accurate at the time of publication. The inclusion of a Web site does not indicate an endorsement by the authors or McGraw-Hill Ryerson, and McGraw-Hill Ryerson does not guarantee the accuracy of the information presented at these sites.

ISBN-13: 978-1-25-965471-8
ISBN-10: 1-25-965471-0

1 2 3 4 5 6 7 8 9 0 TCP 1 2 3 4 5 6 7 8 9

Printed and bound in Canada.

Product Director, Canada: *Rhondda McNabb*
Portfolio Manager: *Alex Campbell*
Senior Marketing Manager: *Patti Rozakos*
Content Developer: *Melissa Hudson*
Senior Product Team Associate: *Stephanie Giles*
Supervising Editor: *Janie Deneau*
Photo/Permissions Editor: *Nadine Bachan*
Copy Editor: *Janice Dyer*
Plant Production Coordinator: *Sarah Strynatka*
Manufacturing Production Coordinator: *Jason Stubner*
Cover Design: *Michelle Losier*
Cover Image: © *Blend Images — Erik Isakson*
Interior Design: *Dianne Reynolds / Liz Harasymczuk*
Page Layout: *MPS Limited*
Printer: *Transcontinental Printing Group*

Brief Contents

Contents

CHAPTER 4

Muscular Strength and Endurance   138

CHAPTER 5

Flexibility and Low-Back Health   210

Contents

Contents

Contents

Wellness in the Digital Age

LABORATORY EXERCISES **connect**

Preface

For today's fitness-conscious university/college student, the fifth Canadian edition of *Fit & Well* combines the best of two worlds. In the area of physical fitness, *Fit & Well* offers expert knowledge based on the latest findings in exercise physiology and nutrition, along with tools for self-assessment and guidelines for becoming fit. In the area of wellness, it offers accurate, current information on today's most important health-related topics and issues, again with self-tests and guidelines for achieving wellness. The text provides comprehensive advice on wellness-related behaviour and practising a healthier way of life, as well as thorough coverage of health-related fitness and nutrition. *Fit & Well* provides the reader with comprehensive advice on making informed choices about food and promotes behavioural change throughout the text. Making informed choices is the *Fit & Well* difference.

Content and Organization of the Fifth Canadian Edition

In the fifth Canadian edition of *Fit & Well,* the organization of the text follows the format of fitness and wellness courses. Instructors do not have to jump around in the text to meet the needs of their course.

Chapter 1 provides an introduction to fitness and wellness and explains the principles of behaviour change. Chapters 2, 3, 4, 5, 6, and 9 focus on the various areas of fitness.

Chapter 2 provides an overview, discussing the components of fitness, the principles of physical training, and the factors involved in designing a well-rounded, personalized exercise program.

Chapter 3 provides basic information on how the cardiorespiratory system functions, how the body produces energy for exercise, and how individuals can create successful cardiorespiratory fitness programs. Information has also been added to Chapter 3 on the benefits of cardiorespiratory endurance exercise for children and adolescents.

Chapters 4, 5, and 6 look at muscular strength and endurance, flexibility and low-back health, and body composition. Sections include core strength training and the physiology of stretching, with added information on training with and without equipment.

Chapters 7 and 8 explore nutrition and weight management and their impact on the physical dimension of wellness. This edition includes information on alternate diets such as First Nations, Métis, and Inuit, and the Vegetarian Food Guide Pyramid.

Chapter 9 "puts it all together," describing the nature of a complete program that develops all the components of fitness. This chapter also includes complete sample exercise programs.

Chapters 10 and 11 focus on two of the most important reasons for making lifestyle changes: cardiovascular disease and cancer. Students learn the basic mechanisms of these diseases, how they are related to lifestyle, and what individuals can do to prevent them.

Chapter 12 discusses stress and its relationship to disease. The chapter also describes ways to manage your stress to reduce your risk for those disease processes.

Finally, Chapter 13 looks at additional wellness topics such as aging, the health care system, and environmental health before finishing with a reminder about wellness for life.

Chapter 14 Substance Use and Misuse, and Chapter 15 Sexually Transmitted Infections (STIs) are now found online.

There are some significant changes to this fifth edition. For example, a revamped **Strengthening Mental Wellness** box has been included in many chapters. This box aims to incorporate information and tips on challenging the mental wellness dimension in each chapter topic. In addition, chapters now include **new and up-to-date photos** that better depict activities for areas such as flexibility and muscle training.

The fifth Canadian edition of *Fit & Well* has also been completely revised to include updated Canadian examples, references, data, and statistics. Coverage of the latest version of Canada's Food Guide has been included, along with information from Canada's Physical Activity Guide, the Canadian Society for Exercise Physiologists, and the Canadian Association for Health, Physical Education, Recreation, and Dance (CAHPERD).

Chapter-by-Chapter Changes

Chapter 1, Introduction to Wellness, Fitness, and Lifestyle Management

- Discussions of dimensions of wellness are expanded to include cultural and occupational wellness.

- The discussions of the National Wellness Goals are refined to focus on the newest round of initiatives to tackle obesity in Canada.

- All of the chapter's considerable statistical material is updated to reflect the latest information on causes of death, life expectancy, and measures of quality of life.

Chapter 2, Basic Principles of Physical Fitness

- Includes the most recent statistics available from Statistics Canada and the Physical Activity Monitors on the physical activity and exercise habits of Canadians.

- A new Fitness Tip on progressive overload is provided.

Chapter 3, Cardiorespiratory Endurance

- A **Take Charge** feature discusses high-intensity training programs.

- Updated coverage of warm-up and cool-down, high-intensity interval training, and cross-training is included.

Chapter 4, Muscular Strength and Endurance

- Discusses the many ways to develop muscular strength and endurance without going to the gym and includes a bank of photos to help students carry out these exercises.

- Expanded information is provided on the use of stability balls and core training.

Chapter 5, Flexibility and Low-Back Health

- Includes a new figure illustrating the core musculature.

- A new **Wellness Tip** discusses the benefits of a rehabilitation program after injury or surgery.

Chapter 6, Body Composition

- Includes newly updated statistics from Statistics Canada on the prevalence of overweight and obesity in Canada.

- Introduces a new **Wellness Tip** feature on Type 2 diabetes.

- A number of new **Strengthening Mental Wellness** boxes are provided in this chapter.

Chapter 7, Nutrition

- The entire chapter has been updated, where applicable, to discuss the Food and Nutrition Board and Health Canada's Guidelines for Canadians.

- A new **Wellness Tip** helps students understand the potential for low fat foods to be unhealthy.

- Health Canada recommendations for fish consumption are provided.

Chapter 8, Weight Management

- Reiterates the latest statistics on overweight and obesity in Canada, and discusses the health implications of overweight and obesity.

- Challenges students to examine their own weight, think of reasons they may have gained weight, and list ways they can begin reducing their weight right away.

- A new **In Focus** feature about nutritional and workout supplementation helps inform decision-making.

Chapter 9, Putting Together a Complete Fitness Program

- A new Evidence for Exercise feature on the importance of reducing sedentary time is included.

- Provides updated coverage of apps for tracking and motivation during a fitness program.

Chapter 10, Cardiovascular Health

- Updated statistics on incidence, prevalence, and deaths reflect the latest available data.

- Updated information on CVD prevention strategies, metabolic syndrome, and drugs and CVD risk factors is included.

Chapter 11, Cancer

- Includes updated statistics on new cases and deaths from the major forms of cancer.

- A new section on detecting and treating cancer informs students about these important aspects of the disease.

Chapter 12, Stress

- Includes updated statistics on stress and stress management techniques.

- New sections on Type D personality and an enhanced discussion of how gender influences stress are provided.

Chapter 13, Wellness for Life

- Updated statistics in this chapter reflect current information.

- Emphasizes the concept of sustainability, including sustainable energy and sustainable development, and the potential positive impact of sustainable practices on the environment.

- Includes an expanded discussion related to air quality and smog, the greenhouse effect, and global warming.

Chapter 14, Substance Use and Misuse (available on ▣ connect)

- Includes updated statistics on alcohol use and abuse based on the latest data from sources such as Health Canada and the Canadian Addictions Survey.

- Statistics on alcohol-related accidents, injuries, deaths, and arrests are updated.

- Statistics on tobacco use are updated based on the latest data from the Canadian Community Health Survey and Health Canada.

Chapter 15, Sexually Transmitted Infections (STIs) (available on ▣ connect)

- Statistics throughout the chapter are updated to reflect the latest available information from sources such as the Public Health Agency of Canada, the World Health Organization, and the Canadian Public Health Association.

- New information on HIV testing and HPV vaccination is included.

Key Features and Learning Aids

The *Fit & Well* learning system continues to provide the information students need to start their journey to fitness and wellness. *Fit & Well's* authoritative, science-based information is written by experts who work and teach in the field of exercise science, physical education, and health education. *Fit & Well* provides accurate, reliable, and current information on key health and fitness topics, while also addressing issues related to mind–body health, research, diversity, gender, and consumer health. Text features and interactive activities include self-assessments and fitness labs, a daily fitness and nutrition log, sample programs, and a wealth of behaviour change tools and tips. If marked in the Table of Contents, additional content for box features can be found on Connect.

Critical Consumer boxes help students navigate the numerous and diverse set of health-related products currently available.

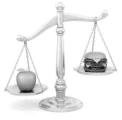

Diversity Matters boxes address the ways in which our personal backgrounds influence our health strengths, risks, and behaviours.

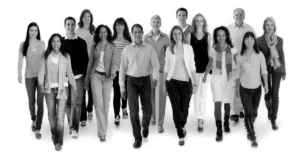

The Evidence for Exercise boxes demonstrate that physical activity and exercise recommendations are based on solid scientific evidence.

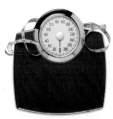

In Focus boxes explore current trends and topics in fitness and wellness, such as high-intensity training and exercising with kettlebells, stability balls, and medicine balls.

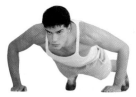

Take Charge boxes distill from the text the practical advice students need to apply information to their own lives.

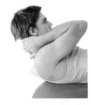

Wellness in the Digital Age boxes focus on the many new fitness and wellness-related devices and applications that are available every day.

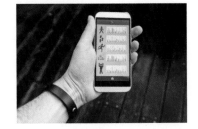

Learning Objectives

Each chapter begins with a list of **Learning Objectives** that preview the main points of the chapter.

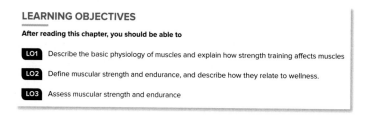

LEARNING OBJECTIVES

After reading this chapter, you should be able to

LO1 Describe the basic physiology of muscles and explain how strength training affects muscles

LO2 Define muscular strength and endurance, and describe how they relate to wellness.

LO3 Assess muscular strength and endurance

Test Your Knowledge

Each chapter opens with **Test Your Knowledge**—a series of three multiple choice and true-false questions, with answers. These self-quizzes facilitate learning by emphasizing key points, highlighting common misconceptions, and sparking debate.

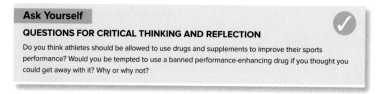

TEST YOUR KNOWLEDGE

1. **For women, weight training typically results in which of the following?**
   a. bulky muscles
   b. significant increases in body weight
   c. improved body image
2. **To maximize strength gains, it is a good idea to hold your breath as you lift a weight.**
   True or false?

Ask Yourself

Ask Yourself questions help students retain what they've learned in each chapter by applying and examining the concepts.

Ask Yourself

QUESTIONS FOR CRITICAL THINKING AND REFLECTION

Do you think athletes should be allowed to use drugs and supplements to improve their sports performance? Would you be tempted to use a banned performance-enhancing drug if you thought you could get away with it? Why or why not?

Fitness and Wellness Tips

Fitness and Wellness Tips catch students' attention and get them thinking—and doing something—about their fitness and wellness.

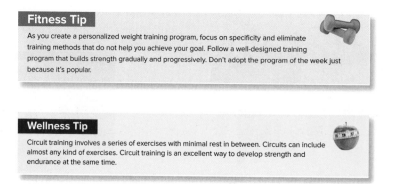

Fitness Tip

As you create a personalized weight training program, focus on specificity and eliminate training methods that do not help you achieve your goal. Follow a well-designed training program that builds strength gradually and progressively. Don't adopt the program of the week just because it's popular.

Wellness Tip

Circuit training involves a series of exercises with minimal rest in between. Circuits can include almost any kind of exercises. Circuit training is an excellent way to develop strength and endurance at the same time.

Strengthening Mental Wellness

The new **Strengthening Mental Wellness** boxes allow students to consider the relationship of their mental dimension with each chapter topic. These boxes serve to reinforce the need to prioritize this dimension whenever possible.

> **Strengthening Mental Wellness**
>
> Another way to contribute toward your behaviour change is to be confident about your ability to create change. Adopt a positive outlook, take pride in your good qualities while recognizing your insecurities, and live in the present. Engage in the process so that you become a participant of change.

Career Options In . . .

Career Options In . . . boxes introduce students to different career paths related to the particular chapter topic.

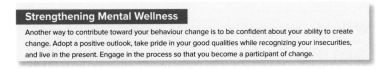

> **CAREER OPTIONS IN...**
>
> **MUSCLE FITNESS**
>
> **Rehabilitation:** kinesiologist, massage therapist, soft-tissue specialist
>
> **Community:** ergonomist/equipment designer, strength coach, fitness consultant

Vital Statistics

Vital Statistics tables and figures highlight issues such as the leading causes of death in Canada and the factors that play a part in each one; the relationship between lifestyle and quality of life; public health achievements of the twentieth century; the most popular fitness activities; the effects of binge drinking on college and university students; and a wealth of other information. For students who learn best when material is displayed graphically or numerically, Vital Statistics tables and figures offer a way to grasp information quickly and directly.

TABLE 1.2

Leading Causes of Death Among Canadians Aged 1 to 24 years, 2013

Rank	Cause of Death	Percentage (of 2622 total deaths)
1	Accidents	36
2	Suicide	16
3	Cancer	11

Glossary

Within each eBook chapter, important terms appear as pop-tip annotations, helping students handle new vocabulary. In the print edition text, important terms are defined in a **running glossary.**

> **slow-twitch fibres**   Red muscle fibres that are fatigue-resistant but have a slow contraction speed and a lower capacity for tension; usually recruited for endurance activities.
> **fast-twitch fibres**   White muscle fibres that contract rapidly and forcefully but fatigue quickly; usually recruited for actions requiring strength and power.
> **intermediate fibres**   A muscled fibre that responds somewhere in between the speed, endurance, and contractile force of slow- and fast-twitch fibres.

Illustrated Exercise Sections

To ensure students understand how to perform important exercises and stretches, the fifth Canadian edition of *Fit & Well* includes three **illustrated exercise sections,** one in Chapter 4 and two in Chapter 5. The section in Chapter 4 covers exercises for developing muscular strength and endurance, as performed with your body weight, with free weights, and using weight machines. One section in Chapter 5 presents stretches for flexibility, and the other presents exercises to stretch and strengthen the lower back. Each exercise is illustrated with one or more full-colour photographs showing proper technique. Digital video clips of the exercises from the text and key lab activities are available online.

Weight Training Exercises: Body Weight

connect

Exercise 1

Air Squats

Instructions:

(photo a) Keep your back straight and head level; stand with feet slightly more than shoulder-width apart and toes pointed slightly outward.

Sample Programs

To help students get started, Chapter 9 offers four complete **sample programs** designed to develop overall fitness. The programs are built around four popular activities: walking/jogging/running, bicycling, swimming, and rowing machine. They include strength training and stretching exercises. Each program includes detailed information about technique and guidelines for using equipment; target intensity, duration, and frequency; record keeping; and adjustments to make as fitness improves. The chapter also includes general guidelines for putting together a personal fitness program: setting goals; selecting activities; setting targets for intensity, duration, and frequency; maintaining a commitment; and recording and assessing progress.

SAMPLE PROGRAMS FOR POPULAR ACTIVITIES

The following sections present sample programs based on different types of cardiorespiratory activities—walking/jogging/running and calisthenics circuit training. Each sample program includes regular cardiorespiratory endurance exercise, resistance training, and stretching. Read the descriptions of the programs you're considering, and decide which will work best for you based on your present routine, the potential for enjoyment, and adaptability to your lifestyle. If you choose one of these programs, complete the personal fitness program plan in Lab 9.1, just as if you had created a program from scratch.

Tips for Today and the Future

Chapter-ending **Tips for Today and the Future** sections provide a very brief distillation of the major message of each chapter, followed by suggestions for a few simple things that students can try right away and in the near future. Tips for Today and the Future are designed to encourage students and to build their confidence by giving them easy steps they can take immediately and in the next few days and weeks to improve their wellness.

Tips for Today and the Future

You don't need a complicated or heavy training program to improve strength: Just one set of 8 to 12 repetitions of 8 to 10 exercises, done 2 to 4 days per week, is enough for general fitness.

RIGHT NOW YOU CAN

• Do a set of static (isometric) exercises. If you're sitting, try tightening your abdominal muscles as you press your lower back into the seat or work your arms by placing the palms of your hands on top of your thighs and pressing down. Hold the contraction for 6 seconds and do 5 to 10 repetitions; don't hold your breath.

• Think of three things you've done in the past 24 hours that would have been easier or more enjoyable if you increased your level of muscular strength and endurance. Visualize improvements in your quality of life that could come from increased muscular strength and endurance.

Common Questions Answered

Sections called **Common Questions Answered** appear at the end of most of the chapters. In these student-friendly sections, the answers to frequently asked questions are presented in easy-to-understand terms. Included are such questions as these: "Do I need more protein in my diet when I train with weights?" "How can I safely increase exercise intensity to build fitness?" "Can physical training limit flexibility?" and "How can I tell if I'm allergic to a food?"

Common Questions ANSWERED

Q I have asthma. Is it OK for me to start an exercise program?
A Probably, but you should see your doctor before you start exercising, especially if you have been sedentary up to this point. Your personal physician can advise you on the type of exercise program that is best for you given the severity of your condition, and how to avoid suffering exercise-related asthma attacks.
Q What should my fitness goals be?
A Begin by thinking about your general overall goals—the benefits you want to obtain by increasing your activity level and/or beginning a formal exercise program. Examples of long-term goals include reducing your risk of chronic diseases, increasing your energy level, and maintaining a healthy body weight.

Chapter Summaries

Chapter summaries offer students a concise review and a way to make sure they have grasped the most important concepts in the chapter.

SUMMARY

- Hypertrophy, or increased muscle fibre size, occurs when weight training causes the number of myofibrils to increase; total muscle size thereby increases. Strength also increases through muscle learning. Most women do not develop large muscles from weight training.
- Improvements in muscular strength and endurance lead to enhanced physical performance, protection against injury, improved body composition, better self-image, improved muscle and bone health with aging, reduced risk of chronic disease, and decreased risk of premature death.

For Further Exploration

End-of-chapter **For Further Exploration** sections offer suggestions for student resources that can be found online to build fitness and wellness.

FOR FURTHER EXPLORATION

Organizations and Websites

Canada's Physical Activity Guide. Offers many suggestions for incorporating physical activity into everyday life.
http://www.phac-aspc.gc.ca/pau-uap/paguide/

Hands-on Laboratory Activities

To help students apply the principles of fitness and wellness to their own lives, *Fit & Well* includes **laboratory activities** for classroom use. These hands-on activities give students the opportunity to assess their current level of fitness and wellness, to create plans for changing their lifestyle to reach wellness, and to monitor their progress. They can assess their daily physical activity, for example, or their level of cardiorespiratory endurance; they can design a program to improve muscular strength or meet weight-loss goals; and they can explore their risk of developing cardiovascular disease or cancer. Many labs end with a section labelled "Using Your Results," which guides students in evaluating their scores, setting goals for change, and moving forward. Labs are found at the end of each chapter and are also available in an interactive format online.

Quick-Reference Appendices

Included at the end of the book are two appendices containing vital information in an easy-to-use format.

Appendix A, **Nutritional Content of Popular Food Items**, provides students with a link to assess their nutritional intake with Health Canada's Canadian Nutrient File. This appendix also lists some common fast food restaurant URLs for students to access nutrition guides.

Appendix B, **Monitoring Your Progress**, is a log that enables students to record and summarize the results of the assessment tests they complete as part of the laboratory activities. With space for preprogram and postprogram assessment results, the log provides an easy way to track the progress of a behaviour change program.

Behaviour Change Workbook (Available on ▣ connect)

The **Behaviour Change Workbook** contains 15 separate activities that complement the lifestyle management model presented in Chapter 1. The workbook guides students in developing a successful program by walking them through each of the steps of behaviour change—from choosing a target behaviour to completing and signing an agreement. It also includes activities to help students overcome common obstacles to behaviour change.

Teaching and Learning Tools

Mc Graw Hill Education connect®

Learn without Limits

McGraw-Hill Connect® is an award-winning digital teaching and learning platform that gives students the means to better connect with their coursework, with their instructors, and with the important concepts that they will need to know for success now and in the future. With Connect, instructors can take advantage of McGraw-Hill Education's trusted content to seamlessly deliver assignments, quizzes, and tests online. McGraw-Hill Connect is a learning platform that continually adapts to each student, delivering precisely what they need, when they need it, so class time is more engaging and effective. Connect makes teaching and learning personal, easy, and proven.

Connect Key Features:

SmartBook®

As the first and only adaptive reading experience, SmartBook is changing the way students read and learn. SmartBook creates a personalized reading experience by highlighting the most important concepts a student needs to learn at that moment in time. While engaging with SmartBook, the reading experience continuously adapts by highlighting content based on what each student knows and doesn't know. This ensures that the student is focused on the content needed to close specific knowledge gaps, while simultaneously promoting long-term learning.

Connect Insight®

Connect Insight is Connect's new one-of-a-kind visual analytics dashboard—now available for instructors—that provides at-a-glance information regarding student performance, which is immediately actionable. By presenting assignment, assessment, and topical performance results together with a time metric that is easily visible for aggregate or individual results, Connect Insight gives instructors the ability to take a just-in-time approach to teaching and learning, which was never before available. Connect Insight presents data that helps instructors improve class performance in a way that is efficient and effective.

Simple Assignment Management

With Connect, creating assignments is easier than ever, so instructors can spend more time teaching and less time managing.

- Assign SmartBook learning modules.
- Edit existing questions and create their own questions.
- Draw from a variety of text specific questions, assignable videos, resources, and test bank material to assign online.
- Streamline lesson planning, student progress reporting, and assignment grading to make classroom management more efficient than ever.

Smart Grading

When it comes to studying, time is precious. Connect helps students learn more efficiently by providing feedback and practice material when they need it, where they need it.

- Automatically score assignments, giving students immediate feedback on their work and comparisons with correct answers.
- Access and review each response; manually change grades or leave comments for students to review.
- Track individual student performance—by question, assignment or in relation to the class overall—with detailed grade reports.
- Reinforce classroom concepts with practice tests and instant quizzes.
- Integrate grade reports easily with Learning Management Systems including Blackboard, D2L, and Moodle.

Mobile Access

Connect makes it easy for students to read and learn using their smartphones and tablets. With the mobile app, students can study on the go – including reading and listening using the audio functionality – without constant need for internet access.

Instructor Library

The Connect Instructor Library is a repository for additional resources to improve student engagement in and out of the class. It provides all the critical resources instructors need to build their course.

- Access Instructor resources.
- View assignments and resources created for past sections.
- Post your own resources for students to use.

Instructor Resources

- *Instructor's Manual*
- *Computerized Test Bank*
- *Microsoft® PowerPoint® Slides*

Superior Learning Solutions and Support

The McGraw-Hill Education team is ready to help instructors assess and integrate any of our products, technology, and services into your course for optimal teaching and learning performance. Whether it's helping your students improve their grades, or putting your entire course online, the McGraw-Hill Education team is here to help you do it. Contact your Learning Solutions Consultant today to learn how to maximize all of McGraw-Hill Education's resources.

For more information, please visit us online: **http://www.mheducation.ca/he/solutions**

Acknowledgments

Extensive feedback from numerous reviews and the valuable suggestions provided through that process helped to develop this fifth Canadian edition. Thank you to the following colleagues for their invaluable advice:

Renee Hober-Rose, *Conestoga College*
Michael Kennedy, *University of Alberta*
Emilio Landolfi, *University of the Fraser Valley*
Julie Rissler, *Algonquin College*

Many thanks to the McGraw-Hill Education team of Alex Campbell, Portfolio Manager and Margaret Greenfield, Senior Marketing Manager; with special mention of Melissa Hudson, Content Developer; Janie Deneau, Supervising Editor; and Janice Dyer, Copy Editor; whose help in navigating the "habitat" we work in has been instrumental in completing this edition. Additional gratitude to Sophie Verzosa and our many students who continue to provide feedback along the way.

Ilsa E. Wong
University of Lethbridge

Fit & Well Disclaimer

The information in this textbook is for general educational purposes only. It does not and is not intended to provide medical advice, recommendations, diagnosis, or treatment. This textbook is a general resource for non-medical university students and does not qualify the reader to provide medical advice, recommendations, diagnosis, or treatment. It is not a substitute for professional medical advice, recommendations, diagnosis, or treatment, and readers should never disregard professional medical advice, or delay seeking such advice, because of information contained in this textbook.

General Disclaimer

While reasonable efforts have been made to ensure the accuracy, timeliness, and completeness of the information contained in this textbook at the time of its preparation, it may contain errors. More recent information may have become available, which may make the information contained in this textbook incomplete or inaccurate.

The information contained in this textbook is provided "as is" without warranty of any kind. Neither McGraw-Hill Ryerson Limited, nor the authors, contributors, and/or editors assume any responsibility for any errors, omissions or inaccuracies in the information contained in this textbook or for the use of any information contained in this textbook. To the fullest extent permitted by law, McGraw-Hill Ryerson Limited and the authors, contributors, and/or editors disclaim all warranties, representations, and conditions of any kind, whether express or implied, including the implied warranties of merchantability and fitness for a particular purpose, with respect to the information contained in the textbook. In no event will McGraw-Hill Ryerson Limited, or any of the authors, editors, or contributors be liable for any damages of any kind (including, without limitation, direct, indirect, incidental, consequential, special, exemplary, and punitive damages), lost profits, personal injury (including death), fines, fees, penalties or other liabilities, resulting from the use of the information contained in this textbook.

This textbook includes references to third party materials, including websites, papers, and other resources, for your convenience. Neither McGraw-Hill Ryerson Limited nor the authors, editors, or contributors is responsible for the content of third-party materials, and makes no representations as to their accuracy, timeliness, or completeness. Any reference to a product or service in this textbook is not an endorsement of or by such product or service.

This textbook may contain information which you may find offensive. Any opinions expressed in this textbook are those of the authors, editors, and/or contributors, and do not reflect the opinion of McGraw-Hill Ryerson Limited and its employees.

CHAPTER 1

Introduction to Wellness, Fitness, and Lifestyle Management

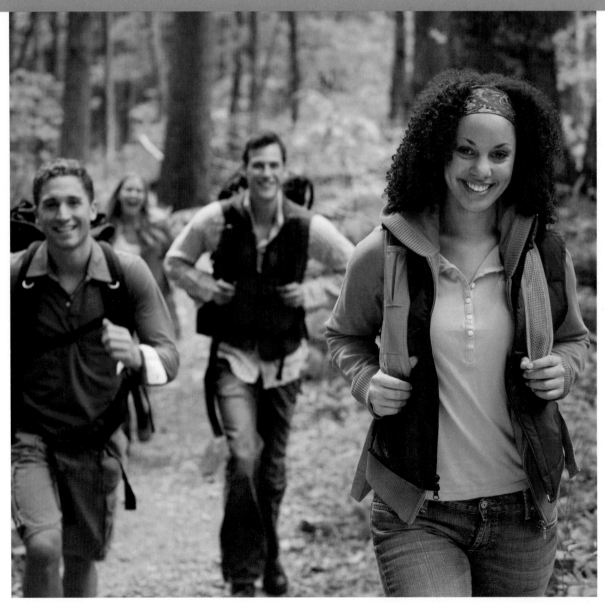

© rubberball / Getty RF

LEARNING OBJECTIVES

After reading this chapter, you should be able to

LO1   Describe the dimensions of wellness

LO2   Identify the major health problems in Canada today and discuss their causes

LO3   Describe the behaviours that are part of a wellness lifestyle

LO4   List some of the available sources of wellness information and explain how to think critically about them

LO5   Explain the steps in creating a behaviour management plan to change a wellness-related behaviour

TEST YOUR KNOWLEDGE

1. **Which of the following lifestyle factors is the leading preventable cause of death for Canadians?**
   a. excess alcohol consumption
   b. cigarette smoking
   c. obesity

2. **The terms *health* and *wellness* mean the same thing.**

   True or false?

3. **Which of the following health-related issues affects the greatest number of university/college students each year?**
   a. stress
   b. colds/flu/sore throat
   c. sleep problems
   d. concern for a friend or family member

ANSWERS

1. **B.** Smoking contributes to more than 37 000 deaths per year; poor diet and inactivity are responsible for about 21 000 deaths; and alcohol contributes to about 4300 deaths.

2. **FALSE.** Although the words are used interchangeably, they actually have different meanings. The term *health* refers to the overall condition of the body or mind and to the presence or absence of illness or injury. The term *wellness* refers to optimal health and vitality, encompassing all the dimensions of well-being.

3. **A.** About 27% of university/college students suffer so much stress that it affects their academic performance. High stress levels affect overall health and wellness, making it important to learn effective stress management techniques.

A university/college student sets the following goals:

- join in new social circles and make new friends whenever possible
- exercise every day
- clean up trash and plant trees in blighted neighbourhoods in the community

These goals may differ, but they have one thing in common: each contributes, in its own way, to this student's health and well-being. Not satisfied merely to be free of illness, this student wants more, and has decided to live actively and fully—not just to be healthy, but to pursue a state of overall wellness.

1.1 Wellness: The New Health Goal

Generations of people have viewed health simply as the absence of disease, and that view largely prevails today. The word **health** typically refers to the overall condition of a person's body or mind. **Wellness** expands this idea of health to include our ability to achieve optimal health. Beyond the simple presence or absence of disease, wellness refers to optimal health and vitality—to living life to its fullest. Although we use the words *health* and *wellness* interchangeably, there are two important differences between them:

- Health—or some aspects of it—can be determined or influenced by factors beyond your control, such as your genes, age, and family history. For example, a man with a strong family history of prostate cancer will have a higher-than-average risk for developing prostate cancer.
- Wellness is largely determined by the decisions you make about how you live. That same man can reduce his risk of cancer by eating sensibly, exercising, and having regular screening tests. Even if he develops the disease, he may still rise above its effects to live a rich, meaningful life. This means not only caring for himself physically, but also maintaining a positive outlook, keeping up his relationships with others, challenging himself intellectually, and nurturing other aspects of his life.

health   The overall condition of body or mind and the presence or absence of illness or injury.
wellness   Optimal health and vitality, encompassing the seven dimensions of well-being.

Enhanced wellness, therefore, involves making conscious decisions to control **risk factors** that contribute to disease or injury. Age and family history are risk factors you cannot control. Behaviours such as choosing not to smoke, exercising, and eating a healthy diet are well within your control.

risk factors   Conditions that increase one's chances of disease or injury.

LO1 The Dimensions of Wellness

Here are nine dimensions of wellness:

- physical
- emotional
- intellectual
- interpersonal
- cultural

- spiritual

- environmental

- financial

- occupational

Each dimension of wellness affects the others. Further, the process of achieving wellness is constant and dynamic (Figure 1.1), involving change and growth. Ignoring any dimension of wellness can have harmful effects on your life. The following sections briefly introduce the dimensions of wellness. Figure 1.2 (on the next page) lists some of the specific qualities and behaviours associated with each dimension. Lab 1.1 will help you learn what wellness means to you and where you fall on the wellness continuum.

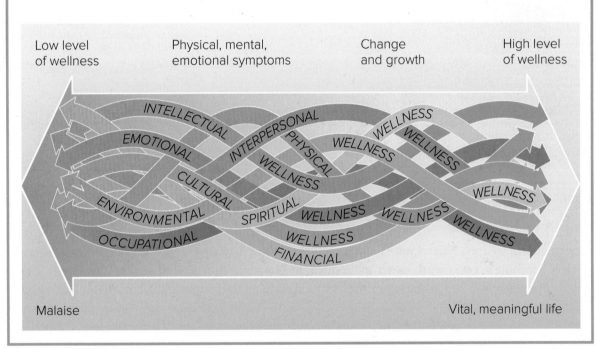

FIGURE 1.1

The wellness continuum. The concept of wellness includes vitality in nine interrelated dimensions, all of which contribute to overall wellness.

Low level of wellness

Physical, mental, emotional symptoms

Change and growth

High level of wellness

Malaise

Vital, meaningful life

Physical Wellness

Your physical wellness includes not just your body's overall condition and the absence of disease, but also your fitness level and your ability to care for yourself. The higher your fitness level (which is discussed throughout this book), the higher your level of physical wellness will be. Similarly, as you develop the ability to take care of your own physical needs, you ensure a greater level of physical wellness. To achieve optimum physical wellness, you need to make choices that will help you avoid illnesses and injuries. The decisions you make now, and the habits you develop over your lifetime, will largely determine the length and quality of your life.

FIGURE 1.2

Qualities and behaviours associated with the dimensions of wellness.

PHYSICAL WELLNESS	EMOTIONAL WELLNESS	INTELLECTUAL WELLNESS
• Eating well • Exercising • Avoiding harmful habits • Practising safer sex • Recognizing symptoms of disease • Getting regular checkups • Avoiding injuries	• Optimism • Trust • Self-esteem • Self-acceptance • Self-confidence • Ability to understand and accept one's feelings • Ability to share feelings with others	• Openness to new ideas • Capacity to question • Ability to think critically • Motivation to master new skills • Sense of humour • Creativity • Curiosity • Lifelong learning
INTERPERSONAL WELLNESS	**CULTURAL WELLNESS**	**SPIRITUAL WELLNESS**
• Communication skills • Capacity for intimacy • Ability to establish and maintain satisfying relationships • Ability to cultivate a support system of friends and family	• Creating relationships with those who are different from you • Maintaining and valuing your own cultural identity • Avoiding stereotyping based on ethnicity, gender, religion, or sexual orientation	• Capacity for love • Compassion • Forgiveness • Altruism • Joy and fulfillment • Caring for others • Sense of meaning and purpose • Sense of belonging to something greater than oneself
ENVIRONMENTAL WELLNESS	**FINANCIAL WELLNESS**	**OCCUPATIONAL WELLNESS**
• Having abundant, clean natural resources • Maintaining sustainable development • Recycling whenever possible • Reducing pollution and waste	• Having a basic understanding of how money works • Living within one's means • Avoiding debt, especially for unnecessary items • Saving for the future and for emergencies	• Enjoying what you do • Feeling valued by your manager • Building satisfying relationships with co-workers • Taking advantage of opportunities to learn and be challenged

Emotional Wellness

Your emotional wellness reflects your ability to understand and deal with your feelings. Emotional wellness involves attending to your own thoughts and feelings, monitoring your reactions, and identifying obstacles to emotional stability. *Self-acceptance* is your personal satisfaction with yourself, which might exclude society's expectations, whereas *self-esteem* relates to the way you think others perceive you. *Self-confidence* can be a part of both acceptance and esteem. Achieving this type of wellness means finding solutions to emotional problems, with professional help if necessary.

Intellectual Wellness

Those who enjoy intellectual (or mental) wellness constantly challenge their minds. An active mind is essential to wellness because it detects problems, finds solutions, and directs behaviour. People who enjoy intellectual wellness never stop learning. They seek out and relish new experiences and challenges.

Interpersonal Wellness

Satisfying and supportive relationships are essential to physical and emotional health. Learning good communication skills, developing the capacity for intimacy, and cultivating a supportive network are all important to interpersonal (or social) wellness. Social wellness requires participating in and contributing to your community and to society.

Wellness Tip

Enhancing one dimension of wellness can have positive effects on others. For example, joining a meditation group can help you enhance your spiritual well-being, but it can also affect the emotional and interpersonal dimensions of wellness by enabling you to meet new people and develop new friendships.

Cultural Wellness

Cultural wellness refers to the way you interact with others who are different from you in terms of ethnicity, religion, gender, sexual orientation, age, and customs (practices). It involves creating relationships with others and suspending judgment of others' behaviour until you have lived with them or "walked in their shoes." It also includes accepting, valuing, and even celebrating the different cultural ways people interact in the world. The extent to which you maintain and value cultural identities is one measure of cultural wellness.

Spiritual Wellness

To enjoy spiritual health is to possess a set of guiding beliefs, principles, or values that give meaning and purpose to your life, especially in difficult times. The well person uses spirituality to focus on positive aspects of life and to fend off negative feelings such as cynicism, anger, and pessimism. Organized religions help many people develop spiritual health. Religion, however, is not the only source or form of spiritual wellness. Many people find meaning and purpose in their lives on their own—through nature, art, meditation, political action, or good works—or with their loved ones.

Environmental Wellness

Your environmental wellness is defined by the livability of your surroundings. Personal health depends on the health of the planet—from the safety of the food supply to the degree of violence in society. To improve your environmental wellness, you can learn about and protect yourself against hazards in your surroundings and work to make your world a cleaner and safer place.

Financial Wellness

Financial wellness refers to your ability to live within your means and manage your money in a way that gives you peace of mind. It includes balancing your income and expenses, staying out of debt, saving for the future, and understanding your emotions about money. For more on this topic, see the box entitled Financial Wellness on the next page.

Occupational Wellness

Occupational wellness refers to the level of happiness and fulfillment you gain through your work. Although high salaries and prestigious titles are nice, they alone do not bring about occupational wellness. Occupationally well people truly like their work, feel a connection with others in the workplace, and have opportunities to learn and be challenged. Another important aspect of occupational wellness is recognition from managers and colleagues. An ideal job draws on your interests and passions, as well as your vocational or professional skills, and allows you to feel that you are contributing to society in your everyday work.

In FOCUS

FINANCIAL WELLNESS

With the news full of stories of home mortgage rates, credit card debt, and personal bankruptcies, it has become painfully clear that many Canadians do not know how to manage their finances. You can avoid stress—and gain financial peace of mind—by developing the skills that contribute to financial wellness.

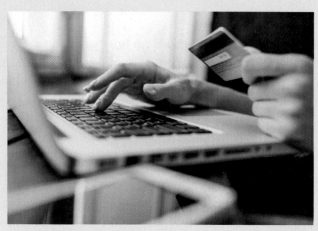

© Shutterstock / Kite_rin

Financial wellness means having a healthy relationship with money. It involves knowing how to manage your money, using self-discipline to live within your means, using credit cards wisely, staying out of debt, meeting your financial obligations, having a long-range financial plan, and saving.

Learn to Budget

Although the word *budget* may conjure up thoughts of deprivation, a budget is really just a way of tracking where your money goes and making sure you're spending it on the things that are most important to you. To start one, list your monthly income and your expenditures. If you aren't sure where you spend your money, track your expenses for a few weeks or a month. Then organize your expenditures into categories, such as housing, food, transportation, entertainment, services, personal care, clothes, books and school supplies, health care, credit card and loan payments, and miscellaneous. Use categories that reflect the way you actually spend your money. Knowing where your money goes is the first step in gaining control of it.

Now total your income and expenditures. Are you taking in more than you spend, or vise versa? Are you surprised by your spending patterns? Use this information to set guidelines and goals for yourself. If your expenses exceed your income, identify ways to make some cuts. For example, instead of paying for cable TV, you can stream news and entertainment shows from the Internet through your television or Blu-ray player. If you have both a cellphone and a land line, consider whether you can give one up. If you're spending money on movies and restaurants, consider less expensive options like having a weekly game night with friends or organizing an occasional potluck dinner.

Be realistic about what you can cut, but also realize that you may have to adjust your mindset about what you can afford. Once you have a balance between income and expenses, don't stop there. Try to have a little left over each month for an emergency fund or savings. You may be surprised by how much peace of mind you can gain by living within your means!

Be Wary of Credit Cards

One recent financial study found that 58% of Canada's post-secondary students aged 18 to 24 are worried about money. Sixty-four percent of the students surveyed expect to graduate with debt, and one quarter of them expected to owe in excess of $25 000 upon graduation. Yet 47% of the students surveyed said the most convenient way to pay for day-to-day expenses is with a credit card.

The best way to avoid credit card debt is to have just one card, to use it only when necessary, and to pay off the entire balance every month. Make sure you understand terms like *APR* (annual percentage rate—the interest you're charged on your balance), *credit limit* (the maximum amount you can borrow at any one time), *minimum monthly payment* (the smallest payment your creditor will accept each month), *grace period* (the number of days you have to pay your bill before interest, late fees, or other penalties are charged), and *over-the-limit* and *late fees* (the amount you'll be charged if your payment is late or you go over your credit limit). Banks make most of their money from fees. Read the fine print!

To see what you really do or don't know about credit cards, take the credit card quiz at http://www.fcac-acfc.gc.ca/eng/resources/toolCalculator/CreditCard/quiz/CreditCardQuiz-eng.asp?sn=0.

Get Out of Debt

If you do have credit card debt, stop using your cards and start paying them off. If you can't pay the whole balance, at least try to pay more than the minimum payment each month. It can take a very long time to pay off a loan by making only the minimum payments. For example, to pay off a credit card balance of $2000 at 10% interest with monthly payments of $20 would take 203 months—17 years. To see for yourself, check out an online credit card payment calculator tool like http://www.fcac-acfc.gc.ca/Eng/resources/toolsCalculators/Pages/CreditCa-OutilsIn.aspx. And remember: By carrying a balance and incurring finance charges, you are also paying back much more than your initial loan.

Become Financially Literate

Although modern life requires financial literacy—which includes everything from basics like balancing a chequebook to more sophisticated endeavours like developing a long-term financial plan—most Canadians have not received any kind of education in financial skills. The consensus is that developing lifelong financial skills should begin in early adulthood, during the university/college years, if not earlier.

If you want to improve your financial literacy, a good way to start is to take a course in personal finance or financial management skills. There are also many magazines that focus on money management, and of course a wealth of information can be found online. Make it a priority to achieve financial wellness, and start now. Money may not buy you love, but having control over your money can buy you a lot of peace of mind.

SOURCES: Financial Consumer Agency of Canada (2017). *Tools, calculators, and educational programs* (https://www.canada.ca/en/services/finance/tools.html); Smith, C. & Barboza, G.A.. 2013. The role of trans-generational financial knowledge and self-reported financial literacy on borrowing practices and debt accumulation of college students. *Social Science Electronic Publishing, Inc.* (http://ssrn.com/abstract=2342168); Plymouth State University. *Student Monetary Awareness and Responsibility Today!* (http://www.plymouth.edu/office/financial-aid/smart/).

LO2 New Opportunities for Taking Charge

A century ago, people considered themselves lucky just to survive to adulthood (see Figure 1.3 on the next page). A child born in the early 1900s, for example, could expect to live only about 57 years. Many people died as a result of common **infectious diseases** (e.g., pneumonia, tuberculosis, diarrhea) and poor environmental conditions (e.g., unrefrigerated food, poor sanitation, air and water pollution).

infectious diseases Diseases that can spread from one person to another; caused by microorganisms such as bacteria and viruses.

Life expectancy has gradually increased since the 1900s, and as of 2017, the average Canadian's life expectancy was 82.2 years. This increase is due largely to the development of vaccines and antibiotics to prevent

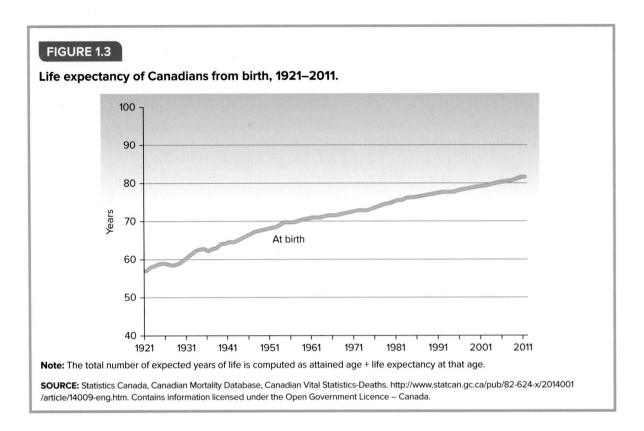

FIGURE 1.3

Life expectancy of Canadians from birth, 1921–2011.

Note: The total number of expected years of life is computed as attained age + life expectancy at that age.

SOURCE: Statistics Canada, Canadian Mortality Database, Canadian Vital Statistics-Deaths. http://www.statcan.gc.ca/pub/82-624-x/2014001 /article/14009-eng.htm. Contains information licensed under the Open Government Licence – Canada.

and fight infectious diseases, and to public health measures to improve living conditions. But even though life expectancy has increased, poor health limits most Canadians' activities during the last few years of their lives, resulting in some sort of impaired life (Figure 1.4).[1]

Today, a different set of diseases has emerged as our major health threat: heart disease, cancer, and stroke are three of the leading causes of death for Canadians (Table 1.1). Treating these and other **chronic diseases** is costly and difficult.

chronic diseases Diseases that develop and continue over a long period of time; usually caused by a variety of factors, including lifestyle factors.

FIGURE 1.4

Quantity of life versus quality of life. Years of healthy life as a proportion of life expectancy in the Canadian population.

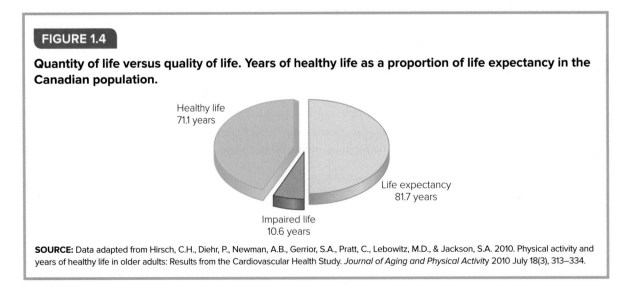

SOURCE: Data adapted from Hirsch, C.H., Diehr, P., Newman, A.B., Gerrior, S.A., Pratt, C., Lebowitz, M.D., & Jackson, S.A. 2010. Physical activity and years of healthy life in older adults: Results from the Cardiovascular Health Study. *Journal of Aging and Physical Activity* 2010 July 18(3), 313–334.

TABLE 1.1

Leading Causes of Death in Canada, 2013

Rank	Cause of Death	Number of Deaths
1	Malignant neoplasms (cancers)	75,112
2	Diseases of heart (heart disease)	49,891
3	Cerebrovascular diseases (stroke)	13,400
4	Chronic lower respiratory diseases	11,976
5	Accidents (unintentional injuries)	11,452
6	Diabetes mellitus (diabetes)	7,045
7	Influenza and pneumonia	6,551
8	Alzheimer's disease	6,345
9	Intentional self-harm (suicide)	4,054
10	Nephritis, nephrotic syndrome, and nephrosis (kidney disease)	2,978

SOURCE: Adapted from Statistics Canada, Health Statistics Division, Leading Causes of Death, by sex, 2013 (Table 13100394; Formerly CANSIM Table 102-0561). Contains information licensed under the Open Government Licence – Canada.

The good news is that we do have some control over whether we develop chronic diseases. We make choices every day that either increase or decrease our risks for such diseases. These lifestyle choices include behaviours such as exercise, diet, and alcohol use. Lifestyle factors contribute to our risk of suffering from chronic diseases, and we can make good choices in an effort to profoundly influence and reduce our own health risks. The need to make good choices is especially true for teens and young adults. For Canadians under the age of 24 years, for example, the top three causes of death are accidents, suicide, and cancer (Table 1.2). Wellness cannot be prescribed; physicians and other health care professionals can provide information, advice, and encouragement—but the rest is up to each individual.

TABLE 1.2

Leading Causes of Death Among Canadians Aged 1 to 24 years, 2013

Rank	Cause of Death	Percentage (of 2622 total deaths)
1	Accidents	36
2	Suicide	16
3	Cancer	11
4	Homicide	4
5	Congenital malformations	4
6	All other causes	27

SOURCE: Adapted from Statistics Canada, Health Statistics Division, Leading Causes of Death, by sex, 2013 (Table 13100394; Formerly CANSIM Table 102-0561). Contains information licensed under the Open Government Licence – Canada.

This chapter provides an overview of a lifestyle that contributes to wellness and describes a method that can help you make lasting changes in your life to promote good health. The chapters that follow provide more detailed information about physical activity, healthy eating habits, and other components of a wellness lifestyle. The book as a whole is designed to be used to help you take charge of your behaviour and improve the quality of your life—to become fit and well.

Fitness Tip

In Tables 1.1 and 1.2, notice how many causes of death are related to lifestyle. This is an excellent motivator for adopting healthy habits and staying in good condition. Maintaining physical fitness and a healthy diet can lead to a longer life. It's a fact!

National Wellness Goals

You may think of health and wellness as personal concerns, goals that you strive for on your own for your own benefit. But the Canadian government also has a vital interest in the health of all Canadians. A healthy population is the nation's greatest resource, the source of its vigour and wealth. Poor health, in contrast, drains the nation's resources and raises national health care costs. In fact, Canada's health care spending was estimated to be $228 billion in 2016, with projections to rise in future years. As the embodiment of our society's values, the federal government also has a humane interest in people's health.

In 2005, the federal, provincial, and territorial health ministers created the Pan-Canadian Public Health Network in an effort to better collaborate on strengthening public health across Canada. One of their key initiatives has been tackling obesity[2] through coordinating efforts in three key areas:

1. **Supportive environments**. Making social and physical environments where children live, learn, and play more supportive of physical activity and healthy eating.

2. **Early action**. Identifying the risk of overweight and obesity in children and addressing it early.

3. **Nutritious foods**. Looking at ways to increase the availability and accessibility of nutritious foods and decrease the marketing of foods and beverages high in fat, sugar, and/or sodium to children.

As part of these initiatives, you can see what your province or territory has done to contribute to these key areas by checking out http://www.phn-rsp.ca/thcpr-vcpsre-2017/index-eng.php, where all provincial initiatives are listed and described.

In an effort to carry out health strategies and achieve their goals, the Canadian government (Public Health Agency of Canada), in conjunction with the Canadian Society for Exercise Physiology (CSEP), has created *Canada's Physical Activity Guide to Healthy Active Living* (2011). These tools identify expectations for levels of physical activity that put Canadians of all ages on a path to wellness. Specific guides are provided with information for children, youth, and older adults. Some provinces have begun to use these and other tools to develop curriculum directed at increasing healthy lifestyle habits in students at the high school level and beyond.

CAREER OPTIONS IN...

WELLNESS

Teaching: university or college-level instructor, junior high or high school teacher

Community-Based: wellness program coordinator, disease-specific agency specialist (e.g., YMCA/YWCA), health promotion

Government Agencies: public health agency, Workers' Compensation Board, health care centre

Self-Employed: health behaviour consultant or workshop presenter, health care writer

SOURCE: Physical and Health Education Canada (http://www.phecanada.ca).

LO3 Behaviours That Contribute to Wellness

A lifestyle based on good choices and healthy behaviours maximizes the quality of life. It helps you avoid disease, remain strong and fit, and maintain your physical and mental health as long as you live.

Be Physically Active

The human body is designed to be active. It readily adapts to nearly any level of activity and exertion. **Physical fitness** is a set of physical attributes that allows the body to respond or adapt to the demands and stress of physical effort. The more we ask of our bodies, the stronger and more fit they become. When our bodies are not kept active, they deteriorate. Bones lose their density, joints stiffen, muscles become weak, and cellular energy systems begin to degenerate. To be truly well, human beings must be active.

> **physical fitness**   A set of physical attributes that allows the body to respond or adapt to the demands and stress of physical effort.

Unfortunately, a **sedentary** lifestyle is common among Canadians today. Close to 70% of Canadians' waking hours are spent in sedentary pursuits,[3] and only slightly more than 2 in 10 Canadian adults meet Canadian physical activity standards.[4] Options for physical activity are vast and range from traditional sports and physical activities (e.g., walking, jogging), to increased activity through video games (e.g., Nintendo Wii) and movement activities (e.g., yoga).

> **sedentary**   Physically inactive; literally, "sitting."

The benefits of physical activity are both physical and mental, immediate and long term (see Figure 1.5). In the short term, being physically fit makes it easier to do everyday tasks, such as lifting; it provides reserve strength for emergencies; and it helps people look and feel good. In the long term, being physically fit offers protection against chronic diseases and lowers the risk of dying prematurely (see the box Does Being Physically Active Make a Difference in How Long You Live? on the next page). Physically active people are less

---

FIGURE 1.5

Benefits of regular physical activity.

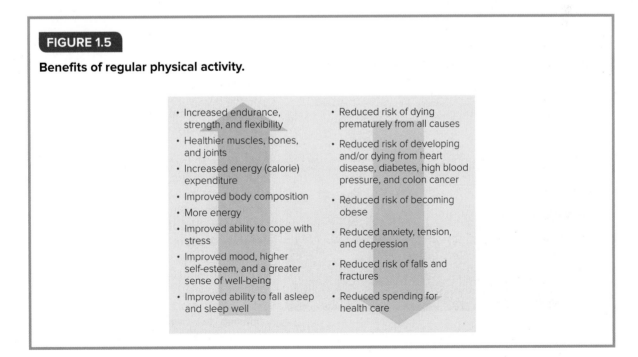

- Increased endurance, strength, and flexibility
- Healthier muscles, bones, and joints
- Increased energy (calorie) expenditure
- Improved body composition
- More energy
- Improved ability to cope with stress
- Improved mood, higher self-esteem, and a greater sense of well-being
- Improved ability to fall asleep and sleep well

- Reduced risk of dying prematurely from all causes
- Reduced risk of developing and/or dying from heart disease, diabetes, high blood pressure, and colon cancer
- Reduced risk of becoming obese
- Reduced anxiety, tension, and depression
- Reduced risk of falls and fractures
- Reduced spending for health care

likely to develop or die from heart disease, respiratory disease, high blood pressure, cancer, osteoporosis, and type 2 diabetes (the most common form of diabetes).[5] As they get older, they may also be able to avoid weight gain, muscle and bone loss, fatigue, and other problems associated with aging.

The Evidence *for* EXERCISE

DOES BEING PHYSICALLY ACTIVE MAKE A DIFFERENCE IN HOW LONG YOU LIVE?

How can we be sure that physical activity and exercise are good for our health? To answer this question, the US Department of Health and Human Services charged a committee with the task of reviewing the scientific literature to discover whether there is sufficient evidence to support providing physical activity recommendations to the public. The committee's report, the *Physical Activity Guidelines Advisory Committee Report, 2008*, summarizes the scientific evidence for the health benefits of habitual physical activity and the risks of sedentary behaviour. The report provides the rationale for government physical activity guidelines that are identical to those of the Public Health Agency of Canada.

The Physical Activity Guidelines Advisory committee started by asking whether physical activity actually helps people live longer. The committee investigated the link between physical activity and all-cause mortality—deaths from all causes—by looking at 73 studies dating from 1995 to 2008. The subjects of the studies were both men and women, from all age groups (16 to 65+ years), and from different racial and ethnic groups.

The data from these studies strongly support an *inverse relation* between physical activity and all-cause mortality; that is, physically active individuals were less likely to die during a study's follow-up period (ranging from 10 months to 28 years). The review found that active people have about a 30% lower risk of dying compared with inactive people. These inverse associations were found not just for healthy adults, but also for older adults (age 65 and older), for people with coronary artery disease and diabetes, for people with impaired mobility, and for people who were overweight or obese. Poor fitness and low physical activity levels were found to be better predictors of premature death than smoking, diabetes, or obesity. The committee also found that about 150 minutes (2–2.5 hours) of physical activity per week is sufficient to decrease all-cause mortality (see Chapter 2 for more details). It appears that the overall volume of energy expended, regardless of what kinds of activities produce the energy expenditure, makes a difference in risk of premature death.

The committee also looked at whether there is a *dose-response* relationship between physical activity and all-cause mortality—that is, whether more activity results in a greater reduction in death rates. Again, the studies showed an inverse relation between these two variables: more activity above and beyond 150 minutes per week produces greater benefits. Surprisingly, for inactive people, benefits are seen at levels below 150 minutes per week. In fact, *any* increase in physical activity resulted in reduced risk of death. The committee refers to this as the "some is good; more is better" message. A target of 150 minutes per week is recommended, but any level of activity below the target is encouraged for inactive individuals.

Looking more closely at this relationship, the committee found that the

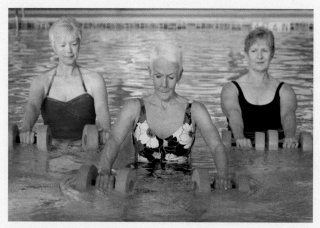

© Terry Vine / Blend Images LLC

greatest risk reduction is seen at the lower end of the physical activity spectrum (30–90 minutes per week). In fact, sedentary people who become more active have the greatest potential for improving health and reducing the risk of premature death. Additional risk reduction occurs as physical activity increases, but at a slower rate. For example, individuals who engaged in physical activity for 90 minutes per week had a 20% reduction in mortality risk compared with inactive people, and individuals who were active for 150 minutes per week, as noted earlier, had a 30% reduction in risk. But to achieve a 40% reduction in mortality, individuals had to be physically active for 420 minutes per week (7 hours).

The message from the research is clear: It doesn't matter what activity you choose or even how much time you can devote to it per week, as long as you get moving. The life you save will be your own!

SOURCE: Physical Activity Guidelines Advisory Committee. 2008. *Physical Activity Guidelines Advisory Committee Report, 2008.* Washington, DC: U.S. Department of Health and Human Services.

Choose a Healthy Diet

In addition to being sedentary, many Canadians have a diet that is too high in calories, unhealthy fats, and added sugars, and too low in fibre, complex carbohydrates, fruits, and vegetables. Like physical inactivity, this diet is linked to a number of chronic diseases. A healthy diet provides necessary nutrients and sufficient energy without also providing too much of the dietary substances linked to diseases. (See Chapter 7 for more detailed discussion of North American diets.)

Maintain a Healthy Body Weight

Overweight and obesity are strongly associated with a number of disabling and potentially fatal conditions and diseases, including heart disease, cancer, and type 2 diabetes. Recent trend (1985–2011) data show that obesity rates in Canada have tripled.[6] Healthy body weight is an important part of wellness—but short-term dieting is not part of a fit and well lifestyle. Maintaining a healthy body weight requires a lifelong commitment to regular exercise, a healthy diet, and effective stress management.

Manage Stress Effectively

Many people cope with stress by eating, drinking, or smoking too much. Others don't deal with it at all. In the short term, inappropriate stress management can lead to fatigue, sleep disturbances, and other unpleasant symptoms. Over longer periods of time, poor management of stress can lead to less efficient functioning of the immune system and increased susceptibility to disease. Learning to incorporate effective stress management techniques into daily life is an important part of a fit and well lifestyle. (See Chapter 12 for a greater understanding of stress, how it affects us, and mechanisms to reduce the effects of stress.)

Avoid Tobacco and Drug Use and Limit Alcohol Consumption

Tobacco use is a risk factor for many of the leading causes of death among Canadians. It is estimated to kill over 37 000 Canadians[7] each year, more than any other behavioural or environmental factor. A hundred years ago, before cigarette smoking was widespread, lung cancer was considered a rare disease. Today, with over 20% of the Canadian population smoking,[8] lung cancer is the most common cause of cancer death among both men and women and is one of the leading causes of death overall.

Certain forms of alcohol consumption can be linked to a shortened lifespan and even death. In 2002, approximately 4300 Canadians lost their lives to alcohol-related diseases and/or accidents.[9] Alcohol or drug intoxication is an especially notable factor in the death and disability of young people, particularly through **unintentional injuries** (such as drownings and car crashes caused by drunk driving) and violence.

> **unintentional injuries**   Injuries that occur without harm being intended.

Protect Yourself from Disease and Injury

The most effective way of dealing with disease and injury is to prevent them. Many of the lifestyle strategies discussed here help protect you against chronic illnesses. In addition, you can take specific steps to avoid infectious diseases, particularly those that are sexually transmitted.

Take Other Steps toward Wellness

Other important behaviours contribute to wellness, including these:

- Develop meaningful relationships.
- Plan for successful aging.
- Learn about the health care system.
- Act responsibly toward the environment.

Labs 1.1 and 1.2 will help you evaluate your behaviours as they relate to wellness.

The Role of Other Factors in Wellness

Heredity, the environment, and adequate health care are other important influences on health. These factors can interact in ways that raise or lower the quality of a person's life and the risk of developing particular diseases. For example, a sedentary lifestyle combined with a genetic predisposition for diabetes can greatly increase a person's risk for developing the disease. If this sedentary, genetically predisposed person also lacks adequate health care, they are much more likely to suffer dangerous complications from diabetes.

But in many cases, behaviour can tip the balance toward health even if heredity or environment is a negative factor. Breast cancer, for example, can run in families, but it is also associated with being overweight and having a sedentary lifestyle. A woman with a family history of breast cancer is less likely to die from the disease if she controls her weight, exercises, performs regular breast self-exams, and consults with her physician about mammograms.

LO4 1.2 Reaching Wellness through Lifestyle Management

Moving in the direction of wellness means cultivating healthy behaviours and working to overcome unhealthy ones. This approach to lifestyle management is sometimes called **behaviour change**. As you may already know from experience, changing an unhealthy habit can be harder than it looks. When you embark on a behaviour change plan, it may seem like too much work at first. But as you make progress, you will gain confidence in your ability to take charge of your life. You will also experience the benefits of wellness—more energy, greater vitality, deeper feelings of appreciation and curiosity, and a higher quality of life.

> **behaviour change**   A lifestyle management process that involves cultivating healthy behaviours and working to overcome unhealthy ones.

The rest of this chapter outlines a general process for changing unhealthy behaviours that is backed by research and that has worked for many people. You will also find many specific strategies and tips for change. For additional support, work through the activities in the Behaviour Change Workbook.

Getting Serious about Your Health

Before you can start changing a wellness-related behaviour, you have to know that the behaviour is problematic and that you *can* change it. To make good decisions, you need information about relevant topics and issues, including what resources are available to help you change.

Examine Your Current Health Habits

Have you considered how your current lifestyle is affecting your health today and how it will affect your health in the future? Do you know which of your current habits enhance your health and which ones may be harmful? Begin your journey toward wellness with self-assessment: Think about your own behaviour, complete the self-assessment in Lab 1.2, and talk with friends and family members about what they've noticed about your lifestyle and your health.

Choose a Target Behaviour

Changing any behaviour can be demanding. This is why it's a good idea to start small, by choosing one behaviour you want to change—called a **target behaviour**—and working on it until you succeed. Your chances of success will be greater if your first goal is simple, such as resisting the urge to snack between classes. As you change one behaviour, make your next goal a little more significant, and build on your success.

> **target behaviour**   An isolated behaviour selected as the object of a behaviour change program.

Learn about Your Target Behaviour

Once you've chosen a target behaviour, you need to know its risks and benefits for you—both now and in the future. As a starting point, use this text and the resources listed in For Further Exploration; refer to the box Evaluating Sources of Health Information (on the next page) for additional guidelines. Ask these questions:

- How is your target behaviour affecting your level of wellness today?
- What diseases or conditions does this behaviour place you at risk for?
- What effect would changing your behaviour have on your health?

Wellness Tip

If you're overweight, losing as little as 2 or 3 kilograms can significantly reduce your risk of developing diabetes. To learn more, visit the Canadian Diabetes Association's website at http://www.diabetes.ca.

Find Help

Have you identified a particularly challenging target behaviour or mood—something like alcohol addiction, binge eating, or depression—that interferes with your ability to function or places you at a serious health risk? You may need help to change behaviours or conditions that are too deeply rooted or too serious for

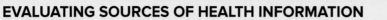

Critical CONSUMER

EVALUATING SOURCES OF HEALTH INFORMATION

Surveys indicate that university/college students are smart about evaluating health information. They trust the health information they receive from health professionals and educators and are skeptical about popular information sources, such as magazine articles and websites.

How smart are you about evaluating health information? Here are some tips.

General Strategies

Whenever you encounter health-related information, take the following steps to make sure it is credible:

- **Go to the original source.** Media reports often simplify the results of medical research. Find out for yourself what a study really reported, and determine whether it was based on good science. What type of study was it? Was it published in a recognized medical journal? Was it an animal study or did it involve people? Did the study include a large number of people? What did the study's authors actually report?
- **Watch for misleading language.** Reports that feature "breakthroughs" or "dramatic proof" are probably hype. A study might state that a behaviour "contributes to" or "is associated with" an outcome; this does not prove a cause-and-effect relationship.
- **Distinguish between research reports and public health advice.** Do not change your behaviour based on the results of a single report or study. If an agency such as Health Canada or the Canadian Cancer Society urges a behaviour change, however, you should follow its advice. Large, funded organizations issue such advice based on many studies, not a single report.
- **Remember that anecdotes are not facts.** A friend may tell you he lost weight on some new diet, but individual success stories do not mean the plan is truly safe or effective. Check with your doctor before making any serious lifestyle changes.
- **Be skeptical.** If a report seems too good to be true, it probably is. Be wary of information contained in advertisements. An ad's goal is to sell a product, even if there is no need for it—and sometimes even if the product has not been proven to be safe or effective.
- **Make choices that are right for you.** Friends and family members can be a great source of ideas and inspiration, but you need to make health-related choices that work best for you.

Internet Resources

Online information sources pose special challenges. When reviewing a health-related website, ask these questions:

- **What is the source of the information?** Websites maintained by government agencies, professional associations, or established academic or medical institutions are likely to provide trustworthy information. Many other groups and individuals post accurate information, but it is important to look at the qualifications of the people who are behind the site. (Check the home page or click the "About Us" link.)
- **How often is the site updated?** Look for sites that are updated frequently. Check the "last modified" date of any webpage.
- **Is the site promotional?** Be wary of information from sites that sell specific products, use testimonials as evidence, appear to have a social or political agenda, or ask for money.
- **What do other sources say about a topic?** Be wary of claims and information that appear at only one site or come from a chat room, bulletin board, or blog.
- **Does the site conform to any set of guidelines or criteria for quality and accuracy?** Look for sites that identify themselves as conforming to some code or set of principles, such as those set forth by the Health on the Net Foundation or the Canadian Medical Association. These codes include criteria such as use of information from respected sources and disclosure of the site's sponsors.

self-management. Don't be discouraged by the seriousness or extent of the problem; many resources are available to help you solve it. On campus, the student health centre or campus counselling centre can provide assistance. To locate community resources, consult your physician or the Internet.

LO5 Building Motivation to Change

Knowledge is necessary for behaviour change, but it isn't usually enough to make people act. Millions of people have sedentary lifestyles, for example, even though they know it's bad for their health. This is particularly true of young adults, who may not be motivated to change because they feel well despite engaging in unhealthy behaviours (see the box Wellness Matters for University/College Students). To succeed at behaviour change, you need strong motivation.

In FOCUS

WELLNESS MATTERS FOR UNIVERSITY/COLLEGE STUDENTS

If you are like most university/college students, you probably feel pretty good about your health right now. Most university/college students are in their late teens or early 20s, lead active lives, have plenty of friends, and look forward to a future filled with opportunity. With all these things going for you, why shouldn't you feel good?

A Closer Look

Although most university/college-age people look healthy, appearances can be deceiving. Each year, thousands of students lose productive academic time to physical and emotional health problems—some of which can continue to plague them for life.

The following table shows the top 10 health issues affecting students' academic performance, according to the Fall 2010 American College Health Association National College Assessment II.

Health Issue	Students Affected (%)
Stress	25.4
Sleep difficulties	17.8
Anxiety	16.4
Cold/flu/sore throat	13.8
Excessive Internet use/computer games	11.6
Work	11.4
Concern for a troubled friend or family member	10.1
Depression	10.0
Relationship difficulties	9.6
Extracurricular activities	8.8

Each of these issues is related to one or more of the nine dimensions of wellness, and most can be influenced by choices students make daily. Although some troubles—such as the death of a friend—cannot be controlled, other physical and emotional concerns can be minimized by choosing

continued

healthy behaviours. For example, there are many ways to manage stress, the top health issue affecting students. By reducing unhealthy choices (such as using alcohol to relax) and by increasing healthy choices (such as using time management techniques), even busy students can reduce the impact of stress on their life.

The survey also estimated that, based on students' reporting of their height and weight, more than 33% of university/college students are either overweight or obese. Although heredity plays a role in determining an individual's weight, lifestyle is also a factor in weight and weight management. In many studies over the past few decades, a large percentage of students have reported behaviours such as these:

- overeating
- snacking on junk food
- frequently eating high-fat foods
- using alcohol and binge drinking

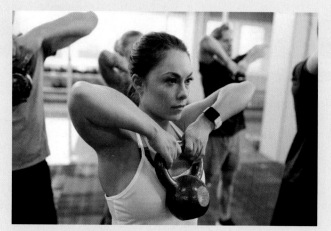

Shutterstock / Syda Productions

Clearly, eating behaviours are often a matter of choice. Although students may not see (or feel) the effects of their dietary habits today, the long-term health risks are significant. Overweight and obese persons run a higher-than-normal risk of developing diabetes, heart disease, and cancer later in life. We now know with certainty that improving your eating habits, even a little, can lead to weight loss and improved overall health.

Other Choices, Other Problems

Students commonly make other unhealthy choices. Here are some examples from the 2004 Canadian Campus Survey:

- Nearly 62% of students had spent money on at least one gambling activity since the school year began.
- About 32% of students had engaged in hazardous or harmful drinking patterns in the past year.
- Almost 17% of students had used cannabis at least once during the past month.

What choices do you make in these situations? Remember: It's never too late to change. The sooner you trade an unhealthy behaviour for a healthy one, the longer you'll be around to enjoy the benefits.

The Transition to University/College

Embarking on a new academic path can often mean moving far away from home, family, and friends and starting anew. A new environment, new academic expectations, and many more responsibilities for first-year students often mean new challenges. Keup and Stolzenberg's (2004) *Your First College Year* survey reported that one-third of the student sample felt "frequently overwhelmed by all they had to do" during their transition to university/college. In addition, more than one-third felt "frequently" or "occasionally" lonely or homesick and worried about meeting new people.

It has recently been suggested that one way to ease the challenges of the transition to university/college is to focus some of your wellness energies on your intrapersonal skills, interpersonal skills, adaptability, stress management skills, and general mood. Enhancing these emotional and social skills have been shown to positively alter academic success and academic retention. Look for specialized programs run by your university/college student groups or counselling centres.

SOURCES: Adlaf, E.M., Demers, A., Gliksman, L. (Eds.). 2005. *Canadian Campus Survey 2004.* Centre for Addiction and Mental Health, Toronto, ON: CAMH; American College Health Association. 2012. *American College Health Association National College Health Assessment* II: *Reference Group Executive Summary Spring 2012.* Hanover, MD: American College Health Association; Parker, J.D.A., & Duffy, J.M. (2005, January 12). *Making a Successful Transition During the First Year of College: Does Emotional Intelligence Matter?* Retrieved October 20, 2011, from University of South Carolina (http://www.sc.edu/fye/resources/assessment/newessay/author /parkerduffy.html).

Examine the Pros and Cons of Change

Health behaviours have short-term and long-term benefits and costs. Consider the benefits and costs of an inactive lifestyle:

- **Short term**. Allows you more time to watch TV and hang out with friends, but leaves you less physically fit and less able to participate in recreational activities.
- **Long term**. Increases the risk of heart disease, cancer, stroke, and premature death.

To successfully change your behaviour, you must believe that the benefits of change outweigh the costs.

Carefully examine the pros and cons of continuing your current behaviour and of changing to a healthier one. Focus on the effects that are most meaningful to you, including those that are tied to your personal identity and values. For example, engaging in regular physical activity and adequate sleep can support an image of yourself as an active person who is a good role model for others. To work toward independence and taking control over your life, quitting smoking can be one way to eliminate dependency. To complete your analysis, ask friends and family members about the effects of your behaviour on them. For example, a younger sister may tell you that your smoking habit influenced her decision to take up smoking.

The short-term benefits of behaviour change can be an important motivating force. Although some people are motivated by long-term goals, such as avoiding a disease that may hit them in 30 years, most are more likely to be moved to action by shorter-term, more personal goals. Feeling better, doing better in school, improving at a sport, reducing stress, and increasing self-esteem are common short-term benefits of health behaviour change. Many wellness behaviours are associated with immediate improvements in quality of life. For example, surveys have found that nonsmokers feel healthy and full of energy more days each month than do smokers, and they report fewer days of sadness and troubled sleep; the same is true when physically active people are compared with sedentary people. Over time, these types of differences add up to a substantially greater quality of life for people who engage in healthy behaviours.

Boost Self-Efficacy

When you start thinking about changing a health behaviour, a big factor in your eventual success is whether you have confidence in yourself and in your ability to change. **Self-efficacy** refers to your belief in your ability to successfully take action and perform a specific task. Strategies for boosting self-efficacy include developing an internal locus of control, using visualization and self-talk, and obtaining encouragement from supportive people.

self-efficacy   The belief in one's ability to take action and perform a specific behaviour.

Locus of Control

Who do you believe is controlling your life? Is it your parents, friends, or school? Is it "fate"? Or is it you? **Locus of control** refers to the figurative "place" a person designates as the source of responsibility for the events in their life. People who believe they are in control of their own lives are said to have an internal locus of control. Those who believe that factors beyond their control—heredity, friends and family, the environment, fate, luck, or other outside forces—are more important in determining the events of their lives are said to have an external locus of control.

> **locus of control** The figurative "place" a person designates as the source of responsibility for the events in their life.

For lifestyle management, an internal locus of control is an advantage because it reinforces motivation and commitment. An external locus of control can sabotage efforts to change behaviour. For example, if you believe you are destined to die of breast cancer because your mother died from the disease, you may view monthly breast self-exams and regular checkups as a waste of time. In contrast, if you believe you can take action to reduce your hereditary risk of breast cancer, you will be motivated to follow guidelines for early detection of the disease.

If you find yourself attributing too much influence to outside forces, gather more information about your wellness-related behaviours. List all the ways that making lifestyle changes will improve your health. If you believe you'll succeed, and if you recognize and accept that you are in charge of your life, you're on your way to wellness.

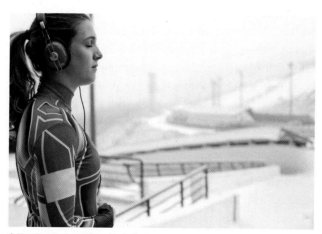

© Hero Images Inc. / Alamy Stock Photo

Visualization and Self-Talk

One of the best ways to boost your confidence and self-efficacy is to visualize yourself successfully engaging in a new, healthier behaviour. For example, imagine yourself going for a regular after-dinner walk or choosing healthier snacks. Also visualize yourself enjoying all the short-term and long-term benefits that your lifestyle change will bring. Create a new self-image: What will you and your life be like when you become a regular exerciser or a nonsmoker?

You can also use **self-talk**, the internal dialogue you carry on with yourself, to increase your confidence in your ability to change. Counter any self-defeating patterns of thought with more positive or realistic thoughts: "I am a strong, capable person, and I can maintain my commitment to change." (See Chapter 12 for more on self-talk.)

> **self-talk** A person's internal dialogue.

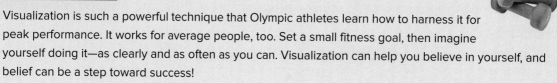

Fitness Tip

Visualization is such a powerful technique that Olympic athletes learn how to harness it for peak performance. It works for average people, too. Set a small fitness goal, then imagine yourself doing it—as clearly and as often as you can. Visualization can help you believe in yourself, and belief can be a step toward success!

Role Models and Other Supportive Individuals

Social support can make a big difference in your level of motivation and your chances of success. Perhaps you know people who have reached the goal you are striving for; they could be role models or mentors for you, providing guidance and support for your efforts. Gain strength from their experiences, and tell yourself, "If they can do it, so can I." In addition, find a buddy who wants to make the same changes you do and who can take an active role in your behaviour change program. For example, an exercise buddy can provide companionship and encouragement for times when you might be tempted to skip your workout.

Identify and Overcome Barriers to Change

Don't let past failures at behaviour change discourage you; they can be a great source of information you can use to boost your chances of future success. Make a list of the problems and challenges you faced in your previous behaviour change attempts; to this, add the short-term costs of behaviour change that you identified in your analysis of the pros and cons of change. Once you've listed these key barriers to change, develop a practical plan for overcoming each one. For example, if you always smoke when you're with certain friends, decide in advance how you will turn down the next cigarette you are offered.

Enhancing Your Readiness to Change

The transtheoretical or "stages of change" model is an effective approach to lifestyle self-management (see Figure 1.6 on the next page). According to this model, you move through distinct stages as you work to change your target behaviours. Research suggests that most people make several attempts before they successfully change a behaviour; four out of five people experience some degree of backsliding. For this reason, the stages of change are best conceptualized as a spiral, in which people cycle back through previous stages but are further along in the process each time they renew their commitment.

The following sections will help you determine what stage you are in for your target behaviours. For tips on changing stages, see the box Tips for Moving Forward in the Cycle of Behaviour Change on page 25.

Precontemplation

People at this stage do not think they have a problem and do not intend to change their behaviour. They may be unaware of the risks associated with their behaviour or may deny them. They may have tried unsuccessfully to change in the past and may now feel demoralized and think the situation is hopeless. They may also blame other people or external factors for their problems. People in the precontemplation stage believe there are more reasons or more important reasons not to change than there are reasons to change.

Contemplation

People at this stage know they have a problem and intend to take action within six months. They acknowledge the benefits that behaviour change will have for them but are also very aware of the costs of changing—to be successful, people must believe that the benefits of change outweigh the costs. People in the contemplation stage wonder about possible courses of action but don't know how to proceed. There may also be specific barriers to change that appear too difficult to overcome.

FIGURE 1.6

The Stages of Change: a spiral model.

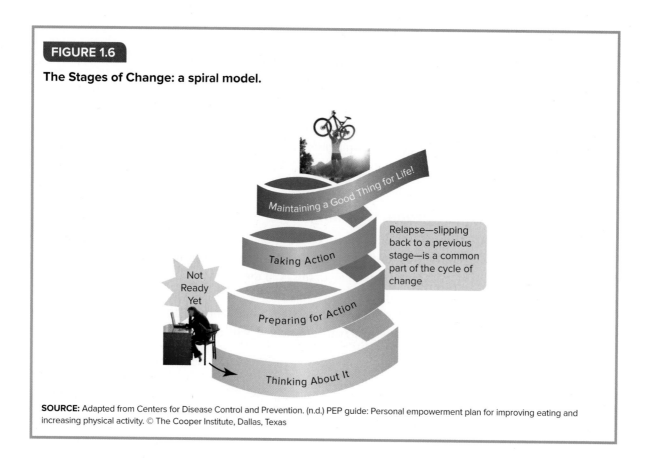

SOURCE: Adapted from Centers for Disease Control and Prevention. (n.d.) PEP guide: Personal empowerment plan for improving eating and increasing physical activity. © The Cooper Institute, Dallas, Texas

Preparation

People at this stage plan to take action within a month or may already have begun to make small changes in their behaviour. They may be engaging in their new, healthier behaviour, but not yet regularly or consistently. They may have created a plan for change but may be worried about failing.

Action

During the action stage, people outwardly modify their behaviour and their environment. The action stage usually requires the greatest commitment of time and energy, and people in this stage are at risk for reverting to old, unhealthy patterns of behaviour.

Maintenance

People at this stage have maintained their new, healthier lifestyle for at least six months. Lapses may have occurred, but people in maintenance have been successful in quickly re-establishing the desired behaviour. The maintenance stage can last for months or years.

Termination

People at this stage have exited the cycle of change and are no longer tempted to lapse back into their old behaviour. They have a new self-image and total self-efficacy with regard to their target behaviour.

Take CHARGE

TIPS FOR MOVING FORWARD IN THE CYCLE OF BEHAVIOUR CHANGE

Precontemplation

- **Raise your awareness.** Research your target behaviour and its effects.
- **Be self-aware.** Look at the mechanisms you use to resist change, such as denial or rationalization. Find ways to counteract these mechanisms.
- **Seek social support.** Ask friends and family members to help you identify target behaviours and understand their impact on the people around you.
- **Identify helpful resources.** Access resources such as exercise classes or stress-management workshops offered by your school.

Contemplation

- **Keep a journal.** Keep a record of your target behaviour and the circumstances that elicit the behaviour to help you plan a change program.
- **Do a cost–benefit analysis.** Identify the costs and benefits (both current and future) of maintaining your behaviour and of changing it. Costs can be monetary, social, emotional, and so on.
- **Identify barriers to change.** Learn your obstacles to change so you can work to overcome them.
- **Engage your emotions.** Watch movies or read books about people with your target behaviour. Imagine what your life will be like if you don't change.
- **Create a new self-image.** Imagine what you'll be like after changing your target behaviour. Try to think of yourself in new terms right now.
- **Think before you act.** Learn why you engage in the target behaviour. Determine what "sets you off," and train yourself not to act reflexively.

Preparation

- **Create a plan.** Include a start date, goals, rewards, and specific steps you will take to change your behaviour.
- **Make change a priority.** Create and sign a contract with yourself.
- **Practise visualization and self-talk.** Use these techniques to help you mentally prepare for challenging situations.
- **Take short steps.** Boost your confidence and motivation by practising your new behaviour for a short time—even a single day.

Action

- **Monitor your progress.** Keep up with your journal entries.
- **Change your environment.** Make changes that will discourage the target behaviour—for example, getting rid of snack foods or not stocking the refrigerator with beer.
- **Find alternatives to your target behaviour.** Make a list of things you can do to replace the behaviour.
- **Reward yourself.** Identify rewards in your change plan. Give yourself lots of praise, and focus on your success.
- **Involve your friends.** Tell them you want to change, and ask for their help.
- **Don't get discouraged.** Remember that real change is difficult.

Maintenance

- **Keep going.** Continue using the positive strategies that worked in earlier stages.
- **Be prepared for lapses.** Don't let slip-ups set you back.
- **Be a role model.** Try helping someone else do the same thing once you have successfully changed your behaviour.

Dealing with Relapse

People seldom progress through the stages of change in a straightforward, linear way. Rather, they tend to move to a certain stage and then slip back to a previous stage before resuming their forward progress. If you experience a lapse (a single slip) or a relapse (a return to old habits), don't give up. Relapse can be demoralizing, but it is not the same as failure; failure means stopping before you reach your goal and never changing your target behaviour. During the early stages of the change process, it's a good idea to plan for relapse so you can avoid guilt and self-blame and get back on track quickly. Follow these steps:

1. **Forgive yourself.** A single setback isn't the end of the world, but abandoning your efforts to change could have negative effects on your life.

2. **Give yourself credit for the progress you have already made.** You can use that success as motivation to continue.

3. **Move on.** You can learn from a relapse and use that knowledge to deal with potential setbacks in the future.

Developing Skills for Change: Creating a Personalized Plan

Once you are committed to making a change, it's time to put together a plan of action. Your key to success is a well-thought-out plan that sets goals, anticipates problems, and includes rewards. This plan includes the five steps outlined in the following sections.

1. Monitor Your Behaviour and Gather Data

Keep a record of your target behaviour and the circumstances surrounding it. Record this information for at least a week or two. Keep your notes in a health journal or notebook or on your computer (see the sample journal entries in Figure 1.7). Record each occurrence of your behaviour, noting the following:

- what the activity was
- when and where it happened
- what you were doing
- how you felt at that time

If your goal is to start an exercise program, track your activities to determine how to make time for workouts. A blank log is provided in Activity 3 in the Behaviour Change Workbook.

2. Analyze the Data and Identify Patterns

After you have collected data on the behaviour, analyze the data to identify patterns. When are you most likely to overeat? To skip a meal? What events trigger your appetite? Perhaps you are especially hungry midmorning or when you put off eating dinner until 9 o'clock at night. Perhaps you overindulge in food and drink when you go to a particular restaurant or when you're with certain friends. Note the connections between your feelings and such external cues as time of day, location, situation, and the actions of others around you.

FIGURE 1.7

Sample health journal entries.

Date	November 5		Day M [TU] W TH F SA SU								

Time of day	M/S	Food eaten	Cals.	H	Where did you eat?	What else were you doing?	How did someone else influence you?	What made you want to eat what you did?	Emotions and feelings?	Thoughts and concerns?
7:30	M	1 C Crispix cereal 1/2 C skim milk coffee, black 1 C orange juice	110 40 — 120	3	home	looking at news headlines on my phone	alone	I always eat cereal in the morning	a little keyed up & worried	thinking about quiz in class today
10:30	S	1 apple	90	1	hall outside classroom	studying	alone	felt tired & wanted to wake up	tired	worried about next class
12:30	M	1 C chili 1 roll 1 pat butter 1 orange 2 oatmeal cookies 1 soda	290 120 35 60 120 150	2	campus food court	talking	eating w/ friends; we decided to eat at the food court	wanted to be part of group	excited and happy	interested in hearing everyone's plans for the weekend
	M/S = Meal or snack			H = Hunger rating (0–3)						

3. Be "Smart" about Setting Goals

If your goals are too challenging, you will have trouble making steady progress and will be more likely to give up altogether. If, for example, you are in poor physical condition, it will not make sense to set a goal of being ready to run a marathon within two months. If you set goals you can live with, it will be easier to stick with your behaviour change plan and be successful.

Experts suggest that your goals meet the SMART criteria; that is, your behaviour change goals should be:

- **Specific.** Avoid vague goals like "eat more fruits and vegetables." Instead, state your objectives in specific terms, such as "eat two cups of fruit and three cups of vegetables every day."

- **Measurable.** Recognize that your progress will be easier to track if your goals are quantifiable, so give your goal a number. You might measure your goal in terms of time (such as "walk briskly for 20 minutes a day"), distance ("run 3 kilometres, three days per week"), or some other amount ("drink 8 glasses of water every day").

- **Attainable.** Set goals that are within your physical limits. For example, if you are a poor swimmer, it might not be possible for you to meet a short-term fitness goal by swimming laps. Walking or biking might be better options.

- **Realistic.** Manage your expectations when you set goals. For example, it may not be possible for a long-time smoker to quit cold turkey. A more realistic approach might be to use nicotine-replacement patches or gum for several weeks while getting help from a support group.

- **Time frame–specific.** Give yourself a reasonable amount of time to reach your goal, state the time frame in your behaviour change plan, and set your agenda to meet the goal within the time frame.

Using these criteria, a sedentary person who wanted to improve their health and build fitness might set a goal of being able to run 5 kilometres in 30 minutes, to be achieved within a time frame of 6 months. To work toward that goal, the person might set a number of smaller, intermediate goals that are easier to achieve. For example, a list of goals might look like this:

Week	Frequency (days/week)	Activity	Duration (minutes)
1	3	Walk < 1.6 km	10–15
2	3	Walk 1.6 km	15–20
3	4	Walk 1.6–3 km	20–25
4	4	Walk 3–5 km	25–30
5–7	3–4	Walk/run 1.6 km	15–20
...			
21–24	4–5	Run 3–5 km	25–30

Of course, it may not be possible to meet these goals, but you never know until you try. As you work toward meeting your long-term goal, you may find it necessary to adjust your short-term goals. For example, you may find that you can start running sooner than you thought, or you may be able to run farther than you originally estimated. In such cases, it may be reasonable to make your goals more challenging. Otherwise, you may want to make them easier in order to stay motivated.

For some goals and situations, it may make more sense to focus on something other than your outcome goal. If your goal involves a long-term lifestyle change, such as reaching a healthy weight, it is better to focus on developing healthy habits than to target a specific weight loss. Your goal in this case might be exercising for 30 minutes every day, reducing portion sizes, or eliminating late-night snacks.

Wellness Tip

Your environment contains powerful cues for both positive and negative lifestyle choices. Parks and running/bike paths encourage physical activity, even in an urban setting. Examine your environment for cues that can support your behaviour-change efforts.

4. Devise a Plan of Action

Develop a strategy that will support your efforts to change. Your plan of action should include the following steps:

Get What You Need

Identify campus and community resources that can help you. For example, you can join a community walking club or sign up for a smoking cessation program. You may also need to buy some new running shoes or nicotine replacement patches. Get the items you need right away; waiting can delay your progress.

Modify Your Environment

If there are cues in your environment that trigger your target behaviour, try to control them. For example, if you normally have alcohol at home, getting rid of it can help prevent you from indulging. If you usually study with a group of friends in an environment that allows smoking, try moving to a nonsmoking area. If you always buy a snack at a certain vending machine, change your route to avoid it.

Control Related Habits

You may have habits that contribute to your target behaviour; modifying these habits can help change the behaviour. For example, if you usually plop down on the sofa while watching TV, try putting an exercise bike in front of the set so you can burn calories while watching your favourite programs.

Reward Yourself

Giving yourself instant, real rewards for good behaviours will reinforce your efforts. Plan your rewards, and decide in advance what each one will be and how you will earn it. Tie rewards to achieving specific goals or subgoals. For example, you might treat yourself to a movie after a week of avoiding snacks. Make a list of items or events to use as rewards. They should be special to you and preferably unrelated to food or alcohol.

Involve the People around You

Tell family and friends about your plan and ask them to help. To help them respond appropriately to your needs, create a specific list of dos and don'ts. For example, ask them to support you when you set aside time to exercise or avoid second helpings at dinner.

Plan for Challenges

Think about situations and people that might derail your program, and develop ways to cope with them. For example, if you think it will be hard to stick to your usual exercise program during exams, schedule short bouts of physical activity (such as a brisk walk) as stress-reducing study breaks.

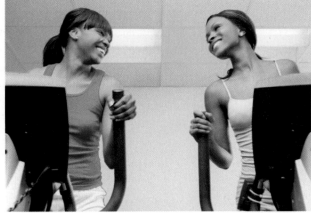

© JGI / Jamie Grill / Blend Images LLC

Help from a committed friend can ensure the success of any behaviour-change program, whether you want to eat better, lose weight, stop smoking, or exercise more.

5. Make a Personal Contract

A serious personal contract—one that commits you to your word—can result in a higher chance of follow-through than a casual, off-hand promise. Your contract can help prevent procrastination by specifying the important dates and can also serve as a reminder of your personal commitment to change.

Your contract should include a statement of your goal and your commitment to reaching it. The contract should also include details, such as the following:

- the date you will start
- the steps you will take to measure your progress
- the strategies you plan to use to promote change
- the date you expect to reach your final goal

Have someone—preferably someone who will be actively helping you with your program—sign your contract as a witness.

Figure 1.8 (on the next page) shows a sample behaviour change contract for someone who is committing to eating more fruit every day. A blank contract is included as Activity 8 in the Behaviour Change Workbook.

FIGURE 1.8

A sample behaviour change contract.

Behaviour Change Contract

1. I, ___Tammy Lau___, agree to _increase my consumption of fruit from_
1 cup per week to 2 cups per day.

2. I will begin on ___10/5___ and plan to reach my goal of _2 cups_
of fruit per day by _12/7_

3. To reach my final goal, I have devised the following schedule of mini-goals.
For each step in my program, I will give myself the reward listed.

I will begin to have ½ cup	10/5	see movie
of fruit with breakfast		
I will begin to have ½ cup	10/26	new cd
of fruit with lunch		
I will begin to substitute fruit	11/16	concert
juice for soda 1 time per day		

My overall reward for reaching my goal will be _trip to beach_

4. I have gathered and analyzed data on my target behaviour and have
identified the following strategies for changing my behaviour: _Keep the_
fridge stocked with easy-to-carry fruit. Pack fruit in my backpack
every day. Buy lunch at place that serves fruit.

5. I will use the following tools to monitor my progress toward my final goal:
Chart on fridge door
Health journal

I sign this contract as an indication of my personal commitment to reach
my goal: ___Tammy Lau___   _9/28_

I have recruited a helper who will witness my contract and also increase
his consumption of fruit; eat lunch with me twice a week.
___Eric March___   _9/28_

Putting Your Plan into Action

The starting date has arrived, and you are ready to put your plan into action. This stage requires commitment and resolve to stick with the plan no matter what temptations you encounter. Remember all the reasons you have to make the change—and remember that *you* are the boss. Use all your strategies to make your plan work. Make sure your environment is change-friendly and obtain as much support and encouragement from others as possible. In addition, keep track of your progress in your health journal and give yourself regular rewards. And don't forget to give yourself a pat on the back—congratulate yourself, notice how much better you look or feel, and feel good about how far you've come and how you've gained control of your behaviour.

Staying with It

As you continue with your program, don't be surprised when you run up against obstacles; they're inevitable. In fact, it's a good idea to expect problems and give yourself time to step back, see how you're doing, and make some changes before going on. If your program is grinding to a halt, identify what is blocking your progress. It may come from one of the sources described in the following sections.

Social Influences

Take a hard look at the reactions of the people you're counting on, and see if they're really supporting you. If they come up short, connect and network with others who will be more supportive. A related trap is trying to get your friends or family members to change *their* behaviours. The decision to make a major behaviour change is something people come to only after intensive self-examination. You may be able to influence someone by tactfully providing facts or support, but that's all. Focus on yourself. If you succeed, you may become a role model for others.

Levels of Motivation and Commitment

You won't make real progress until an inner drive leads you to the stage of change at which you are ready to make a personal commitment to the goal. If commitment is your problem, you may need to wait until the behaviour you're dealing with makes your life more unhappy or unhealthy; then your desire to change it will be stronger. Or you may find that changing your goal will inspire you to keep going. For more ideas, refer to Activity 9 in the Behaviour Change Workbook.

Strengthening Mental Wellness

Another way to contribute toward your behaviour change is to be confident about your ability to create change. Adopt a positive outlook, take pride in your good qualities while recognizing your insecurities, and live in the present. Engage in the process so that you become a participant of change.

Believe that you can participate in behaviour change by doing the following:

- Know what your motivators are; how do your values and goals become your motivators?
- Understand how your level of willpower can influence those motivators.
- Be confident that you can direct yourself toward positive change.

Choice of Techniques and Level of Effort

If your plan is not working as well as you thought it would, make changes where you're having the most trouble. If you've lagged on your running schedule, for example, maybe it's because you don't like running; an aerobics class might suit you better. There are many ways to move toward your goal. Or you may not be trying hard enough. You do have to push toward your goal. If it were easy, you wouldn't need to have a plan.

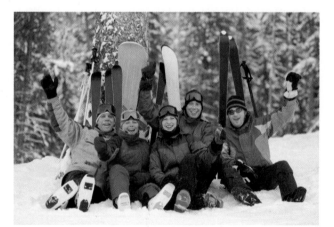

Design Pics / Don Hammond

A convenient setting and a friendly companion help make exercise a satisfying and pleasurable experience. Choosing the right activity and doing it the right way are important elements in a successful behaviour change program.

Stress Barrier

If you've hit a wall in your program, look at the sources of stress in your life. If the stress is temporary, such as catching a cold or having a term paper due, you may want to wait until it passes before strengthening your efforts. If the stress is ongoing, find healthy ways to manage it (see Chapter 12). You may even want to make stress management your highest priority for behaviour change.

Procrastinating, Rationalizing, and Blaming

Be alert to games you might be playing with yourself, so you can stop them. Such games include the following:

- **Procrastinating.** If you tell yourself, "It's Friday already; I might as well wait until Monday to start," you're procrastinating. Break your plan into smaller steps that you can accomplish one day at a time.

- **Rationalizing.** If you tell yourself, "I wanted to go swimming today but wouldn't have had time to wash my hair afterward," you're making excuses by rationalizing.

- **Blaming.** If you tell yourself, "I couldn't exercise because Dave was hogging the elliptical trainer," you're blaming others for your own failure to follow through. Blaming is a way of taking your focus off the real problem and denying responsibility for your own actions.

Be Fit and Well for Life

Your first attempts at making behaviour changes may never go beyond the contemplation or preparation stage. Those that do may not all succeed. But as you experience some success, you'll start to have more positive feelings about yourself. You may discover new physical activities and sports you enjoy, and you may encounter new situations and meet new people. Perhaps you'll surprise yourself by accomplishing things you didn't think were possible—breaking a longstanding nicotine habit, competing in a race, climbing a mountain, or developing a leaner body. Most of all, you'll discover the feeling of empowerment that comes from taking charge of your health. Being healthy takes extra effort, but the paybacks in energy and vitality are priceless.

Once you've started, don't stop. Assume that health improvement is forever. Take on the easier problems first, and then use what you learn to tackle more difficult problems later. When you feel challenged, remind yourself that you are creating a lifestyle that minimizes your health risks and maximizes your enjoyment of life. You can take charge of your health in a dramatic and meaningful way. *Fit and Well* will show you how.

Tips for Today and the Future

You are in charge of your health! Many of the decisions you make every day have an impact on the quality of your life, both now and in the future.

RIGHT NOW YOU CAN

- Go for a 15-minute walk.

- Have a piece of fruit for a snack.

- Call a friend and arrange for a time to catch up with each other.

- Start thinking about whether you have a health behaviour you'd like to change. If you do, consider the elements of a behaviour change strategy. For example, begin a mental list of the pros and cons of the behaviour, or talk to someone who can support you in your attempts to change.

IN THE FUTURE YOU CAN

- Stay current on health- and wellness-related news and issues.

- Participate in health awareness and promotion campaigns in your community—for example, support smoking restrictions in local venues.

- Be a role model for someone else who is working on a health behaviour you have successfully changed.

SUMMARY

- Wellness is the ability to live life fully, with vitality and meaning. Wellness is dynamic and multidimensional; it incorporates physical, emotional, intellectual, interpersonal, cultural, spiritual, environmental, financial, and occupational dimensions.

- People today have greater control over and greater responsibility for their health than ever before.

- Behaviours that promote wellness include being physically active; choosing a healthy diet; maintaining a healthy body weight; managing stress effectively; avoiding use of tobacco and limiting alcohol use; and protecting yourself from disease and injury.

- Although heredity, environment, and health care all play roles in wellness and disease, behaviour can mitigate their effects.

- To make lifestyle changes, you need information about yourself, your health habits, and the resources available to help you change.

- You can increase your motivation for behaviour change by examining the benefits and costs of change, boosting self-efficacy, and identifying and overcoming key barriers to change.

- The stages of change model describes six stages that people may move through as they try to change their behaviour: precontemplation, contemplation, preparation, action, maintenance, and termination.

- A specific plan for change can be developed by (1) collecting data on your behaviour and recording it in a journal; (2) analyzing the recorded data; (3) setting specific goals; (4) devising strategies for modifying the environment, rewarding yourself and involving others, and; (5) making a personal contract.

- To start and maintain a behaviour change program, you need commitment, a well-developed and manageable plan, social support, and strong stress-management techniques. It is also important to monitor the progress of your program, revising it as necessary.

FOR FURTHER EXPLORATION

Organizations and Websites

The Internet addresses (also called uniform resource locators, or URLs) listed here were accurate at the time of publication. These websites include comprehensive information on a number of areas related to wellness. Some of the websites also include a search function.

continued

Center for Science in the Public Interest Nutrition Action Health Letter

http://www.cspinet.org/nah/index.htm

Harvard Health Letter

http://www.health.harvard.edu

Mayo Clinic Housecall

http://www.mayoclinic.com/health/housecall/HouseCall)

Tufts University Health & Nutrition Newsletter

http://www.tuftshealthletter.com

University of California at Berkeley Wellness Letter

http://www.berkeleywellness.com/

Laboratory Activities

Name _____ **Section** _____ **Date** _____

Lab 1.1 Your Wellness Profile

connect

Consider how your lifestyle, attitudes, and characteristics relate to each of the nine dimensions of wellness. Fill in your strengths for each dimension (examples of strengths are listed with each dimension). Once you've completed your lists, choose what you believe are your five most important strengths and circle them.

Physical wellness: To maintain overall physical health and engage in appropriate physical activity (e.g., stamina, strength, flexibility, healthy body composition).

_____

_____

_____

Emotional wellness: To have a positive self-concept, deal constructively with your feelings, and develop positive qualities (e.g., optimism, trust, self-confidence, determination).

_____

_____

_____

Intellectual wellness: To pursue and retain knowledge, think critically about issues, make sound decisions, identify problems, and find solutions (e.g., common sense, creativity, curiosity).

_____

_____

_____

Interpersonal/Social wellness: To develop and maintain meaningful relationships with a network of friends and family members, and to contribute to your community (e.g., friendly, good-natured, compassionate, supportive, good listener).

_____

_____

_____

Cultural wellness: To accept, value, and even celebrate personal and cultural differences (e.g., refuse to stereotype based on ethnicity, gender, religion, or sexual orientation; create relationships with those who are different from you; maintain and value your own cultural identity).

_____

_____

_____

Spiritual wellness: To develop a set of beliefs, principles, or values that give meaning or purpose to one's life; to develop faith in something beyond oneself (e.g., religious faith, service to others).

_____

_____

_____

Environmental wellness: To protect yourself from environmental hazards and to minimize the negative impact of your behaviour on the environment (e.g., carpooling, recycling).

_____

_____

_____

Financial wellness: To live within your means and manage your money in a way that gives you peace of mind (e.g., budget planning and saving).

_____

_____

_____

Occupational wellness: To gain a measure of happiness and fulfillment through your work (e.g., enjoy what you do, feel valued by your manager, build positive relationships with co-workers, take advantage of opportunities to learn and be challenged).

_____

_____

_____

Next, think about where you fall on the wellness continuum for each of the dimensions of wellness. Indicate your placement for each—physical, emotional, intellectual, interpersonal/social, cultural, spiritual, environmental, financial, and occupational—by placing Xs on the continuum below.

| Low level of wellness | Physical, psychological, emotional symptoms | Change and growth | High level of wellness |

Based on both your current lifestyle and your goals for the future, what do you think your placement on the wellness continuum will be in 10 years? What new health behaviours would you have to adopt to achieve your goals? Which of your current behaviours would you need to change to maintain or improve your level of wellness in the future?

_____

_____

_____

Does the description of wellness given in this chapter encompass everything you believe is part of wellness for you? Write your own definition of wellness, and include any additional dimensions that are important to you. Then rate your level of wellness based on your own definition.

_____
_____
_____

Using Your Results

How did you score? Are you satisfied with your current level of wellness—overall and in each dimension? In which dimension(s) would you most like to increase your level of wellness?

_____
_____
_____

What should you do next? As you consider possible target behaviours for a behaviour change program, choose things that will maintain or increase your level of wellness in one of the dimensions you listed as an area of concern. Remember to consider health behaviours such as smoking or eating a high-fat diet that may threaten your level of wellness in the future. Below, list several possible target behaviours and the wellness dimensions that they influence.

_____
_____
_____

For additional guidance in choosing a target behaviour, complete the lifestyle self-assessment in Lab 1.2.

Name _____ Section _____ Date _____

Lab 1.2 Lifestyle Evaluation

connect

How does your current lifestyle compare with the lifestyle recommended for wellness? For each question, choose the answer that best describes your behaviourol; then add up your score for each section.

Exercise/Fitness	Almost Always	Sometimes	Never
1. I engage in moderate exercise, such as brisk walking or swimming, for the equivalent of at least 150 minutes per week.	4	1	0
2. I do exercises to develop muscular strength and endurance at least twice a week.	2	1	0
3. I spend some of my leisure time participating in individual, family, or team activities, such as gardening, bowling, or softball.	2	1	0
4. I maintain a healthy body weight, avoiding overweight and underweight.	2	1	0
Exercise/Fitness Score: _____			

Nutrition	Almost Always	Sometimes	Never
1. I eat a variety of foods each day, including 5 or more servings of fruits and/or vegetables.	3	1	0
2. I limit the amount of saturated and trans fat in my diet.	3	1	0
3. I avoid skipping meals.	2	1	0
4. I limit the amount of salt and added sugars I eat.	2	1	0
Nutrition Score: _____			

Tobacco Use	Almost Always	Sometimes	Never
1. I avoid smoking cigarettes.	4	1	0
2. I avoid using a pipe or cigars.	2	1	0
3. I avoid spit tobacco.	2	1	0
4. I limit my exposure to environmental tobacco smoke.	2	1	0
Tobacco Use Score: _____			

Alcohol and Drugs	Almost Always	Sometimes	Never
1. I avoid alcohol, or I drink no more than 1 (women) or 2 (men) drinks a day.	4	1	0
2. I avoid using alcohol or other drugs as a way of handling stressful situations or the problems in my life.	2	1	0
3. I am careful not to drink alcohol when taking medications (such as cold or allergy medications) or when pregnant.	2	1	0
4. I read and follow the label directions when using prescribed and over-the-counter drugs.	2	1	0
Alcohol and Drugs Score: _____			

Emotional Health	Almost Always	Sometimes	Never
1. I enjoy being a student, and I have a job or do other work that I enjoy.	2	1	0
2. I find it easy to relax and express my feelings freely.	2	1	0
3. I manage stress well.	2	1	0
4. I have close friends, relatives, or others whom I can talk to about personal matters and call on for help when needed.	2	1	0
5. I participate in group activities (such as community or spiritual organizations) or hobbies that I enjoy.	2	1	0
Emotional Health Score: _____			

Safety	Almost Always	Sometimes	Never
1. I wear a seat belt while riding in a car.	2	1	0
2. I avoid driving while under the influence of alcohol or other drugs.	2	1	0
3. I obey traffic rules and the speed limit when driving.	2	1	0
4. I read and follow instructions on the labels of potentially harmful products or substances, such as household cleaners, poisons, and electrical appliances.	2	1	0
5. I avoid using a cell phone while driving.	2	1	0

Safety Score: _____

Disease Prevention	Almost Always	Sometimes	Never
1. I know the warning signs of cancer, heart attack, and stroke.	2	1	0
2. I avoid overexposure to the sun and use sunscreen.	2	1	0
3. I get recommended medical screening tests (such as blood pressure and cholesterol checks and Pap tests), immunizations, and booster shots.	2	1	0
4. I practise monthly skin and breast/testicle self-exams.	2	1	0
5. I am not sexually active or I have sex with only one mutually faithful, uninfected partner or I always engage in "safer sex" (using condoms) and I do not share needles to inject drugs.	2	1	0

Disease Prevention Score: _____

Scores of 9 and 10. Excellent! Your answers show that you are aware of the importance of this area to your health. More important, you are putting your knowledge to work for you by practising good health habits. As long as you continue to do so, this area should not pose a serious health risk.

Scores of 6 to 8. Your health practices in this area are good, but there is room for improvement.

Scores of 3 to 5. Your health risks are showing.

Scores of 0 to 2. You may be taking serious and unnecessary risks with your health.

Using Your Results

How did you score? In which areas did you score the lowest? Are you satisfied with your scores in each area? In which areas would you most like to improve your scores?

_____

_____

_____

What should you do next? To improve your scores, look closely at any item to which you answered "sometimes" or "never." Identify and list at least three possible targets for a health behaviour change program. (If you are aware of other risky health behaviours you currently engage in, but which were not covered by this assessment, you may include those in your list.) For each item on your list, identify your current "stage of change" and one strategy you could adopt to move forward. Possible strategies might be obtaining information about the behaviour, completing an analysis of the pros and cons of change, or beginning a written record or your target behaviour.

Behaviour	Stage	Strategy
1. _____	_____	_____
2. _____	_____	_____
3. _____	_____	_____

SOURCE: Adapted from *Healthstyle: A Self-Test,* developed by the U.S. Public Health Service. The behaviours covered in this test are recommended for most North Americans, but some may not apply to people with certain chronic diseases or disabilities or to pregnant women, who may require special advice from their physician.

CHAPTER 2

Basic Principles of Physical Fitness

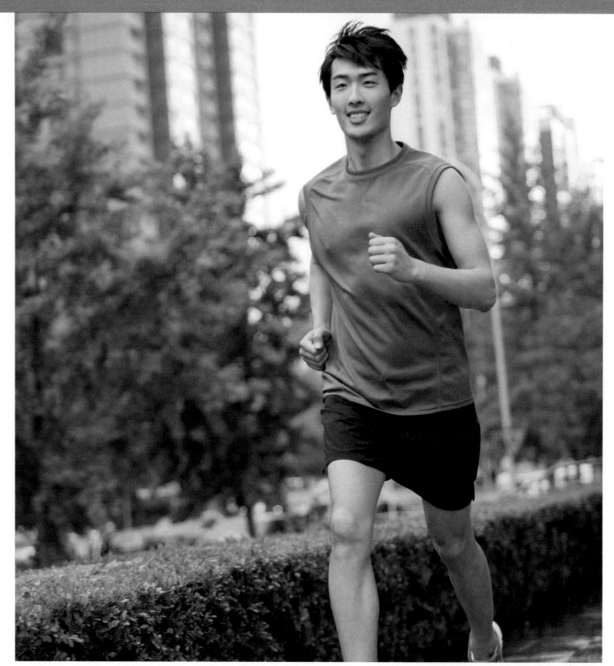

© Lane Oatey / Blue Jean Images / Getty Images RF

LEARNING OBJECTIVES

After reading this chapter, you should be able to

LO1 Describe how much exercise is recommended for developing health and fitness

LO2 Identify the components of physical fitness and the way each component affects wellness

LO3 Explain the goal of physical training and the basic principles of training

LO4 Describe the principles involved in designing a well-rounded exercise program

LO5 List the steps that can be taken to make an exercise program safe, effective, and successful

TEST YOUR KNOWLEDGE

1. **To improve your health, you must exercise vigorously for at least 30 consecutive minutes, five or more days per week.**

   True or false?

2. **Which of the following activities uses about 150 calories?**
   a. washing a car for 45 to 60 minutes
   b. shooting a basketball for 30 minutes
   c. jumping rope for 15 minutes

3. **Regular exercise can make a person smarter.**

   True or false?

ANSWERS

1. **FALSE.** Experts recommend 150 minutes of moderate-intensity physical activity or 75 minutes of vigorous-intensity physical activity per week. This activity can be accomplished in short bouts—multiple 10-minute sessions, for example—spread out over the course of the day.

2. **ALL THREE.** The more intense an activity is, the more calories it burns in a given amount of time. This is one reason why people who exercise vigorously can get the same benefits in less time than people who exercise longer at a moderate intensity.

3. **TRUE.** Regular exercise (even moderate-intensity exercise) benefits the human brain and nervous system in a variety of ways. For example, exercise improves cognitive function—that is, the brain's ability to learn, remember, think, and reason.

Any list of the benefits of physical activity is impressive. Although people vary greatly in terms of physical fitness and performance ability, the benefits of regular physical activity are available to everyone. Much of the increased health benefits from exercise occur when going from no activity (sedentary) to some moderate-intensity activity (see Figure 2.1 on the next page). Further health benefits occur when exercising harder or longer. The relative risk of death from all causes and the risk of heart disease decrease by as much as 65% when comparing the least and most active men and women. In Figure 2.1, relative risk of death refers to the risk of death per year of sedentary people compared to people in various activity levels.

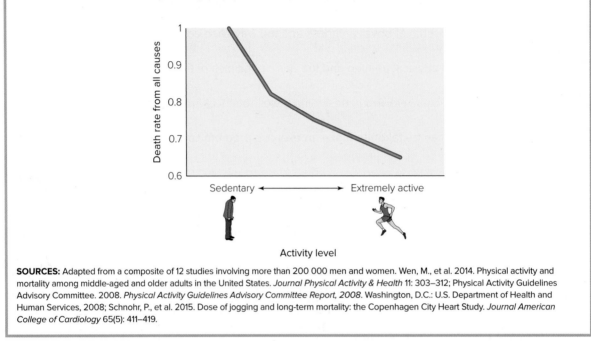

SOURCES: Adapted from a composite of 12 studies involving more than 200 000 men and women. Wen, M., et al. 2014. Physical activity and mortality among middle-aged and older adults in the United States. *Journal Physical Activity & Health* 11: 303–312; Physical Activity Guidelines Advisory Committee. 2008. *Physical Activity Guidelines Advisory Committee Report, 2008*. Washington, D.C.: U.S. Department of Health and Human Services, 2008; Schnohr, P., et al. 2015. Dose of jogging and long-term mortality: the Copenhagen City Heart Study. *Journal American College of Cardiology* 65(5): 411–419.

This chapter provides an overview of physical fitness. It explains how lifestyle physical activity and more formal exercise programs contribute to wellness. It also describes the components of fitness, the basic principles of physical training, and the essential elements of a well-rounded exercise program. Chapters 3 to 6 provide an in-depth look at each of the elements of a fitness program; Chapter 9 will help you put all these elements together into a complete, personalized program.

2.1 Physical Activity and Exercise for Health and Fitness

Despite the fact that two-thirds of Canadians strongly agree that leading a healthy lifestyle can lead to long-term health benefits, levels of physical inactivity in Canada are still too high. According to Statistics Canada (2015), only 2 in 10 Canadian adults and 1 in 10 Canadian children are active enough to meet Canada's Physical Activity Guidelines.

The 2008 Physical Activity Monitors[1] (sponsored by the Canadian Fitness and Lifestyle Research Institute) report that factors such as gender, age, and income level may impact our level of physical activity. For example:

- Women of all age groups are less likely to be physically active than men; the older women become, the wider the gap between the genders.

- Those with higher incomes are more likely to be at least moderately active than those with lower incomes.

Possible barriers to increased activity include lack of time and resources, social and environmental influences, and—most important—lack of motivation and commitment (see Lab 2.2 for more on barriers). Some people also fear injury. Although physical activity carries some risks, the risks of inactivity are far greater. Increased physical activity may be the single most important lifestyle behaviour change for promoting health and well-being.

Physical Activity on a Continuum

Physical activity is a movement carried out by the skeletal muscles and requiring energy. Different types of physical activity can vary by ease of intensity. Standing up or walking down a hallway requires little energy or effort, but each is a higher level of activity than sitting or lying down. More intense and sustained activities, such as cycling 10 kilometres or running in a race, require considerably more effort.

physical activity   Body movement carried out by the skeletal muscles that requires energy.

Exercise refers to a planned, structured, repetitive movement intended specifically to improve or maintain physical fitness. As discussed in Chapter 1, physical fitness is a set of physical attributes that allows the body to respond or adapt to the demands and stress of physical effort—to perform moderate to vigorous levels of physical activity without becoming overly tired. Levels of fitness depend on such physiological factors as the heart's ability to pump blood and the energy-generating capacity of the cells. These factors depend on both *genetics*—a person's inborn potential for physical fitness—and *behaviour*—getting enough physical activity to stress the body and cause long-term physiological changes.

exercise   Planned, structured, repetitive movement intended to improve or maintain physical fitness.

Physical activity is essential to health and confers wide-ranging health benefits (see also the box Exercise is Good For Your Brain), but exercise is necessary to significantly improve physical fitness. This important distinction between physical activity, which improves health and wellness, and exercise, which improves fitness, is a key concept in understanding the guidelines discussed in this section.

The Evidence *for* EXERCISE

EXERCISE IS GOOD FOR YOUR BRAIN

Some scientists call exercise the new "brain food." Studies show that even moderate physical activity can improve brain health and function and may delay the decline in cognitive function that occurs for many people as they age. Regular physical activity has the following positive effects on the human brain:

- Improves cognitive function—the brain's ability to learn, remember, think, and reason.
- Helps overcome the negative effects of a poor diet on brain health.
- Promotes the creation of new nerve cells (neurons) throughout the nervous system. By promoting this process (called *neurogenesis*), exercise provides some protection against injury and degenerative conditions that destroy neurons. Physical activity is less effective for promoting brain health when exercising in polluted air.

continued

- Enhances the entire nervous system's *plasticity*—its ability to change and adapt. In the brain, spinal cord, and nerves, this can mean developing new pathways for transmitting sensory information or motor commands.
- Appears to have a protective effect on the brain as people age, helping to delay or even prevent the onset of neurodegenerative disorders such as Alzheimer's disease.

Although most people consider brain health to be a concern for the elderly, it is vital to wellness throughout life. For this reason, many studies on exercise and brain health include children as well as older adults. Targeted research has also focused on the impact of exercise on people with disorders such as cerebral palsy, multiple sclerosis, and developmental disabilities. Generally speaking, these studies all reach a similar conclusion: Exercise enhances brain health, at least to some degree, in people of all ages and a wide range of health statuses.

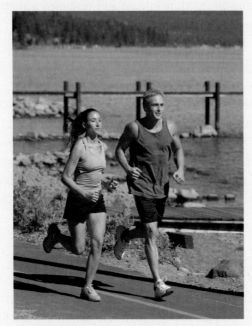

© moodboard / Alamy

Along with the brain's physical health, mental health is also enhanced by exercise. Even modest activity, such as taking a daily walk, can help combat a variety of mental health disorders and improve mood.

It's hard to understate the impact of physical and mental disorders related to brain health. According to the Alzheimer's Society (http://www.alzheimer.ca), almost 750 000 Canadians currently suffer from cognitive impairment—and the number is increasing steadily. People with depression, anxiety, or other mental disorders are more likely to suffer from chronic physical conditions. Taken together, these and other brain-related disorders cost untold millions of dollars in health care costs and lost productivity, as well as thousands of years of productive lifetime lost.

For the sake of your brain—as well as your muscles, bones, and heart—start creating your exercise program soon. You'll be healthier, and you may even feel a little smarter.

SOURCES: Guiney, H., and L. Machado. 2013. Benefits of regular aerobic exercise for executive functioning in healthy populations. *Psychonomic Bulletin and Review* 20(1): 73–86; Garber, C.E., et al. 2011. Quantity and quality of exercise for developing and maintaining cardiorespiratory, musculoskeletal, and neuromotor fitness in apparently healthy adults: Guidance for prescribing exercise. *Medicine and Science in Sports and Exercise* 43(7): 1334–1359; Bos, I., et al. 2013. Subclinical effects of aerobic training in urban environment. *Medicine Science in Sports and Exercise* 45(3): 439–447; Siette, J., et al. 2013. Age-specific effects of voluntary exercise on memory and the older brain. *Biological Psychiatry* 73(5): 435–442.

Wellness Tip

Do you set aside blocks of time every day for studying? If so, your schedule probably makes it easier to get your work done. The same is true of exercising. Make it a part of your daily routine, like studying.

Lifestyle Physical Activity for Health Promotion

The Public Health Agency of Canada, in conjunction with the Canadian Society for Exercise Physiology (CSEP), conclude that optimal health benefits are within reach for Canadians if they achieve minimum standards for physical activity. The Canadian Physical Activity Guidelines suggest that each age demographic should attain the following levels of physical activity:

- Children aged 5 to 11 years and youth aged 12 to 17 should accumulate at least 60 minutes of moderate- to vigorous-intensity physical activity daily.

- Adults aged 18 and older should accumulate at least 150 minutes of moderate- to vigorous-intensity aerobic physical activity per week, in bouts of 10 minutes or more.

In addition to guidelines for the amount of physical activity that Canadians should be achieving, CSEP also recommends that each group participate in muscle- and bone-strengthening activities. The guidelines can be downloaded for free at http://csepguidelines.ca.

In the lifestyle approach to physical activity, people can choose activities that they find enjoyable and that fit into their daily routine. In addition, everyday tasks at school, work, and home can be structured to contribute to the daily activity total. The daily total of lifestyle activity can be accumulated in multiple short bouts, such as two 10-minute bicycle rides to and from class and a brisk 15-minute walk to the post office. Figure 2.2 provides more examples of activities that Canadians can perform in achieving acceptable levels of physical activity. See also the box Classifying Activity Levels on the next page.

FIGURE 2.2

Activities to increase Canadians' physical activity.

Very light effort	Light effort	Moderate effort	Vigorous effort	Maximum effort
	60 Minutes	30–60 Minutes	20–30 Minutes	
• Strolling	• Light walking	• Brisk walking	• Aerobics	• Sprinting
• Dusting	• Easy gardening	• Biking	• Jogging	• Racing
	• Stretching	• Raking leaves	• Hockey	
		• Swimming	• Basketball	
		• Dancing	• Fast swimming	
		• Water aerobics	• Fast dancing	
		Range Needed to Stay Healthy		

SOURCE: Based on Canada's Physical Activity Guide to Healthy Active Living from Public Health Agency of Canada and the Canadian Society for Exercise Physiology. Cat. No. H39-429/1998-1E ISBN 0-662-866. (http://www.physicalactivityplan.org/resources/CPAG.pdf).

By increasing lifestyle physical activity, you can expect to significantly improve your health and well-being. If all the Canadians who are now completely sedentary were to adopt a more active lifestyle, there would be an enormous benefit to the public's health and to individual well-being.

In FOCUS

CLASSIFYING ACTIVITY LEVELS

Assessing your physical activity level is easier if you know how to classify different kinds of activities. Fitness experts categorize activities into the following three levels:

- **Light activity** includes the routine tasks associated with typical day-to-day life, such as vacuuming, walking slowly, shopping, or stretching. You probably perform dozens of light activities every day without even thinking about it. You can gain significant health benefits by turning light activities into moderate activities—by walking briskly instead of slowly, for example.
- **Moderate activity** causes your breathing and heart rate to accelerate but still allows for comfortable conversation, such as walking at a rate of 4 to 6 kilometres per hour. It is sometimes described as activity that can be performed comfortably for about 45 minutes. Examples of moderate physical activity include brisk walking, social dancing, and cycling moderately on level terrain.
- **Vigorous activity** elevates your heart and breathing rates considerably and has other physical effects that improve your fitness level. Examples include jogging, hiking uphill, swimming laps, and playing most competitive sports.

Fitness Tip

To make your workouts more effective, find an exercise buddy. You can help each other set goals, stay on track, keep time, and count reps. Exercising with a friend makes working out more enjoyable, too.

LO1 How Much Physical Activity Is Enough?

Some experts feel that people get most of the health benefits of an exercise program simply by becoming more active over the course of the day; the amount of activity needed depends on an individual's health status and goals. Other experts feel that the activity goal set by the lifestyle approach is too low; they argue that people should exercise long enough and intensely enough to improve their body's capacity for exercise—that is, to improve physical fitness. There is probably truth in both of these positions.

Regular physical activity, regardless of the intensity, makes you healthier and can help protect you from many chronic diseases. Although you get many of the health benefits of exercise simply by being more active, you obtain even more benefits when you are physically fit. In addition to long-term health benefits, fitness also contributes significantly to quality of life. Fitness can give you freedom to move your body the way you want. Fit people have more energy and better body control. They can enjoy a more active lifestyle than their more sedentary counterparts. Even if you don't like sports, you need physical energy and stamina in your daily life and for many non-sport leisure activities such as visiting museums, playing with children, and gardening.

Where does this leave you? Most experts agree that some physical activity is better than none, but that more—as long as it does not result in injury—is better than some. To set a personal goal for physical activity and exercise, consider your current activity level, your health status, and your overall goals. At the very least, strive to become more active and do 30 minutes of moderate-intensity activity at least five days per week.

Choose to be active whenever you can. If weight management is a concern for you, begin by achieving the goal of 30 minutes of activity per day and then try to raise your activity level further, to 60 to 90 minutes per day or more. For even better health and well-being, participate in a structured exercise program that develops physical fitness. Any increase in physical activity will contribute to your health and well-being—now and in the future.

LO2 2.2 Components of Physical Fitness

Some components of fitness relate to specific skill activities, such as tennis and skiing, and others to general health. **Health-related fitness** includes the following components:

- cardiorespiratory endurance
- muscular strength
- muscular endurance
- flexibility
- body composition

health-related fitness   Physical capacities that contribute to health: cardiorespiratory endurance, muscular strength, muscular endurance, flexibility, and body composition.

Health-related fitness helps you withstand physical challenges and protects you from disease.

Fitness Tip

Very few activities build all the health-related components of fitness at the same time. This is why variety is important. Create a routine that lets you build one or two fitness components every day. Variety also keeps your workouts enjoyable.

Cardiorespiratory Endurance

Cardiorespiratory endurance is the ability to perform prolonged, large-muscle, dynamic exercise at moderate to high levels of intensity. It depends on such factors as the ability of the lungs to deliver oxygen from the environment to the bloodstream, the capacity of the heart to pump blood, the ability of the nervous system and blood vessels to regulate blood flow, and the capability of the cell's chemical systems to use oxygen and process fuels for exercise and rest.

cardiorespiratory endurance   The ability of the body to perform prolonged, large-muscle, dynamic exercise at moderate to high levels of intensity.

When cardiorespiratory fitness is low, the heart has to work hard during normal daily activities and may not be able to work hard enough to sustain high-intensity physical activity in an emergency. As cardiorespiratory fitness improves, related physical functions also improve. For example:

- The heart pumps more blood per heartbeat.
- Resting heart rate slows.
- Blood volume increases.
- Blood supply to tissues improves.

- The body can cool itself better.

- Blood vessels become more pliable.

- Resting blood pressure decreases.

- Metabolism in skeletal muscle is enhanced, which improves fuel use.

- The level of antioxidant chemicals in the body increases and oxidation decreases. During metabolism, the body naturally produces chemicals called free radicals (oxidative stress) that cause cell damage. Exercise training increases the production of antioxidants that help neutralize free radicals.

A healthy heart can better withstand the strains of everyday life, the stress of occasional emergencies, and the wear and tear of time.

Cardiovascular endurance training also improves the functioning of the body's chemical systems, particularly in the muscles and liver. These changes enhance the body's ability to derive energy from food, allow the body to perform more exercise with less effort, increase sensitivity to insulin, and prevent type 2 diabetes. Exercise reduces blood vessel inflammation, which is linked to coronary artery disease, heart attack, and stroke.

Physically fit people also have healthier, more resilient genes. Exercise preserves gene structures called telomeres, which form the ends of the DNA strands and hold them together. Over time the telomeres shorten, reducing their effectiveness, which triggers illness and death. Exercise helps to keep them from getting too short.

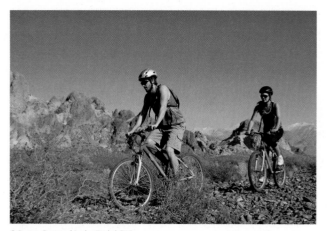

© Image Source / Javier Perini CM

Cardiorespiratory endurance is a key component of health-related fitness. These mountain bikers are conditioning their hearts and lungs as well as gaining many other health benefits.

Cardiorespiratory endurance is a central component of health-related fitness because heart and lung function is so essential to overall good health. A person can't live very long or very well without a healthy heart or healthy lungs. Poor cardiorespiratory fitness is linked with heart disease, type 2 diabetes, colon cancer, stroke, depression, and anxiety. A moderate level of cardiorespiratory fitness can even help compensate for certain health risks, including excess body fat. In fact, people with higher levels of body fat but who are otherwise fit have been found to have lower death rates than those who are lean but who have low cardiorespiratory fitness.[2]

You can develop cardiorespiratory endurance through activities that involve continuous, rhythmic movements of large-muscle groups, such as the legs. Such activities include walking, jogging, cycling, and aerobic dancing.

Ask Yourself

QUESTIONS FOR CRITICAL THINKING AND REFLECTION

Does your current lifestyle include enough physical activity—30 minutes of moderate-intensity activity five or more days a week—to support health and wellness? Does your lifestyle go beyond this level to include enough vigorous physical activity and exercise to build physical fitness? What changes could you make in your lifestyle to develop physical fitness?

Muscular Strength

Muscular strength is the amount of force a muscle can produce with a single maximum effort. It depends on such factors as the size of muscle cells and the ability of nerves to activate muscle cells. Strong muscles are important for the smooth and easy performance of everyday activities, such as climbing stairs, as well as for emergency situations. They help keep the skeleton in proper alignment, preventing back and leg pain and providing the support necessary for good posture. Muscular strength has obvious importance in recreational activities. Strong people can hit a tennis ball harder, kick a soccer ball farther, and ride a bicycle uphill more easily.

> **muscular strength** The amount of force a muscle can produce with a single maximum effort.

Muscle tissue is an important element of overall body composition. Greater muscle mass means faster energy use and a higher rate of **metabolism**, the sum of all the vital processes by which food energy and nutrients are made available to and used by the body. Greater muscle mass reduces markers of oxidative stress and maintains mitochondria (the "powerhouses" of the cell); both of these benefits are important for metabolic health and long life. Training to build muscular strength can also help people manage stress and boost their self-confidence.

> **metabolism** The sum of all the vital processes by which food energy and nutrients are made available to and used by the body.

Maintaining strength and muscle mass is vital for healthy aging. Stronger people live longer. Older people tend to experience a decrease in both number and size of muscle cells, a condition called *sarcopenia*. Many of the remaining muscle cells become slower, and some become nonfunctional because they lose their attachment to the nervous system. Strength training (also known as *resistance training* or *weight training*) increases antioxidant enzymes and lowers oxidative stress. It also helps maintain muscle mass and function and possibly helps decrease the risk of osteoporosis (bone loss) in older people, greatly enhancing their quality of life and preventing life-threatening injuries.

Muscular Endurance

Muscular endurance is the ability to resist fatigue and sustain a given level of muscle tension—that is, to hold a muscle contraction for a long period of time or to contract a muscle over and over again. It depends on such factors as the size of muscle cells, the ability of muscles to store fuel, blood supply, and the metabolic capacity of muscles.

> **muscular endurance** The ability of a muscle to remain contracted or to contract repeatedly for a long period of time.

Muscular endurance is important for good posture and for injury prevention. For example, if abdominal and back muscles cannot support and stabilize the spine correctly when you sit or stand for long periods, the chances of low-back pain and back injury are increased. Good muscular endurance in the trunk muscles is more important than muscular strength for preventing back pain. Muscular endurance helps people cope with daily physical demands and enhances performance in sports and work.

Flexibility

Flexibility is the ability to move the joints through their full range of motion. It depends on joint structure, the length and elasticity of connective tissue, and nervous system activity. Flexible, pain-free joints are important for good health and well-being. Inactivity causes the joints to become stiffer with age. Stiffness, in

> **flexibility** The ability to move joints through their full range of motion.

turn, often causes older people to assume unnatural body postures that can stress joints and muscles. Stretching exercises can help ensure a healthy range of motion for all major joints.

Body Composition

Body composition refers to the proportion of fat and **fat-free mass** (muscle, bone, and water) in the body. Healthy body composition involves a high proportion of fat-free mass and an acceptably low level of body fat, adjusted for age and gender. A person with excessive body fat—especially fat in the abdomen—is more likely to experience health problems, including heart disease, insulin resistance, high blood pressure, stroke, joint problems, type 2 diabetes, gallbladder disease, blood vessel inflammation, some types of cancer, back pain, and premature death.

> **body composition** The proportion of fat and fat-free mass (muscle, bone, and water) in the body.
> **fat-free mass** The nonfat component of the human body, consisting of skeletal muscle, bone, and water.

The best way to lose fat is through a lifestyle that includes a sensible diet and exercise. The best way to add muscle mass is through resistance training. Large changes in body composition are not necessary to improve health; even a small increase in physical activity and a small decrease in body fat can lead to substantial health improvements.

Wellness Tip

The words "over time" are key to realizing the benefits of physical activity. If you get in the habit of being active, you'll notice the benefits over time. After a few weeks of exercise, you'll breathe with less effort and recover faster, and you'll feel stronger and more flexible. In time, exercise and lifestyle changes will result in your clothes fitting differently, and you may even notice changes in the mirror. Practise patience and watch the rewards pile up!

Skill (Neuromuscular)-Related Components of Fitness

In addition to the five health-related components of physical fitness, the ability to perform a particular sport or activity may depend on **skill (neuromuscular)-related fitness**. Neuromuscular refers to the complex control of muscles and movement by the brain and spinal column. The components of skill-related fitness include the following:

> **skill (neuromuscular)-related fitness** Physical capacities that contribute to performance in a sport or an activity: speed, power, agility, balance, coordination, and reaction time.

- **Speed.** The ability to perform a movement in a short period of time.
- **Power.** The ability to exert force rapidly based on a combination of strength and speed.
- **Agility.** The ability to change the position of the body quickly and accurately.

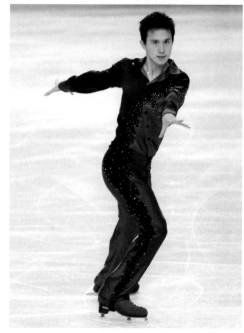

© Olga Besnard / GetStock.com

Elite athletes like Patrick Chan demonstrate sport-specific skills such as speed, power, agility, coordination, and reaction time.

- **Balance.** The ability to maintain equilibrium while moving or while stationary.
- **Coordination.** The ability to perform motor tasks accurately and smoothly using body movements and the senses.
- **Reaction and movement time.** The ability to respond or react quickly to a stimulus.

Skill-related fitness tends to be sport-specific and is best developed through practice. For example, playing basketball can develop the speed, coordination, and agility needed to engage in the sport. Participating in sports is fun, can help build fitness, and contributes to other areas of wellness. Young adults often find it easier to exercise regularly when they participate in sports and activities they enjoy, such as dancing, tennis, snowboarding, or basketball. Older adults can develop balance by practising exercises such as yoga and tai chi. Skill-related activities are particularly important for older adults to help prevent life-threatening falls.

LO3 2.3 Principles of Physical Training: Adaptation to Stress

The human body is very adaptable. The greater the demands made on it, the more it adjusts to meet those demands. Over time, immediate, short-term **adaptations** or adjustments translate into long-term changes and improvements. When breathing and heart rate increase during exercise, for example, the heart gradually develops the ability to pump more blood with each beat. Then, during exercise, it doesn't have to beat as fast to meet the cells' demands for oxygen. The goal of **physical training** is to produce these long-term changes and improvements in the body's functioning and fitness. Although people differ in the maximum levels of physical fitness and performance they can achieve through training, the wellness benefits of exercise are available to everyone (see the box Fitness and Disability).

adaptation The physiological changes that occur with exercise training.
physical training The performance of different types of activities that cause the body to adapt and improve its level of fitness.

DIVERSITY Matters

FITNESS AND DISABILITY

Physical fitness and athletic achievement are not limited to the able-bodied. People with disabilities can also attain high levels of fitness and performance. Elite athletes compete in the Paralympics, the premier event for athletes with disabilities, which is held in the same year and city as the Olympics. The performance of these skilled athletes makes it clear that people with disabilities can be active, healthy, and extraordinarily fit. Just like able-bodied athletes, athletes with disabilities strive for excellence and can serve as role models.

Currently, some 3.8 million Canadians are estimated to have chronic, significant disabilities. Some disabilities are the result of injury, such as spinal cord injuries sustained in car crashes. Other disabilities result from illness, such as the blindness that sometimes occurs as a complication of diabetes or the joint stiffness that accompanies arthritis. And some disabilities are present at birth, as in the case of

continued

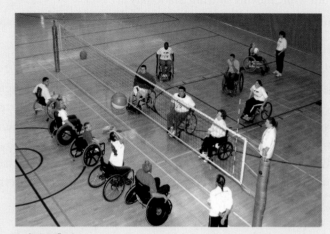
Realistic Reflections

congenital limb deformities or cerebral palsy.

Exercise and physical activity are as important for people with disabilities as for able-bodied individuals—if not *more* important. Being active helps prevent secondary conditions that may result from prolonged inactivity, such as circulatory or muscular problems. It provides an emotional boost that helps support a positive attitude as well as opportunities to make new friends, increase self-confidence, and gain a sense of accomplishment. However, Canadians with disabilities are less likely to be physically active than other Canadians.

People with disabilities don't have to be elite athletes to participate in sports and lead an active life. Many health clubs, fitness centres, city recreation centres, and universities/colleges offer activities and events geared for people of all ages and types of disabilities. They may have modified aerobics classes, special weight training machines, classes involving mild exercise in warm water, and other activities adapted for people with disabilities. Popular sports and recreational activities include adapted horseback riding, golf, swimming, and skiing. Competitive sports are also available—for example, there are wheelchair versions of billiards, tennis, weight lifting, hockey, and basketball, as well as sports for people with hearing, visual, or intellectual impairments. For those who prefer to get their exercise at home, special videos are available that are geared to individuals who use wheelchairs or who have arthritis, hearing impairments, metabolic diseases, or many other disabilities.

In addition, as part of a Canada 150 initiative, the Rick Hansen Foundation and the Government of Canada recently awarded 55 Canadian communities Access4All Barrier Buster grants. These monies will help break down accessibility barriers across the country.

If you have a disability and want to be more active, check with your physician about what's appropriate for you. Contact your local community centre, university/college, YMCA/YWCA, independent living centre, or fitness centre to locate potential facilities. Look for a facility with experienced personnel and appropriate adaptive equipment. For specialized information, check with hospitals and health associations that are geared to specific disabilities, such as the Canadian Arthritis Society.

SOURCES: Active Living Alliance for Canadians with a Disability (http://www.ala.ca); Rick Hansen Foundation. Access4All Program. Available online at http://access4all.rickhansen.com/; Statistics Canada. (Revised 2017). A profile of persons with disabilities among Canadians aged 15 or older, 2012. Available online at: http://www.statcan.gc.ca/pub/89-654-x/89-654-x2015001-eng.htm. Catalogue no. 89-654-X. Published by authority of the Minister responsible for Statistics Canada. © 2015 Minister of Industry. Reproduced and distributed on an "as is" basis with the permission of Statistics Canada.

Particular types and amounts of exercise are most effective in developing the various components of fitness. To put together an effective exercise program, you should first understand the basic principles of physical training, including the following:

- specificity
- progressive overload

- reversibility
- individual differences

All of these rest on the larger principle of adaptation.

Specificity—Adapting to Type of Training

To develop a particular fitness component, you must perform exercises designed specifically for that component. This is the principle of **specificity**. Weight training develops muscular strength, for example, but is less effective for developing cardiorespiratory endurance or flexibility. Specificity also applies to the skill-related fitness components (e.g., to improve at tennis, you must practise tennis) and to the different parts of the body (e.g., to develop stronger arms, you must exercise your arms). A well-rounded exercise program includes exercises geared to each component of fitness, to different parts of the body, and to specific activities or sports.

> **specificity**   The training principle that the body adapts to the particular type and amount of stress placed on it.

Sports science pioneer Franklin Henry from the University of California, Berkeley, developed the principle of specificity of training. His studies show that a specific movement performed at a specific speed develops a unique skill. In addition, motor control studies have shown that practice reinforces motor patterns in the brain that are specific to a given movement. In other words, there is no general coordination, agility, balance, and accuracy; the balance required in skiing is different from the balance required to stand on one foot or do tricks on a skateboard, and requires its own specific training.

Progressive Overload—Adapting to Amount of Training and the FITT Principle

The body adapts to the demands of exercise by improving its functioning. When the amount of exercise (also called *overload* or *stress*) is increased progressively, fitness continues to improve. This is the principle of **progressive overload**.

> **progressive overload**   The training principle that placing increasing amounts of stress on the body causes adaptations that improve fitness.

The amount of overload is very important: Too little exercise will have no effect on fitness (although it may improve health); too much may cause injury and problems with the body's immune or endocrine (hormone) systems. The point at which exercise becomes excessive is highly individual. For example, it occurs at a much higher level in an Olympic athlete than in a sedentary person. For every type of exercise, there is a training threshold at which fitness benefits begin to occur, a zone within which maximum fitness benefits occur, and an upper limit of safe training.

The amount of exercise needed depends on the individual's current level of fitness, genetically determined capacity to adapt to training, and fitness goals, as well as the component being developed. A novice, for example, might experience fitness benefits from jogging a kilometre in six minutes, but this level of exercise would not benefit trained distance runners. Beginners should start at the lower end of the fitness benefit zone, while fitter individuals will make more rapid gains by exercising at the higher end of the fitness benefit zone. Progressive overload is critical. Exercising at the same intensity every training session will maintain fitness but will not increase it because the training stress is below the threshold required to produce adaptation. Fitness increases only if the volume and intensity of workouts increase.

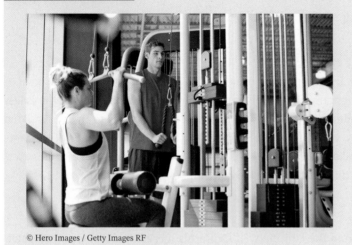

Fitness Tip

Progressive overload is important because the body adapts to overload (increased volume and intensity of exercise) by becoming more fit. This is true even if your starting level of fitness is low. At the gym, don't be intimidated by people who seem to be in better shape than you are. Remember that they got in shape by focusing on themselves, not by worrying about what other people thought about them.

© Hero Images / Getty Images RF

The amount of overload needed to maintain or improve a particular level of fitness for a particular fitness component is determined through four dimensions, represented by the acronym FITT:

- **F**requency—how often
- **I**ntensity—how hard
- **T**ime—how long (duration)
- **T**ype—mode of activity

Some experts use the acronym FITTE, where the *E* stands for enjoyment—a key component of a successful, long-term fitness program. Chapter 3, Chapter 4, and Chapter 5 show you how to apply the FITT principle to exercise programs for cardiorespiratory endurance, muscular strength and endurance, and flexibility, respectively.

Frequency

Developing fitness requires regular exercise. Optimum exercise frequency, expressed in number of days per week, varies with the component being developed and the individual's fitness goals. For most people, three to five days per week of cardiorespiratory endurance exercise and two or more days per week of resistance and flexibility training are appropriate for a general fitness program.

An important consideration in determining appropriate exercise frequency is recovery time. The amount of time required to recover from exercise is highly individual and depends on factors such as training experience, age, and intensity of training. For example, 24 hours of rest between highly intensive workouts that involve heavy weights or track sprints is not enough recovery time for safe and effective training in most cases. Intense workouts need to be spaced out during the week to allow for sufficient recovery time. On the other hand, you can exercise every day if your program consists of moderate-intensity walking or cycling. Learn to "listen to your body" to get enough rest between workouts. Chapters 3 to 5 provide more detailed information about training techniques and recovery periods for workouts focused on different fitness components.

Intensity

Fitness benefits occur when you exercise harder than your normal level of activity. The appropriate exercise intensity varies with each fitness component. To develop cardiorespiratory endurance, for example, you must raise your heart rate above normal. To develop muscular strength, you must lift a heavier weight than normal. To develop flexibility, you must stretch muscles beyond their normal length.

Time (Duration)

Fitness benefits occur when you exercise for an extended period of time:

- For cardiorespiratory endurance exercise, 20 to 60 minutes is recommended. Exercise can take place in a single session or in several sessions of 10 or more minutes. The greater the intensity of exercise, the less time needed to obtain fitness benefits.
- For high-intensity exercise, such as running, for example, 20 to 30 minutes is appropriate.
- For more moderate-intensity exercise, such as walking, 45 to 60 minutes may be needed. High-intensity exercise poses a greater risk of injury than lower-intensity exercise, so if you are a nonathletic adult, it's probably best to emphasize lower- to moderate-intensity activity of longer duration.

To build muscular strength, muscular endurance, and flexibility, similar amounts of time are advisable, but these exercises are more commonly organized in terms of a specific number of *repetitions* of a particular exercise. For resistance training, for example, a recommended program includes one or more sets of 8 to 12 repetitions of 8 to 10 different exercises that work the major muscle groups. Older adults should do 10 to 15 repetitions per set with lighter weights.

Type (Mode of Activity)

The type of exercise in which you should engage varies with each fitness component and with your personal fitness goals. To develop cardiorespiratory endurance, you need to engage in continuous activities involving large-muscle groups—walking, jogging, cycling, or swimming, for example. Resistive exercises develop muscular strength and endurance, while stretching exercises build flexibility. The frequency, intensity, and time of the exercise will be different for each type of activity. See the section Guidelines for Training in this chapter for more on choosing appropriate activities for your fitness program.

Reversibility—Adapting to a Reduction in Training

Fitness is a reversible adaptation. The body adjusts to lower levels of physical activity in the same way it adjusts to higher levels. This is the principle of **reversibility**. When a person stops exercising, some fitness improvements are lost in as little as two weeks' time.[3] However, not all fitness levels reverse at the same rate. Strength fitness is very resilient, so a person can maintain strength fitness by doing resistive exercise as infrequently as once a week. On the other hand, cardiovascular and cellular fitness reverse themselves more quickly—sometimes within just a few days or weeks. If you must temporarily reduce the frequency or duration of your training, you can maintain much of your fitness improvement by keeping the intensity of your workouts constant.

---

reversibility   The training principle that fitness improvements are lost when demands on the body are lowered.

Individual Differences—Limits on Adaptability

Anyone watching the Olympics can see that, from a physical standpoint, we are not all created equal. There are large individual differences in our ability to improve fitness, achieve a desirable body composition, and learn and perform sports skills. Some people are able to run longer distances, lift more weight, or kick a soccer ball more skillfully than others will ever be able to, no matter how much they train. People respond to training at different rates, so a program that works for one person may not be right for another person.

There are limits on the adaptability—the potential for improvement—of any human body. The body's ability to transport and use oxygen, for example, can only be improved by about 5–25% through endurance training.[4] An endurance athlete must therefore inherit a large metabolic capacity in order to reach competitive performance levels. In the past few years, scientists have identified specific genes that influence body fat, strength, and endurance. For example, more than 800 genes are associated with endurance performance, and 100 of those determine individual differences in exercise capacity. However, physical training improves fitness regardless of heredity, and the average person's body can improve enough to achieve reasonable fitness goals.

LO4 2.4 Designing Your Own Exercise Program

Physical training works best when you have a plan. A plan helps you make gradual but steady progress toward your goals. First, determine that exercise is safe for you; then assess how fit you are, decide what your goals are, and choose the right activities to help you get there.

Getting Medical Clearance

Participating in exercise and sports is usually a wonderful experience that improves wellness in both the short and the long term. In rare instances, however, vigorous exertion is associated with sudden death. It may seem difficult to understand that although regular exercise protects people from heart disease, exercise also increases the risk of sudden death for some.

Exercise and Cardiac Risk

Overall, the risk of death from exercise is small—and people are much safer exercising than engaging in many other common activities, including driving a car. One study of joggers found 1 death for every 396 000 hours of jogging; another study of men involved in a variety of physical activities found 1 death per 1.5 million hours of exercise.

In people under the age of 35, congenital heart defects (i.e., heart abnormalities present at birth) are the most common cause of exercise-related sudden death. In nearly all other cases, coronary artery disease is responsible. In this condition, fat and other substances build up in the arteries that supply blood to the heart. Death can result if an artery becomes blocked or if the heart's rhythm and pumping action are disrupted. Exercise, particularly intense exercise, may trigger a heart attack in someone with underlying heart disease.

The riskiest scenario may involve the middle-aged or older individual who suddenly begins participating in a vigorous sport or activity after being sedentary for a long time. Engaging in very vigorous exercise over the long term can also be risky for some individuals due to stress on the cardiovascular system. For example, a study of joggers in Denmark found the lowest mortality rate among those who jogged a moderate amount (2 to 3 workouts for a total of 60 to 150 minutes per week); higher rates of death were found among non-joggers and those who jogged at a very intense level and/or for long distances (even moderate jogging is high-intensity exercise).

Where does this leave you? Overall, exercise causes many positive changes in the body—in healthy people as well as those with heart disease—that more than make up for the slightly increased short-term risk of sudden death. People who exercise regularly have an overall risk of sudden death only about two-thirds that of non-exercisers. Active people who stop exercising can expect their heart attack risk to increase by 300%. The risk of heart-related sudden death in middle-aged and older adults is least in people who exercise approximately 150 minutes per week—the activity level recommended by the Canadian Society for Exercise Physiology (CSEP) and the Public Health Agency of Canada.

Medical Clearance Recommendations

People of any age who are not at high risk for serious health problems can safely exercise at a moderate intensity (60% or less of maximum heart rate) without a prior medical evaluation. (See Chapter 3 for a discussion of maximum heart rate.) Likewise, if you are male and under 40 or female and under 50 and in good health, exercise is probably safe for you. If you do not fit into these age groups, or if you have health problems—especially high blood pressure, heart disease, muscle or joint problems, or obesity—see your physician before starting a vigorous exercise program. The CSEP recommends using the Physical Activity Readiness Questionnaire (PAR-Q) to help evaluate exercise safety; it is included in Lab 2.1. Completing it should alert you to any potential problems you may have. If a physician isn't sure whether exercise is safe for you, they may recommend an **exercise stress test** or a **graded exercise test (GXT)** to see whether you show symptoms of heart disease during exercise. For most people, however, it's far safer to exercise than to remain sedentary.

exercise stress test A test usually administered on a treadmill or cycle ergometer using an electrocardiogram (EKG or ECG) to analyze changes in electrical activity in the heart during exercise; used to determine if any heart disease is present and to assess current fitness level.
graded exercise test (GXT) An exercise test that starts at an easy intensity and progresses to maximum capacity.

Assessing Yourself

The first step in creating a successful fitness program is to assess your current level of physical activity and fitness for each of the five health-related fitness components. The results of the assessment tests will help you set specific fitness goals and plan your fitness program. Lab 2.3 gives you the opportunity to assess your current overall level of activity and determine if it is appropriate. Assessment tests in Chapter 3, Chapter 4, Chapter 5, and Chapter 6 will help you evaluate your cardiorespiratory endurance, muscular strength, muscular endurance, flexibility, and body composition.

Setting Goals

The ultimate general goal of every health-related fitness program is the same—wellness that lasts a lifetime. That lifelong goal might include the specific goals of walking 30 to 60 minutes every day or doing a few calisthenic exercises every morning. Whatever your specific goals, they must be important enough to you to keep you motivated. Most sports psychologists believe that setting and achieving goals is the most effective way to stay motivated about exercise. (Refer to Chapter 1 for more on goal setting, as well as the Common Questions

Answered in this chapter.) After you complete the assessment tests in Chapter 3, Chapter 4, Chapter 5, and Chapter 6, you will be able to set goals directly related to each fitness component, such as working toward a 5 kilometre jog or doing 20 push-ups. First, though, think carefully about your overall goals, and be clear about why you are starting a program.

Strengthening Mental Wellness

Remember that there are many benefits to creating a balanced physical activity program. Find out more about the mental and emotional benefits from the HealthLinkBC Fact Sheet, "Mental and Emotional Benefits of Physical Activity," found at https://www.healthlinkbc.ca/physical-activity/mental-and-emotional -benefits. You can also receive daily motivational emails from ParticipACTION by signing up at https:// www.participaction.com/en-ca/GetStarted.

Choosing Activities for a Balanced Program

An ideal fitness program combines a physically active lifestyle with a systematic exercise program to develop and maintain physical fitness. This basis for a program is detailed in Canada's Physical Activity Guidelines for Canadians (see the guidelines for adults in Figure 2.3). Full details for all age groups can be found on the Public Health Agency website (http://www.phac-aspc.gc.ca/hp-ps/hl-mvs/pa-ap/03paap-eng.php). If you are currently sedentary, your goal is to focus on activities that will gradually increase the amount of moderate-intensity physical activity in your daily life. Appropriate activities include brisk walking, climbing stairs, yard work, and washing your car. You don't have to exercise vigorously, but you should experience a moderate increase in your heart and breathing rates. As described earlier, your activity time can be broken up into small blocks over the course of a day.

These guidelines have proven to be universal and are included in CSEP's Physical Activity Training for Health (PATH) protocols (see the box Physical Activity Training for Health (CSEP-PATH) on page 60). A balanced program includes activities to develop all the health-related components of fitness:

- **Cardiorespiratory endurance** is developed by continuous rhythmic movements of large-muscle groups in activities such as walking, jogging, cycling, swimming, and aerobic dance and other forms of group exercise. High-intensity interval training (HIIT)—short bouts of high-intensity exercise followed by rest—also builds endurance quickly. The advantage of HIIT is that it does not take as much time as traditional endurance training. The disadvantage is that it can be painful and uncomfortable. The safety of HIIT has not been determined. Choose activities that you enjoy and that are convenient. Popular choices are inline skating, skiing, dancing, and backpacking. Start-and-stop activities such as tennis, racquetball, and soccer can also develop endurance if your skill level is sufficient to enable periods of continuous play. (Training for cardiorespiratory endurance is discussed in Chapter 3.)

- **Muscular strength and endurance** can be developed through resistance training—training with weights or performing calisthenic exercises such as push-ups, planks, and curl-ups. (Training for muscular strength and endurance is discussed in Chapter 4.)

- **Flexibility** is developed by stretching the major muscle groups, regularly and with proper technique. (Flexibility is discussed in Chapter 5.)

- **Healthy body composition** can be developed through a sensible diet and a program of regular exercise. Cardiorespiratory endurance exercise is best for reducing body fat; resistance training builds muscle

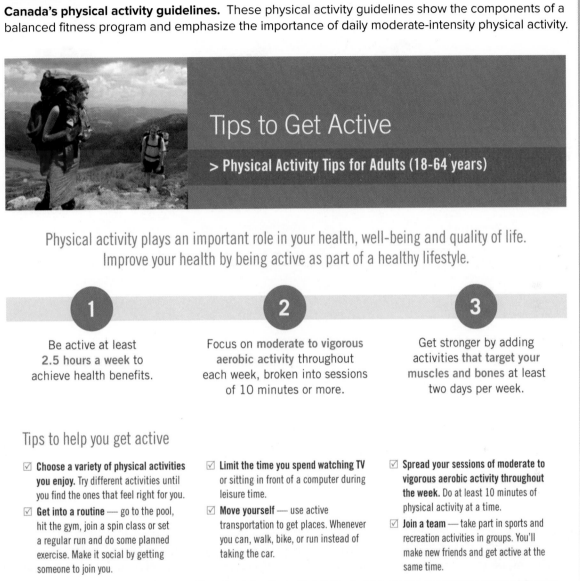

FIGURE 2.3

Canada's physical activity guidelines. These physical activity guidelines show the components of a balanced fitness program and emphasize the importance of daily moderate-intensity physical activity.

Tips to Get Active

> Physical Activity Tips for Adults (18-64 years)

Physical activity plays an important role in your health, well-being and quality of life. Improve your health by being active as part of a healthy lifestyle.

1

Be active at least 2.5 hours a week to achieve health benefits.

2

Focus on **moderate to vigorous aerobic activity** throughout each week, broken into sessions of 10 minutes or more.

3

Get stronger by adding activities **that target your muscles and bones** at least two days per week.

Tips to help you get active

☑ **Choose a variety of physical activities you enjoy.** Try different activities until you find the ones that feel right for you.

☑ **Get into a routine** — go to the pool, hit the gym, join a spin class or set a regular run and do some planned exercise. Make it social by getting someone to join you.

☑ **Limit the time you spend watching TV** or sitting in front of a computer during leisure time.

☑ **Move yourself** — use active transportation to get places. Whenever you can, walk, bike, or run instead of taking the car.

☑ **Spread your sessions of moderate to vigorous aerobic activity throughout the week.** Do at least 10 minutes of physical activity at a time.

☑ **Join a team** — take part in sports and recreation activities in groups. You'll make new friends and get active at the same time.

SOURCE: Canadian Physical Activity Guidelines. Tips to Get Active: Physical Activity Tips for Adults (18–64 years). Canadian Society for Exercise Physiology/Public Health Agency of Canada, 2011. Reproduced with permission from the Minister of Health, 2016.

mass, which, to a small extent, helps increase metabolism. (Body composition is discussed in Chapter 6 and weight management in Chapter 8.)

Refer to Figure 2.4 on the next page for a summary of the health and fitness benefits of different levels of physical activity. (Chapter 9 provides guidelines to help you choose activities and put together a complete exercise program that suits your goals and preferences.)

Although sedentary activities are often unavoidable—attending class, studying, working in an office, and so on—many people *choose* inactivity over activity during their leisure time. You can change sedentary patterns by becoming more active whenever you can. In other words, move more and sit less.

FIGURE 2.4

Health and fitness benefits of different amounts of physical activity and exercise.

	Lifestyle physical activity	Moderate exercise program	Vigorous exercise program
Description	Moderate physical activity (150 minutes per week; muscle-strengthening exercises 2 or more days per week)	Cardiorespiratory endurance exercise (20–60 minutes, 3–5 days per week); strength training (2–3 nonconsecutive days per week); and stretching exercises (2 or more days per week)	Cardiorespiratory endurance exercise (20–60 minutes, 3–5 days per week); interval training; strength training (3–4 nonconsecutive days per week); and stretching exercises (5–7 days per week)
Sample activities or program	• Walking to and from work, 15 minutes each way • Cycling to and from class, 10 minutes each way • Doing yard work for 30 minutes • Dancing (fast) for 30 minutes • Playing basketball for 20 minutes • Muscle exercises such as push-ups, squats, or back exercises	• Jogging for 30 minutes, 3 days per week • Weight training, 1 set of 8 exercises, 2 days per week • Stretching exercises, 3 days per week	• Running for 45 minutes, 3 days per week • Intervals, running 400 m at high effort, 4 sets, 2 days per week • Weight training, 3 sets of 10 exercises, 3 days per week • Stretching exercises, 6 days per week
Health and fitness benefits	Better blood cholesterol levels, reduced body fat, better control of blood pressure, improved metabolic health, and enhanced glucose metabolism; improved quality of life; reduced risk of some chronic diseases Greater amounts of activity can help prevent weight gain and promote weight loss	All the benefits of lifestyle physical activity, plus improved physical fitness (increased cardiorespiratory endurance, muscular strength and endurance, and flexibility) and even greater improvements in health and quality of life and reductions in chronic disease risk	All the benefits of lifestyle physical activity and a moderate exercise program, with greater increases in fitness and somewhat greater reductions in chronic disease risk Participating in a vigorous exercise program may increase risk of injury and overtraining

(left), RubberBall Productions, (centre), © Royalty-Free/Corbis, (right), © Thinkstock Images/Jupiterimages

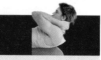

Take CHARGE

PHYSICAL ACTIVITY TRAINING FOR HEALTH (CSEP-PATH)

The PATH is a resource manual created by the Canadian Society for Exercise Physiologists (CSEP) that serves as a support tool for the training and certification of CSEP Certified Personal Trainers (CSEP-CPTs), CSEP Certified Exercise Physiologists (CSEP-CEPs), and other qualified exercise professionals in Canada.

There are many levels of assessment and counselling to choose from, as CSEP certification continues to be a client-centred approach. For example, you could complete a full appraisal, a partial appraisal, or seek advice only. The CSEP-PATH and CSEP certifications focus on health enhancement and creating a guideline for a physical activity/exercise program. In addition, active living and lifestyle habits that relate to overall health status are examined, and in many cases an individualized exercise program can be prescribed (with a personal trainer).

Many of the physical assessments in this text are adapted from the CSEP protocols. When considering your initial assessment results, you may want to consider a full appraisal (or even a partial appraisal)

from a CSEP-certified professional. At the very least, a visit with a CSEP-certified personal trainer may help you develop a program that is right for you.

Qualifications

A CSEP-certified health/fitness professional (i.e., a CSEP Certified Personal Trainer® or CSEP Certified Exercise Physiologist®) is all three: health/fitness counsellor, fitness appraiser, and personal trainer. They are the only fitness professionals in Canada that have acquired their skills, knowledge/abilities, and training through some formal academic training (i.e., university/college coursework). The CSEP further qualifies their professional status by having candidates complete a vigorous examination process in the subject matter. To contact a CSEP professional (CSEP-CPT or CSEP-CEP) in your area, search the CSEP Online Member Directory (http://csep.ca/view.asp?ccid=645) or contact one of their provincial/regional offices.

SOURCE: Canadian Society for Exercise Physiologists (http://www.csep.ca/home).

CAREER OPTIONS FOR...

PRINCIPLES OF PHYSICAL TRAINING

Fitness and wellness: certified fitness consultant, strength and conditioning specialist, health club director

Recreation: sport and fitness program coordinator, community sports administrator, special event coordinator

Rehabilitation: athletic injury trainer, kinesiologist, special population adaptive specialist

SOURCE: Physical and Health Education Canada.

LO5 Guidelines for Training

The following guidelines will make your exercise program more effective and successful.

Train the Way You Want Your Body to Change

Stress your body so it adapts in the desired direction. For example, to have a more muscular build, lift weights; to be more flexible, do stretching exercises; and to improve performance in a particular sport, practise that sport or its movements.

Train Regularly

Consistency is the key to improving fitness. Fitness improvements are lost if too much time is allowed to pass between exercise sessions.

Start Slowly and Get in Shape Gradually

As Figure 2.5 (on the next page) shows, an exercise program can be divided into three phases:

- **Beginning phase.** The body adjusts to the new type and level of activity.

- **Making progress phase.** Fitness increases.
- **Maintenance phase.** The targeted level of fitness is sustained over the long term.

Progression of an exercise program. This figure shows how the amount of overload is increased gradually over time in a walking and running program. Regardless of the activity chosen, it is important that an exercise program begin slowly and progress gradually. Once you achieve the desired level of fitness, you can maintain it by exercising three to five days a week.

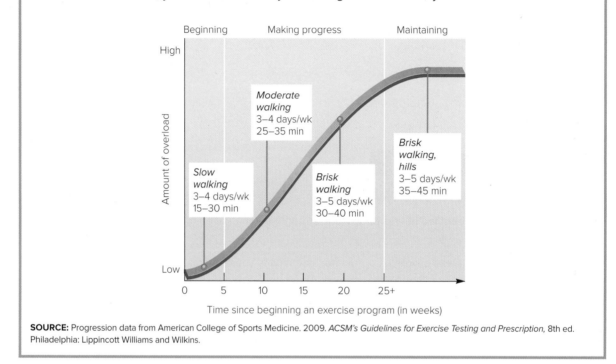

SOURCE: Progression data from American College of Sports Medicine. 2009. *ACSM's Guidelines for Exercise Testing and Prescription,* 8th ed. Philadelphia: Lippincott Williams and Wilkins.

When beginning a program, start slowly to give your body time to adapt to the stress of exercise. Choose activities carefully according to your fitness status. If you have been sedentary or are overweight, try an activity such as walking or swimming that won't jar the body or strain the joints.

As you progress, increase the duration and frequency of the activity before increasing its intensity. If you train too much or too intensely, you are more likely to suffer injuries or become **overtrained**, a condition characterized by lack of energy, aching muscles and joints, and decreased physical performance. Injuries and overtraining slow down an exercise program and impede motivation. The goal is not to get in shape as quickly as possible, but to gradually become and remain physically fit.

overtraining A condition caused by training too much or too intensely, characterized by lack of energy, decreased physical performance, and aching muscles and joints.

Wellness Tip

Moderation is important, especially if you're just starting to get physically active. Work at a pace that's comfortable and enjoyable, with a goal of making gradual improvements. This will help you get into the habit of being active and will help you avoid burnout.

Warm Up before Exercise

Warming up can decrease your chances of injury by helping your body gradually progress from rest to activity. A good warm-up can increase muscle temperature, reduce joint stiffness, bathe the joint surfaces in lubricating fluid, and increase blood flow to the muscles, including the heart. Some studies suggest that warming up may also enhance muscle metabolism and mentally prepare you for a workout.

A warm-up should include low-intensity, whole-body movements similar to those used in the activity. For example, runners may walk and jog slowly prior to running at full-speed, while a tennis player might hit forehands and backhands at a low intensity before playing a vigorous set of tennis. A warm-up is not the same thing as a stretching workout. For safety and effectiveness, it is best to stretch *after* an endurance or strength-training workout, when muscles are warm—and not as part of a warm-up. (Appropriate and effective warm-ups are discussed in greater detail in Chapter 3, Chapter 4, and Chapter 5.)

Cool Down after Exercise

During exercise, as much as 90% of circulating blood is directed to the muscles and skin, up from as little as 20% during rest. If you suddenly stop moving after exercise, the amount of blood returning to your heart and brain may be insufficient, and you may experience dizziness, a drop in blood pressure, or other problems. Cooling down at the end of a workout helps safely restore circulation to its normal resting condition. After you exercise, cool down before sitting, lying down, or jumping into the shower by continuing to move at a slow pace—walking for 5 to 10 minutes, for example—as your heart and breathing rate slowly return to normal. At the end of the cool-down period, do stretching exercises while your muscles are still warm. Cool down longer after intense exercise sessions.

Exercise Safely

Physical activity can cause injury or even death if you don't consider safety. For example, you should always do the following:

- Wear a helmet when biking, skiing, or rock climbing.
- Wear eye protection when playing racquetball or squash.
- Wear bright clothing when exercising on a public street.
- Walk or run with a partner in a park or on a deserted track.
- Give vehicles plenty of leeway, even when you have the right of way.
- Be aware of people exercising near you in the weight room, and use spotters and collars when appropriate.

Overloading your muscles and joints can lead to serious injury, so train within your capacity. Use high-quality equipment and keep it in good repair. Report broken gym equipment to the health club manager or physical education instructor.

Listen to Your Body and Get Adequate Rest

Rest can be as important as exercise for improving fitness. Fitness reflects an adaptation to the stress of exercise. Building fitness involves a series of exercise stresses, recuperation, and adaptation leading to improved fitness, followed by further stresses. Build rest into your training program, and don't exercise if it doesn't feel right. Sometimes you need a few days of rest to recover enough to train with the intensity required for improving fitness. Getting enough sleep is an important part of the recovery process. On the other hand, you also can't train sporadically. If you listen to your body and it always tells you to rest, you won't make any progress.

Cycle the Volume and Intensity of Your Workouts

To add enjoyment and variety to your program, and to further improve fitness, don't train at the same intensity during every workout. Train intensely on some days and train lightly on others. Proper management of the level of workout intensity is a key to improved physical fitness. Use cycle training, also known as *periodization*, to provide enough recovery for intense training; by training lightly one workout, you can train harder the next. However, take care to increase the volume and intensity of your program gradually—never more than 10% per week.

Vary Your Activities

Change your exercise program from time to time to keep things fresh and help develop a higher degree of fitness. The body adapts quickly to an exercise stress, such as walking, cycling, or swimming. Gains in fitness in a particular activity become more difficult with time. Varying the kinds of exercises in your program allows you to adapt to many types of exercise and develops fitness in a variety of activities (see the box Vary Your Activities). Changing activities may also help reduce your risk of injury.

Take CHARGE

VARY YOUR ACTIVITIES

Do you have a hard time thinking of new activities to try? Check the boxes next to the activities listed here that interest you. Then look for resources and facilities on your campus or in your community.

Outdoor Exercises		
☐ Walking	☐ Swimming	☐ Cycling
☐ Inline skating	☐ Horseback riding	☐ Rowing
☐ Hiking	☐ Fly fishing	☐ Ice skating
☐ Running	☐ Skateboarding	☐ Backpacking

Exercises You Can Do at Home and Work		
☐ Desk exercises	☐ Sweeping	☐ Rope skipping
☐ Yard work	☐ Walking the dog	☐ Housework
☐ Painting the walls	☐ Gardening	☐ Shovelling snow
☐ Calisthenics	☐ Exploring on foot	

Sports and Games		
☐ Basketball	☐ Tennis	☐ Volleyball
☐ Softball	☐ Hockey	☐ Windsurfing
☐ Bowling	☐ Surfing	☐ Dancing
☐ Golf	☐ Badminton	☐ Snow skiing
☐ Soccer	☐ Ultimate Frisbee	☐ Gymnastics

Health Club Exercises		
☐ Weight training	☐ Circuit training	☐ Group exercise
☐ Ski machine	☐ Supine bike	☐ Rowing machine
☐ Elliptical trainer	☐ Medicine ball	☐ Punching bag
☐ Treadmill	☐ Plyometrics	☐ Racquetball
☐ Stationary bike	☐ Water aerobics	

Train with a Partner

People who train together can motivate and encourage each other through rough spots and help each other develop proper exercise techniques. Training with a partner can make exercising seem easier and more fun. It can also help you keep motivated and on track. A commitment to a friend is a powerful motivator.

If you can afford it, you may benefit from a certified personal trainer who can give you instruction in exercise techniques and help provide motivation. This is a central principle in cross-training exercise techniques such as CrossFit, a commercial exercise program that uses a variety of training methods to improve fitness (e.g., running, swimming, climbing, gymnastics, functional training, Olympic weight lifting, kettlebells, rope climbing, and calisthenics).

Train Your Mind

Becoming fit requires commitment, discipline, and patience. These qualities come from understanding the importance of exercise and having clear and reachable goals. Use the lifestyle management techniques discussed in Chapter 1 to keep your program on track. Believe in yourself and your potential, and you *will* achieve your goals!

Fuel Your Activity Appropriately

Good nutrition, including rehydration and resynthesis of liver and muscle carbohydrate stores, is part of optimal recuperation from exercise. Consume enough calories to support your exercise program without gaining body fat. Many studies show that consuming carbohydrates and protein before or after exercise promotes restoration of stored fuels and helps heal injured tissues so that you can exercise intensely again shortly. (Nutrition for exercise is discussed in greater detail in Chapter 3 and Chapter 7.)

Have Fun

You are more likely to stick with an exercise program if it's fun. Choose a variety of activities that you enjoy. Some people like to play competitive sports, such as pickleball, golf, or volleyball. Competition can boost motivation, but remember that sports are competitive, whereas training for fitness is not. Other people like more solitary activities, such as jogging, walking, or swimming. Still others like high-skill individual sports, such as skiing, surfing, or skateboarding. Many activities can help you get fit, so choose the ones you enjoy. You can also boost your enjoyment and build your social support network by exercising with friends and family.

Track Your Progress

Monitoring the progress of your program can help keep you motivated and on track. Depending on the activities you've included in your program, you may track different measures of your program—minutes of jogging, kilometres of cycling, laps of swimming, number of push-ups, amount of weight lifted, and so on. If your program is focused on increasing daily physical activity, consider using an inexpensive pedometer or exercise GPS app to monitor the number of steps you take each day. See Lab 2.3 for more information on setting goals and monitoring activity with a pedometer; see the box Digital Workout Aids (on the next page) for an introduction to products and apps that can help you track your progress. (Specific examples of program monitoring can be found in the labs for Chapter 3, Chapter 4, and Chapter 5.)

A qualified personal trainer can also help you get started in an exercise program or a new form of training. Make sure this person has proper qualifications, such as certification by CSEP or the ACSM, National Strength and Conditioning Association (NSCA). Don't seek out a person for advice simply because they look fit. UCLA researchers found that 60% of the personal trainers in their study couldn't pass a basic exam on training methods, exercise physiology, or biomechanics. Trainers who performed best had college degrees in exercise physiology, physical education, or physical therapy. So choose your trainer carefully and don't get caught up with fads or appearances.

Wellness *in the* DIGITAL AGE

DIGITAL WORKOUT AIDS

When you're just starting to get physically active, you can wind up with a lot of questions. How many kilometres did you walk? How many sit-ups did you do? How many minutes did you run? When your mind is completely focused on just *doing* an activity, it's easy to lose count of time, distance, and reps. But it's important to keep track of these things: Move too little and you won't see any progress; move too much and you run the risk of injury or burnout. Either outcome is bad news for your exercise program.

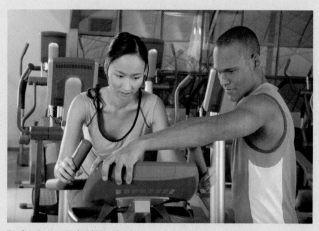

Denkou Images GmbH / SuperStock

Luckily, we live in a digital age, and the fitness industry is providing an ever-growing array of high-tech tools and applications (apps) that can track your progress for you. For example, you can track your distance (Runkeeper) or the number of steps you run/walk (FitBit), or map out your route and record it for reference (Map My Run). Advanced trackers can even record changes in elevation, speed, and acceleration you encounter during your workout. Heart rate monitors can help you reach and maintain the right exercise intensity. If calisthenics are your choice, some systems and apps work for specific exercises to count reps, assess your form, and challenge you to push yourself harder.

Smartphone programs, such as Coach's Eye, Hudl Technique, and Dartfish, can help you analyze your golf swing or tennis forehand in slow motion. The programs even make it possible to compare your progress by showing several performances side-by-side.

You can track more than just your exercise habits with digital assistance. Here some some examples of the many aspects of wellness and electronic devices and smart programs that can help you track them:

- Dietary habits—Nutrition Quiz Pro, Lifesum
- Calories consumed and burned—Calorie Counter & Diet Tracker by MyFitnessPal
- Stress management—BreathPacer
- Meditation and spirituality—myMeditation
- Heart rate and respiration—Heart Rate Monitor by LogYourRun
- Menstrual cycles—Period Tracker Lite
- Family medical history—My Medical
- Journaling—Lume Personal Tracker

And these are just a few of the options that are available. We'll introduce a variety of these digital devices and apps in later chapters in the "Wellness in the Digital Age" feature boxes like this one. You may find one or more digital apps (many of which are free) that appeal to you and can help you make progress toward your own fitness and wellness goals.

Keep Your Exercise Program in Perspective

As important as physical fitness is, it is only part of a well-rounded life. You have to have time for work and school, family and friends, relaxation, and hobbies. Some people become overinvolved in exercise and neglect other parts of their lives. They think of themselves as runners, dancers, swimmers, or triathletes rather than as people who participate in those activities. Balance and moderation are the key ingredients of a fit and well life.

Where Do You Go from Here?

Now that you have an awareness of the basics behind lifestyle change, take some time to learn about the physical changes that can happen when you engage in a fitness training program. Chapter 3, Chapter 4, and Chapter 5 will guide you through the development of specific programs for the cardiovascular, muscle, and flexibility systems, while Chapter 6 helps you to understand the overall effect that these systems can have on our body composition. You can then use the information in Chapter 1 and Chapter 2 to help create an overall general fitness training program in Chapter 9.

Tips for Today and the Future

Physical activity and exercise offer benefits in nearly every area of wellness. Even a low-to-moderate level of activity provides valuable health benefits. The important thing is to get moving!

RIGHT NOW YOU CAN

- Look at your calendar for the rest of the week and write in some physical activity—such as walking, running, biking, skating, swimming, hiking, or playing Frisbee—on as many days as you can. Schedule the activity for a specific time and stick to it.
- Call a friend and invite them to start planning a regular exercise program with you.
- Download a fitness app on your phone and keep track of your daily activity.

IN THE FUTURE YOU CAN

- Schedule a session with a qualified personal trainer who can evaluate your current fitness level and help you set personalized fitness goals.
- Create seasonal workout programs for the summer, spring, fall, and winter. Develop programs that are varied but consistent with your overall fitness goals.

Common Questions ANSWERED

Q I have asthma. Is it OK for me to start an exercise program?

A Probably, but you should see your doctor before you start exercising, especially if you have been sedentary up to this point. Your personal physician can advise you on the type of exercise program that is best for you given the severity of your condition, and how to avoid suffering exercise-related asthma attacks.

Q What should my fitness goals be?

A Begin by thinking about your general overall goals—the benefits you want to obtain by increasing your activity level and/or beginning a formal exercise program. Examples of long-term goals include reducing your risk of chronic diseases, increasing your energy level, and maintaining a healthy body weight.

continued

To help shape your fitness program, set specific, short-term goals based on measurable factors. These specific goals should be an extension of your overall goals—the specific changes to your current activity and exercise habits needed to achieve your general goals. In setting short-term goals, be sure to use the SMART criteria described in Chapter 1: Make sure your goals are **S**pecific, **M**easurable, **A**ttainable, **R**ealistic, and **T**ime frame–specific.

You need information about your current levels of physical activity and physical fitness in order to set appropriate goals. The labs in this chapter will help you determine your physical activity level, such as how many minutes per day you engage in moderate or vigorous activity or how many daily steps you take. Using this information, you can set goals for lifestyle physical activity to help you meet your overall goals. For example, if your general long-term goals are to reduce the risk of chronic disease and prevent weight gain, the Dietary Guidelines recommend 60 minutes of moderate physical activity daily. If you currently engage in 30 minutes of moderate activity daily, then your behaviour change goal would be to add 30 minutes of daily physical activity (or an equivalent number of additional daily steps—about 3500 to 4000); your time frame for the change might be 8 to 12 weeks.

Labs in Chapter 3, Chapter 4, Chapter 5, and Chapter 6 provide opportunities to assess your fitness status for all the health-related components of fitness. The results of these assessments can guide you in setting specific fitness goals. For instance, if the labs in Chapter 4 indicate that you have good muscular strength and endurance in your lower body but poor strength and endurance in your upper body, then setting a specific goal for improving upper-body muscle fitness would be an appropriate goal—increasing the number of push-ups you can do from 22 to 30, for example. Chapters 3 to 6 include additional advice for setting appropriate goals.

After you start your behaviour change program, you may discover that your goals aren't quite appropriate; perhaps you were overly optimistic, or maybe you set the bar too low. There are limits to the amount of fitness you can achieve, but within the limits of your genes, health status, and motivation, you can make significant improvements in fitness. Adjust your goals as needed.

Q Should I follow my exercise program if I'm sick?

A If you have a mild head cold or feel one coming on, it is probably OK to exercise moderately. Just begin slowly and see how you feel. However, if you have symptoms of a more serious illness— fever, swollen glands, nausea, extreme tiredness, muscle aches—wait until you have fully recovered before resuming your exercise program. Continuing to exercise while suffering from an illness more serious than a cold can compromise your recovery and may even be dangerous.

SUMMARY

- Moderate daily exercise contributes substantially to good health. Even without a formal, vigorous exercise program, you can get many of the same health benefits by becoming more physically active.

- If you are already active, you will benefit even more by increasing the intensity or duration of your activity.

- The five components of physical fitness that are most important for health are cardiorespiratory endurance, muscular strength, muscular endurance, flexibility, and body composition.

- Physical training is the process of producing long-term improvements in the body's functioning through exercise. All training is based on the fact that the body adapts to physical stress.

- According to the principle of *specificity*, bodies change specifically in response to the type of training received.

- Bodies also adapt to *progressive overload*. Therefore, when you progressively increase the frequency, intensity, and time (duration) of the right type of exercise, you become increasingly fit.

- Bodies adjust to lower levels of activity by losing fitness, a principle known as *reversibility*. To counter the effects of reversibility, keep training at the same intensity, even if you reduce the number or length of sessions.

- According to the principle of *individual differences*, people vary in the maximum level of fitness they can achieve and in the rate of change they can expect from an exercise program.

- When designing an exercise program, determine if medical clearance is needed, assess your current level of fitness, set realistic goals, and choose activities that develop all components of fitness.

- Train regularly, get in shape gradually, warm up and cool down, maintain a structured but flexible program, get enough rest, exercise safely, vary activities, consider training with a partner or personal trainer, train your mind, eat sensibly, have fun, monitor your progress, and keep exercise in perspective.

FOR FURTHER EXPLORATION

Journals

ACSM Health and Fitness Journal

https://journals.lww.com/acsm-healthfitness/pages/default.aspx

Applied Physiology, Nutrition and Metabolism

http://www.nrcresearchpress.com/loi/apnm

Physician and Sportsmedicine

http://www.physsportsmed.com

Organizations and Websites

American College of Sports Medicine (ACSM). Provides brochures, publications, and audio- and videotapes.

http://www.acsm.org

American Council on Exercise (ACE). Promotes exercise and fitness; features fact sheets on many consumer topics, including choosing shoes, cross-training, and steroids.

http://www.acefitness.org

Canada's Physical Activity Guide. Offers many suggestions for incorporating physical activity into everyday life.

http://www.phac-aspc.gc.ca/pau-uap/paguide/

Canadian Association for Health, Physical Education, Recreation, and Dance (CAHPERD). Promotes quality health and physical education programs.

http://www.cahperd.org

Canadian Kinesiology Alliance. Promotes the advancement of the profession of kinesiology, the study of human movement.

http://www.cka.ca

continued

Canadian Society for Exercise Physiology. Promotes human performance through research related to exercise physiology.

http://www.csep.ca

Certified Personal Trainers Network. Includes current research, education, and professional development for personal trainers.

http://www.cptn.com

CDC Physical Activity Information. Provides information on the benefits of physical activity and suggestions for incorporating moderate physical activity into daily life.

http://www.cdc.gov/nccdphp/dnpa/physical

MedlinePlus: Exercise and Physical Fitness. Provides links to news and reliable information about fitness and exercise from government agencies and professional associations.

http://www.nlm.nih.gov/medlineplus/exercisephysicalfitness.html

ParticipACTION. Includes current Canadian initiatives aimed at encouraging movement.

https://www.participaction.com/en-ca/home

Laboratory Activities

Name _____ Section _____ Date _____

Lab 2.1 Safety of Exercise Participation

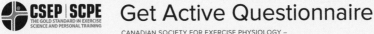

Get Active Questionnaire (GAQ)

The Get Active Questionnaire is endorsed by the Canadian Society for Exercise Physiology as a tool that will help you decide if you should discuss exercise with a health care provider or qualified exercise professional before beginning a program. Complete the questionnaire and follow the instructions before starting an exercise program.

CSEP | SCPE
THE GOLD STANDARD IN EXERCISE SCIENCE AND PERSONAL TRAINING

Get Active Questionnaire

CANADIAN SOCIETY FOR EXERCISE PHYSIOLOGY –
PHYSICAL ACTIVITY TRAINING FOR HEALTH (CSEP-PATH®)

Physical activity improves your physical and mental health. Even small amounts of physical activity are good, and more is better.

For almost everyone, the benefits of physical activity far outweigh any risks. For some individuals, specific advice from a Qualified Exercise Professional (QEP – has post-secondary education in exercise sciences and an advanced certification in the area – see csep.ca/certifications) or health care provider is advisable. **This questionnaire is intended for all ages – to help move you along the path to becoming more physically active.**

☐ I am completing this questionnaire for myself.

☐ I am completing this questionnaire for my child/dependent as parent/guardian.

PREPARE TO BECOME MORE ACTIVE

YES | **NO**

The following questions will help to ensure that you have a safe physical activity experience. Please answer **YES** or **NO** to each question <u>before</u> you become more physically active. If you are unsure about any question, answer **YES**.

1 Have you experienced **ANY** of the following (A to F) **within the past six months**?

   A A diagnosis of/treatment for heart disease or stroke, or pain/discomfort/pressure in your chest during activities of daily living or during physical activity?

   B A diagnosis of/treatment for high blood pressure (BP), or a resting BP of 160/90 mmHg or higher?

   C Dizziness or lightheadedness during physical activity?

   D Shortness of breath at rest?

   E Loss of consciousness/fainting for any reason?

   F Concussion?

2 Do you currently have pain or swelling in any part of your body (such as from an injury, acute flare-up of arthritis, or back pain) that affects your ability to be physically active?

3 Has a health care provider told you that you should avoid or modify certain types of physical activity?

4 Do you have any other medical or physical condition (such as diabetes, cancer, osteoporosis, asthma, spinal cord injury) that may affect your ability to be physically active?

NO to all questions: go to Page 2 – ASSESS YOUR CURRENT PHYSICAL ACTIVITY

YES to any question: go to Reference Document – ADVICE ON WHAT TO DO IF YOU HAVE A YES RESPONSE

PAGE 1 OF 2

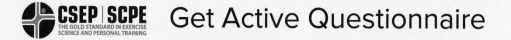

ASSESS YOUR CURRENT PHYSICAL ACTIVITY

Answer the following questions to assess how active you are now.

1 During a typical week, on how many days do you do moderate- to vigorous-intensity aerobic physical activity (such as brisk walking, cycling or jogging)?

> DAYS/ WEEK

2 On days that you do at least moderate-intensity aerobic physical activity (e.g., brisk walking), for how many minutes do you do this activity?

> MINUTES/ DAY

For adults, please multiply your average number of days/week by the average number of minutes/day:

> MINUTES/ WEEK

Canadian Physical Activity Guidelines recommend that adults accumulate at least 150 minutes of moderate- to vigorous-intensity physical activity per week. For children and youth, at least 60 minutes daily is recommended. Strengthening muscles and bones at least two times per week for adults, and three times per week for children and youth, is also recommended (see csep.ca/guidelines).

GENERAL ADVICE FOR BECOMING MORE ACTIVE

Increase your physical activity gradually so that you have a positive experience. Build physical activities that you enjoy into your day (e.g., take a walk with a friend, ride your bike to school or work) and reduce your sedentary behaviour (e.g., prolonged sitting).

If you want to do **vigorous-intensity physical activity** (i.e., physical activity at an intensity that makes it hard to carry on a conversation), and you do not meet minimum physical activity recommendations noted above, consult a Qualified Exercise Professional (QEP) beforehand. This can help ensure that your physical activity is safe and suitable for your circumstances.

Physical activity is also an important part of a healthy pregnancy.

Delay becoming more active if you are not feeling well because of a temporary illness.

DECLARATION

To the best of my knowledge, all of the information I have supplied on this questionnaire is correct.
If my health changes, I will complete this questionnaire again.

I answered NO to all questions on Page 1	**I answered YES to any question on Page 1**
▼	Check the box below that applies to you:
Sign and date the Declaration below	☐ I have consulted a health care provider or Qualified Exercise Professional (QEP) who has recommended that I become more physically active.
▼	☐ I am comfortable with becoming more physically active on my own without consulting a health care provider or QEP.

Name (+ Name of Parent/Guardian if applicable) [Please print]   Signature (or Signature of Parent/Guardian if applicable)   Date of Birth

Date   Email (optional)   Telephone (optional)

With planning and support you can enjoy the benefits of becoming more physically active. A QEP can help.

☐ Check this box if you would like to consult a QEP about becoming more physically active.
(This completed questionnaire will help the QEP get to know you and understand your needs.)

General Health Profile

To help further assess the safety of exercise for you, complete as much of this health profile as possible.

General Information

Age: _____ Total cholesterol: _____ Blood pressure: _____ / _____

Height: _____ HDL: _____ Triglycerides: _____

Weight: _____ LDL: _____ Blood glucose level: _____

Are you currently trying to _____ gain or _____ lose weight? (check one if appropriate)

Medical Conditions/Treatments

Check any of the following that apply to you and add any other conditions that might affect your ability to exercise safely.

_____ heart disease   _____ depression, anxiety, or   _____ other injury or joint

_____ lung disease   another psychological   problem: _____

_____ diabetes   disorder   _____ substance abuse problem

_____ allergies   _____ eating disorder   _____ other: _____

_____ asthma   _____ back pain   _____ other: _____

                                 _____ arthritis   _____ other: _____

_____ Do you have a family history of cardiovascular disease (CVD) (a parent, sibling, or child who had a heart attack or stroke before age 55 for men or 65 for women)?

List any medications or supplements you are taking or any medical treatments you are undergoing. Include the name of the substance or treatment and its purpose. Include both prescription and over-the-counter drugs and supplements.

_____

_____

_____

Lifestyle Information

Check any of the following that is true for you, and fill in the requested information.

_____ I usually eat high-fat foods (fatty meats, cheese, fried foods, butter, full-fat dairy products) every day.

_____ I consume fewer than 5 servings of fruits and vegetables on most days.

_____ I smoke cigarettes or use other tobacco products. If true, describe your use of tobacco (type and frequency):

_____

_____ I regularly drink alcohol. If true, describe your typical weekly consumption pattern:

_____

_____ I often feel as if I need more sleep. (I need about hours _____ per day; I get about _____ hours per day.)

_____ I feel as though stress has reduced my level of wellness during the past year.

Describe your current activity pattern. What types of moderate physical activity do you engage in on a daily basis? Are you involved in a formal exercise program or do you regularly participate in sports or recreational activities?

_____

_____

_____

Using Your Results

How did you score? Did the GAQ indicate that exercise is likely to be safe for you? Is there anything in your health profile that you think may affect your ability to exercise safely? Have you had any problems with exercise in the past?

_____

_____

What should you do next? If the assessments in this lab indicate that you should see a physician before beginning an exercise program, or if you have any questions about the safety of exercise for you, make an appointment to talk with your health care provider to address your concerns.

Name _____ Section _____ Date _____

Lab 2.2 Overcoming Barriers to Being Active

McGraw Hill Education **connect**

Barriers to Being Active Quiz

Directions: Listed below are reasons that people give to describe why they do not get as much physical activity as they think they should. Read each statement and indicate how likely you are to say each one.

How likely are you to say this?	Very likely	Somewhat likely	Somewhat unlikely	Very unlikely
1. My day is so busy now, I just don't think I can make the time to include physical activity in my regular schedule.	3	2	1	0
2. None of my family members or friends like to do anything active, so I don't have a chance to exercise.	3	2	1	0
3. I'm just too tired after work to get any exercise.	3	2	1	0
4. I've been thinking about getting more exercise, but I just can't seem to get started.	3	2	1	0
5. I'm getting older so exercise can be risky.	3	2	1	0
6. I don't get enough exercise because I have never learned the skills for any sport.	3	2	1	0
7. I don't have access to jogging trails, swimming pools, bike paths, etc.	3	2	1	0
8. Physical activity takes too much time away from other commitments—like work, family, etc.	3	2	1	0
9. I'm embarrassed about how I will look when I exercise with others.	3	2	1	0
10. I don't get enough sleep as it is. I just couldn't get up early or stay up late to get some exercise.	3	2	1	0
11. It's easier for me to find excuses not to exercise than to go out and do something.	3	2	1	0
12. I know of too many people who have hurt themselves by overdoing it with exercise.	3	2	1	0
13. I really can't see learning a new sport at my age.	3	2	1	0
14. It's just too expensive. You have to take a class or join a club or buy the right equipment.	3	2	1	0
15. My free times during the day are too short to include exercise.	3	2	1	0
16. My usual social activities with family or friends do not include physical activity.	3	2	1	0
17. I'm too tired during the week and I need the weekend to catch up on my rest.	3	2	1	0
18. I want to get more exercise, but I just can't seem to make myself stick to anything.	3	2	1	0
19. I'm afraid I might injure myself or have a heart attack.	3	2	1	0
20. I'm not good enough at any physical activity to make it fun.	3	2	1	0
21. If we had exercise facilities and showers at work, then I would be more likely to exercise.	3	2	1	0

Scoring

- Enter the circled number in the spaces provided, putting the number for statement 1 on line 1, statement 2 on line 2, and so on.
- Add the scores for the three questions on each line below. Your barriers to physical activity fall into one or more of seven categories: lack of time, social influence, lack of energy, lack of willpower, fear of injury, lack of skill, and lack of resources. A score of 5 or above in any category shows that this is an important barrier for you to overcome.

<u>1</u>	+	<u>8</u>	+	<u>15</u>	= Lack of time
<u>2</u>	+	<u>9</u>	+	<u>16</u>	= Social influences
<u>3</u>	+	<u>10</u>	+	<u>17</u>	= Lack of energy
<u>4</u>	+	<u>11</u>	+	<u>18</u>	= Lack of willpower
<u>5</u>	+	<u>12</u>	+	<u>19</u>	= Fear of injury
<u>6</u>	+	<u>13</u>	+	<u>20</u>	= Lack of skill
<u>7</u>	+	<u>14</u>	+	<u>21</u>	= Lack of resources

Using Your Results

How did you score? How many key barriers did you identify? Are they what you expected?

_____

_____

_____

What should you do next? For your key barriers, try the strategies listed below and/or develop additional strategies that work for you. Check off any strategy that you try.

Suggestions for Overcoming Physical Activity Barriers

Lack of Time

_____   Identify available time slots. Monitor your daily activities for one week. Identify at least three 30-minute time slots you could use for physical activity.

_____   Add physical activity to your daily routine. For example, walk or ride your bike to work or shopping, organize social activities around physical activity, walk the dog, exercise while you watch TV, park farther from your destination, etc.

_____   Make time for physical activity. For example, walk, jog, or swim during your lunch hour, or take fitness breaks instead of coffee breaks.

_____   Other:

_____

Social Influence

_____   Explain your interest in physical activity to friends and family. Ask them to support your efforts.

_____   Invite friends and family members to exercise with you. Plan social activities involving exercise.

_____   Develop new friendships with physically active people. Join a group, such as the YMCA or a hiking club.

_____   Other:

_____

Lack of Energy

_____ Schedule physical activity for times in the day or week when you feel energetic.

_____ Convince yourself that if you give it a chance, exercise will increase your energy level; then, try it.

_____ Other:

_____

Lack of Willpower

_____ Plan ahead. Make physical activity a regular part of your daily or weekly schedule and write it on your calendar.

_____ Invite a friend to exercise with you on a regular basis and write it on *both* your calendars.

_____ Join an exercise group or class.

_____ Other:

_____

Fear of Injury

_____ Learn how to warm up and cool down to prevent injury.

_____ Learn how to exercise appropriately considering your age, fitness level, skill level, and health status.

_____ Choose activities involving minimal risk.

_____ Other:

_____

Lack of Skill

_____ Select activities requiring no new skills, such as walking, climbing stairs, or jogging.

_____ Exercise with friends who are at the same skill level as you are.

_____ Find a friend who is willing to teach you some new skills.

_____ Take a class to develop new skills.

_____ Other:

_____

Lack of Resources

_____ Select activities that require minimal facilities or equipment, such as walking, jogging, jumping rope, or calisthenics.

_____ Identify inexpensive, convenient resources available in your community (e.g., community education programs, park and recreation programs, work site programs, etc.).

_____ Other:

_____

Are any of the following additional barriers important for you? If so, try some of the strategies listed here or create your own.

Weather Conditions

_____ Develop a set of regular activities that are always available regardless of weather (e.g., indoor cycling, aerobic dance, indoor swimming, calisthenics, stair climbing, rope skipping, mall walking, dancing, gymnasium games, etc.).

_____ Consider outdoor activities that depend on weather conditions (e.g., cross-country skiing, outdoor swimming, outdoor tennis, etc.) as "bonuses"—extra activities possible when weather and circumstances permit.

_____ Other:

Travel

_____ Put a jump rope in your suitcase and jump rope.

_____ Walk the halls and climb the stairs in hotels.

_____ Stay in places with swimming pools or exercise facilities.

_____ Join the YMCA/YWCA (ask about reciprocal membership agreement).

_____ Visit the local shopping mall and walk for half an hour or more.

_____ Bring your favourite aerobic exercise video on your phone or tablet.

_____ Other:

Family Obligations

_____ Trade babysitting time with a friend, neighbour, or family member who also has small children.

_____ Exercise with the kids—go for a walk together, play tag or other running games, download an aerobic dance or exercise video and exercise together. You can spend time together and still get your exercise.

_____ Hire a babysitter and look at the cost as a worthwhile investment in your physical and mental health.

_____ Jump rope, do calisthenics, ride a stationary bicycle, or use other home gymnasium equipment while the kids watch TV or when they are sleeping.

_____ Try to exercise when the kids are not around (e.g., during school hours or their nap time).

_____ Other:

Retirement Years

_____ Look on your retirement as an opportunity to become more active instead of less. Spend more time gardening, walking the dog, and playing with your grandchildren. Children with short legs and grandparents with slower gaits are often great walking partners.

_____ Learn a new skill you've always been interested in, such as ballroom dancing, square dancing, or swimming.

_____ Now that you have the time, make regular physical activity a part of every day. Go for a walk every morning or every evening before dinner. Treat yourself to an exercycle and ride every day during a favourite TV show.

_____ Other:

SOURCE: Adapted from CDC Division of Nutrition and Physical Activity. 2010. *Promoting Physical Activity: A Guide for Community Action*, 2nd ed. Champaign, Ill.: Human Kinetics.

Name _____ Section _____ Date _____

Lab 2.3 Using a Pedometer to Track Physical Activity

connect

How physically active are you? Would you be more motivated to increase daily physical activity if you had an easy way to monitor your level of activity? If so, consider wearing a pedometer to track the number of steps you take each day—a rough but easily obtainable reflection of daily physical activity. Smartphone pedometer apps use sensors that can provide reasonably accurate step measure counts. These apps are either low cost or free.

Determine Your Baseline

Wear the pedometer for a week to obtain a baseline average daily number of steps.

	M	Tu	W	Th	F	Sa	Su	Average
Steps								

Set Goals

Set an appropriate goal for increasing steps. The goal of 10 000 steps per day is widely recommended, but your personal goal should reflect your baseline level of steps. For example, if your current daily steps are far below 10 000, a goal of walking 2000 additional steps each day might be appropriate. If you are already close to 10 000 steps per day, choose a higher goal. Also consider the following guidelines from health experts:

- To reduce the risk of chronic disease, aim to accumulate at least 150 minutes of moderate physical activity per week.

- To help manage body weight and prevent gradual, unhealthy weight gain, engage in 60 minutes of moderate- to vigorous-intensity activity on most days of the week.

- To sustain weight loss, engage daily in at least 60 to 90 minutes of moderate-intensity physical activity.

To help gauge how close you are to meeting these time-based physical activity goals, you might walk for 10 to 15 minutes while wearing your pedometer to determine how many steps correspond with the time-based goals.

Once you have set your overall goal, break it down into several steps. For example, if your goal is to increase daily steps by 2000, set mini-goals of increasing daily steps by 500, allowing two weeks to reach each mini-goal. Smaller goals are easier to achieve and can help keep you motivated and on track. Having several interim goals also gives you the opportunity to reward yourself more frequently. Note your goals below:

Mini-goal 1: _____ Target date: _____ Reward: _____

Mini-goal 2: _____ Target date: _____ Reward: _____

Mini-goal 3: _____ Target date: _____ Reward: _____

Overall goal: _____ Target date: _____ Reward: _____

Develop Strategies for Increasing Steps

What can you do to become more active? This text includes a variety of suggestions, including walking when you do errands, getting off one stop from your destination on public transportation, parking an extra block or two away from your destination, and doing at least one chore every day that requires physical activity.

If weather or neighbourhood safety is an issue, look for alternative locations to walk. For example, find an indoor gym or shopping mall or even a long hallway. Check out locations that are near or on the way to your campus, workplace, or residence. If you think walking indoors will be dull, walk with friends or family members or wear headphones (if safe) and listen to music, audiobooks, or podcasts.

Are there any days of the week for which your baseline steps are particularly low and/or it will be especially difficult because of your schedule to increase your number of steps? Be sure to develop specific strategies for difficult situations.

Below, list at least five strategies for increasing daily steps:

_____

_____

_____

_____

_____

Track Your Progress

Based on the goals you set, fill in your goal portion of the progress chart with your target average daily steps for each week. Then wear your pedometer every day and note your total daily steps. Track your progress toward each mini-goal and your final goal. Every few weeks, stop and evaluate your progress. If needed, adjust your plan and develop additional strategies for increasing steps. In addition to the chart on this worksheet, you might also want to graph your daily steps to provide a visual reminder of how you are progressing toward your goals. Make as many copies of this chart as you need.

Week	Goal	M	Tu	W	Th	F	Sa	Su	Average
1									
2									
3									

Progress Checkup

How close are you to meeting your goal? How do you feel about your program and your progress?

_____

_____

If needed, describe changes to your plan and additional strategies for increasing steps:

_____

_____

_____

Week	Goal	M	Tu	W	Th	F	Sa	Su	Average
4									
5									
6									

Week 5 to 8 Progress Checkup

How close are you to meeting your goal? How do you feel about your program and your progress?

_____

_____

_____

If needed, describe changes to your plan and additional strategies for increasing steps:

_____

_____

_____

Week	Goal	M	Tu	W	Th	F	Sa	Su	Average
7									
8									
9									

Week 9 to 12 Progress Checkup

How close are you to meeting your goal? How do you feel about your program and your progress?

_____

_____

_____

If needed, describe changes to your plan and additional strategies for increasing steps:

_____

_____

_____

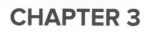

CHAPTER 3

Cardiorespiratory Endurance

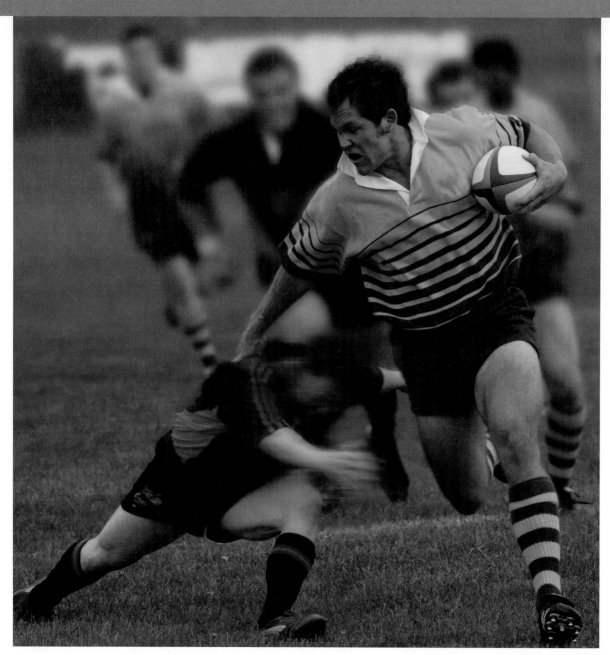

Design Pics / Don Hammond

LEARNING OBJECTIVES

After reading this chapter, you should be able to

LO1 Describe how the body produces the energy it needs for exercise

LO2 List the major effects and benefits of cardiorespiratory endurance exercise

LO3 Explain how cardiorespiratory endurance is measured and assessed

LO4 Describe how frequency, intensity, time (duration), and type of exercise affect the development of cardiorespiratory endurance

LO5 Explain the best ways to prevent and treat common exercise injuries

TEST YOUR KNOWLEDGE

1. **Compared to sedentary people, those who engage in regular moderate endurance exercise are likely to**
   a. have fewer colds
   b. be less anxious and depressed
   c. fall asleep more quickly and sleep better
   d. be more alert and creative

2. **About how much blood does the heart pump during each minute of aerobic exercise?**
   a. 4 to 5 litres
   b. 8 to 10 litres
   c. 18 to 20 litres

3. **During an effective 30-minute cardiorespiratory endurance workout, you should lose 0.5 to 1 kilogram.**

   True or false?

ANSWERS

1. **ALL FOUR.** Endurance exercise has many immediate benefits that affect all the dimensions of wellness and improve overall quality of life.

2. **C.** During exercise, cardiac output increases to 18 to 20 litres or more per minute, compared to 4 to 5 litres at rest.

3. **FALSE.** Any weight loss during an exercise session is due to fluid loss that needs to be replaced to prevent dehydration and enhance performance. It's best to drink enough during exercise to match fluid loss in sweat; weigh yourself before and after a workout to make sure you are drinking enough.

Cardiorespiratory endurance—the ability of the body to perform prolonged, large-muscle, dynamic exercise at moderate-to-high levels of intensity—is a key health-related component of fitness. As explained in Chapter 2, a healthy cardiorespiratory system is essential to high levels of fitness and wellness.

This chapter reviews the short- and long-term effects and benefits of cardiorespiratory endurance exercise. It then describes several tests that are commonly used to assess cardiorespiratory fitness. Finally, it provides guidelines for creating your own cardiorespiratory endurance program, one that is geared to your current level of fitness and built around activities you enjoy.

LO1 3.1 Basic Physiology of Cardiorespiratory Endurance Exercise

Having a basic understanding of the body processes involved in cardiorespiratory endurance exercise can help you design a safe and effective fitness program.

The Cardiorespiratory System

The **cardiorespiratory system** consists of the heart, the blood vessels, and the respiratory system (i.e., air passages, trachea, bronchi, and lungs). This system circulates blood through the body, transporting oxygen, nutrients, and other key substances to the organs and tissues that need them. It also carries away waste products so they can be used or expelled.

> **cardiorespiratory system**   The system that circulates blood through the body; consists of the heart, blood vessels, and respiratory system.

The Heart

The heart is a four-chambered, fist-sized muscle located just beneath the ribs under the sternum (breastbone). Its role is to pump oxygen-poor blood to the lungs and oxygenated (oxygen-rich) blood to the rest of the body. Blood actually travels through two separate circulatory systems: The right side of the heart pumps blood to the lungs in **pulmonary circulation**, and the left side pumps blood through the rest of the body in **systemic circulation**.

> **pulmonary circulation**   The part of the circulatory system that moves blood between the heart and the lungs; controlled by the right side of the heart.
> **systemic circulation**   The part of the circulatory system that moves blood between the heart and the rest of the body; controlled by the left side of the heart.

The following steps describe the path that blood follows as it travels through the heart and the cardiorespiratory system (Figure 3.1):

1. Waste-laden, oxygen-poor blood travels through large vessels, called **venae cavae**, into the heart's right upper chamber, or **atrium**.
2. After the right atrium fills, it contracts and pumps blood into the heart's right lower chamber, or **ventricle**.
3. When the right ventricle is full, it contracts and pumps blood through the pulmonary artery into the lungs.
4. In the lungs, blood picks up oxygen and discards carbon dioxide. Oxygen moves from the lungs to the blood and carbon dioxide moves from the blood to the lungs by a process called **diffusion**. During exercise, you breathe faster to promote diffusion of these gases.

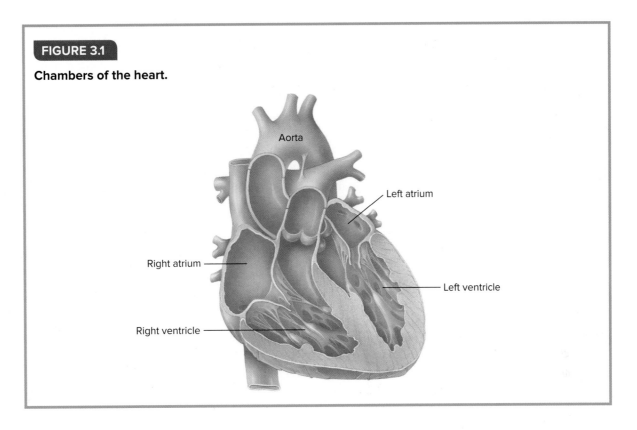

FIGURE 3.1

Chambers of the heart.

5. The cleaned, oxygenated blood flows from the lungs through the pulmonary veins and into the heart's left atrium.

6. After the left atrium fills, it contracts and pumps blood into the left ventricle.

7. When the left ventricle is full, it pumps blood through the **aorta**—the body's largest artery—for distribution to the rest of the body's blood vessels.

venae cavae   The large veins through which blood is returned to the right atrium of the heart.
atrium   One of the two upper chambers of the heart in which blood collects before passing to the ventricles (pl. atria).
ventricle   One of the two lower chambers of the heart, from which blood flows through arteries to the lungs and other parts of the body.
diffusion   The process by which oxygen moves from the lungs to the blood and carbon dioxide moves from the blood to the lungs; faster breathing concentrates oxygen and decreases carbon dioxide in the lungs and promotes diffusion.
aorta   The body's large artery; receives blood from the left ventricle and distributes it to the body.

The period of the heart's contraction is called **systole**; the period of relaxation is called **diastole**. During systole, the atria contract first, pumping blood into the ventricles. A fraction of a second later, the ventricles contract, pumping blood to the lungs and the body. During diastole, blood flows into the heart. **Blood pressure**, the force exerted by blood on the walls of the blood vessels, is created by the pumping action of the heart. Blood pressure is greater during systole than during diastole.

systole   Contraction of the heart.
diastole   Relaxation of the heart.
blood pressure   The force exerted by the blood on the walls of the blood vessels; created by the pumping action of the heart.

The heartbeat—the split-second sequence of contractions of the heart's four chambers—is controlled by nerve impulses. These signals originate in a bundle of specialized cells in the right atrium called the *pacemaker* or *sinoatrial (SA) node*. The heart produces nerve impulses at a steady rate—unless it is speeded up or slowed down by the brain in response to stimuli such as exercise.

The Blood Vessels

Blood vessels are classified by size and function. **Veins** carry blood to the heart; **arteries** carry it away from the heart. Veins have thin walls, while arteries have thick elastic walls that enable them to expand and relax with the volume of blood being pumped through them.

> **veins**   Vessels that carry blood to the heart.
> **arteries**   Vessels that carry blood away from the heart.

The blood vessels are lined with **endothelial cells** that secrete **nitric oxide**, a chemical messenger regulating blood flow. Inflammation, physical inactivity, poor diet, smoking, high blood pressure, or insulin resistance can promote blood vessel disease, which has a wide range of negative effects ranging from erectile dysfunction to heart disease. Regular physical activity helps maintain healthy blood vessels.

> **endothelial cells**   Cells lining the blood vessels.
> **nitric oxide**   A gas released by the endothelial cells to promote blood flow. The capacity of these cells to release nitric oxide is an important marker of good health.

After leaving the heart, the aorta branches into smaller and smaller vessels. The smallest arteries branch still further into **capillaries**, tiny vessels only one cell thick. The capillaries deliver oxygen and nutrient-rich blood to the tissues and pick up oxygen-poor, waste-laden blood. From the capillaries, this blood empties into small veins (*venules*) and then into larger veins that return it to the heart to repeat the cycle.

> **capillaries**   Very small blood vessels that distribute blood to all parts of the body.

Blood pumped through the heart doesn't reach the cells of the heart, so the organ has its own network of arteries, veins, and capillaries. Two large vessels, the right and left coronary arteries, branch off the aorta and supply the heart muscle with oxygenated blood. The fit and well lifestyle helps prevent coronary artery disease.

The Respiratory System

The **respiratory system** supplies oxygen to the body, carries off carbon dioxide—a waste product of body processes—and helps regulate acid produced during metabolism. Air passes in and out of the lungs as a result of pressure changes brought about by the contraction and relaxation of the diaphragm and rib muscles. As air is inhaled, it passes through the nasal passages, throat, larynx, trachea (windpipe), and bronchi into the lungs. The lungs consist of many branching tubes that end in tiny, thin-walled air sacs called **alveoli**.

> **respiratory system**   The lungs, air passages, and breathing muscles; supplies oxygen to the body and removes carbon dioxide.
> **alveoli**   Tiny air sacs in the lungs that allow the exchange of oxygen and carbon dioxide between the lungs and blood.

Carbon dioxide and oxygen are exchanged between alveoli and capillaries in the lungs. Carbon dioxide passes from blood cells into the alveoli, where it is carried up and out of the lungs (exhaled). Oxygen from inhaled air passes from the alveoli into blood cells; these oxygen-rich blood cells then return to the heart and are pumped throughout the body. Oxygen is an important component of the body's energy-producing system, so the cardiorespiratory system's ability to pick up and deliver oxygen is critical for the functioning of the body.

The Cardiorespiratory System at Rest and during Exercise

At rest and during light activity, the cardiorespiratory system functions at a fairly steady pace. Your heart beats at a rate of about 50 to 90 beats per minute, and you take about 12 to 20 breaths per minute. Optimal blood pressure readings for a young, healthy male are approximately 120 mm Hg (systolic) and 80 mm Hg (diastolic). Women typically display blood pressure readings (both systolic and diastolic) that average 10 to 20 mm HG below that of men. These differences are likely related to height; blood pressure is higher in taller individuals and males are typically taller than females.[1]

During exercise, the demands on the cardiorespiratory system increase. Body cells, particularly working muscles, need to obtain more oxygen and fuel and eliminate more waste products. To meet these demands, your body makes the following changes:

- Heart rate increases, up to 170 to 210 beats per minute during intense exercise.
- The heart's **stroke volume** increases, meaning that the heart pumps out more blood with each beat.
- The heart pumps and circulates more blood per minute, primarily as a result of a faster heart rate and greater stroke volume. During exercise, this **cardiac output** increases to 18 to 23 litres per minute, compared to about 4.5 to 6 litres per minute at rest.

stroke volume   The amount of blood the heart pumps with each beat.
cardiac output   The amount of blood pumped by the heart each minute; a function of heart rate and stroke volume.

- Blood flow changes, so as much as 85–90% of the blood may be delivered to working muscles. At rest, about 15–20% of blood is distributed to the skeletal muscles.
- Systolic blood pressure increases, while diastolic blood pressure holds steady or declines slightly. A typical exercise blood pressure might be 175/65.
- To oxygenate this increased blood flow, you take deeper breaths and breathe faster, up to 40 to 60 breaths per minute.

All of these changes are controlled and coordinated by special centres in the brain, which use the nervous system and chemical messengers to control the process.

LO1 Energy Production

Metabolism is the sum of all the chemical processes necessary to maintain the body. Energy is required to fuel vital body functions—to build and break down tissue, contract muscles, conduct nerve impulses, regulate body temperature, and so on. The rate at which your body uses energy—its **metabolic rate**—depends on your level of activity. At rest, you have a low metabolic rate; if you begin to walk, your metabolic rate increases. If you jog, your metabolic rate may increase more than 800% above its resting level. Olympic-calibre distance runners can increase their metabolic rate by 2000% or more.

metabolic rate   The rate at which the body uses energy.

Energy from Food

The body converts chemical energy from food into substances that cells can use as fuel. These fuels can be used immediately or stored for later use. The body's ability to store fuel is critical; if all the energy from food was released immediately, much of it would be wasted.

The three classes of energy-containing nutrients in food are carbohydrates (e.g., sugar, wheat flour, honey), fats (e.g., meat, nuts, fried foods), and proteins (e.g., seafood, poultry, dairy food). During digestion, most carbohydrates are broken down into the simple sugar **glucose**. Some glucose remains circulating in the blood ("blood sugar"), where it can be used as a quick source of fuel to produce energy. Glucose may also be converted to **glycogen** and stored in the liver and muscles. If glycogen stores are full and the body's immediate need for energy is met, the remaining glucose is converted to fat and stored in the body's fatty tissues. Excess energy from dietary fat is also stored as body fat. Protein in the diet is used primarily to build new tissue, but it can be broken down for energy or incorporated into fat stores. Glucose, glycogen, and fat are important fuels for the production of energy in the cells, while protein is a significant energy source only when other fuels are lacking. (See Chapter 7 for more on the other roles of carbohydrate, fat, and protein in the body.)

> **glucose** A simple sugar that circulates in the blood and can be used by cells to fuel adenosine triphosphate (ATP) production.
>
> **glycogen** A complex carbohydrate stored principally in the liver and skeletal muscles; the major fuel source during most forms of intense exercise. Glycogen is the storage form of glucose.

ATP: The Energy "Currency" of Cells

The basic form of energy used by cells is **adenosine triphosphate**, or **ATP**. When a cell needs energy, it breaks down ATP, a process that releases energy in the only form the cell can use directly. Cells store a small amount of ATP; when they need more, they create it through chemical reactions that use the body's stored fuels—glucose, glycogen, and fat. When you exercise, your cells need to produce more energy. Consequently, your body mobilizes its stores of fuel to increase ATP production.

> **adenosine triphosphate (ATP)** The energy source for cellular processes.

Exercise and the Three Energy Systems

The muscles in your body use three energy systems to create ATP and fuel cellular activity. These systems use different fuels and chemical processes and perform different, specific functions during exercise (Table 3.1).

The Immediate Energy System

The **immediate ("explosive") energy system** provides energy rapidly but for only a short period of time. It is used to fuel activities that last for about 10 or fewer seconds, such as sports like weight lifting or shot-put, or daily life activities like rising from a chair or picking up a bag of groceries. The components of this energy system include existing cellular ATP stores and creatine phosphate (CP), a chemical that cells can use to make ATP. CP levels are depleted rapidly during exercise, so the maximum capacity of this energy system is reached within a few seconds. Cells must then switch to the other energy systems to restore levels of ATP and CP. Without adequate ATP, muscles will stiffen and become unusable.

> **immediate ("explosive") energy system** The system that supplies energy to muscle cells through the breakdown of cellular stores of ATP and creatine phosphate (CP).

TABLE 3.1

TABLE 3.1

Characteristics of the Body's Energy Systems

	Anaerobic-Alactic (Immediate)	Energy System* Anaerobic-Lactic	Oxidative (Aerobic)
Resistance to fatigue	Low	Intermediate	High
Intensity of activity for which system predominates	High	High	Low to moderately high
Rate of ATP production	Immediate, very rapid	Rapid	Slower, but prolonged
Fuel	Adenosine triphosphate (ATP), creatine phosphate (CP)	Muscle stores of glycogen and glucose	Body stores of glycogen, glucose, fat, and protein
Oxygen used for energy production?	No	No	Yes
Sample exercises	Weight lifting, picking up a bag of groceries	400-metre run, running up several flights of stairs	1500-metre run, 30-minute walk, standing in line for a long time

*For most activities, all three systems contribute to energy production; the duration and intensity of the activity determine which system predominates.

SOURCE: Adapted from Boone, T. 2014. *Introduction to Exercise Physiology,* 1st ed. Burlington, MA: Jones and Bartlett Learning, 2014.

The Nonoxidative Energy System

The **nonoxidative (anaerobic) energy system** is used at the start of an exercise session and for high-intensity activities lasting for about 10 seconds to 2 minutes, such as the 400-metre run. During daily activities, this system may be called on to help you run to catch a bus or dash up several flights of stairs. The nonoxidative energy system creates ATP by breaking down glucose and glycogen. The system doesn't require oxygen to produce energy, which is why it is referred to as the **anaerobic** system. This system's capacity to produce energy is limited, but it can generate a great deal of ATP in a short period of time. For this reason, it is the most important energy system for very intense exercise.

> **nonoxidative (anaerobic) energy system** The system that supplies energy to muscle cells through the breakdown of muscle stores of glucose and glycogen; also called the *anaerobic system* or the *lactic acid system* because chemical reactions take place without oxygen and produce lactic acid.
> **anaerobic** Occurring in the absence of oxygen.

There are two key limiting factors for the anaerobic-lactic energy system. First, the body's supply of glucose and glycogen is limited. If these are depleted, a person may experience fatigue and dizziness, and judgment may be impaired. (The brain and nervous system rely on carbohydrates as fuel.) Second, the rapid metabolism caused by this energy system increases hydrogen and potassium ions that interfere with metabolism and muscle contraction and cause fatigue. During heavy exercise, such as sprinting, large increases in hydrogen and potassium ions cause muscles to fatigue rapidly.

The anaerobic energy system also creates metabolic acids. Fortunately, exercise training increases the body's ability to cope with metabolic acid. Improved fitness allows you to exercise at higher intensities before the abrupt build-up of metabolic acids—a point that scientists call the *lactate threshold*. One metabolic acid, called **lactic acid** (lactate), is often linked to fatigue during intense exercise. Lactic acid does not last long in blood. It breaks down into lactate and hydrogen ion (acid) as soon as it is produced. Lactate is an important fuel at rest and during exercise.

lactic acid A metabolic acid resulting from the metabolism of glucose and glycogen; an important source of fuel for many tissues of the body, its accumulation may produce fatigue.

The Oxidative Energy System

The **oxidative (aerobic) energy system** operates during any physical activity that lasts longer than about two minutes, such as distance running, swimming, hiking, or even standing in line. The oxidative system requires oxygen to generate ATP, which is why it is considered an **aerobic** system. The oxidative system cannot produce energy as quickly as the other two systems, but it can supply energy for much longer periods of time. It provides energy during most daily activities.

oxidative (aerobic) energy system The system that supplies energy to cells through the breakdown of glucose, glycogen, and fats; also called the *aerobic system* because chemical reactions require oxygen.
aerobic Dependent on the presence of oxygen.

In the oxidative energy system, ATP production takes place in cellular structures called **mitochondria**. Because mitochondria can use carbohydrates (glucose and glycogen) or fats to produce ATP, the body's stores of fuel for this system are much greater than those for the other two energy systems. The actual fuel used depends on the intensity and duration of exercise and on the fitness status of the individual. Carbohydrates are favoured during more intense exercise (over 65% of maximum capacity); fats are used for mild, low-intensity activities. During a prolonged exercise session, carbohydrates are the predominant fuel at the start of the workout, but fat use increases over time. Fit individuals use a greater proportion of fat as fuel because increased fitness allows people to do activities at lower intensities. This is an important adaptation because glycogen depletion is one of the limiting factors for the oxidative energy system. By being able to use more fat as fuel, a fit individual can exercise for a longer time before glycogen is depleted and muscles become fatigued. Aerobic exercise and high-intensity interval training increase the number and capacity of mitochondria. Increased mitochondrial capacity is the most important benefit of exercise. Mitochondrial health and fitness are linked to a reduced risk of disease and improved longevity.

mitochondria Intracellular structures containing enzymes used in the chemical reactions that convert the energy in food to a form the body can use.

Oxygen is another factor limiting exercise capacity. The oxygen requirement of this energy system is proportional to the intensity of exercise. As intensity increases, so does oxygen consumption. The body's ability to increase oxygen use is limited; this limit is referred to as **maximal oxygen consumption,** or $\dot{V}O_{2max}$. $\dot{V}O_{2max}$ refers to the highest rate of oxygen consumption an individual is capable of during maximum physical effort. It is expressed in millilitres of oxygen per minute per kilogram of body weight per minute. In the symbol, the $\dot{V}$ stands for volume, the dot over the $\dot{V}$ means per minute, the O_2 stands for oxygen, and the max means maximum. $\dot{V}O_{2max}$ determines how intensely a person can perform endurance exercise and for how long, and it is considered the best overall measure of the capacity of the cardiorespiratory system. Table 3.2 (on the next page) shows the different levels of $\dot{V}O_{2max}$ that those who participate and excel in a variety of physical activities may display. (The assessment tests described later in the chapter are designed to help you predict your $\dot{V}O_{2max}$.)

maximal oxygen consumption $\dot{V}O_{2max}$ The highest rate of oxygen consumption an individual is capable of during maximum physical effort, reflecting the body's ability to transport and use oxygen; measured in millilitres of oxygen used per minute per kilogram of body weight.

The Energy Systems in Combination

Your body typically uses all three energy systems when you exercise; the intensity and duration of the activity determine which system predominates. For example, when you play tennis, you use the immediate energy system when hitting the ball, but you replenish cellular energy stores using the nonoxidative and oxidative systems. When cycling, the oxidative system predominates. However, if you must suddenly exercise intensely—ride up a steep hill, for example—the other systems become important because the oxidative system is unable to supply ATP fast enough to sustain high-intensity effort.

Physical Fitness and Energy Production

Physically fit people can increase their metabolic rate substantially, generating the energy needed for powerful or sustained exercise. People who are not fit cannot respond to exercise in the same way. Their bodies are less capable of delivering oxygen and fuel to exercising muscles; they can't burn as many calories during or after exercise, and they are also less able to cope with lactic acid and other substances produced during intense physical activity that contribute to fatigue. Because of this, they become fatigued more rapidly; their legs hurt and they breathe heavily walking up a flight of stairs, for example. Regular physical training can substantially improve the body's ability to produce energy and meet the challenges of increased physical activity.

In designing an exercise program, focus on the energy system most important to your goals. Because improving the functioning of the cardiorespiratory system is critical to overall wellness, endurance exercise that uses the oxidative energy system—activities performed at moderate to high intensities for a prolonged duration—is a key component of any health-related fitness program.

Ask Yourself

QUESTIONS FOR CRITICAL THINKING AND REFLECTION

When you think about the types of physical activity you engage in during your typical day or week, which ones use the immediate energy system? The nonoxidative energy system? The oxidative energy system? How can you increase activities that use the oxidative energy system?

TABLE 3.2

Maximal Oxygen Uptake (mL/kg/min) in Various Population Groups

	Age	Males	Females
Nonathletes	10–19	47–56	38–46
	20–29	43–52	33–42
	30–39	39–48	30–38
	40–49	36–44	26–35
	50–59	34–41	24–33
	60–69	31–38	22–30
	70–79	28–35	20–27
Athletes			
Baseball/softball	18–32	48–56	52–57
Basketball	18–30	40–60	43–60
Bicycling	18–26	62–74	47–57
Canoeing	22–28	55–67	48–52
Football	20–36	42–60	
Gymnastics	18–22	52–58	36–50
Ice hockey	10–30	50–63	
Jockey	20–40	50–60	
Orienteering	20–60	47–53	46–60
Racquetball	20–35	55–62	50–60
Rowing	20–35	60–72	58–65
Skiing, alpine	18–30	57–68	50–55
Skiing, Nordic	20–28	65–94	60–75
Ski jumping	18–24	58–63	
Soccer	22–28	54–64	50–60
Speed skating	18–24	56–73	44–55
Swimming	10–25	50–70	40–60
Track & field, discus	22–30	42–55	
Track & field, running	18–39	60–85	50–75
	40–75	40–60	35–60
Track & field, shot put	22–30	40–46	
Volleyball	18–22		40–56
Weightlifting	20–30	38–52	
Wrestling	20–30	52–65	

SOURCE: Reprinted with permission from W.L. Kenney, J.H. Wilmore, and D.C. Costill, 2012. *Physiology of Sport and Exercise,* 5th edition. (Champaign, IL: Human Kinetics). p. 269.

LO2 3.2 Benefits of Cardiorespiratory Endurance Exercise

Cardiorespiratory endurance exercise helps the body become more efficient and better able to cope with physical challenges. It also lowers risk for many chronic diseases.

Improved Cardiorespiratory Functioning

Earlier in this chapter, we described some of the major changes that occur in the cardiorespiratory system when you exercise, such as increases in cardiac output and blood pressure, breathing rate, and blood flow to the skeletal muscles. In the short term, all these changes help the body respond to the challenge of exercise. When performed regularly, endurance exercise also leads to permanent adaptations in the cardiorespiratory system (Figure 3.2). These improvements reduce the effort required to do everyday tasks and make the body better able to respond to physical challenges. This, in a nutshell, is what it means to be physically fit.

FIGURE 3.2

Immediate and long-term effects of regular cardiorespiratory endurance exercise. When endurance exercise is performed regularly, short-term changes in the body develop into more permanent adaptations; these include improved ability to exercise, reduced risk of many chronic diseases, and improved psychological and emotional well-being.

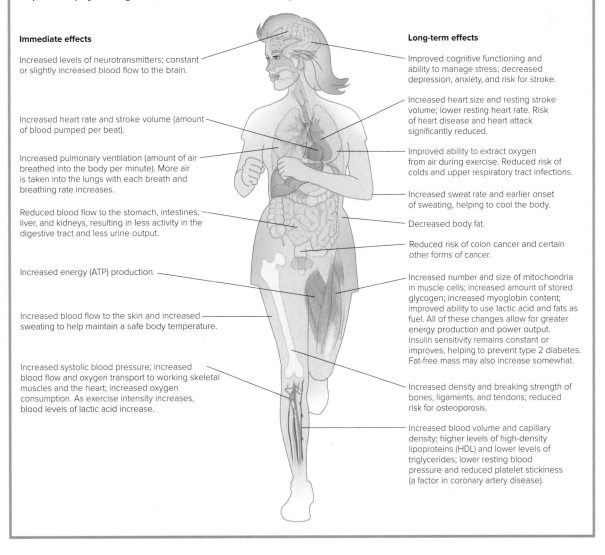

Immediate effects

Increased levels of neurotransmitters; constant or slightly increased blood flow to the brain.

Increased heart rate and stroke volume (amount of blood pumped per beat).

Increased pulmonary ventilation (amount of air breathed into the body per minute). More air is taken into the lungs with each breath and breathing rate increases.

Reduced blood flow to the stomach, intestines, liver, and kidneys, resulting in less activity in the digestive tract and less urine output.

Increased energy (ATP) production.

Increased blood flow to the skin and increased sweating to help maintain a safe body temperature.

Increased systolic blood pressure; increased blood flow and oxygen transport to working skeletal muscles and the heart; increased oxygen consumption. As exercise intensity increases, blood levels of lactic acid increase.

Long-term effects

Improved cognitive functioning and ability to manage stress; decreased depression, anxiety, and risk for stroke.

Increased heart size and resting stroke volume; lower resting heart rate. Risk of heart disease and heart attack significantly reduced.

Improved ability to extract oxygen from air during exercise. Reduced risk of colds and upper respiratory tract infections.

Increased sweat rate and earlier onset of sweating, helping to cool the body.

Decreased body fat.

Reduced risk of colon cancer and certain other forms of cancer.

Increased number and size of mitochondria in muscle cells; increased amount of stored glycogen; increased myoglobin content; improved ability to use lactic acid and fats as fuel. All of these changes allow for greater energy production and power output. Insulin sensitivity remains constant or improves, helping to prevent type 2 diabetes. Fat-free mass may also increase somewhat.

Increased density and breaking strength of bones, ligaments, and tendons; reduced risk for osteoporosis.

Increased blood volume and capillary density; higher levels of high-density lipoproteins (HDL) and lower levels of triglycerides; lower resting blood pressure and reduced platelet stickiness (a factor in coronary artery disease).

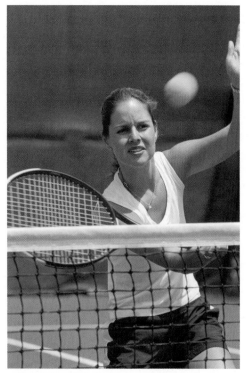

© Bill Varie / Workbook Stock / Getty Images

Exercise offers both long-term health benefits and immediate pleasures. Many popular sports and activities develop cardiorespiratory endurance.

Endurance exercise enhances the heart's health in the following ways:

- Maintains or increases the heart's own blood and oxygen supply.

- Increases the heart muscle's function so it pumps more blood per beat. This improved function keeps the heart rate lower both at rest and during exercise. The resting heart rate of a fit person is often 10 to 20 beats per minute lower than that of an unfit person. This translates into as many as 10 million fewer beats in the course of a year.

- Strengthens the heart's contractions.

- Increases the heart's cavity size (in young adults).

- Increases blood volume so the heart pushes more blood into the circulatory system during each contraction (larger stroke volume). Increased blood volume also improves temperature regulation, which reduces the load on the heart.

- Reduces blood pressure.

Improved Cellular Metabolism

Regular endurance exercise also improves the body's metabolism, down to the cellular level, enhancing your ability to produce and use energy efficiently. Cardiorespiratory training improves metabolism in the following ways:

- Increases the number of capillaries in the muscles. Additional capillaries supply the muscles with more fuel and oxygen and more quickly eliminate waste products. Greater capillary density also helps heal injuries and reduce muscle aches.

- Trains muscles to make the most of oxygen and fuel so they work more efficiently.

- Increases the size of and number of mitochondria in muscle cells, increasing cells' energy capacity.

- Prevents glycogen depletion and increases the muscles' ability to use lactic acid and fat as fuels.

Regular exercise may also help protect your cells from chemical damage caused by agents called *free radicals*. (See Chapter 7 for more on free radicals and special enzymes the body uses to fight them.)

Fitness programs that best develop metabolic efficiency include both long-duration, moderately intense endurance exercise and brief periods of more intense effort. For example, climbing a small hill while jogging or cycling introduces the kind of intense exercise that leads to more efficient use of lactic acid and fats.

Reduced Risk of Chronic Disease

Regular endurance exercise lowers your risk of many chronic, disabling diseases. It can also help people with those diseases improve their health (see the box Benefits of Exercise for Older Adults). The most significant health benefits occur when someone who is sedentary becomes moderately active.

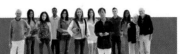

DIVERSITY Matters

BENEFITS OF EXERCISE FOR OLDER ADULTS

Research has shown that most aspects of physiological functioning peak when people are about 30 years old, then decline at a rate of about 0.5–1.0% per year. This decline in physical capacity shows up in decreases in maximal oxygen consumption, cardiac output, muscular strength, fat-free mass, joint mobility, and other factors. However, regular exercise can substantially alter the rate of decline and promote both longevity and improved quality of life.

Regular endurance exercise can improve maximal oxygen consumption in older adults by up to 15–30%—the same degree of improvement seen in younger adults. In fact, studies have shown that Masters athletes in their seventies have $\dot{V}O_{2max}$ values equivalent to those of sedentary 20-year-olds.

At any age, endurance training can improve cardiorespiratory functioning, cellular metabolism, body composition, and psychological and emotional well-being. Older adults who exercise regularly have better balance and greater bone density and are less likely than their sedentary peers to suffer injuries as a result of falls. Regular endurance training also substantially reduces the risk of many chronic and disabling diseases, including heart disease, cancer, diabetes, osteoporosis, and dementia.

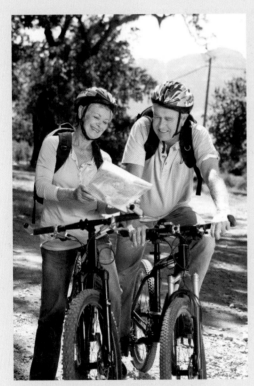

Shutterstock / Monkey Business Images

Other forms of exercise training are also beneficial for older adults. Resistance training, a safe and effective way to build strength and fat-free mass, helps people remain independent as they age. Lifting weights also benefits older people; improvements in strength appear quickly and are easily applied to everyday tasks such as climbing stairs and carrying groceries. Flexibility exercises can improve the ranges of motion in joints, another aid in helping people maintain functional independence as they age.

It's never too late to start exercising. Even those over 80 can see improved physical functioning and quality of life after beginning an exercise program. Most older adults can participate in moderate walking and strengthening and stretching exercises, and modified programs can be created for people with chronic conditions and other special health concerns. The wellness benefits of exercise are available to people of all ages and levels of ability.

Cardiovascular Diseases

Sedentary living is a key contributor to cardiovascular disease (CVD). CVD is a general category that encompasses several diseases of the heart and blood vessels, including coronary heart disease (which can cause heart attacks), stroke, and high blood pressure (see the box Combine Aerobic Exercise with Strength Training on the next page). Sedentary people are significantly more likely to die of CVD than are fit individuals.

Cardiorespiratory endurance exercise lowers your risk of CVD by doing the following:

- Promotes a healthy balance of fats in the blood. High concentrations of blood fats such as cholesterol and triglycerides are linked to CVD. Exercise raises levels of "good cholesterol" (high-density *lipoproteins,* or HDL) and may lower levels of "bad cholesterol" (low-density lipoproteins, or LDL).

- Reduces high blood pressure, which is a contributing factor to several kinds of CVD.
- Enhances the capacity of cell mitochondria.
- Enhances the function of the cells that line the arteries (endothelial cells).
- Reduces chronic inflammation.
- Prevents obesity and type 2 diabetes, both of which contribute to CVD.

(Details on various types of CVD, their associated risk factors, and lifestyle factors that can reduce your risk for developing CVD are discussed in Chapter 10.)

The Evidence *for* EXERCISE

COMBINE AEROBIC EXERCISE WITH STRENGTH TRAINING

Emphasizing one aspect of fitness at the expense of others may be a special concern for weight trainers who don't do enough cardiorespiratory conditioning. Although exercise experts universally agree that resistance training is beneficial for a variety of reasons (as we will discuss in Chapter 4), it also has a downside.

A number of global studies have tracked the impact of weight-training exercises on the cardiovascular system to determine whether resistance training is helpful or harmful to the heart and blood vessels. These studies have shown that strength training poses short- and long-term risks to cardiovascular health, especially to arterial health. Aside from the risk of injury, lifting weights has been shown to have the following adverse effects on the cardiovascular system:

- Promotes short-term stiffness of the blood vessels, which could promote hypertension (high blood pressure) over time and increase the load on the heart.

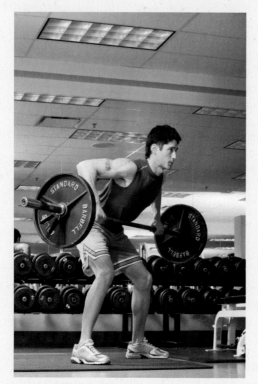

© Paul Burns / Getty Images

- Causes extreme short-term boosts in blood pressure, especially when lifting heavy weights; one Canadian study revealed that blood pressure can reach 480/350 mm Hg during heavy lifting. Over the long term, sharp elevations in blood pressure can damage arteries, even if each pressure increase lasts only a few seconds.
- Places stress on the endothelial cells that line blood vessels. Because these cells secrete nitrous oxide (a chemical messenger involved in a variety of bodily functions), this stress can contribute to a wide range of negative effects, from erectile dysfunction to heart disease.

A variety of studies have shown that the best way to offset cardiovascular stress caused by strength training is to do cardiorespiratory endurance exercise (such as brisk walking or using an elliptical machine) immediately after a weight-training session. Groundbreaking Japanese research showed that following resistance training with aerobic exercise prevents the stiffening of blood vessels and its associated damage. In this eight-week study, participants did aerobics before lifting weights, after lifting weights, or not at all.

The group that did aerobics after weight training saw the greatest positive impact on arterial health; participants who did aerobics before lifting weights did not see any improvement in the health of their blood vessels.

Strength training does promote endurance fitness by improving nervous control of the muscles and increasing tendon strength. These changes increase muscle strength and the rate of force development, enhance the economy of movement, and increase the speed that blood cells travel through the muscles.

The bottom line of all this research? Resistance training and cardiorespiratory exercise are both good for you, if you do them in the right order. So, when you plan your workouts, be sure to do 15 to 60 minutes of aerobic exercise after each weight-training session.

SOURCES: Ashor, A. W., et al. 2014. Effects of exercise modalities on arterial stiffness and wave reflection: A systematic review and meta-analysis of randomized controlled trials. *PLoS ONE* 9(10): e110034; Okamoto, T. M. Masuhara, and K. Ikuta. 2006. Effects of eccentric and concentric resistance training on arterial stiffness. *Journal of Human Hypertension* 20(5): 348–354; Okamoto, T. M. Masuhara, and K. Ikuta. 2007. Combined aerobic and resistance training and vascular function: Effect of aerobic exercise before and after resistance training. *Journal of Applied Physiology* 103(5): 1655–1661; Physical Activity Guidelines Advisory Committee. 2008. *Physical Activity Guidelines Advisory Committee Report, 2008.* Washington, D.C.: U.S. Department of Health.

Cancer

Although the findings are not conclusive, some studies have shown a relationship between increased physical activity and a reduction in the risk of cancer. Exercise reduces the risk of colon cancer in men and women,[2] and there is promising data indicating that it reduces the risk of cancer of the breast[3] and reproductive organs[4] in women. Exercise may also reduce the risk of lung cancer, endometrial cancer, pancreatic cancer, and prostate cancer. (See Chapter 11 for more information on various types of cancer and the impact of exercise on the risk for developing cancer.)

Type 2 Diabetes

Regular exercise helps prevent the development of type 2 diabetes, the most common form of diabetes.[5] Physical activity is also an important part of treating the disease. Obesity is a key risk factor for diabetes, and exercise helps keep body fat at healthy levels. But even without fat loss, exercise improves control of blood sugar levels in many people with diabetes. Exercise metabolizes (burns) excess sugar and makes cells more sensitive to the hormone insulin, which is involved in the regulation of blood sugar levels. (See Chapter 6 for a more detailed discussion on diabetes and insulin resistance.)

Osteoporosis

A special benefit of exercise, especially for women, is protection against osteoporosis, a disease that results in loss of bone density and poor bone strength. Weight-bearing exercise helps build bone during the teens and 20s. People with denser bones can better endure the bone loss that occurs with aging. With stronger bones and muscles and better balance, fit people are less likely to experience debilitating falls and bone fractures. (See Chapter 7 for more on osteoporosis.)

Inflammation

Inflammation is the body's response to tissue and cell damage (e.g., from injury, high blood pressure, or intense exercise), environmental poisons (e.g., cigarette smoke), or poor metabolic health (e.g., high blood fats, poor blood sugar control). Acute inflammation is a short-term response to exercise and is an important way that the body improves physical fitness. For example, short-term inflammation triggers increased muscle protein synthesis that promotes muscle fitness and recovery from exercise. Chronic inflammation, on the other hand, is a prolonged, abnormal process that causes tissue breakdown and diseases such as atherosclerosis, cancer, and rheumatoid arthritis.

While exercise increases acute inflammation during and shortly after a workout, it reduces chronic levels of inflammation—if the training program is not too severe. For example, practising endurance training three to five days a week will reduce inflammation. Training excessively, such as running a marathon several times a month or doing severe cross-training workouts five to seven days per week, will cause overtraining and chronic inflammation. We could call this the Goldilocks effect: the training program should not be too much or too little; it should be just right.

Deaths from All Causes

Physically fit people have a reduced risk of dying from all causes, with the greatest benefits found for people with the highest levels of fitness (see Figure 3.3 for the results of one recent study). Physical inactivity is a good predictor of premature death and is as important a risk factor as smoking, high blood pressure, obesity, and diabetes.

FIGURE 3.3

Survival rates for older adults doing vigorous, moderate, or no exercise, 1992–2008. The Health and Retirement Study—a long-term study of older adults—found that people who exercised vigorously over a 16-year period (1992–2008) had a lower death rate than those who exercised at moderate intensities or did no physical activity. After 16 years, the survival rate was 84% for those doing vigorous exercise, 78% for those doing moderate-intensity physical activity, and only 65% for those doing no physical activity. Exercising longer or more intensely reduces the risk of dying prematurely from a variety of causes.

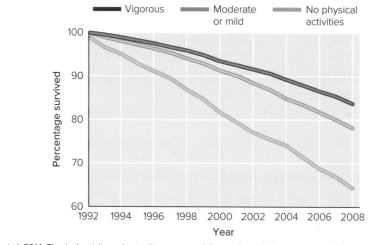

SOURCE: Wen, M., et al. 2014. Physical activity and mortality among middle-aged and older adults in the United States. *Journal of Physical Activity & Health,* 11(2): 303–312.

Better Control of Body Fat

Too much body fat is linked to a variety of health problems, including CVD, cancer, and type 2 diabetes. Healthy body composition can be difficult to achieve and maintain—especially for someone who is sedentary—because a diet that contains all essential nutrients can be relatively high in calories. Excess calories are stored in the body as fat. Regular exercise increases daily calorie expenditure so that a healthy diet is less likely to lead to weight gain. Endurance exercise burns calories directly and, if intense enough, continues to do so by raising resting metabolic rate for several hours following an exercise session. A higher metabolic rate means that it is easier for a person to maintain a healthy weight or to lose weight. However, exercise alone cannot ensure a healthy body composition. As described in Chapters 6 through 8, you will lose more weight more rapidly and keep it off longer if you decrease your calorie intake and boost your calorie expenditure through exercise.

Improved Immune Function

Exercise can have either positive or negative effects on the immune system, the physiological processes that protect us from diseases such as colds, bacterial infections, and even cancer. Moderate-endurance exercise boosts immune function, whereas excessive training (overtraining) depresses it, at least temporarily. Physically fit people get fewer colds and upper respiratory tract infections than people who are not fit.

Exercise affects immune function by influencing levels of specialized cells and chemicals involved in the immune response. As discussed in Chapter 2, physically active people also have healthier, more resilient genes, which promotes immunity. Exercise preserves the telomeres, which form the ends of the DNA strands and hold them together. Without exercise, the telomeres shorten over time, eventually reducing the effectiveness of the immune system. In addition to regular moderate exercise, the immune system can be strengthened by eating a well-balanced diet, managing stress, and getting seven to eight hours of sleep every night.

Improved Psychological and Emotional Well-Being

Most people who participate in regular endurance exercise experience social, psychological, and emotional benefits. Skill mastery and self-control enhance a person's self-image. Recreational sports provide an opportunity to socialize, have fun, and strive to excel. Endurance exercise lessens anxiety, depression, stress, anger, and hostility, thereby improving mood and boosting cardiovascular health. Regular exercise also improves sleep.

LO3 3.3 Assessing Cardiorespiratory Fitness

The body's ability to maintain a level of exertion (exercise) for an extended period of time is a direct reflection of cardiorespiratory fitness. It is determined by the body's ability to take up, distribute, and use oxygen during physical activity. As explained earlier, the best quantitative measure of cardiorespiratory endurance is maximal oxygen consumption, expressed as $\dot{V}O_{2max}$, the amount of oxygen the body uses when a person reaches maximum ability to supply oxygen during exercise. Maximal oxygen consumption can be measured precisely in an exercise physiology laboratory through analysis of the air a person inhales and exhales when exercising to a level of exhaustion (maximum intensity). This procedure can be expensive and time-consuming, making it impractical for the average person.

Choosing an Assessment Test

Fortunately, several simple assessment tests provide reasonably good estimates of maximal oxygen consumption (within plus or minus 10–15% of the results of a laboratory test). Four commonly used assessments are the following:

- **The 1.6-Kilometre Walk Test.** This test estimates your level of cardiorespiratory fitness (maximal oxygen consumption) based on the amount of time it takes you to complete 1.6 kilometres of brisk walking and your exercise heart rate at the end of the walk. A fast time and a low heart rate indicate a high level of cardiorespiratory endurance.

- **The 3-Minute Step Test.** The rate at which the pulse returns to normal after exercise is also a good measure of cardiorespiratory capacity; heart rate remains lower and recovers faster in people who are more physically fit. For the step test, you step continually at a steady rate and then monitor your heart rate during recovery.

- **The 2.4-Kilometre Run-Walk Test.** Oxygen consumption increases with speed in distance running, so a fast time on this test indicates high maximal oxygen consumption.

- **The Beep Test.** This test predicts maximal oxygen consumption and is excellent for people who are physically fit and wish to measure their capacity for high-intensity exercise, such as sprints. A prerecorded series of "beeps" (tones) sound off at faster and faster intervals. Your task is to keep up with the beeps during the exercise.

Lab 3.1 provides detailed instructions for each of these tests. An additional assessment, the 12-minute swim test, is also provided. To assess yourself, choose one of these methods based on your access to equipment, your current physical condition, and your own preference.

Don't take any of these tests without checking with your physician if you are ill or have any of the risk factors for exercise discussed in Chapter 2 and Lab 2.1.

Additional assessments for cardiorespiratory fitness include cycle ergometer and swimming tests and a distance test for people who use wheelchairs. Occupationally, you can use cardiorespiratory tests such as the Physical Ability Requirement Evaluation (PARE) and the Physical Readiness Evaluation for Police (PREP) to evaluate your potential for physical readiness to work. Check with your local or federal workplace association for physical/cardiorespiratory tests that may be required of your chosen profession.

Strengthening Mental Wellness

Participating in moderate amounts of physical activity have been proven to result in improved mood and emotional states. Other common psychological benefits resulting from exercise include the following:

- reduced stress and an improved ability to cope with stress
- feelings of increased energy
- improved body image
- greater confidence in physical abilities

These benefits only serve to increase motivation to continue exercising, leading to greater psychological benefits. In order to experience some of these results, you may need to do the following:

- Participate in as little as 10 minutes of aerobic exercise each day, such as a light jog or brisk walk.
- Continue to exercise at levels that reach Health Canada's recommended 150 minutes per week of moderate exercise. This will allow you to see long-term benefits.

Monitoring Your Heart Rate

Each time your heart beats, it pumps blood into your arteries. You can measure your heart rate—the number of heart contractions per minute—by using a heart rate monitor or counting your pulse beats. Modern heart rate monitors are inexpensive and accurate. Several companies make heart rate monitor apps that are used with Smartphones to measure heart rate, distances, route maps, running or cycling speed, and calories burned. Counting your pulse is the traditional method of measuring heart rate. Each contraction of the heart produces a surge of blood that causes a pulse you can feel by holding your fingers against an artery. Heart rate can also be used to monitor exercise intensity during a workout. (Intensity is described in more detail in the next section.)

The two most common sites for monitoring heart rate are the carotid artery in the neck and the radial artery in the wrist (see Figure 3.4). To take your pulse, press your index and middle fingers gently on the correct site. (Use your middle and ring finger if you have a strong pulse in your index finger.) You may have to

FIGURE 3.4

Checking your pulse. The pulse can be taken at the carotid artery in the neck (top) or at the radial artery in the wrist (bottom).

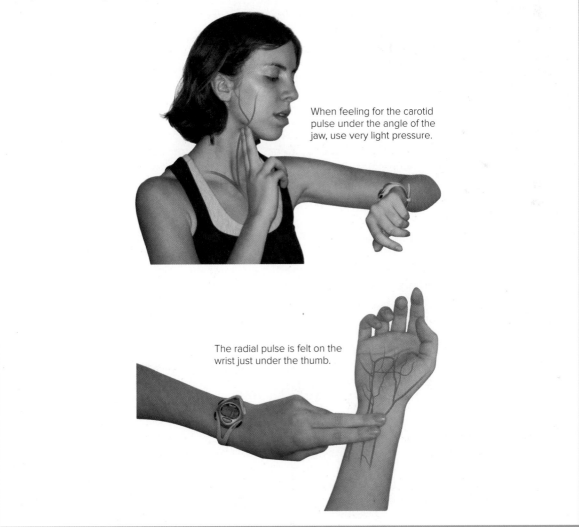

When feeling for the carotid pulse under the angle of the jaw, use very light pressure.

The radial pulse is felt on the wrist just under the thumb.

shift position several times to find the best place to feel your pulse. Do not use your thumb to check your pulse; it has a pulse of its own that can confuse your count. Be careful not to push too hard, particularly when taking your pulse in the carotid artery; strong pressure on this artery may cause a reflex that slows the heart rate.

Heart rates are usually assessed in beats per minute (bpm). But counting your pulse for an entire minute isn't practical when you're exercising. And because heart rate slows rapidly when you stop exercising, a full minute's worth of counting can give inaccurate results. It's best to do a shorter count, such as 15 seconds, and then multiply the result by 4 to get your heart rate in beats per minute. You can also use a heart rate monitor to check your pulse (see the box Fitness Trackers, Heart Rate Monitors, and GPS Devices for more information).

Wellness *in the* DIGITAL AGE

FITNESS TRACKERS, HEART RATE MONITORS, AND GPS DEVICES

Technology has transformed the market for trackers and monitors. It is difficult to keep up with the latest exercise monitors designed as stand-alone units, Smartphone apps, and GPS accessories. A heart rate monitor is an electronic device that checks your pulse, either continuously or on demand. These devices make it easy to monitor your heart rate before, during, and after exercise. Some include global positioning system (GPS) receivers that help you track the distance you walk, run, or bike. Wearable fitness trackers, made by Adidas, Nike, FitBit, Withings, and BodyMedia, among others, measure distance and steps covered, calories burned, and exercise intensity.

Fitness Trackers

High-tech monitors such as the Nike Fuelband, Nike+Sensor, and Adidas miCoach track daily activities, including running and walking and sports like basketball. They track steps taken, distance covered, and calories burned. Fitness trackers allow you to keep track of your progress, compete against other people, and meet challenges.

Wearable Monitors

Most consumer-grade monitors have two pieces: a strap that wraps around your chest and a wrist strap. The chest strap contains one or more small electrodes, which detect changes in the heart's electrical voltage. A transmitter in the chest strap sends this data to a receiver in the wrist strap. A small computer in the wrist strap calculates your heart rate and displays it on a small screen.

In a few low-cost monitors, the chest and wrist straps are connected together by a wire, but the most popular monitors use wireless technology to transmit data between the straps. In advanced wireless monitors, data is encoded so it cannot be read by any other monitors that may be nearby, as is often the case in a crowded gym. A one-piece (or "strapless") heart rate monitor does not include a chest strap; the wrist-worn device contains sensors that detect a pulse in your hand.

Monitors in Gym Equipment

Many pieces of workout equipment—including newer-model treadmills, stationary bikes, and elliptical trainers—feature built-in heart rate monitors. The monitor is usually mounted into the device's handles. To check your heart rate at any time while working out, simply grip the handles in the appropriate place; within a few seconds, your current heart rate will appear on the device's console.

Other Features

Heart rate monitors can do more than just check your pulse. For example, most monitors can also estimate the following kinds of information:

- highest and lowest heart rate during a session
- average heart rate
- target heart range, based on your age, weight, and other factors
- time spent within the target range
- number of calories burned during a session

Some monitors can upload their data to a computer, so information can be stored and analyzed. The analytical software can help you track your progress over a period of time or a number of workouts. AliveECG is a phone app that can send an electrocardiogram instantly to a physician via email. Monitors with GPS option can record the distance you have travelled during a workout or over an entire day.

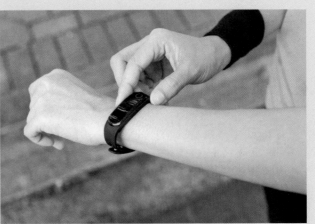

Shutterstock / Sasils

Choosing and using monitors

Heart rate monitors are useful if very close tracking of heart rate is important in your program. They offer several advantages:

- They are accurate, and they reduce the risk of mistakes when checking your own pulse. (Note, however, that chest-strap monitors are considered more accurate than strapless models. If you use a monitor built into gym equipment, its accuracy will depend on how well the device is maintained.)
- They are easy to use, although a sophisticated, multifunction monitor may take some time to master.
- They do the monitoring for you, so you don't have to worry about checking your own pulse.

When shopping for a heart rate, fitness tracker, or exercise GPS monitor, do your homework. Quality, reliability, and warranties vary. Ask personal trainers in your area for their recommendations, and look for product reviews in consumer magazines or online.

Interpreting Your Score

Once you've completed one or more of the assessment tests, use the table under "Rating Your Cardiovascular Fitness" at the end of Lab 3.1 to determine your current level of cardiorespiratory fitness. As you interpret your score, remember that field tests of cardiorespiratory fitness are not precise scientific measurements and do have a 10–15% margin of error.

You can use the assessment tests to monitor the progress of your fitness program by retesting yourself from time to time. Always compare scores for the *same* test: Your scores on different tests may vary considerably because of differences in skill and motivation and weaknesses in the tests themselves.

3.4 Developing a Cardiorespiratory Endurance Program

Cardiorespiratory endurance exercises are best for developing the type of fitness associated with good health, so they should serve as the focus of your exercise program. To create a successful endurance exercise program, follow these guidelines:

- Set realistic goals.
- Set your starting frequency, intensity, and duration of exercise at appropriate levels.
- Choose suitable activities.
- Warm up and cool down.
- Adjust your program as your fitness improves.

Setting Goals

You can use the results of cardiorespiratory fitness assessment tests to set a specific oxygen consumption goal for your cardiorespiratory endurance program. Your goal should be high enough to ensure a healthy cardio-respiratory system, but not so high that it will be impossible to achieve. Scores in the fair and good ranges for maximal oxygen consumption suggest good fitness; scores in the excellent and superior ranges indicate a high standard of physical performance.

Through endurance training, you may be able to improve maximal oxygen consumption $\dot{V}O_{2max}$ by about 10–30%. The amount of improvement possible depends on age, health status, and initial fitness level. People who start at a very low fitness level can improve by a greater percentage than elite athletes because the latter are already at a much higher fitness level, one that may approach their genetic physical limits. If you are tracking $\dot{V}O_{2max}$ using the field tests described in this chapter, you may be able to increase your score by more than 30% due to improvements in other physical factors, such as muscle power, which can affect your performance on the tests.

Another physical factor you can track to monitor progress is resting heart rate—your heart rate at complete rest, measured in the morning before you get out of bed and move around. Resting heart rate may decrease by as much as 10 to 15 beats per minute in response to endurance training. Changes in resting heart rate may be noticeable after only four to six weeks of training.

You may want to set other types of goals for your fitness program. For example, if you walk, jog, or cycle as part of your fitness program, you may want to set a time or distance goal, such as working up to walking up to 10 kilometres in one session, completing a 5 kilometre run in 28 minutes, or cycling a total of 50 kilometres per week. A more modest goal might be to achieve Health Canada's minimum activity level of doing at least 150 minutes of moderate to vigorous activity per week. Although it's best to base your program on SMART goals (those that are **S**pecific, **M**easurable, **A**ttainable, **R**ealistic, and **T**ime frame-specific), you may also want to set some more qualitative goals, such as becoming more energetic, sleeping better, and improving the fit of your clothes.

LO4 Applying the FITT Equation

As described in Chapter 2, you can use the acronym FITT to remember key parameters of your fitness program: **F**requency, **I**ntensity, **T**ime (duration), and **T**ype of activity.

Frequency of Training

Accumulating at least 150 minutes per week of moderate to vigorous physical activity is enough to promote health. Most experts recommend that people exercise three to five days per week to build cardiorespiratory endurance. Training more than five days per week can lead to injury and isn't necessary for the typical person on an exercise program designed to promote wellness. It is safe to do moderate-intensity activity such as walking and gardening every day. Training fewer than three days per week makes it difficult to improve your fitness (unless exercise intensity is very high) or to use exercise to lose weight. Remember, however, that some exercise is better than none.

Intensity of Training

Intensity is the most important factor for increasing aerobic fitness. You must exercise intensely enough to stress your body so that fitness improves. Four methods of monitoring exercise intensity are described here; choose the method that works best for you. Be sure to make adjustments in your intensity levels for environmental or individual factors. For example, on a hot and humid day or on your first day back to your program after an illness, you should decrease your intensity level.

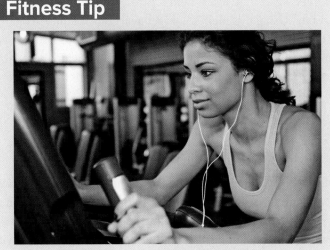

Fitness Tip

Listen to fast-paced music for a better workout! In a recent study, students rode a stationary bike while listening to music at different tempos. The subjects rode harder when listening to faster music and performed less exercise in response to slower music.

© Blend Images / Alamy

Target Heart Rate Zone

One of the best ways to monitor the intensity of cardiorespiratory endurance exercise is to measure your heart rate. It isn't necessary to exercise at your maximum heart rate to improve maximal oxygen consumption. Fitness adaptations occur at lower heart rates with a much lower risk of injury.

According to the American College of Sports Medicine, your **target heart rate zone**—the range of heart rates at which you should exercise to experience cardiorespiratory benefits—is between 65% and 90% of your maximum heart rate. To calculate your target heart rate zone, follow these steps:

target heart rate zone The range of heart rates that should be reached and maintained during cardiorespiratory endurance exercise to obtain training effects.

1. Estimate your maximum heart rate (MHR) by subtracting your age from 220, or have it measured precisely by undergoing an exercise stress test in a doctor's office, hospital, or sports medicine lab. (Note: The formula to estimate MHR carries an error of about plus or minus 10 to 15 beats per minute and can be very inaccurate for some people, particularly older adults and young children. If your exercise heart rate seems inaccurate—that is, exercise within your target zone seems either too easy or too difficult—then use the perceived exertion method described in the next section or have your maximum heart rate measured precisely.) You can get a reasonable estimate of maximal heart rate by exercising at maximal intensities on a stationary bike, treadmill, or elliptical trainer that has a built-in heart rate monitor. This method is not recommended unless you are physically fit and accustomed to intense exercise.

2. Multiply your MHR by 65% and 90% to calculate your target heart rate zone. Very unfit people should use 55% of MHR for their training threshold.

For example, a 19-year-old would calculate her target heart rate zone as follows:

$$MHR = 220 - 19 = 201$$
$$65\% \text{ training intensity} = 0.65 \times 201 = 131 \text{ bpm}$$
$$90\% \text{ training intensity} = 0.90 \times 201 = 181 \text{ bpm}$$

To gain fitness benefits, the young woman in our example would have to exercise at an intensity that raises her heart rate to between 131 and 181 bpm.

An alternative method for calculating target heart rate uses **heart rate reserve**, the difference between maximum heart rate and resting heart rate. Using this method, target heart rate is equal to resting heart rate plus between 50% (40% for very unfit people) and 85% of heart rate reserve. Although some people will obtain more accurate results using this more complex method, both methods provide reasonable estimates of an appropriate target heart rate zone. Lab 3.2 gives formulas for both methods of calculating target heart rate.

heart rate reserve The difference between maximum heart rate and resting heart rate; used in one method for calculating target heart rate range.

If you have been sedentary, start by exercising at the lower end of your target heart rate range (65% of maximum heart rate or 50% of heart rate reserve) for at least four to six weeks. Fast and significant gains in maximal oxygen consumption can be made by exercising closer to the top of the range, but you may increase your risk of injury and overtraining. You *can* achieve significant health benefits by exercising at the bottom of your target range, so don't feel pressured into exercising at an unnecessarily intense level. If you exercise at a lower intensity, you can increase the duration or frequency of training to obtain as much benefit as possible to your health, as long as you are above the 65% training threshold. For people with a very low initial level of fitness, a lower training intensity, 55–64% of maximum heart rate or 40–49% of heart rate reserve, may be sufficient to achieve improvements in maximal oxygen consumption, especially at the start of an exercise program. Intensities of 70–85% of maximum heart rate are appropriate for individuals with average levels of fitness.

By monitoring your heart rate, you will know if you are working hard enough to improve, not hard enough, or too hard. As your program progresses and your fitness improves, you will need to jog, cycle, or walk faster to reach your target heart rate zone. To monitor your heart rate during exercise, count your pulse while you're still moving or immediately after you stop exercising. Count beats for 15 seconds, and then multiply that number by 4 to see if your heart rate is in your target zone. Table 3.3 shows target heart rate ranges and 15-second counts based on the maximum heart rate formula.

TABLE 3.3

Target Heart Rate Range and 15-Second Counts

Age (years)	Target Heart Rate Range (bpm)*	10-Second Count (beats)*
20–24	127–180	32–45
25–29	124–176	31–44
30–34	121–171	30–43
35–39	118–167	30–42
40–44	114–162	29–41
45–49	111–158	28–40
50–54	108–153	27–38
55–59	105–149	26–37
60–64	101–144	25–36
65+	97–140	24–35

*Target heart rates lower than those shown here are appropriate for individuals with a very low initial level of fitness. Ranges are based on the following formula: Target heart rate = 0.65 to 0.90 of maximum heart rate, assuming maximum heart rate = 220 − age. The heart rate range values shown here correspond to RPE values of about 12 to 18.

METs

One way in which scientists describe fitness is in terms of the capacity to increase metabolism (energy usage level) above rest. Scientists use METs to measure the metabolic cost of an exercise. One **MET** represents the body's resting metabolic rate—that is, the energy or calorie requirement of the body at rest. Exercise intensity is expressed in multiples of resting metabolic rate. For example, an exercise intensity of 2 METs is twice the resting metabolic rate.

> **MET**   A unit of measure that represents the body's resting metabolic rate—that is, the energy requirement of the body at rest.

METs are used to describe exercise intensities for occupational activities and exercise programs. Exercise intensities of less than 3 to 4 METs are considered low. Household chores and most industrial jobs fall into this category. Exercise at these intensities does not improve fitness for most people, but it will improve fitness for people with low physical capacities. Activities that increase metabolism by 6 to 8 METs are classified as moderate-intensity exercises and are suitable for most people beginning an exercise program. Vigorous exercise increases metabolic rate by more than 10 METs. Fast running or cycling, as well as intense play in sports like racquetball, can place people in this category. Table 3.4 lists the MET ratings for various activities.

TABLE 3.4

Approximate MET and Caloric Costs of Selected Activities for a 70-Kilogram Person

Activity	METs	Caloric Expenditure
Rest	1	1.2
Light housework	2–4	2.4–4.8
Bowling	2–4	2.5–5
Walking	2–7	2.5–8.5
Archery	3–4	3.7–5
Dancing	3–7	3.7–8.5
Hiking	3–7	3.7–8.5
Horseback riding	3–8	3.7–10
Cycling	3–8	3.7–10
Basketball (recreational)	3–9	3.7–11
Swimming	4–8	5–10
Tennis	4–9	5–11
Fishing (fly, stream)	5–6	6–7.5
In-line skating	5–8	6–10
Skiing (downhill)	5–8	6–10
Rock climbing	5–10	6–12
Scuba diving	5–10	6–12
Skiing (cross-country)	6–12	7.5–15
Jogging	8–12	10–15

Note: Intensity varies greatly with effort, skill, and motivation.

SOURCE: Adapted from American College of Sports Medicine. 2013. *ACSM's Guidelines for Exercise Testing and Prescription,* 9th ed. Philadelphia: Wolters Kluwer/Lippincott Williams & Wilkins Health.

METs are intended to be only an approximation of exercise intensity. Skill, body weight, body fat, and environment affect the accuracy of METs. As a practical matter, however, we can disregard these limitations. METs are a good way to express exercise intensity because this system is easy for people to remember and apply.

Ratings of Perceived Exertion

Another way to monitor intensity is to monitor your perceived level of exertion. Repeated pulse counting during exercise can become a nuisance if it interferes with the activity. As your exercise program progresses, you will probably become familiar with the amount of exertion required to raise your heart rate to target levels. In other words, you will know how you feel when you have exercised intensely enough. If this is the case, you can use the scale of **ratings of perceived exertion (RPE)** shown in Figure 3.5 to monitor the intensity of your exercise session without checking your pulse.

ratings of perceived exertion (RPE) A system of monitoring exercise intensity based on assigning a number to the subjective perception of target intensity.

FIGURE 3.5

Ratings of perceived exertion (RPE). Experienced exercisers may use this subjective scale to estimate how near they are to their target heart rate zone.

RPE scale	
6	
7	Extremely light
8	
9	Very light
10	
11	Light
12	
13	Somewhat hard
14	
15	Hard (heavy)
16	
17	Very hard
18	
19	Extremely hard
20	Maximal exertion

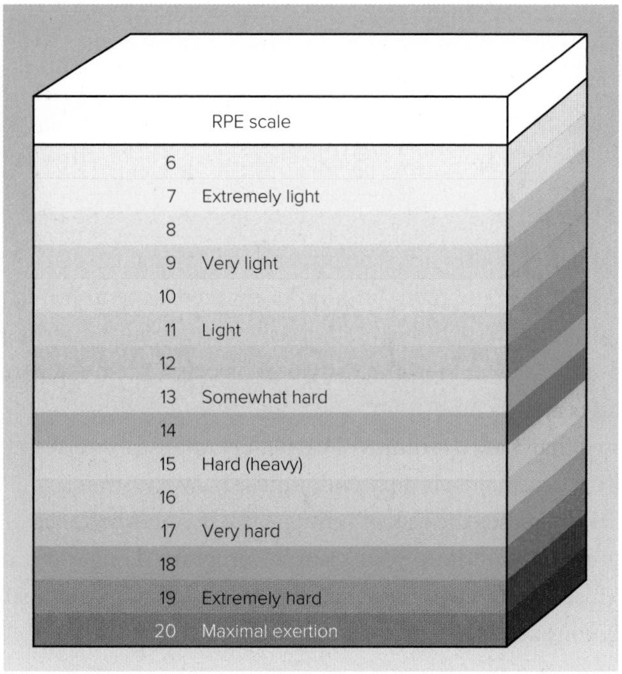

SOURCE: *Psychology from Research to Practice* (1978), ed. H.L. Pick. Kluwer Academic/Plenum Publishing Corporation. Reprinted with kind permission of Springer Science and Business Media and the author.

To use the RPE scale, select a rating that corresponds to your subjective perception of how hard you are exercising when you are training in your target heart rate zone. For example, if your target zone is about 135 to 155 bpm, exercise intensely enough to raise your heart rate to that level, and then associate a rating—such as "somewhat hard" or "hard" (14 or 15)—with how hard you feel you are working. To reach and maintain intensity in future workouts, exercise hard enough to reach what you feel is the same level of exertion. You should periodically check your RPE against your target heart rate zone to make sure it's correct. RPE is an accurate means of monitoring exercise intensity, and you may find it easier and more convenient than pulse counting.

Talk Test

Another easy method of monitoring exercise exertion—in particular, to prevent overly intense exercise—is the talk test. Although your breathing rate will increase during cardiorespiratory endurance exercise, you should not work out so intensely that you cannot speak comfortably. Speech is limited to short phrases during vigorous-intensity exercise. The talk test is an effective gauge of intensity for many types of activities.[6,7]

Table 3.5 (on the next page) provides a quick reference for each of the three methods of estimating exercise intensity discussed here.

TABLE 3.5

Estimating Exercise Intensity

Method	Moderate Intensity	Vigorous Intensity
Percent of maximum heart rate	55–69%	70–90%
Heart rate reserve	40–59%	60–85%
Rating of perceived exertion	12–13 (somewhat hard)	14–16 (hard)
Talk test	Speech with some difficulty	Speech limited to short phrases

Time (Duration) of Training

A total duration of 30 to 60 minutes of exercise is recommended, taking place in a single session or in multiple sessions lasting 10 or more minutes. The total duration of exercise depends on its intensity. To improve cardiorespiratory endurance during a low- to moderate-intensity activity such as walking or slow swimming, you should exercise for 45 to 60 minutes. For high-intensity exercise performed at the top of your target heart rate zone, a duration of 20 minutes is sufficient.

Some studies have shown that 5 to 10 minutes of extremely intense exercise (greater than 90% of maximal oxygen consumption) improves cardiorespiratory endurance. However, training at this intensity, particularly during high-impact activities, increases the risk of injury. Also, if you experience discomfort in high-intensity exercise, you are more likely to discontinue your exercise program. Longer-duration, low- to moderate-intensity activities generally result in more gradual gains in maximal oxygen consumption. In planning your program, start with less vigorous activities and gradually increase intensity.

Type of Activity

Cardiorespiratory endurance exercises include activities that involve the rhythmic use of large muscle groups for an extended period of time, such as jogging, walking, cycling, aerobic dancing and other forms of group exercise, cross-country skiing, and swimming. Start-and-stop sports, such as tennis and racquetball, also qualify if you have enough skill to play continuously and intensely enough to raise your heart rate to target levels. Other important considerations are access to facilities, expense, equipment, and the time required to achieve an adequate skill level and workout.

Warming Up and Cooling Down

As we saw in Chapter 2, it's important to warm up before every session of cardiorespiratory endurance exercise and to cool down afterward. Because the body's muscles work better when their temperature is slightly above resting level, warming up enhances performance and decreases the chance of injury. It gives the body time to redirect blood to active muscles and the heart time to adapt to increased demands. Warming up also helps spread protective fluid throughout the joints, preventing injury to their surfaces.

A warm-up session should include low-intensity, whole-body movements similar to those in the activity that will follow, such as walking slowly before beginning a brisk walk. An active warm-up of 5 to 10 minutes is adequate for most types of exercise; however, warm-up time will depend on your level of fitness, experience, and individual preferences.

What about stretching as part of a warm-up? Performing *static* stretches—those in which you move a joint to the end of the range of motion and hold the position—as part of your pre-exercise warm-up has not been found to prevent injury and has little or no effect on post-exercise muscle soreness. Static stretching before exercise may also adversely affect strength, power, balance, reaction time, and movement time by interfering with muscle and joint receptors that are used in the performance of sport and movement skills. For these reasons, it is often recommended that static stretches be performed at the end of your workout, after your cool-down but while your muscles are still warm and your joints are lubricated.

On the flip side, *dynamic* stretches—those involving continuous movement of joints through a range of motion—can be an appropriate part of a warm-up. Slow and controlled movements such as walking lunges, heel kicks, and arm circles can raise muscle temperature while moving joints through their range of motion. (See Chapter 5 for a detailed discussion of stretching and flexibility exercises.)

Cooling down after exercise is important for returning the body to a nonexercising state. A cool-down helps maintain blood flow to the heart and brain and redirects blood from working muscles to other areas of the body; it helps prevent a large drop in blood pressure, dizziness, and other potential cardiovascular complications. A cool-down, consisting of 5 to 10 minutes of reduced activity, should follow every workout to allow heart rate, breathing, and circulation to return to normal. Decrease the intensity of exercise gradually during your cool-down. For example, following a running workout, begin your cool-down by jogging at half speed for 30 seconds to a minute; then do several minutes of walking, reducing your speed slowly. A good rule of thumb is to cool down at least until your heart rate drops below 100 beats per minute.

The general pattern of a safe and successful workout for cardiorespiratory fitness is illustrated in Figure 3.6.

FIGURE 3.6

The FITT principle for a cardiorespiratory endurance workout. Longer-duration exercise at lower intensities can often be as beneficial for promoting health as shorter-duration, high-intensity exercise.

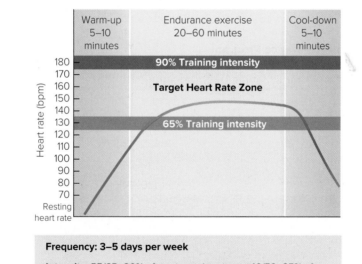

Frequency: 3–5 days per week

Intensity: 55/65–90% of maximum heart rate, 40/50–85% of heart rate reserve plus resting heart rate, or an RPE rating of about 12–18 (lower intensities—55–64% of maximum heart rate and 40–49% of heart rate reserve—are applicable to people who are quite unfit; for average individuals, intensities of 70–85% of maximum heart rate are appropriate)

Time (duration): 20–60 minutes (one session or multiple sessions lasting 10 or more minutes)

Type of activity: Cardiorespiratory endurance exercises, such as walking, jogging, biking, swimming, cross-country skiing, and rope skipping

Building Cardiorespiratory Fitness

Building fitness is as much an art as a science. Your fitness improves when you overload your body. However, you must carefully increase the intensity, frequency, and duration of exercise to avoid injury and overtraining.

General Program Progression

For the initial phase of your program, which may last anywhere from three to six weeks, exercise at the low end of your target heart rate zone. Begin with a frequency of 2 to 4 days per week, and choose a duration appropriate for your fitness level: 12 to 15 minutes if you are very unfit, 20 minutes if you are sedentary but otherwise healthy, and 30 to 40 minutes if you are an experienced exerciser. Use this phase of your program to allow both your body and your schedule to adjust to your new exercise routine. Once you can exercise at the upper levels of frequency (4 or 5 days per week) and duration (30 to 40 minutes) without excessive fatigue or muscle soreness, you are ready to progress.

The next phase of your program is the improvement phase, lasting from four to six months. During this phase, slowly and gradually increase the amount of overload until you reach your target level of fitness (see the sample training progression in Table 3.6). Take care not to increase overload too quickly. It is usually best to avoid increasing intensity and duration during the same session or all three training variables in one week. Increasing duration in increments of 5 to 10 minutes every 2 to 3 weeks is usually appropriate. Signs of a too-rapid progression in overload include muscle aches and pains, lack of usual interest in exercise, extreme fatigue, and inability to complete a workout. Keep an exercise log or training diary to help monitor your workouts and progress.

TABLE 3.6

Sample Progression for an Endurance Program

Stage/Week	Frequency (days/week)	Intensity* (beats/minute)	Time (duration in minutes)
Initial stage			
1	3	120–130	15–20
2	3	120–130	20–25
3	4	130–145	20–25
4	4	130–145	25–30
Improvement stage			
5–7	3–4	145–160	25–30
8–10	3–4	145–160	30–35
11–13	3–4	150–165	30–35
14–16	4–5	150–165	30–35
17–20	4–5	160–180	35–40
21–24	4–5	160–160	35–40
Maintenance stage			
25+	3–5	160–180	20–60

*The target heart rates shown here are based on calculations for a healthy 20-year-old; the program progresses from an initial target heart rate of 50% to a maintenance range of 70–85% of maximum heart rate.

SOURCE: Adapted from American College of Sports Medicine. 2009. *ACSM's Guidelines for Exercise Testing and Prescription,* 8th ed. Philadelphia: Lippincott Williams and Wilkins. Reprinted with permission from the publisher.

Interval Training

You will not improve your fitness indefinitely. The more fit you become, the harder you must work to improve. Few exercise techniques are more effective at improving fitness rapidly than *high-intensity interval training (HIIT)*—a series of very brief, high-intensity exercise sessions interspersed with short rest periods. The four components of interval training are distance, repetition, intensity, and rest, defined as follows:

- **Distance** refers to either the distance or the time of the exercise interval.
- **Repetition** is the number of times the exercise is repeated.
- **Intensity** is the speed at which the exercise is performed.
- **Rest** is the time spent recovering between exercises.

You can use interval training in your favourite aerobic exercises. In fact, the type of exercise you select is not important as long as you exercise at a high intensity and rest for 3 to 5 minutes between repetitions. You can even use HIIT training to help develop sports skills. For example, a runner might do 4 to 8 repetitions of 200-metre sprints at near-maximum effort; a tennis player might practise volleys against a wall as fast as possible for 4 to 8 repetitions lasting 30 seconds each; and a swimmer might swim 4 to 8 repetitions of 50 metres at 100% effort.

If you add HIIT to your exercise program, do not practise interval training more than three days per week. Intervals are exhausting and easily lead to injury. Let your body tell you how many days you can tolerate. If you become overly tired after doing interval training three days per week, cut back to two days. If you feel good, try increasing the intensity or number of intervals (but not the number of days per week) and see what happens. As with any kind of exercise program, begin HIIT training slowly and progress conservatively. Although HIIT training produces substantial fitness improvements, it is best to integrate it into your total exercise program.

Pros

Canadian researchers found that six sessions of high-intensity interval training on a stationary bike increased muscle oxidative capacity by 38%, muscle glycogen by 20%, and cycle endurance capacity by 100%. The subjects made these amazing improvements by exercising only 15 minutes over a period of two weeks. Each workout consisted of 4 to 7 repetitions of high-intensity exercise (each repetition consisted of 30 seconds at near maximum effort) on a stationary bike. Follow-up studies showed that practising HIIT 1 to 3 times per week improved endurance and aerobic capacity just as well as training 5 times per week for 60 minutes for 6 weeks. These studies (and more than 50 others) show the value of high-intensity training for building aerobic capacity and endurance.

Cons

High-intensity interval training appears to be safe and effective in the short term, but there are concerns about the long-term safety and effectiveness of this type of training, so consider the following issues:

- High-intensity training could be dangerous for some people. A physician might be reluctant to give certain patients the green light for this type of exercise.
- Always warm up with several minutes of low-intensity exercise before practising HIIT. High-intensity exercise without a warm-up can cause cardiac arrhythmias (abnormal heart rhythms), even in healthy people.
- HIIT might trigger overuse injuries in unfit people. For this reason, it is essential to start gradually, especially for someone at a low level of fitness. Exercise at submaximal intensities for at least four to six weeks before starting high-intensity interval training. Cut back on interval training or rest if you feel overly fatigued or develop overly sore joints or muscles.

Other types of high-intensity training may combine intervals with other types of exercises and training techniques; see the box High-Intensity Conditioning Programs on the next page.

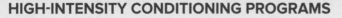

In FOCUS

HIGH-INTENSITY CONDITIONING PROGRAMS

In recent years, high-intensity power-based "extreme" conditioning programs, such as CrossFit, Gym Jones, and Insanity, have grown in popularity. These programs typically incorporate a range of activity types and may include high-intensity aerobic exercise, interval training, free-weight exercises, and gymnastics moves. The programs may be geared toward developing whole-body fitness, limiting workout time by using short but high-intensity sessions, and/or adding a competitive aspect to fitness training.

CrossFit is a popular example of a high-intensity program that emphasizes use of broad and constantly changing training stimuli. It includes activities designed to develop not only cardiorespiratory endurance, but also strength, power, speed, coordination, ability, balance, and accuracy. Workouts are short and intense, but should be tailored to an individual's current fitness level and age. They may include aerobic activities such as running and rope skipping, plus whole-body strength training activities such as power lifts, plyometrics, sled pulls, and kettlebell exercises.

The sample workouts below provide a flavour of this type of high-intensity training.

Sample Workouts

Complete three circuits (series) of the activities, but do not exceed 20 to 30 minutes for the workout. Break the exercises into sets if you cannot complete all the repetitions (e.g., 20 pull-ups). Record your time. Train as hard and as fast as you can while maintaining good technique. Select a weight that allows you to complete the reps in the sets. (Principles of resistance exercise are described in Chapter 4.) Change the exercises with every workout.

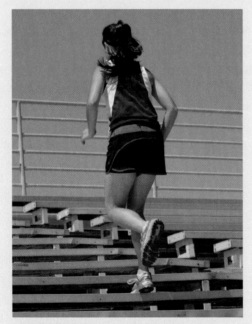

Courtesy Tom Fahey

Workout 1
40 push-ups
10 standing long jumps
40 squats with hands on your hips
20 dumbbell or kettlebell swings
Skip rope rapidly for three minutes
Rest three minutes; repeat circuit 2 more times

Workout 2
20 pull-ups
20 dumbbell thrusters (front squat with barbell or dumbbells, then immediately perform an overhead press)
20 overhead squats
10 kettlebell snatches (10 for each arm)
2 minutes spinning on bike while standing, maximum intensity
Rest 3 minutes; repeat circuit 2 more times

Cautions and Guidelines

High-intensity training programs have their critics, who point to the increased risk of severe injury and lack of concern for the principle of specificity (training the way you want your body to adapt) with this type of training. Good technique is essential; the emphasis on speed and intensity can make it difficult to achieve good technique, but performing high-speed cleans and squats improperly can lead to severe injury.

Performing high-speed, high-repetition sit-ups or squats often pushes muscles and joints to failure, causing severe knee or back injury or muscle destruction (rhabdomyolysis or "rhabdo"). Until recently, physicians only encountered rhabdo after extreme trauma from automobile accidents. These days, rhabdo may becoming more common because of the popularity of "feel the burn" high-intensity training programs. Biomechanical studies suggest that high-speed sit-ups and squats can damage the spine. The benefits of high levels of fitness are counterbalanced by the risk of injury.

In spite of the potential risks of high-intensity training, it can be a suitable option for fit individuals who enjoy and are motivated by varied, high-intensity workouts that require little time or equipment. If you are considering this type of training, consider the following:

- Follow general guidelines for medical clearance for exercise (see Chapter 2).
- Use good form and appropriate safety equipment for all exercises and activities; do not sacrifice form for speed, number of repetitions, or any other goal.
- Drink plenty of water and avoid exercising in hot and humid environments.
- Don't push yourself beyond the limits of your strength or conditioning level. Monitor yourself for signs of overtraining (unusual fatigue or muscle soreness), injuries, and rhabdomyolysis (severe muscle pain or weakness; dark, red, or cola-coloured urine).
- Get advice from a qualified professional; when choosing a class, fitness facility, or trainer, follow the guidelines presented in Chapter 2.

SOURCES: Smith, M. M., A. J. Sommer, B. E. Starkoff, and S. T. Devor. 2013. CrossFit-based high intensity power training improves maximal aerobic fitness and body composition. *Journal of Strength Conditioning Research.* 27(11): 3159—3172; Heinrich, K. M. 2014. High-intensity compared to moderate-intensity training for exercise initiation, enjoyment, adherence, and intentions: an intervention study. *BMC Public Health* 14: 789; Bergeron N. F., et al. 2011. *CHAMP/ACSM Executive Summary: High-Intensity Training Workshop.* (http://hprc-online.org /physical-fitness/training-exercise/exercise/guidelines/champ-acsm-high-intensity-training-conference); Skelly L E., et al. 2014. High-intensity interval exercise induces 24-h energy expenditure similar to traditional endurance exercise despite reduced time commitment. *Applied Physiology Nutrition Metabolism* 39(7): 845–848.

Maintaining Cardiorespiratory Fitness

You will not improve your fitness indefinitely and if you increase intensity and duration indefinitely, you are likely to become injured or overtrained. After a progression phase of four to six months, you may reach your goal of an acceptable level of fitness. You can then maintain fitness by continuing to exercise at the same intensity at least three nonconsecutive days every week. If you stop exercising, you lose your gains in fitness fairly rapidly. If you take time off for any reason, start your program again at a lower level and rebuild your fitness in a slow and systematic way.

When you reach the maintenance phase, you may want to set new goals for your program and make some adjustments to maintain your motivation. For example, you might set a new goal of participating in a local 5K race, or you might add new buddies to your program or mix up your exercise sessions by working out in a new setting. Adding variety to your program can be a helpful strategy.

Engaging in multiple types of endurance activities, an approach known as **cross-training**, can help boost enjoyment and prevent some types of injuries. For example, instead of jogging five days a week, try changing your program so that you jog three days a week, play tennis one day a week, and go for a bike ride one day a week. While all these activities build endurance, alternating between them reduces the strain on specific joints and muscles. Varying your activities also offers new physical and mental challenges that can keep your fitness program fresh and fun.

cross-training   Alternating two or more activities to improve a single component of fitness.

LO5 3.5 Exercise Safety and Injury Prevention

Exercising safely and preventing injuries are two important challenges for people who engage in cardiorespiratory endurance exercise. This section provides basic safety guidelines that can be applied to a variety of fitness activities. (Chapter 4 and Chapter 5 include additional advice specific to strength training and flexibility training.)

Hot Weather and Heat Stress

Human beings require a relatively constant body temperature to survive. A change of just a few degrees in body temperature can quickly lead to distress and even death. If you lose too much water or if your body temperature gets too high, you may suffer from heat stress. Problems associated with heat stress include dehydration, heat cramps, heat exhaustion, and heatstroke.

In a high-temperature environment, exercise safety depends on the body's ability to dissipate heat and maintain blood flow to active muscles. The body releases heat from exercise through the evaporation of sweat. This process cools the skin and the blood circulating near the body's surface. Sweating is an efficient process as long as the air is relatively dry. As humidity increases, however, the sweating mechanism becomes less efficient because extra moisture in the air inhibits the evaporation of sweat from the skin. This is why it takes longer to cool down in humid weather than in dry weather.

You can avoid significant heat stress by staying fit, avoiding overly intense or prolonged exercise for which you are not prepared, drinking adequate fluids before and during exercise, and wearing clothes that allow heat to dissipate.

Dehydration

Your body needs water to carry out many chemical reactions and to regulate body temperature. Sweating during exercise depletes your body's water supply and can lead to **dehydration** if fluids aren't replaced. Although dehydration is most common in hot weather, it can occur even in comfortable temperatures if fluid intake is insufficient. Dehydration increases body temperature and decreases sweat rate, plasma volume, cardiac output, maximal oxygen consumption, exercise capacity, muscular strength, and stores of liver glycogen. You may begin to feel thirsty when you have a fluid deficit of about 1% of total body weight.

dehydration Excessive loss of body fluid.

Drinking fluids before and during exercise is important to prevent dehydration and enhance performance. As a general rule, drink about 500 millilitres (about 16 ounces or 2 cups) of fluid four hours before exercise, and 250 to 350 millilitres (about 8–12 ounces) 15 minutes immediately before exercise. During exercise lasting less than 60 minutes, drink 150 to 250 millilitres (about 3–8 ounces) of water every 15 to 20 minutes. Consume a sports drink with electrolytes every 15 to 20 minutes when exercising longer than 60 minutes.

Don't drink more than 1.5 litres of water per hour. Very rarely, athletes consume too much water and develop *hyponatremia*, a condition characterized by lung congestion, muscle weakness, and nervous system problems. Following the guidelines presented here can help prevent this condition.

To determine if you're drinking enough fluid, weigh yourself before and after an exercise session; any weight loss is due to fluid loss that needs to be replaced. Urine colour is a good marker of hydration (see Figure 3.7); a dark colour means that you might be dehydrated. Note that diet and supplements can affect urine colour, which affects the accuracy of the test.

Bring a water bottle when you exercise so you can replace your fluids when they're being depleted. For exercise sessions lasting less than 60 to 90 minutes, cool water is an excellent fluid replacement. For longer

Urine Chart to Assess Hydration. A large amount of light-coloured urine means you are well hydrated. The darker the colour, the more dehydrated you are. Vitamins and some foods can make urine darker.

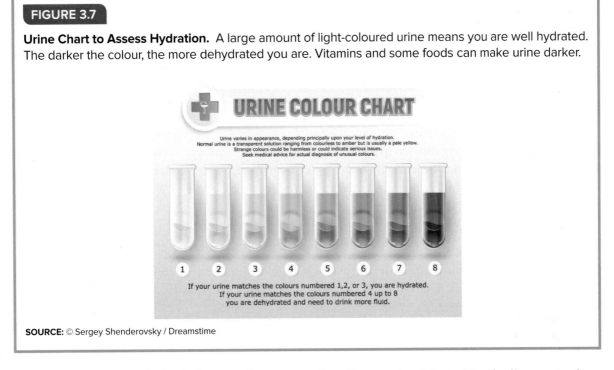

SOURCE: © Sergey Shenderovsky / Dreamstime

workouts, choose a sports drink that contains water and small amounts of electrolytes (sodium, potassium, and magnesium) and simple carbohydrates ("sugar," usually in the form of sucrose, glucose, lactate, or glucose polymers). Electrolytes, which are lost from the body in sweat, are important because they help regulate the balance of fluids in body cells and the bloodstream. The carbohydrates in typical sports drinks are rapidly digestible and can thus help maintain blood glucose levels. Choose a beverage with no more than 8 grams of simple carbohydrate per 100 millilitres. Nonfat milk and chocolate milk, for those who can tolerate dairy products, are excellent fluid replacement beverages because they promote long-term hydration. (See Chapter 7 for more on diet and fluid recommendations for active people.)

Heat Cramps

Involuntary cramping and spasms in the muscle groups used during exercise are sometimes called **heat cramps**. While depletion of sodium and potassium from the muscles is involved with the problem, the primary cause of cramps is muscle fatigue. Children are particularly susceptible to heat cramps, but the condition can also occur in adults, even those who are fit. The best treatment for heat cramps is a combination of gentle stretching, replacement of fluid and electrolytes, and rest.

heat cramps Sudden muscle spasms and pain associated with intense exercise in hot weather.

Heat Exhaustion

Symptoms of **heat exhaustion** include the following:

- a rapid, weak pulse
- low blood pressure

heat exhaustion Heat illness resulting from exertion in hot weather.

- headache
- faintness, weakness, dizziness
- profuse sweating
- pale face
- psychological disorientation (in some cases)
- normal or slightly elevated core body temperature

Heat exhaustion occurs when an insufficient amount of blood returns to the heart because so much of the body's blood volume is being directed to working muscles (for exercise) and to the skin (for cooling). Treatment for heat exhaustion includes resting in a cool area, removing excess clothing, applying cool or damp towels to the body, and drinking fluids. An affected individual should rest for the remainder of the day and drink plenty of fluids for the next 24 hours.

Heatstroke

Heatstroke is a major medical emergency involving the failure of the brain's temperature regulatory centre. The body does not sweat enough, and body temperature rises dramatically to extremely dangerous levels. In addition to high body temperature, symptoms can include the following:

- hot, flushed skin (dry or sweaty), red face
- chills, shivering
- very high or very low blood pressure
- confusion, erratic behaviour
- convulsions, loss of consciousness

heatstroke   A severe and often fatal heat illness characterized by significantly elevated core body temperature.

A heatstroke victim should be cooled as rapidly as possible and immediately transported to a hospital. To lower body temperature, get out of the heat, remove excess clothing, drink cold fluids, and apply cool or damp towels to the body or immerse the body in cold water. People experiencing heatstroke during exercise may still be sweating.

Cold Weather

In extremely cold conditions, problems can occur if a person's body temperature drops or if particular parts of the body are exposed. If the body's ability to warm itself through shivering or exercise can't keep pace with heat loss, the core body temperature begins to drop. This condition, known as **hypothermia**, depresses the central nervous system, resulting in sleepiness and a lower metabolic rate. As metabolic rate drops, body temperature declines even further, and coma and death can result. The risk of hypothermia is particularly severe in cold water.

hypothermia   Low body temperature due to exposure to cold conditions.

Frostbite—the freezing of body tissues—is another potential danger of exercise in extremely cold conditions. Frostbite most commonly occurs in exposed body parts like earlobes, fingers, and the nose, and it can cause permanent circulatory damage. Hypothermia and frostbite both require immediate medical treatment.

frostbite   Freezing of body tissues characterized by pallor, numbness, and a loss of cold sensation.

To exercise safely in cold conditions, don't stay out in very cold temperatures for too long. Take both the temperature and the wind into account when planning your exercise session. Frostbite is possible within 30 minutes in calm conditions when the temperature is colder than −20°C or in windy conditions (50 km/h) if the temperature is below −12°C. **Wind chill** values that reflect both the temperature and the wind speed are available as part of a local weather forecast and from Environment Canada (http://www.weatheroffice.gc.ca /canada_e.html).

> **wind chill**   A measure of how cold it feels based on the rate of heat loss from exposed skin caused by cold and wind; the temperature that would have the same cooling effect on a person as a given combination of temperature and wind speed.

Appropriate clothing provides insulation and helps trap warm air next to the skin. Dress in layers so you can remove them as you warm up and can put them back on if you get cold. A substantial amount of heat loss comes from the head and neck, so keep these areas covered. In subfreezing temperatures, protect the areas of your body most susceptible to frostbite—fingers, toes, ears, nose, and cheeks—with warm socks, mittens or gloves, and a cap, hood, or ski mask. Wear clothing that breathes and will wick moisture away from your skin to avoid being cooled or overheated by trapped perspiration. Many types of comfortable, lightweight clothing are available that provide good insulation. It's also important to warm up thoroughly and to drink plenty of fluids.

Poor Air Quality

Air pollution can decrease exercise performance and negatively affect health, particularly if you smoke or have respiratory problems such as asthma, bronchitis, or emphysema. The effects of smog are worse during exercise than at rest because air enters the lungs faster. Polluted air may also contain carbon monoxide, which displaces oxygen in the blood and reduces the amount of oxygen available to working muscles. One study found that exercise in polluted air can decrease lung function to the same extent as heavy smoking. Another study found that training in a polluted environment counteracted the normally beneficial effects of exercise on the brain. Symptoms of poor air quality include eye and throat irritations, difficulty breathing, and possibly headache and malaise.

Do not exercise outdoors during a smog alert or if air quality is very poor. If you have any type of cardiorespiratory difficulty, you should also avoid exertion outdoors when air quality is poor. You can avoid some smog and air pollution by exercising in indoor facilities, in parks, near water (e.g., riverbanks, lakeshores, and ocean beaches), or in residential areas with less traffic—areas with stop-and-go traffic will have lower air quality than areas where traffic moves quickly. Air quality is also usually better in the early morning and late evening, before and after the commute hours. Environment Canada forecasts the air quality in many major cities through the Air Quality Health Index (https://weather.gc.ca/airquality/ pages/index_e.html).

Exercise Injuries

Most injuries are annoying rather than serious or permanent. However, an injury that isn't cared for properly can escalate into a chronic problem, sometimes serious enough to permanently curtail the activity. It's important to learn how to deal with injuries so they don't derail your fitness program. Strategies for the care of common exercise injuries and discomforts appear in Table 3.7 (on the next page); some general guidelines are given in the following sections.

TABLE 3.7

Care of Common Exercise Injuries and Discomforts

Injury	Symptoms	Treatment
Blister	Accumulation of fluid in one spot under the skin	Don't pop or drain it unless it interferes too much with your daily activities. If it does pop, clean the area with antiseptic and cover with a bandage. Do not remove the skin covering the blister.
Bruise (contusion)	Pain, swelling, and discolouration	R-I-C-E: rest, ice, compression, elevation.
Fracture and/or dislocation	Pain, swelling, tenderness, loss of function, and deformity	Seek medical attention, immobilize the affected area, and apply cold.
Joint sprain	Pain, tenderness, swelling, discolouration, and loss of function	R-I-C-E; apply heat when swelling has disappeared. Stretch and strengthen affected area.
Muscle cramp	Painful, spasmodic muscle contractions	Gently stretch for 15–30 seconds at a time and/or massage the cramped area. Drink fluids and increase dietary salt intake if exercising in hot weather.
Muscle soreness or stiffness	Pain and tenderness in the affected muscle	Stretch the affected muscle gently; exercise at a low intensity; apply heat. Nonsteroidal anti-inflammatory drugs, such as ibuprofen, help some people.
Muscle strain	Pain, tenderness, swelling, and loss of strength in the affected muscle	R-I-C-E; apply heat when swelling has disappeared. Stretch and strengthen the affected area.
Plantar fasciitis	Pain and tenderness in the connective tissue on the bottom of your feet	Apply ice, take nonsteroidal anti-inflammatory drugs, and stretch. Wear night splints when sleeping.
Shin splint	Pain and tenderness on the front of the lower leg; sometimes also pain in the calf muscle	Rest; apply ice to the affected area several times a day and before exercise; wrap with tape for support. Stretch and strengthen muscles in the lower legs. Purchase good-quality footwear and run on soft surfaces.
Side stitch	Pain on the side of the abdomen	Stretch the arm on the affected side as high as possible; if that doesn't help, try bending forward while tightening the abdominal muscles.
Tendinitis	Pain, swelling, and tenderness of the affected area	R-I-C-E; apply heat when swelling has disappeared. Stretch and strengthen the affected area.

When to Call a Physician

Some injuries require medical attention. Consult a physician for the following:

- head and eye injuries
- possible ligament injuries
- broken bones
- internal disorders—chest pain, fainting, elevated body temperature, intolerance to hot weather

Also seek medical attention for ostensibly minor injuries that do not get better within a reasonable amount of time. You may need to modify your exercise program for a few weeks to allow an injury to heal.

Managing Minor Exercise Injuries

For minor cuts and scrapes, stop the bleeding and clean the wound. Treat injuries to soft tissue (muscles and joints) with the R-I-C-E principle: **R**est, **I**ce, **C**ompression, and **E**levation.

- **Rest.** Stop using the injured area as soon as you experience pain. Avoid any activity that causes pain.
- **Ice.** Apply ice to the injured area to reduce swelling and alleviate pain. Apply ice immediately for 10 to 20 minutes, and repeat every few hours until the swelling disappears. Let the injured part return to normal temperature between icings, and do not apply ice to one area for more than 20 minutes. An easy method for applying ice is to freeze water in a paper cup, peel some of the paper away, and rub the exposed ice on the injured area. If the injured area is large, surround it with several bags of crushed ice or ice cubes, or with bags of frozen vegetables. Place a thin towel between the bag and your skin. If you use a cold gel pack, limit application time to 10 minutes. Some experts recommend regular icing for up to about 6 hours after an injury, while others suggest continuing as long as swelling persists.
- **Compression.** Wrap the injured area firmly with an elastic or compression bandage between icings. If the area starts throbbing or begins to change colour, the bandage may be wrapped too tightly. Do not sleep with the wrap on.
- **Elevation.** Raise the injured area above heart level to decrease the blood supply and reduce swelling. Use pillows, books, or a low chair or stool to raise the injured area.

The day after the injury, some experts recommend also taking an over-the-counter medication such as aspirin, ibuprofen, or naproxen to decrease inflammation. To rehabilitate your body, follow the steps listed in the box Rehabilitation Following a Minor Athletic Injury.

Take CHARGE

REHABILITATION FOLLOWING A MINOR ATHLETIC INJURY

- Reduce the initial inflammation using the R-I-C-E principle (see above).
- After 36 to 48 hours, apply heat *if the swelling has disappeared completely.* Immerse the affected area in warm water or apply warm compresses, a hot water bottle, or a heating pad. As soon as it's comfortable, begin moving the affected joints slowly. If you feel pain, or if the injured area begins to swell again, reduce the amount of movement. Continue gently stretching and moving the affected area until you have regained normal range of motion.
- Gradually begin exercising the injured area to build strength and endurance. Depending on the type of injury, weight training, walking, and resistance training can all be effective.
- Gradually reintroduce the stress of an activity until you can return to full intensity. Don't progress too rapidly or you'll reinjure yourself. Before returning to full exercise participation, ensure you have a full range of motion in your joints, normal strength and balance among your muscles, normal coordinated patterns of movement (with no injury compensation movements, such as limping), and little or no pain.

Preventing Injuries

The best method for dealing with exercise injuries is to prevent them. If you choose activities for your program carefully and follow the training guidelines described here and in Chapter 2, you should be able to avoid most types of injuries. Important guidelines for preventing athletic injuries include the following:

- Train regularly and stay in condition.
- Gradually increase the intensity, duration, or frequency of your workouts.
- Avoid or minimize high-impact activities; alternate them with low-impact activities.
- Get proper rest between exercise sessions.
- Drink plenty of fluids.
- Warm up thoroughly before you exercise and cool down afterward.
- Achieve and maintain a normal range of motion in your joints.
- Use proper body mechanics when lifting objects or executing sports skills.
- Don't exercise when you are ill or overtrained.
- Use proper equipment, particularly shoes, and choose an appropriate exercise surface. If you exercise on a grass field, soft track, or wooden floor, you are less likely to be injured than on concrete or a hard track.
- Don't return to your normal exercise program until any athletic injuries have healed. Restart your program at a lower intensity and gradually increase the amount of overload.

Tips for Today and the Future

Regular, moderate exercise, even in short bouts spread through the day, can build and maintain cardiorespiratory fitness.

RIGHT NOW YOU CAN

- Assess your cardiorespiratory fitness by using one of the methods discussed in this chapter and in Lab 3.1.
- Do a short bout of endurance exercise: 10 to 15 minutes of walking, jogging, or cycling.
- If you have physical activity planned for later in the day, drink some fluids now to make sure you are fully hydrated for your workout.

IN THE FUTURE YOU CAN

- Graduate to a different, more challenging fitness assessment as your cardiorespiratory fitness improves.
- Incorporate different types of exercises into your cardiorespiratory endurance training to keep yourself challenged and motivated.

Common Questions ANSWERED

Q Do I need a special diet for my endurance exercise program?

A No. For most people, a nutritionally balanced diet contains all the energy and nutrients needed to sustain an exercise program. Don't waste your money on unnecessary vitamins, minerals, and protein supplements. (Chapter 7 has information about putting together a healthy diet.)

Q How can I measure how far I walk or run?

A The simplest way to measure distance is with a GPS-based Smartphone app, which measures your distance, speed, and change in elevation. You can also use a pedometer, which counts your steps. Although stride length varies among individuals, 2000 steps typically equals about 1.6 kilometres, and 10 000 steps equals about 8 kilometres. To track your distance and your progress using a pedometer, follow the guidelines in Lab 2.3.

Q How can I avoid being sore when I start an exercise program?

A For both athletes and nonathletes, it is extremely important to increase intensity very gradually and to rest between exercise sessions. If you train too hard and/or don't rest enough, you are more likely to be injured—and be discouraged from continuing with your fitness program. For endurance training, overload techniques such as interval training and wind sprints can help you build fitness quickly, but they also pose a greater risk of injury or overtraining. Start off with a few high-intensity bouts of exercise and build up gradually. Don't practise interval training or wind sprints more than two or three days per week unless you have a high fitness level.

Q Is it OK to do cardiorespiratory endurance exercise while menstruating?

A Yes. There is no evidence that exercise during menstruation is unhealthy or that it has negative effects on performance. If you have headaches, backaches, and abdominal pain during menstruation, you may not feel like exercising; for some women, exercise helps relieve these symptoms. Listen to your body, and exercise at whatever intensity is comfortable for you.

SUMMARY

- The cardiorespiratory system consists of the heart, blood vessels, and respiratory system; it picks up and transports oxygen, nutrients, and waste products.

- The body takes chemical energy from food and uses it to produce ATP and fuel cellular activities. ATP is stored in the body's cells as the basic form of energy.

- During exercise, the body supplies ATP and fuels cellular activities by combining three energy systems: immediate, for short periods of energy; non-oxidative (anaerobic), for intense activity; and oxidative (aerobic), for prolonged activity. Which energy system predominates depends on the duration and intensity of the activity.

- Cardiorespiratory endurance exercise improves cardiorespiratory functioning and cellular metabolism; it reduces the risk of chronic disease such as heart disease, cancer, type 2 diabetes, obesity, and osteoporosis; and it improves immune function and psychological and emotional well-being.

- Cardiorespiratory fitness is measured by seeing how well the cardiorespiratory system transports and uses oxygen. The upper limit of this measure is called maximal oxygen consumption, or $\dot{V}O_{2max}$. It can be measured precisely in a laboratory, or it can be estimated reasonably well through self-assessment tests.

- To create a successful exercise program, set realistic goals, choose suitable activities, begin slowly, and always warm up and cool down. As fitness improves, exercise more often, longer, and/or harder.

continued

- Intensity of training can be measured through target heart rate zone, METs, ratings of perceived exertion, or the talk test.

- With careful attention to fluid intake, clothing, duration of exercise, and exercise intensity, endurance training can be safe in hot and cold weather conditions.

- Serious injuries require medical attention. Application of the R-I-C-E principle (Rest, Ice, Compression, Elevation) is appropriate for treating many types of muscle or joint injuries.

FOR FURTHER EXPLORATION

Organizations and Websites

Canadian Society for Exercise Physiology. Includes information on a variety of topics related to the study of exercise physiology, exercise biochemistry, fitness, and health.

> http://www.csep.ca

Franklin Institute Science Museum/The Heart: An Online Exploration. Contains information on the structure and function of the heart, blood vessels, and respiratory system.

> https://www.fi.edu/heart-engine-of-life

Health Canada. Provides the latest statistics on Canadian participation levels and information on risk factors and the cardiovascular system.

> http://www.hc-sc.gc.ca/index-eng.php

Heart and Stroke Foundation of Canada. Provides information on the benefits of exercise for a healthy heart.

> http://www.heartandstroke.ca

Industry Canada—Office of Consumer Affairs. Offers practical information for consumers interested in purchasing fitness equipment.

> http://strategis.ic.gc.ca/

MedlinePlus: Exercise and Physical Fitness. Provides links to news and reliable information about fitness from government agencies and professional associations.

> https://medlineplus.gov/exerciseandphysicalfitness.html

Runner's World Online. Contains a wide variety of information about running, including tips for beginning runners, advice about training, and a shoe buyer's guide.

> http://www.runnersworld.com

Women's Sports Foundation. Provides information and links about training and about many specific sports activities.

> https://www.womenssportsfoundation.org/

Yahoo/Recreation. Includes links to many sites with practical advice on many sports and activities.

> http://dir.yahoo.com/recreation/sports

See also the listings in Chapter 2 and Chapter 10.

Laboratory Activities

Name _____ Section _____ Date _____

Lab 3.1 Assessing Your Current Level of Cardiorespiratory Endurance

Mc Graw Hill Education connect®

The conditions for exercise safety given in Chapter 2 apply to all fitness assessment tests. Talk to a physician if needed, and if you experience any unusual symptoms while taking a test, stop exercising and discuss your condition with your instructor. Additional cautions and prerequisites for the five test options presented in this lab are described below.

1.6-Km Walk Test	Recommended for anyone who meets the criteria for safe exercise. This test can be used by people who cannot perform other tests because of low fitness level or injury.
3-Minute Step Test	If you suffer from joint problems in your ankles, knees, or hips or are significantly overweight, check with your physician before taking this test. People with balance problems or for whom a fall would be particularly dangerous, including older adults and pregnant women, should use special caution or avoid this test.
2.4-Km Run-Walk Test	Recommended for people who are healthy and at least moderately active. If you have been sedentary, you should participate in a 4- to 8-week walk-run program before taking the test. Don't take this test in extremely hot or cold weather or if you aren't used to exercising under those conditions.
Beep Test	Recommended for fit individuals; the test is highly strenuous and requires the ability to jog, run, and sprint. Don't take this test unless you can complete at least 10 sets of 50-metre sprints.
12-Minute Swim Test	Recommended for relatively strong swimmers who are confident in the water; if needed, ask a qualified swimming instructor to evaluate your swimming ability before attempting this test.

Choose one of the tests based on your fitness level and available facilities. For best results, don't exercise strenuously or consume caffeine the day of the test, and don't smoke or eat a heavy meal within about 3 hours of the test.

The 1.6-Km Walk Test

Equipment

1. A track or course that allows for measurement of 1.6 kilometres
2. A stopwatch, clock, or watch with a second hand
3. A weight scale

Preparation

Measure your body weight (in pounds) before taking the test.

Body weight: _____ lbs

Instructions

1. Warm up before taking the test. Do some walking, easy jogging, or callisthenics and some stretching exercises.
2. Cover the 1.6-kilometre course as quickly as possible. Walk at a pace that is brisk but comfortable. You must raise your heart rate above 120 beats per minute (bpm).

3. As soon as you complete the distance, note your time and take your pulse for 15 seconds.

   Walking time: _____ min _____ sec

   15-second pulse count: _____ beats

4. Cool down after the test by walking slowly for several minutes.

Determining Maximal Oxygen Consumption

1. Convert your 15-second pulse count into a value for exercise heart rate by multiplying it by 4.

   Exercise heart rate:_____ × 4 = _____ bpm
   <u>15-sec pulse count</u>

2. Convert your walking time from minutes and seconds to a decimal figure. For example, a time of 14 minutes and 45 seconds would be 14 + (45/60), or 14.75 minutes.

   Walking time: _____ min + (_____ sec ÷ 60 sec/min) = _____ min

3. Insert values for your age, gender, weight, walking time, and exercise heart rate in the following equation, where

   W = your weight (in pounds)

   A = your age (in years)

   G = your gender (male = 1; female = 0)

   T = your time to complete the 1.6-kilometre course (in minutes)

   H = your exercise heart rate (in beats per minute)

   $$\dot{V}O_{2max} = 132.853 - (0.0769 \times W) - (0.3877 \times A) + (6.315 \times G) - (3.2649 \times T) - (0.1565 \times H)$$

   For example, a 20-year-old, 190-pound male with a time of 14.75 minutes and an exercise heart rate of 152 bpm would calculate maximal oxygen consumption as follows:

   $$\dot{V}O_{2max} = 132.853 - (0.0769 \times 190) - (0.3877 \times 20) + (6.315 \times 1) - (3.2649 \times 14.75) - (0.1565 \times 152)$$

   $$= 45 \ mL/kg/min$$

   $\dot{V}O_{2max} = 132.853 - (0.0769 \times$ _____ $) - (0.3877 \times$ _____ $) + (6.315 \times$ _____ $)$
                                         weight (lb)   **age (years)**   **Gender**

      $- (3.2649 \times$ _____ $) - (0.1565 \times$ _____ $) =$ _____ mL/kg/min
                  walking time (min)   **exercise heart rate (bpm)**

4. Copy this value for $\dot{V}O_{2max}$ into the appropriate place in the chart at the end of this lab.

The 3-Minute Step Test

Equipment

1. A step, bench, or bleacher step that is about 41 centimetres from ground level

2. A stopwatch, clock, or watch with a second hand

3. A metronome

Preparation

Practise stepping up onto and down from the step before you begin the test. Each step has four beats: up-up-down-down. Males should perform the test with the metronome set for a rate of 96 beats per minute, or 24 steps per minute. Females should set the metronome at 88 beats per minute, or 22 steps per minute.

Instructions

1. Warm up before taking the test. Do some walking, easy jogging, and dynamic stretching exercises.

2. Set the metronome at the proper rate. Your instructor or a partner can call out starting and stopping times; otherwise, have a clock or watch within easy viewing during the test.

3. Begin the test and continue to step at the correct pace for 3 minutes.

4. Stop after 3 minutes. Remain standing and count your pulse for the 15-second period from 5 to 20 seconds into recovery. 15-second pulse count: _____ beats.

5. Cool down after the test by walking slowly for several minutes.

Determining Maximal Oxygen Consumption

1. Convert your 15-second pulse count to a value for recovery heart rate by multiplying by 4.

   Recovery heart rate: $\underbrace{}_{\textbf{15-sec pulse count}} \times 4 = $ _____ bpm

2. Insert your recovery heart rate in the equation below, where

   H = recovery heart rate (in beats per minute)

   Males: $\dot{V}O_{2max} = 111.33 - (0.42 \times H)$

   Females: $\dot{V}O_{2max} = 65.81 - (0.1847 \times H)$

   For example, a man with a recovery heart rate of 162 bpm would calculate maximal oxygen consumption as follows:

   $\dot{V}O_{2max} = 111.33 - (0.42 \times 162) = 43 \ mL/kg/min$

   Males: $\dot{V}O_{2max} = 111.33 - (0.42 \times \underbrace{}_{\textbf{recovery heart rate (bpm)}}) = $ _____ mL/kg/min

   Females: $\dot{V}O_{2max} = 65.81 - (0.1847 \times \underbrace{}_{\textbf{recovery heart rate (bpm)}}) = $ _____ mL/kg/min

3. Copy this value for $\dot{V}O_{2max}$ into the appropriate place in the chart at the end of this lab.

The 2.4-Km Run-Walk Test

Equipment

1. A running track or course that is flat and provides exact measurements of up to 2.4 kilometres

2. A stopwatch, clock, or watch with a second hand

Preparation

You may want to practise pacing yourself prior to taking the test to avoid going too fast at the start and becoming prematurely fatigued. Allow yourself a day or two to recover from your practice run before taking the test.

Instructions

1. Warm up before taking the test. Do some walking, easy jogging, and dynamic stretching exercises.

2. Try to cover the distance as fast as possible without overexerting yourself. If possible, monitor your own time, or have someone call out your time at various intervals of the test to determine whether your pace is correct.

3. Record the amount of time it takes you to complete the 2.4-kilometre distance, in minutes and seconds. Running-walking time: _____ min _____ sec.

4. Cool down after the test by walking or jogging slowly for about 5 minutes.

Determining Maximal Oxygen Consumption

1. Convert your running time from minutes and seconds to a decimal figure. For example, a time of 14 minutes and 25 seconds would be 14 + (25/60), or 14.4 minutes.

   Running-walking time: _____ min + (_____ sec ÷ 60 sec/min) = _____ min

2. Insert your running time in the equation below, where

   T = running time (in minutes)

   $$\dot{V}O_{2max} = (483 \div T) + 3.5$$

   For example, a person who completes 2.4 kilometres in 14.4 minutes would calculate maximal oxygen consumption as follows:

   $$\dot{V}O_{2max} = (483 \div 14.4) + 3.5 = 37 \text{ mL/kg/min}$$

   $$\dot{V}O_{2max} = (483 \div \underline{\hspace{3cm}} + 3.5 = \underline{\hspace{2cm}} \textbf{ mL/kg/min}$$

   run-walk time (min)

3. Copy this value for $\dot{V}O_{2max}$ into the appropriate place in the chart on the final page of this lab.

The Beep Test

This is also called the Multi-Stage Fitness Test, Pacer Test, Yo Yo test, or 20-Metre Shuttle Run Test.

Description

The Beep Test involves running a series of 20-metre shuttles at a specified pace. The pace gets faster each minute as you go to another level. For example, the series begins at a speed of 8.5 kilometres per hour and then increases by 0.5 kilometres per hour with each advancing level. The MP3 audio recording or phone app signals the end of a shuttle with a single beep and the start of the next level with three beeps. The object of the test is to keep up with the beeps as long as possible.

Facilities and Equipment

1. Running track, open field, or gymnasium

2. Two cones or field markers set 20 metres (21 yards, 32 inches) apart (use four cones if testing a large group)

3. Beep Test app or MP3 recording of beeps (widely available free on the Internet—e.g., http://www .beeptestacademy.com; free Beep Test apps are also available for the iPhone and Android Smartphones)

4. Method of playing Beep Test: MP3 player with speaker, Smartphone with speaker, iPad with speaker. You could run this test by yourself if you have an MP3 player with earphones.

Preparation

Don't take this test until you are prepared. A good technique is to run intervals on a track or playing field. For example, run 50 metres, rest 30 seconds, repeat. Gradually, increase the speed and number of repetitions until you can complete at least 10 sets of 50-metre sprints.

Instructions

1. Set up the audio alert system for the test (MP3 player with speaker, or personal MP3 player, or Smartphone with headphones).

2. In this test you will run back and forth between two lines spaced 20 metres apart, keeping pace with an audio beep that plays during the test. The test is arranged in levels. The beeps get faster with each increasing stage. A single beep will sound at the end of the time for each shuttle. A triple beep sounds at the end of each level. The triple beep is a signal that the pace will get faster. Do not stop when you hear the triple beat; continue running toward the other field marker or cone.

3. The test ends when you can't keep pace with the beeps for two consecutive shuttles.

4. Note your level and the total number of shuttles you completed. Record your maximal oxygen consumption and enter it on the chart labelled "Rating Your Cardiovascular Fitness."

Level	Speed (miles per hour)	Minutes per mile	Total Shuttles	Predicted $\dot{V}O_{2max}$ (millilitres oxygen per kilogram body weight)
1	5.3	11.4	2	16.6
1	5.3	11.4	4	17.5
1	5.3	11.4	6	18.5
2	5.6	10.7	8	20.0
2	5.6	10.7	10	20.9
2	5.6	10.7	12	21.8
2	5.6	10.7	14	22.6
3	5.9	10.2	16	23.4
3	5.9	10.2	18	24.3
3	5.9	10.2	20	25.1
3	5.9	10.2	22	26.0
4	6.2	9.7	24	26.8
4	6.2	9.7	26	27.6
4	6.2	9.7	28	28.3
4	6.2	9.7	31	29.5
5	6.5	9.2	33	30.2
5	6.5	9.2	35	31.0
5	6.5	9.2	37	31.8
5	6.5	9.2	40	32.9
6	6.8	8.8	42	33.6
6	6.8	8.8	44	34.3
6	6.8	8.8	46	35.0
6	6.8	8.8	48	35.7
6	6.8	8.8	50	36.4

continued

Level	Speed (miles per hour)	Minutes per mile	Total Shuttles	Predicted $\dot{V}O_{2max}$ (millilitres oxygen per kilogram body weight)
7	7.2	8.4	52	37.1
7	7.2	8.4	54	37.8
7	7.2	8.4	56	38.5
7	7.2	8.4	58	39.2
7	7.2	8.4	60	39.9
8	7.5	8.0	62	40.5
8	7.5	8.0	64	41.1
8	7.5	8.0	66	41.8
8	7.5	8.0	68	42.4
8	7.5	8.0	71	43.3
9	7.8	7.7	73	43.9
9	7.8	7.7	75	44.5
9	7.8	7.7	76	45.2
9	7.8	7.7	78	45.8
9	7.8	7.7	81	46.8
10	8.1	7.4	83	47.4
10	8.1	7.4	85	48.0
10	8.1	7.4	87	48.7
10	8.1	7.4	89	49.3
10	8.1	7.4	92	50.2
11	8.4	7.2	94	50.8
11	8.4	7.2	96	51.4
11	8.4	7.2	98	51.9
11	8.4	7.2	100	52.5
11	8.4	7.2	102	53.1
11	8.4	7.2	104	53.7
12	8.7	6.9	106	54.3
12	8.7	6.9	108	54.8
12	8.7	6.9	110	55.4
12	8.7	6.9	112	56.0
12	8.7	6.9	114	56.5
12	8.7	6.9	116	57.1
13	9.0	6.7	118	57.6
13	9.0	6.7	120	58.2
13	9.0	6.7	122	58.7
13	9.0	6.7	124	59.3
13	9.0	6.7	126	59.8
13	9.0	6.7	129	60.6

Level	Speed (miles per hour)	Minutes per mile	Total Shuttles	Predicted $\dot{V}O_{2max}$ (millilitres oxygen per kilogram body weight)
14	9.3	6.4	131	61.1
14	9.3	6.4	133	61.7
14	9.3	6.4	135	62.2
14	9.3	6.4	137	62.7
14	9.3	6.4	139	63.2
14	9.3	6.4	142	64.0
15	9.6	6.2	144	64.6
15	9.6	6.2	146	65.1
15	9.6	6.2	148	65.6
15	9.6	6.2	150	66.2
15	9.6	6.2	152	66.7
15	9.6	6.2	154	67.5
16	9.9	6.0	156	68.0
16	9.9	6.0	158	68.5
16	9.9	6.0	160	69.0
16	9.9	6.0	162	69.5
16	9.9	6.0	164	69.9
16	9.9	6.0	166	70.5
16	9.9	6.0	168	70.9
17	10.3	5.9	170	71.4
17	10.3	5.9	172	71.9
17	10.3	5.9	174	72.4
17	10.3	5.9	176	72.9
17	10.3	5.9	178	73.4
17	10.3	5.9	180	73.9
17	10.3	5.9	182	74.4
18	10.6	5.7	184	74.8
18	10.6	5.7	186	75.3
18	10.6	5.7	188	75.8
18	10.6	5.7	190	76.2
18	10.6	5.7	192	76.7
18	10.6	5.7	194	77.2
18	10.6	5.7	197	77.9

continued

Level	Speed (miles per hour)	Minutes per mile	Total Shuttles	Predicted $\dot{V}O_{2max}$ (millilitres oxygen per kilogram body weight)
19	10.9	5.5	199	78.3
19	10.9	5.5	201	78.8
19	10.9	5.5	203	79.2
19	10.9	5.5	205	79.7
19	10.9	5.5	207	80.2
19	10.9	5.5	209	80.6
19	10.9	5.5	212	81.3
20	11.2	5.4	214	81.8
20	11.2	5.4	216	82.2
20	11.2	5.4	218	82.6
20	11.2	5.4	220	83.0
20	11.2	5.4	222	83.5
20	11.2	5.4	224	83.9
20	11.2	5.4	226	84.8

Record your score. Copy this value for $\dot{V}O_{2max}$ into the appropriate place in the chart below:

Highest level: _____

Total shuttles run: _____

Predicted $\dot{V}O_{2max}$: _____

SOURCE: Adapted from Ramsbottom, R., J. Brewer, and C. Williams. 1988. A progressive shuttle run test to estimate maximal oxygen uptake. *British Journal of Sports Medicine* 22(4): 141–144.

Once you have calculated your score, place your value in the table below and find your rating on the following chart. Place that rating in the table.

Rating Your Cardiovascular Fitness

Record your $\dot{V}O_{2max}$ score(s) and the corresponding fitness rating from the table below.

Women		Very Poor	Poor	Fair	Good	Excellent	Superior
Age:	18–29	Below 31.6	31.6–35.4	35.5–39.4	39.5–43.9	44.0–50.1	Above 50.1
	30–39	Below 29.9	29.9–33.7	33.8–36.7	36.8–40.9	41.0–46.8	Above 46.8
	40–49	Below 28.0	28.0–31.5	31.6–35.0	35.1–38.8	38.9–45.1	Above 45.1
	50–59	Below 25.5	25.5–28.6	28.7–31.3	31.4–35.1	35.2–39.8	Above 39.8
	60–69	Below 23.7	23.7–26.5	26.6–29.0	29.1–32.2	32.3–36.8	Above 36.8
Men							
Age:	18–29	Below 38.1	38.1–42.1	42.2–45.6	45.7–51.0	51.1–56.1	Above 56.1
	30–39	Below 36.7	36.7–40.9	41.0–44.3	44.4–48.8	48.9–54.2	Above 54.2
	40–49	Below 34.6	34.6–38.3	38.4–42.3	42.4–46.7	46.8–52.8	Above 52.8
	50–59	Below 31.1	31.1–35.1	35.2–38.2	38.3–43.2	43.3–49.6	Above 49.6
	60–69	Below 27.4	27.4–31.3	31.4–34.9	35.0–39.4	39.5–46.0	Above 46.0

SOURCE: Ratings based on norms from the Cooper Institute for Aerobics Research, Dallas, Texas, *The Physical Fitness Specialist Manual*, Revised 2002.

	$\dot{V}O_{2max}$	Cardiovascular Fitness Rating
1.6-km walk test		
3-minute step test		
2.4-km run-walk test		
Beep Test		

The 12-minute Swim Test

If you enjoy swimming and prefer to build a cardiorespiratory training program around this type of exercise, you can assess your cardiorespiratory endurance by taking the 12-Minute Swim Test. You will receive a rating based on the distance you can swim in 12 minutes. (A complete fitness program based on swimming is presented in Chapter 7.)

Note, however, that this test is appropriate only for relatively strong swimmers who are confident in the water. If you are unsure about your swimming ability, this test may not be appropriate for you. If necessary, ask your school's swim coach or a qualified swimming instructor to evaluate your ability in the water before attempting this test.

Equipment

1. A swimming pool that provides measurements in yards
2. A wall clock that is clearly visible from the pool, or someone with a watch who can time you

Preparation

You may want to practise pacing yourself before taking the test to avoid going too fast at the start and becoming prematurely fatigued. Allow yourself a day or two to recover from your practice swim before taking the test.

Instructions

1. Warm up before taking the test. Do some walking or light jogging before getting in the pool. Once in the water, swim a lap or two at an easy pace to make sure your muscles are warm and you are comfortable.
2. Try to cover the distance as fast as possible without overexerting yourself. If possible, monitor your own time, or have someone call out your time at various intervals of the test to determine whether your pace is correct.
3. Record the distance, in yards, that you were able to cover during the 12-minute period.
4. Cool down after the test by swimming a lap or two at an easy pace.
5. Use the following chart to gauge your level of cardiorespiratory fitness.

Distance In Yards

Women		Needs Work	Better	Fair	Good	Excellent
Age:	13-19	Below 500	500–599	600–699	700–799	Above 800
	20–29	Below 400	400–499	500–599	600–699	Above 700
	30–39	Below 350	350–449	450–549	550–649	Above 650
	40–49	Below 300	300–399	400–499	500–599	Above 600
	50–59	Below 250	250–349	350–449	450–549	Above 550
	60 and over	Below 200	250–299	300–399	400–499	Above 500

continued

		Distance In Yards				
Men		*Needs Work*	*Better*	*Fair*	*Good*	*Excellent*
Age:	13-19	Below 400	400–499	500–599	600–699	Above 700
	20–29	Below 300	300–399	400–499	500–599	Above 600
	30–39	Below 250	250–349	350–449	450–549	Above 550
	40–49	Below 200	200–299	300–399	400–499	Above 500
	50–59	Below 150	150–249	250–349	350–449	Above 450
	60 and over	Below 150	150–199	200–299	300–399	Above 400

100 yards = 91 metres

SOURCE: Cooper, K. H. 1982. *The Aerobics Program for Total Well-Being*. New York: Bantam Books.

Record your fitness rating:

	Cardiovascular Fitness Rating
12-Minute Swim Test	

Using Your Results

How did you score? Are you surprised by your rating for cardiovascular fitness? Are you satisfied with your current rating? If you're not satisfied, set a realistic goal for improvement:

_____

_____

_____

Are you satisfied with your current level of cardiovascular fitness as evidenced in your daily life—your ability to walk, run, bicycle, climb stairs, do yard work, engage in recreational activities? If you're not satisfied, set some realistic goals for improvement, such as completing a 5K run or 40K bike ride:

_____

_____

_____

What should you do next? Enter the results of this lab in the Preprogram Assessment column in Appendix B. If you've set goals for improvement, begin planning your cardiorespiratory endurance exercise program by completing the plan in Lab 3.2. After several weeks of your program, complete this lab again, and enter the results in the Postprogram Assessment column of Appendix B. How do the results compare? (Remember, it's best to compare $\dot{V}O_{2max}$ scores for the same test.)

_____

_____

_____

SOURCES: Kline, G.M., et al. 1987. Estimation of $\dot{V}O_{2max}$ from a one-mile track walk, gender, age, and body weight. *Medicine and Science in Sports and Exercise* 19(3): 253–259: McArdle, W.D., F.I. Katch, and V.L. Katch. 2007. *Exercise Physiology: Energy, Nutrition, and Human Performance*. Philadelphia: Lea and Febiger, pp. 225–226; Brooks, G.A., and T.D. Fahey. 1987. *Fundamentals of Human Performance*. New York: Macmillan; Leger, L. and Gadoury, C., 1989. Validity of the 20 m shuttle run test with 1 minute stages to predict $\dot{V}O_{2max}$ in adults. *Canadian Journal of Sport Science* (14)1: 21–26.

Name _____ Section _____ Date _____

Lab 3.2 Developing an Exercise Program
for Cardiorespiratory Endurance

![McGraw Hill Education] connect®

1. **Goals.** List the goals for your cardiorespiratory endurance exercise program. Your goals can be specific or general, short or long term. In the first section, include specific, measurable goals that you can use to track the progress of your fitness program. These goals might be things like raising your cardiorespiratory fitness rating from fair to good or swimming laps for 30 minutes without resting. In the second section, include long-term and more qualitative goals, such as improving self-confidence and reducing your risk for chronic disease.

    Specific Goals: Current Status   Final Goal

    _____   _____

    _____   _____

    Other goals: _____

    _____

2. **Type of Activities.** Choose one or more endurance activities for your program. These can include any activity that uses large-muscle groups, can be maintained continuously, and is rhythmic and aerobic in nature. Examples include walking, jogging, cycling, group exercise such as aerobic dance, rowing, rope skipping, stair climbing, cross-country skiing, swimming, skating, and endurance game activities such as soccer and tennis. Choose activities that are both convenient and enjoyable. Fill in the activity names on the program plan.

    _____

    _____

    _____

3. **Frequency.** On the program plan, fill in how often you plan to participate in each activity; CSEP recommends participating in cardiorespiratory endurance exercise three to five days per week.

Program Plan									
Type of Activity	Frequency (check ✓)							Intensity (bpm or RPE)	Time (min)
	M	Tu	W	Th	F	Sa	Su		

4. **Intensity.** Determine your exercise intensity using one of the following methods, and enter it on the program plan. You should begin your program at a lower intensity and slowly increase intensity as your fitness improves, so select a range of intensities for your program.

   a. **Target heart rate zone.** Calculate target heart rate zone in beats per minute and then calculate the corresponding 15-second exercise count by dividing the total count by 4. For example, the 15-second exercise counts corresponding to a target heart rate zone of 122 to 180 bpm would be 31 to 45 beats.

   Maximum heart rate: 220 − _____ = _____ bpm
   age (years)

   Maximum Heart Rate Method

   65% training intensity = _____ bpm × 0.65 = _____ bpm
   maximum heart rate

   90% training intensity = _____ bpm × 0.90 = _____ bpm
   maximum heart rate

   Target heart rate zone = _____ **to** _____ **bpm 15-second count =** _____ **to** _____

   Heart Rate Reserve Method

   Resting heart rate:_____ bpm (taken after 10 minutes of complete rest)

   Heart rate reserve = _____ bpm − _____ bpm = _____ bpm
   maximum heart rate   resting heart rate

   50% training intensity = (_____ bpm × 0.50) + _____ bpm = _____ bpm
   heart rate reserve   resting heart rate

   85% training intensity = _____ bpm × 0.85) + _____ bpm = _____ bpm
   heart rate reserve   resting heart rate

   Target heart rate zone = _____ **to** _____ **bpm 15-second count =** _____ **to** _____

   b. Ratings of perceived exertion (RPE): If you prefer, determine an RPE value that corresponds to your target heart rate range (see Table 3.3 and Figure 3.5).

5. **Time (duration).** A total time of 30 to 60 minutes is recommended; your duration of exercise will vary with intensity. For developing cardiorespiratory endurance, higher-intensity activities can be performed for a shorter duration; lower intensities require a longer duration. Enter a duration (or a range of duration) on the program plan.

6. **Monitoring your program.** Complete a log like the one shown here to monitor your program and track your progress. Note the date on top, and fill in the intensity and time (duration) for each workout. If you prefer, you can also track other variables such as distance. For example, if your cardiorespiratory endurance program includes walking and swimming, you may want to track kilometres walked and metres swum in addition to the duration of each exercise session.

Activity/Date												
1	Intensity											
	Time											
	Distance											
2	Intensity											
	Time											
	Distance											
3	Intensity											
	Time											
	Distance											
4	Intensity											
	Time											
	Distance											

7. **Making progress.** Follow the guidelines in the chapter and Table 3.6 to slowly increase the amount of overload in your program. Continue keeping a log, and periodically evaluate your progress.

Progress Check-Up: Week _____ of program

Goals: Original Status   *Current Status*

_____   _____

_____   _____

_____   _____

List each activity in your program and describe how satisfied you are with the activity and with your overall progress. List any problems you've encountered or any unexpected costs or benefits of your fitness program so far.

_____

_____

_____

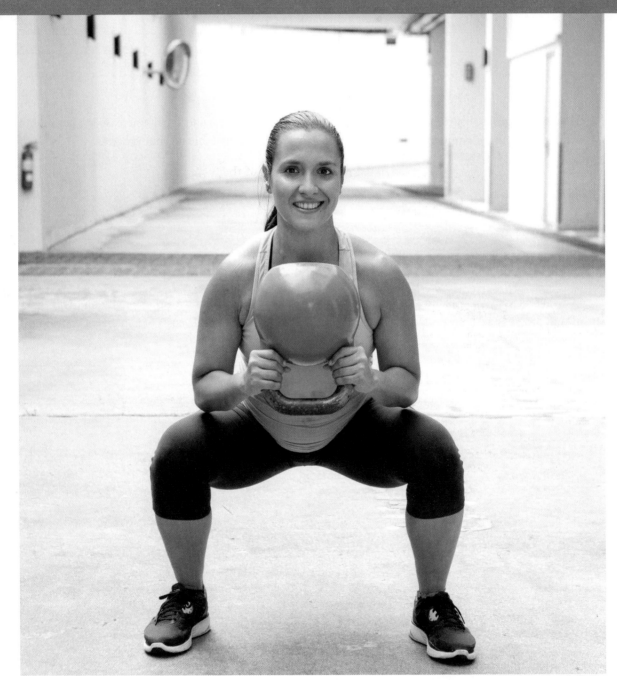

LEARNING OBJECTIVES

After reading this chapter, you should be able to

LO1   Describe the basic physiology of muscles and explain how strength training affects muscles

LO2   Define muscular strength and endurance, and describe how they relate to wellness.

LO3   Assess muscular strength and endurance

LO4   Apply the FITT principle to create a safe and successful strength training program

LO5   Describe the effects of supplements and drugs that are marketed to active people and athletes

LO6   Explain how to safely perform common strength training exercises using body weight, free weights, and weight machines

TEST YOUR KNOWLEDGE

1. **For women, weight training typically results in which of the following?**
   a. bulky muscles
   b. significant increases in body weight
   c. improved body image

2. **To maximize strength gains, it is a good idea to hold your breath as you lift a weight.**

   True or false?

3. **Regular strength training is associated with which of the following benefits?**
   a. denser bones
   b. reduced risk of heart disease
   c. improved body composition
   d. fewer injuries
   e. improved metabolic health
   f. increased longevity

ANSWERS

1. **C.** Because the vast majority of women have low levels of testosterone, they do not develop large muscles or gain significant amounts of weight in response to a moderate weight training program. Men have higher levels of testosterone, so they can build large muscles more easily.

2. **FALSE.** In general, holding your breath while lifting weights, called the Valsalva manoeuvre, can significantly (and possibly dangerously) elevate blood pressure; it also reduces blood flow to the heart and may cause faintness. Unless you are training as a performance athlete, you should breathe smoothly and normally while weight training.

3. **ALL SIX.** Regular strength training has many benefits for both men and women.

Muscles make up more than 40% of your body mass. You depend on them for movement, and, because of their mass, they are the site of a large portion of the energy reactions (metabolism) that take place in your body. Strong, well-developed muscles help you perform daily activities with greater ease, protect you from injury, and enhance your well-being in other ways.

As described in Chapter 2, muscular strength is the ability to generate force during a maximal effort; muscular endurance is the ability to hold or repeat a muscular contraction for a long time. This chapter explains the benefits of *strength training* (also called *resistance training* or *weight training*) and describes methods of assessing muscular strength and endurance. It then explains the basics of weight training and provides guidelines for setting up your own training program.

LO1 4.1 Basic Muscle Physiology and the Effects of Strength Training

Muscles move the body and enable it to exert force. When a muscle contracts (shortens), it moves a bone by pulling on the tendon that attaches the muscle to the bone.

Muscle Fibres

Muscles consist of individual muscle cells, or **muscle fibres**, connected in bundles called fascicles (Figure 4.1). A single muscle is made up of many bundles of muscle fibres and is covered by layers of connective tissue that hold the fibres together. Muscle fibres, in turn, are made up of smaller protein structures called **myofibrils**. Myofibrils are made up of a series of contractile units called *sarcomeres*, which are composed largely of actin and myosin molecules. Muscle cells contract when the myosin molecules glide across the actin molecules in

> **muscle fibre** A single muscle cell, usually classified according to strength, speed of contraction, and energy source.
> **myofibrils** Protein structures that make up muscle fibres.

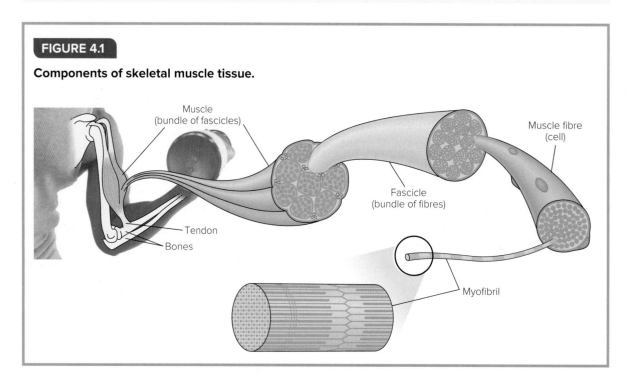

FIGURE 4.1

Components of skeletal muscle tissue.

Muscle (bundle of fascicles)

Tendon

Bones

Fascicle (bundle of fibres)

Muscle fibre (cell)

Myofibril

a ratchet-like movement. Each muscle cell has many **nuclei** containing genes that direct the production of enzymes and structural proteins required for muscle contraction.

> **nucleus** A cell structure containing DNA and genes that direct the production of proteins; plural, *nuclei*.

Strength training increases the size and number of myofibrils, resulting in larger individual muscle fibres. Larger muscle fibres mean a larger and stronger muscle. The development of large muscle fibres is called **hypertrophy**; inactivity causes **atrophy**, the reversal of this process. In some species, muscles can increase in size through a separate process called **hyperplasia**, which involves an increase in the *number* of muscle fibres rather than the *size* of muscle fibres. In humans, hyperplasia is not thought to play a significant role in determining muscle size.

> **hypertrophy** An increase in the size of a muscle fibre, usually stimulated by muscular overload, as occurs during strength training.
> **atrophy** A decrease in the size of muscle fibres, usually attributable to inactivity.
> **hyperplasia** An increase in the number of muscle fibres.

Muscle fibres are classified as slow-twitch, fast-twitch, or intermediate fibres according to their strength, speed of contraction, and energy source.

- **Slow-twitch fibres** are relatively fatigue resistant, but they don't contract as rapidly or strongly as fast-twitch fibres. The principal energy system that fuels slow-twitch fibres is aerobic (oxidative). Slow-twitch muscle fibres are typically reddish in colour.

- **Fast-twitch fibres** contract more rapidly and forcefully than slow-twitch fibres, but they also fatigue more quickly. Although oxygen is important in the energy system that fuels fast-twitch fibres, they rely more on anaerobic (nonoxidative) metabolism than do slow-twitch fibres (see Chapter 3 for a discussion of energy systems). Fast-twitch muscle fibres are typically whitish in colour (e.g., white meat versus dark meat in a turkey).

- **Intermediate fibres** contain a mixture of the qualities of both slow- and fast-twitch fibres. These fibres are less quick to contract than fast-twitch, but they are quicker than slow-twitch fibres. They also endure longer than fast-twitch, but not as long as slow-twitch fibres. Intermediate fibres rely on a combination of anaeorobic and aerobic energy sources and produce less force than fast-twitch fibres, but more than slow-twitch.

> **slow-twitch fibres** Red muscle fibres that are fatigue-resistant but have a slow contraction speed and a lower capacity for tension; usually recruited for endurance activities.
> **fast-twitch fibres** White muscle fibres that contract rapidly and forcefully but fatigue quickly; usually recruited for actions requiring strength and power.
> **intermediate fibres** A muscled fibre that responds somewhere in between the speed, endurance, and contractile force of slow- and fast-twitch fibres.

Most muscle contains a mixture of the fibre types. The proportion of the types of fibres varies significantly among different muscles and different individuals. That proportion is largely fixed at birth, although fibres can contract faster or slower following a period of training or a period of inactivity. The type of fibre that acts during a particular activity depends on the type of work required. Endurance activities like jogging tend to use slow-twitch fibres, whereas strength and **power** activities like sprinting use faster-twitch fibres. Strength training can increase the size and strength of both fast-twitch and slow-twitch fibres, although fast-twitch fibres are preferentially increased.

> **power** The ability to exert force rapidly.

Motor Units

To exert force, the body recruits one or more motor units to contract. A **motor unit** is made up of a nerve connected to a number of muscle fibres. The number of muscle fibres in a motor unit varies from two to hundreds. Small motor units contain slow-twitch fibres, whereas large motor units contain fast-twitch fibres. When a motor nerve calls on its fibres to contract, all fibres contract to their full capacity. The number of motor units recruited depends on the amount of strength required: You use fewer motor units when you pick up a small weight than when you pick up a large weight.

> **motor unit** A motor nerve (one that initiates movement) connected to a number of muscle fibres.

Strength training improves the body's ability to recruit motor units—a phenomenon called **muscle learning**—which increases strength even before muscle size increases. The physiological changes and benefits that result from strength training are summarized in Table 4.1; see the box Gender Differences in Muscular Strength for additional information on hormonal and nervous system influences on muscle tissue.

> **muscle learning** The improvement in the body's ability to recruit motor units, brought about through strength training.

TABLE 4.1

Physiological Changes and Benefits from Strength Training

Change	Benefits
Increased muscle mass* and strength	Increased muscular strength Improved body composition Higher rate of metabolism Toned, healthy-looking muscles Decreased risk of premature death Improved quality of life
Increased use of motor units during muscle contractions	Increased muscular strength and power
Improved coordination of motor units	Increased muscular strength and power
Increased strength of tendons, ligaments, and bones	Lower risk of injury to these tissues
Increased storage of fuel in muscles	Increased resistance to muscle fatigue
Increased size of fast-twitch muscle fibres (from a high-resistance program)	Increased muscular strength and power
Increased size of slow-twitch muscle fibres (from a high-repetition program)	Increased muscular endurance
Increased blood supply to muscles (from a high-repetition program) and improved blood vessel health	Increased delivery of oxygen and nutrients Increased elimination of wastes
Biochemical improvements (e.g., increased sensitivity to insulin)	Enhanced metabolic health
Improved blood fat levels	Reduced risk of heart disease
Increased muscle endurance	Enhanced ability to exercise for long periods and maintain good body posture

*Due to genetic and hormonal differences, men will build more muscle mass than women, but both genders make about the same percent gains in strength through a good program.

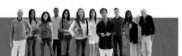

DIVERSITY Matters

GENDER DIFFERENCES IN MUSCULAR STRENGTH

Men are generally stronger than women because they typically have larger bodies overall and a larger proportion of their total body mass is made up of muscle. But when strength is expressed per unit of cross-sectional area of muscle tissue, men are only 1–2% stronger than women in the upper body and about equal to women in the lower body. Because of the larger proportion of muscle tissue in the upper male body, men can more easily build upper-body strength than women can. Individual muscle fibres are larger in men, but the metabolism of cells within those fibres is the same in both sexes.

Two factors that help explain these disparities are testosterone levels and the speed of nervous control of muscle. Testosterone promotes the growth of muscle tissue in both males and females, but testosterone levels are about 5 to 10 times higher in men than in women, allowing men to have larger muscles. Also, because the male nervous system can activate muscles faster, men tend to have more power.

Women are often concerned that they will develop large muscles from strength training. Because of hormonal differences, most women do not develop big muscles unless they train intensely over many years or take anabolic steroids. Women do gain muscle and improve body composition through strength training, but they don't develop bulky muscles or gain significant amounts of weight. A study of average women who weight trained two or three days per week for eight weeks found that the women gained about 0.8 kilogram of muscle and lost about 1.6 kilograms of fat. Losing muscle over time is a much greater health concern for

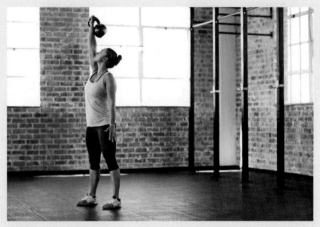
© kupicoo / Getty Images

women than small gains in muscle weight, especially because any gains in muscle weight are typically more than offset by loss of fat weight. Both men and women lose muscle mass and power as they age, but because men start out with more muscle they don't lose power as quickly, and older women tend to have greater impairment of muscle function than older men. This may partially account for the higher incidence of life-threatening falls in older women.

The bottom line is that both men and women can increase strength through strength training. Women may not be able to lift as much weight as men, but kilogram for kilogram of muscle, they have nearly the same capacity to gain strength as men.

As a person ages, motor nerves can become disconnected from the portion of muscle they control. By age 70, 15% of the motor nerves in most people are no longer connected to muscle tissue. Aging and inactivity also cause muscles to become slower and therefore less able to perform quick, powerful movements. Strength training helps maintain motor nerve connections and the quickness of muscles. See the box Benefits of Muscular Strength and Endurance for more information on the importance of improving muscular strength throughout the lifespan.

LO2

The Evidence *for* EXERCISE

BENEFITS OF MUSCULAR STRENGTH AND ENDURANCE

Enhanced muscular strength and endurance can lead to improvements in the areas of performance, injury prevention, body composition, self-image, lifetime muscle and bone health, and metabolic health. Most important, greater muscular strength and endurance reduce the risk of premature death. Stronger people—particularly men—have a lower death rate due to all causes, including cardiovascular disease and cancer. The link between strength and death rate is independent of age, physical activity, smoking, alcohol intake, body composition, and family history of cardiovascular disease.

Improved Performance of Physical Activities

A person with a moderate to high level of muscular strength and endurance can perform everyday tasks—such as climbing stairs and carrying groceries—with ease. Increased strength can enhance enjoyment of recreational sports by making it possible to achieve high levels of performance and to handle advanced techniques. Strength training also results in modest improvements in maximal oxygen consumption. People with poor muscle strength tire more easily and are less effective in both everyday and recreational activities.

Injury Prevention

Increased muscular strength and endurance help protect you from injury in two key ways:

- They enable you to maintain good posture. Good muscle strength and endurance help stabilize the spine, which protects against back and neck injuries.
- They encourage proper body mechanics during everyday activities such as walking and lifting.

Good muscle strength, particularly in the abdomen, hips, lower back, and legs, maintain the spine in proper alignment and help prevent low-back pain, which afflicts more than 80% of Canadians at some time in their lives. (Prevention of low-back pain is discussed in Chapter 5.)

Training for muscular strength and endurance also makes the tendons, ligaments, and cartilage cells stronger and less susceptible to injury. Resistance exercise best prevents injuries when the training program is gradual and progressive and builds all the major muscle groups.

Improved Body Composition

Healthy body composition means the body has a high proportion of fat-free mass and a relatively small proportion of fat. Strength training improves body composition by increasing muscle mass, thereby tipping the body composition ratio toward fat-free mass and away from fat.

Building muscle mass through strength training also helps with losing fat because metabolic rate is related to muscle mass: the greater your muscle mass, the higher your metabolic rate. A high metabolic rate means that a nutritionally sound diet, coupled with regular exercise, will not lead to an increase in body fat. Strength training can boost resting metabolic rate by up to 15%, depending on how hard you train. Resistance exercise also increases muscle temperature, which in turn slightly increases the rate at which you burn calories over the hours following a weight training session.

Enhanced Self-Image and Quality of Life

Strength training leads to an enhanced self-image in both men and women by providing stronger, firmer muscles and a toned, healthy-looking body. Women tend to lose centimetres, increase strength, and develop greater muscle definition. Men tend to build larger, stronger muscles. The larger muscles in men combine with high levels of the hormone testosterone for a strong tissue-building effect.

Because strength training involves measurable objectives (kilograms lifted, repetitions accomplished), you can easily recognize improved performance, leading to greater self-confidence and self-esteem. Strength training also improves quality of life by increasing energy, preventing injuries, and making daily activities easier and more enjoyable.

Improved Muscle and Bone Health with Aging

Research has shown that good muscular strength helps people live healthier lives. A lifelong program of regular strength training prevents muscle and nerve degeneration that can compromise the quality of life and increase the risk of hip fractures and other potentially life-threatening injuries.

Osteoporosis (bone loss) is common in people over age 55, particularly postmenopausal women. Osteoporosis leads to fractures that can be life-threatening. Hormonal changes from aging account for much of the bone loss that occurs, but lack of bone mass due to inactivity and a poor diet are contributing factors. Strength training can lessen bone loss even if it is taken up later in life; if practised regularly, strength training may even build bone mass in postmenopausal women and older men. Increased muscle strength can also help prevent falls, which are a major cause of injury in people with osteoporosis.

In the general population, people begin to lose muscle mass after age 30, a condition called *sarcopenia*. At first they may notice that they cannot play sports as well as they could in high school. After more years of inactivity and strength loss, people may have trouble performing even the simple movements of daily life, such as walking up a flight of stairs or doing yard work. By age 75, about 25% of men and 75% of women cannot lift more than 4.5 kilograms over their head. Although aging contributes to decreased strength, inactivity causes most of the loss. Poor strength makes it much more likely that a person will be injured during everyday activities.

Increased Longevity

Strength training helps you live longer. A number of studies have associated greater muscular strength with lower rates of death from all causes, including cancer and cardiovascular disease. A study of more than 9000 men showed that compared to men with the lowest levels of muscular strength, stronger men were 1.5 times less likely to die from all causes; 1.6 times less likely to die from cardiovascular disease; and 1.25 times less likely to die from cancer. The results were particularly striking in men age 60 and older with low levels of muscular strength, who were more than four times more likely to die from cancer than similar-age men with greater muscular strength.

SOURCES: Physical Activity Guidelines Advisory Committee. 2008. *Physical Activity Guidelines Advisory Committee Report*, 2008. Washington, D.C.: U.S. Department of Health and Human Services; Ruiz, J. R., et al. 2008. Association between muscular strength and mortality in men: Prospective cohort study. *BMJ* 337: a439; Ruiz, J. R., et al. 2009. Muscular strength and adiposity as predictors of adulthood cancer mortality in men. *Cancer Epidemiology, Biomarkers, and Prevention* 18: 1468; Rantanen, T., et al. 2011. Midlife muscle strength and human longevity up to age 100 years: A 44-year prospective study among a decedent cohort. Published online: DOI 10.1007/s11357-011-9256-y.

Metabolic and Heart Health

Strength training helps prevent and manage both cardiovascular disease (CVD) and diabetes by:

- improving glucose metabolism
- increasing maximal oxygen consumption
- reducing blood pressure
- increasing HDL cholesterol and reducing LDL cholesterol (in some people)
- improving blood vessel health

Stronger muscles reduce the demand on the heart during ordinary daily activities such as lifting and carrying objects. The benefits of resistive exercise to the heart are so great that the Canadian Heart and Stroke Foundation recommends that healthy adults and many low-risk cardiac patients do strength training two to four days per week.[1] Resistance training, however, may not be appropriate for people with some types of heart disease.

Wellness Tip

Circuit training involves a series of exercises with minimal rest in between. Circuits can include almost any kind of exercises. Circuit training is an excellent way to develop strength and endurance at the same time.

LO3 4.2 Assessing Muscular Strength and Endurance

Muscular strength is usually assessed by measuring the maximum amount of weight a person can lift in a single effort. This single maximal movement is called a **repetition maximum (RM)**. You can assess the strength of your major muscle groups by taking one-repetition maximum (1 RM) tests for the bench press and by taking functional leg strength tests. You can measure 1 RM directly or estimate it by doing multiple repetitions with a submaximal (lighter) weight. See Lab 4.1 for some of the tests you can perform to estimate your 1 RM.

repetition maximum (RM) The maximum amount of resistance that can be moved a specified number of times; 1 RM is the maximum weight that can be lifted once. 5 RM is the maximum weight that can be lifted five times.

It is best to train for at least several weeks before attempting a direct 1 RM test; once you have a baseline value, you can retest after 6 to 12 weeks to check your progress. Refer to Lab 4.1 for guidelines on taking these tests. Instructions for assessing grip strength using a dynamometer are also included in Lab 4.1. For more accurate results, avoid any strenuous weight training for 48 hours beforehand.

Muscular endurance is usually assessed by counting the maximum number of **repetitions** of a muscular contraction a person can do (such as push-ups or kettlebell snatches) or the maximum amount of time a person can hold a muscular contraction (such as the flexed-arm hang). You can test the muscular endurance of major muscle groups in your body by taking the curl-up test, the push-up test, and the squat endurance test. See Lab 4.2 for complete instructions on taking these assessment tests.

repetitions The number of times an exercise is performed continuously during one set.

4.3 Creating a Successful Strength Training Program

When the muscles are stressed by a greater load than they are used to, they adapt and improve their function. The type of adaptation that occurs depends on the type of stress applied.

Static versus Dynamic Strength Training Exercises

Strength training exercises are generally classified as static or dynamic. Each involves a different way of using and strengthening muscles.

Static Exercise

Also called **isometric** exercise, **static exercise** causes a muscle contraction without a change in the length of the muscle or the angle in the joint on which the muscle acts. In isometrics, the muscle contracts, but there is no movement. To perform an isometric exercise, use an immovable object like a wall to provide resistance, or just tighten a muscle while remaining still (e.g., tighten the abdominal muscles while sitting at a desk). The spine extension and the side bridge, shown in Weight Training Exercises: Body Weight later in this chapter, are both isometric exercises.

static (isometric) exercise   Exercise involving a muscle contraction without a change in the length of the muscle.

Static exercises are particularly important for developing stiff core or torso muscles that support the spine and provide a firm foundation for whole body motions. During almost all movements, some muscles contract statically to support the skeleton so other muscles can contract dynamically. For example, when you throw something, hit a ball, or ski, the core muscles in the abdomen and back stabilize the spine. This stability allows more powerful contractions in the lower- and upper-body muscles. The core muscles also contract statically during dynamic exercises such as squats, lunges, and overhead presses.

Static exercises are useful in strengthening muscles after an injury or surgery, when movement of the affected joint could delay healing. Isometrics are also used to overcome weak points in an individual's range of motion. Statically strengthening a muscle at its weakest point will allow more weight to be lifted with that muscle during dynamic exercise. Certain types of calisthenics and Pilates exercises (described in more detail later in the chapter) also provide static contractions. For maximum strength gains, hold the isometric contraction maximally for 6 seconds and do 2 to 10 repetitions.

Dynamic Exercise

Also called **isotonic** exercise, **dynamic exercise** involves a muscle contraction with a change in the length of the muscle and the angle of the join. Dynamic exercises are the most popular type of exercises for increasing muscle strength and seem to be most valuable for developing strength that can be transferred to other forms of physical activity. They can be performed with weight machines, free weights, or a person's own body weight (as in sit-ups or push-ups).

dynamic (isotonic) exercise   Exercise involving a muscle contraction with a change in the length of the muscle.

There are two kinds of dynamic muscle contractions:

- A **concentric muscle contraction** (also called a *miometric contraction*) occurs when the muscle applies enough force to overcome resistance and shortens as it contracts.

- An **eccentric muscle contraction** (also called *a pliometric contraction*) occurs when the resistance is greater than the force applied by the muscle and the muscle lengthens as it contracts.

concentric muscle contraction   An isotonic contraction in which the muscle gets shorter as it contracts.
eccentric muscle contraction   An isotonic contraction in which the muscle lengthens as it contracts.

For example, in an arm curl, the biceps muscle works concentrically as the weight is raised toward the shoulder and eccentrically as the weight is lowered.

Constant and Variable Resistance

Two of the most common dynamic exercise techniques are constant resistance exercise and variable resistance exercise. Both exercises are extremely effective for building muscular strength and endurance.

- **Constant resistance exercise** uses a constant load (weight) throughout a joint's entire range of motion. Training with free weights is a form of constant resistance exercise. A problem with this technique is that, because of differences in leverage, there are points in a joint's range of motion where

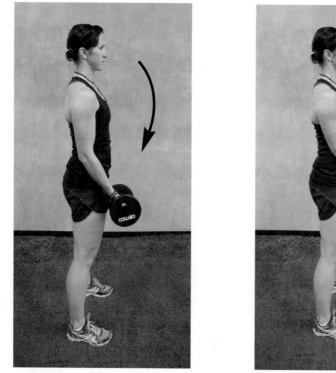

An eccentric contraction
Courtesy of Paula J Gorman

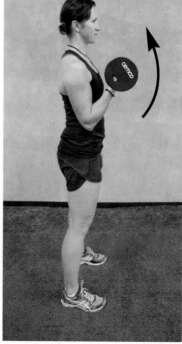

A concentric contraction

the muscle controlling the movement is stronger and points where it is weaker. The amount of weight a person can lift is limited by the weakest point in the range.

- In **variable resistance exercise**, the load is changed to provide maximum load throughout the entire range of motion. This form of exercise uses machines that place more stress on muscles at the end of the range of motion, where a person has better leverage and can exert more force. You can use elastic bands and chains with free weights to add variable resistance to the exercises.

constant resistance exercise   A type of dynamic exercise that uses a constant load throughout a joint's entire range of motion.
variable resistance exercise   A type of dynamic exercise that uses a changing load, providing a maximum load throughout the joint's entire range of motion.

Other Dynamic Exercise Techniques

Athletes use four other kinds of isotonic techniques, primarily for training and rehabilitation.

- **Eccentric (pliometric) loading** places a load on a muscle as it lengthens. The muscle contracts eccentrically to control the weight. Eccentric loading is practised during most types of resistance training. For example, you are performing an eccentric movement as you lower the weight to your chest during a bench press in preparation for the active movement. You can also perform exercises designed specifically to overload muscle eccentrically, a technique called *negatives*.

eccentric (pliometric) loading   Loading the muscle while it is lengthening; sometimes called *negatives*.

- **Plyometrics** is the sudden eccentric loading and stretching of muscles followed by a forceful concentric contraction—a movement that scientists call the stretch-shortening cycle. An example would be the action of the lower-body muscles when jumping from a bench to the ground and then jumping back onto the bench. This type of exercise is used to develop explosive strength; it also helps build and maintain bone density.

plyometrics   Rapid stretching of a muscle group that is undergoing eccentric stress, followed by a rapid concentric contraction.

- In **speed loading** you move a weight as rapidly as possible in an attempt to approach the speeds used in movements like throwing a softball or sprinting. In the bench press, for example, speed loading might involve doing five repetitions as fast as possible using a weight that is half the maximum load you can lift. You can gauge your progress by timing how fast you can perform the repetitions. Training with a **kettlebell**—an iron ball with a handle—is a type of speed loading. Kettlebell training is highly ballistic, meaning that many exercises involve fast, pendulum-type motions, extreme decelerations, and high-speed eccentric muscle contractions. Kettlebell swings require dynamic concentric muscle contractions during the upward phase of the exercise, followed by high-speed eccentric contractions to control the movement when returning to the starting position.

speed loading   Moving a load as rapidly as possible.
kettlebell   A large iron weight with a connected handle; used for ballistic weight training exercises such as swings and one-arm snatches.

- **Isokinetic** exercise involves exerting force at a constant speed against an equal force exerted by a special strength training machine. The isokinetic machine provides variable resistance at different points in the joint's range of motion, matching the effort applied by the individual, while keeping the speed of the movement constant. Isokinetic exercises are excellent for building strength and endurance.

isokinetic   The application of force at a constant speed against an equal force.

Comparing Static and Dynamic Exercises

Static exercises require no equipment, so they can be done virtually anywhere. They build strength rapidly and are useful for rehabilitating injured joints and stabilizing joints in the shoulder and spine. On the other hand, they have to be performed at several different angles for each joint to improve strength throughout its entire range of motion. Dynamic exercises can be performed without equipment (calisthenics) or with equipment (weight lifting). Not only are they excellent for building strength and endurance, they also tend to

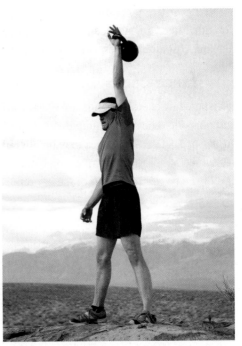

© Jordan Siemens / Getty RF

Kettlebells are growing in popularity. They provide a fast, effective workout when used properly.

build strength through a joint's full range of motion. Most people develop muscular strength and endurance using dynamic exercises. Ultimately, however, the type of exercise you choose depends on individual goals, preferences, and access to equipment.

Weight Machines, Free Weights, and Body Weight Exercises

Muscles get stronger if you make them work against a resistance. Resistance can be provided by free weights, your own body weight, or exercise machines. Many people prefer weight machines because they are safe, convenient, and easy to use. You just set the resistance, sit down at the machine, and start working. Machines make it easy to isolate and work specific muscles. You don't need a **spotter**—someone who stands by to assist when free weights are used—and you don't have to worry about dropping a weight on yourself. Many machines also provide support for the back.

spotter A person who assists with a weight training exercise done with free weights.

Free weights, such as barbells and kettlebells, require more care, balance, and coordination to use than machines, but they strengthen your body in ways that are more adaptable to real life. They are also more popular with athletes for developing functional strength for sports, especially sports that require a great deal of strength. Free weights are widely available, inexpensive, and convenient for home use.

Exercises that use body weight, elastic bands, rocks, or soup cans as resistance enable you to do workouts at home. You can purchase elastic bands at sporting good stores or any home improvement or hardware store. A basic principle of resistant exercise is to "train movements and not muscles." This means that you can overload the body in everyday movements like sitting and standing from a chair, climbing a fence, getting out of a swimming pool without a ladder, and standing after lying on the ground.

Other Training Methods and Types of Equipment

You don't need a fitness centre or expensive equipment to strength train. If you prefer to train at home or you like low-cost alternatives, consider the following options.

Resistance Bands

Resistance or exercise bands are elastic strips or tubes of rubber material that are inexpensive, lightweight, and portable. They are available in a variety of styles and levels of resistance. Some are sold with instructional guides or DVDs, and classes may be offered at fitness centres. Many free weight exercises can be adapted for resistance bands. For example, you can do bicep curls by standing on the centre of the band and holding one end of the band in each hand; the band provides resistance when you stretch it to perform the curl.

Fitness Tip

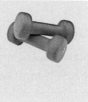

Think resistance bands are just for beginners? Think again. Many serious weight trainers use elastic bands to provide variable resistance during large muscle lifts such as the squat and bench press. Bands can help increase power, rate of force development, and speed.

Exercise (Stability) Balls

The exercise or stability ball is an extra-large inflatable ball. Originally developed for use in physical therapy, it has become a popular piece of exercise equipment for use in the home or gym. It can be used to work the entire body, but it is particularly effective for working the core stabilizing muscles in the abdomen, chest, and back—muscles that are important for preventing back problems. The ball's instability forces the exerciser to use the stability muscles to balance the body, even when just sitting on the ball. The "stir the pot" exercise—a plank position with elbows resting on the ball, which is then moved in small circles—is an example of a core-building exercise that uses the stability ball.

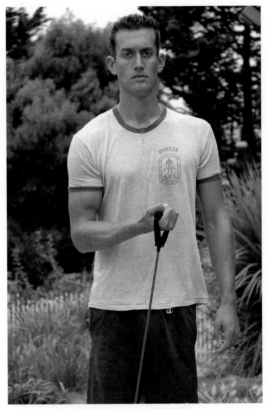

© The McGraw-Hill Companies, Inc. / John Flournoy, photographer

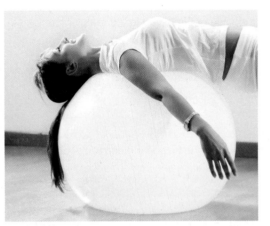

© Ingram Publishing

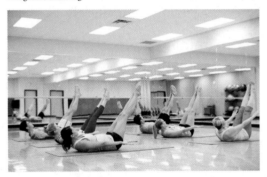

© Hero Images / Getty Images

Resistance for strength training can be provided by many different techniques and types of equipment. Shown here are resistance bands (left), a stability ball (top right), and a Pilates mat exercise (bottom right) that uses body weight for resistance.

There are many ways to incorporate a stability ball into a typical workout. For example, you can perform crunches or curl-ups while lying on a ball instead of on the floor. Lying facedown across a ball provides different leverage points for push-ups. You can also perform a variety of resistance training exercises on a stability ball, but experts recommend using dumbbells rather than barbells when lifting weights on a ball.

When selecting a ball, make sure your thighs are parallel to the ground when you sit on it; if you are a beginner or have back problems, choose a larger ball so your thighs are at an angle, with hips higher than knees. Beginners should use caution until they feel comfortable with the movements and take care to avoid poor form due to fatigue. Table 4.2 (on the next page) outlines the pros and cons of using stability balls.

Pilates

Pilates (*pil LAH teez*) was developed by German gymnast and boxer Joseph Pilates early in the twentieth century. Pilates focuses on strengthening and stretching the core muscles in the back, abdomen, and buttocks to create a solid base of support for whole-body movement; the emphasis is on concentration, control, movement flow, and breathing. Pilates often makes use of specially designed resistance training devices, although some

TABLE 4.2

The Pros and Cons of Stability Balls

Pros	Cons
They activate muscle and nerve groups that might not otherwise get involved in a particular exercise.	Muscle activation when training on unstable surfaces is less effective than traditional training for building strength in muscle groups responsible for a movement or in trunk-stabilizing muscle groups.
Some exercises, such as the stir the pot exercise, can enhance the stability of supporting joints throughout the body.	Some exercises (such as curl-ups) can be more stressful to certain joints and muscles and promote back or shoulder pain in susceptible people.
They can be useful for some older adults because they require balance and can enhance overall stability.	Falling off an unstable surface, especially while holding weights, can cause serious injury.
They add variety and challenge to a workout.	

classes feature just mat or floor work. Mat exercises can be done at home, but because there are hundreds of Pilates exercises, some of them strenuous, it is best to begin with some qualified instruction.

Vibration Training

Vibration training consists of doing basic exercises, such as squats, push-ups, lunges, and modified pull-ups, on a vibrating platform. Vibration is transferred to whichever part of the body is in contact with the vibrating plate or handlebars. Vibration activates stretch receptors in the muscles, which triggers thousands of small reflex muscle contractions. Most studies have found that vibration training causes little or no additional effects above weight training alone.

Medicine Balls, Suspension Training, Stones, and Carrying Exercises

Almost anything that provides resistance to movement will develop strength. Rubber medicine balls weigh up to 23 kilograms and can be used for a variety of functional movements, such as squats and overhead throws.

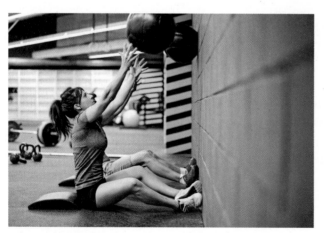

xavierarnau / Getty Images

Medicine balls can be used in many ways to get an effective resistance workout.

Suspension training (e.g., TRX system) uses body weight as the resistance in exercises using ropes or cords attached to a hook, bar, door jam, or sturdy tree branch. You can train with a stone from your backyard or local riverbank when performing exercises such as squats, presses, and carries. Walking while carrying dumbbells, farmer's bars, or heavy stones is an easy and effective way to develop whole-body strength. Carrying exercises are particularly useful for building the core muscles.

Power-Based Conditioning Programs

This type of training combines aerobics, weight training, gymnastics, and high-intensity interval training. Programs such as CrossFit and GymJones employ different exercises every day. More traditional circuit training methods often use the same exercises set up in series. (See the box High Intensity Conditioning Programs in Chapter 3.)

CAREER OPTIONS IN...

MUSCLE FITNESS

Rehabilitation: kinesiologist, massage therapist, soft-tissue specialist

Community: ergonomist/equipment designer, strength coach, fitness consultant

Administration: corporate fitness/educational consultant, sport and fitness program coordinator

SOURCE: Physical and Health Education Canada (http://www.phecanada.ca).

LO4 Applying the FITT Principle: Selecting Exercises and Putting Together a Program

A complete weight training program works all the major muscle groups. It usually takes about 8 to 10 different exercises to get a complete workout. Use the FITT principle—Frequency, Intensity, Time, and Type—to set the parameters of your program.

Frequency of Exercise

For general fitness, Health Canada and the Canadian Society for Exercise Physiology (CSEP) recommend a frequency of two to four days per week for weight training. Allow your muscles at least one day of rest between workouts; if you train too often, your muscles won't be able to work at a high enough intensity to improve their fitness, and soreness and injury are more likely to result. If you enjoy weight training and would like to train more often, try working different muscle groups on alternate days—a training plan called a *split routine.* For example, work your arms and upper body one day, work your lower body the next day, and then return to upper-body exercises on the third day.

Intensity of Exercise: Amount of Resistance

The amount of weight (resistance) you lift in weight training exercises is as important as intensity in cardiorespiratory endurance training (HR or RPE). It determines the way your body will adapt to weight training and how quickly these adaptations will occur.

Choose weights based on your current level of muscular fitness and your fitness goals. Choose a weight heavy enough to fatigue your muscles, but light enough for you to complete the repetitions with good form. (For tips on perfecting your form, see the box Improving Your Technique with Video on the next page.) To build strength rapidly, you should lift weights as heavy as 80% of your maximum capacity (1 RM). If you're more interested in building endurance, choose a lighter weight (perhaps 40–60% of 1 RM) and do more repetitions. New research has found that you can stimulate muscle hypertrophy using only 30–50% of maximum capacity if you stress the muscles adequately.

For example, if your maximum capacity for the leg press is 100 kilograms, you might lift 80 kilograms to build strength and 50 kilograms to build endurance. For a general fitness program to develop both strength and endurance, choose a weight in the middle of this range, perhaps 70% of 1 RM. Or you can create a program that includes both higher-intensity exercise (80% of 1 RM for 5–6 repetitions) and lower-intensity exercise (60% of 1 RM for 15–20 repetitions); this routine will develop both fast-twitch and slow-twitch muscle fibres.

Because it can be tedious and time-consuming to continually reassess your maximum capacity for each exercise, you might find it easier to choose a weight based on the number of repetitions of an exercise you can perform with a given resistance.

Wellness *in the* DIGITAL AGE

IMPROVING YOUR TECHNIQUE WITH VIDEO

Want to get stronger? Then you need to focus on developing your skills at least as much as you focus on lifting more weight. Improving skill is the best way to increase strength during movements such as hitting a tennis ball or baseball, performing a bench press, driving a golf ball, skiing down a slope, or carrying a bag of groceries up a flight of stairs. In the world of weight training, skill means lifting weights with proper form; the better your form, the better your results.

The brain develops precise neural pathways as you learn a skill. As you improve, the pathways conduct nervous impulses faster and more precisely until the movement almost becomes reflexive. The best way to learn a skill is through focused practice that involves identifying mistakes, correcting them, and practising the refined movement many times. However, simply practising the skill is not enough if you want to improve and perform more powerful movements. You must perform the movements correctly rather than practising mistakes or poor form over and over again.

Here's where technology can help. Watch videos of people performing weight-training movements correctly. You may be able to borrow videos from your instructor, purchase low-cost training videos through magazines and sporting goods stores, or find them on the Internet. If you watch training videos online, make sure they were produced by an authoritative source on weight training. Otherwise, you may be learning someone else's mistakes.

Film your movements using a phone camera or inexpensive video camera. Compare your movements with those of a more skilled person performing them correctly. Make a note of poor movement patterns and try to change your technique to make it more mechanically correct. Share your videos with your instructor or a certified personal trainer, who can help you identify poor form and teach you ways to correct your form. Smartphone apps such as Coaches' Eye, Hudl, and Dartfish allow you to analyze movements in slow motion, compare movements side by side, and share your videos with others.

Time of Exercise: Repetitions and Sets

To improve fitness, you must do enough repetitions of each exercise to fatigue your muscles. The number of repetitions needed to cause fatigue depends on the amount of resistance: the heavier the weight, the fewer repetitions to reach fatigue. In general, a heavy weight and a low number of repetitions (5–6) build strength and overload primarily fast-twitch fibres, whereas a light weight and a high number of repetitions (15–20) build endurance and primarily overload slow-twitch fibres.

For a general fitness program to build both strength and endurance, try to do about 8 to 12 repetitions of each exercise; a few exercises, such as abdominal crunches and calf raises, may require more. To avoid injury, older (those 50 to 60 years of age and above) and frailer people should perform more repetitions (10–15) using a lighter weight.

In weight training, a **set** refers to a group of repetitions of an exercise followed by a rest period. To develop strength and endurance for general fitness, you can make gains doing a single set of each exercise—provided you use enough resistance to fatigue your muscles. You should just barely be able to complete the 8 to 12 repetitions, using good form, for each exercise. Doing more than one set of each exercise will increase strength development, and most serious weight trainers do at least three sets of each exercise. (See the section More Advanced Strength Training Programs for guidelines on more advanced programs.)

> **set**   A group of repetitions followed by a rest period.

If you perform more than one set of an exercise, you need to rest long enough between sets to allow your muscles to work at a high enough intensity to increase fitness. The length of the rest interval depends on the amount of resistance. In a program to develop a combination of strength and endurance for wellness, a rest period of one to three minutes between sets is appropriate; if you are lifting heavier loads to build maximum strength, rest three to five minutes between sets. You can save time in your workouts by alternating sets of different exercises so that one muscle group can rest between sets while you work on other muscles.

Overtraining—doing more exercise than your body can recover from—can occur in response to heavy resistance training. Possible signs of overtraining include lack of progress or decreased performance, chronic fatigue, decreased coordination, and chronic muscle soreness. The best remedy for overtraining is rest; add more days of recovery between workouts. With extra rest, chances are you'll be refreshed and ready to train again. Adding variety to your program, as discussed later in the chapter, can also help you avoid overtraining with resistance exercise.

Type or Mode of Exercise

For overall fitness, you need to include exercises for your neck, upper back, shoulders, arms, chest, abdomen, lower back, thighs, buttocks, and calves—about 8 to 10 exercises in all. If you are also training for a particular sport, include exercises to strengthen the muscles important for optimal performance *and* the muscles most likely to be injured. Weight training exercises for general fitness are presented later in this chapter.

Balance Exercises for Opposing Muscle Groups

It is important to balance exercises between **agonist** and **antagonist** muscle groups. When a muscle contracts, the opposing muscle must relax. Whenever you do an exercise that moves a joint in one direction, also select an exercise that works the joint in the opposite direction. For example, if you do knee extensions to develop the muscles on the front of your thighs, also do leg curls to develop the antagonistic muscles on the back of your thighs.

> **agonist**   A muscle in a state of contraction, opposed by the action of another muscle, its antagonist.
> **antagonist**   A muscle that opposes the action of another muscle, its agonist.

Setting Order of Exercises

The order of exercises can also be important. Do exercises for large-muscle groups or for more than one joint before you do exercises that use small-muscle groups or single joints. This allows for more effective overload of the larger, more powerful muscle groups. Small-muscle groups fatigue more easily than larger ones, and small-muscle fatigue limits your capacity to overload larger-muscle groups. For example, lateral raises, which work the shoulder muscles, should be performed after bench presses, which work the chest and arms in addition to the shoulders. If you fatigue your shoulder muscles by doing lateral raises first, you won't be able to lift as much weight and effectively fatigue all the key muscle groups used during the bench press.

Also, order exercises so that you work agonist and antagonist muscle groups in sequence, one after the other. For example, follow biceps curls, which work the biceps, with triceps extensions, which exercise the triceps—the antagonist muscle to the biceps.

The Warm-Up and Cool-Down

As with cardiorespiratory endurance exercise, you should warm up before every weight training session and cool down afterward (Figure 4.2). You should do both a general warm-up—several minutes of walking or easy jogging—and a warm-up for the weight training exercises you plan to perform. For example, if you plan to do one or more sets of 10 repetitions of bench presses with 57 kilograms (125 pounds), you might do one set of 10 repetitions with 23 kilograms (50 pounds) as a warm-up. Do similar warm-up exercises for each exercise in your program.

FIGURE 4.2

The FITT principle for a strength training workout.

Warm-up 5–10 minutes	Strength training exercises for major muscle groups (8–10 exercises)		Cool-down 5–10 minutes
	Sample program		
	Exercise	*Muscle group(s) developed*	
	Bench press	Chest, shoulders, triceps	
	Pull-ups	Lats, biceps	
	Shoulder press	Shoulders, trapezius, triceps	
	Upright rowing	Deltoids, trapezius	
	Biceps curls	Biceps	
	Lateral raises	Shoulders	
	Squats	Gluteals, quadriceps	
	Heel raises	Calves	
	Abdominal curls	Abdominals	
	Spine extensions	Low- and mid-back spine extensors	
Start	Side bridges	Obliques, quadratus lumborum	*Stop*

Frequency: 2–4 nonconsecutive days per week

Intensity/Resistance: Weights heavy enough to cause muscle fatigue when exercises are performed with good form for the selected number of repetitions

Time: Repetitions: 8–12 of each exercise (10–15 with a lower weight for people over age 50–60); **Sets:** 1 (doing more than 1 set per exercise may result in faster and greater strength gains); rest 1–2 minutes between exercises

Type of activity: 8–10 strength training exercises that focus on major muscle groups

---

To cool down after weight training, relax for 5 to 10 minutes after your workout. Although this is controversial, a few studies have suggested that including a period of post-exercise stretching may help prevent muscle soreness; warmed-up muscles and joints make this a particularly good time to work on flexibility.

Wellness Tip

A standard push-up is equivalent to bench-pressing 60% of your body weight. A set of 12 push-ups is a quick, effective upper-body workout. No gym required!

Getting Started and Making Progress

The first few sessions of weight training should be devoted to learning the movements and allowing your nervous system to practise communicating with your muscles so you can develop strength effectively. To start, choose a weight that you can move easily through 8 to 12 repetitions, do only one set of each exercise, and rest one to two minutes between exercises. Gradually add weight and (if you want) sets to your program over the first few weeks until you are doing one to three sets of 8 to 12 repetitions of each exercise.

As you progress, add weight according to the "two-for-two" rule: When you can perform two additional repetitions with a given weight on two consecutive training sessions, increase the load. For example, if your target is to perform 8 to 10 repetitions per exercise, and you performed 12 repetitions in your previous two workouts, it would be appropriate to increase your load. If adding weight means you can do only seven or eight repetitions, stay with that weight until you can again complete 12 repetitions per set. If you can do only four to six repetitions after adding weight, or if you can't maintain good form, you've added too much and should take some off.

You can add more resistance in large muscle exercises, such as squats and bench presses, than you can in smaller muscle exercises, such as curls. For example, when you can complete 12 repetitions of squats with good form, you may be able to add 4.5 to 9 kilograms (10–20 pounds) of additional resistance; for curls, on the other hand, you might add only 1.4 to 2.3 kilograms (3–5 pounds). As a general guideline, try increases of approximately 5%, which is 0.22 kilograms (0.5 pounds) of additional weight for each 4.5 kilograms (10 pounds) you are currently lifting.

You can expect to improve rapidly during the first 6 to 10 weeks of training: a 10–30% increase in the amount of weight lifted. Gains will then come more slowly. Your rate of improvement will depend on how hard you work and how your body responds to resistance training. Factors such as age, motivation, and heredity will affect your progress.

After you have achieved the level of strength and muscularity that you want, you can maintain your gains by training two or three days per week. Monitor the progress of your program by recording the amount of resistance and the number of repetitions and sets you perform on a workout card like the one shown in Figure 4.3 on the next page.

More Advanced Strength Training Programs

The program just described is sufficient to develop and maintain muscular strength and endurance for general fitness. Performing more sets and fewer repetitions with a heavier load will cause greater increases in strength. Such a program might include three to five sets of four to six repetitions each; the load used should be heavy enough to cause fatigue with the smaller number of repetitions. Rest long enough after a set (3–5 minutes) to allow your muscles to recover and to work intensely during the next set.

Experienced weight trainers often practise some form of cycle training, also called *periodization*, in which they vary the exercises, number of sets and repetitions, and intensity within a workout and/or between workouts. For example, you might do a particular exercise more intensely during sets or on some days than others; you might also vary the exercises you perform for particular muscle groups. For more detailed information on these more advanced training techniques, consult a strength coach certified by the National Strength and

FIGURE 4.3

A sample workout card for a general fitness strength training program.

	3G	7:41 AM	
Session date: March 5			

Exercise	Wt	Sets	Reps/secs
Bench press	45	2	10
Pull-ups (assisted)	0	2	7
Shoulder press	25	2	10
Upright rowing	10	2	10
Biceps curls	15	2	8
Lateral raise	5	2	12
Squats	45	2	12
Heel raises	45	2	11
Abdominal curls	0	2	25
Spine extensions	0	2	10
Side bridge	0	2	65

overview   Exercises   Workouts   More

Conditioning Association or another reliable source. If you decide to adopt a more advanced training regimen, start off slowly to give your body a chance to adjust and to minimize the risk of injury.

Weight Training Safety

Injuries happen in weight training. Maximum physical effort, elaborate machinery, rapid movements, and heavy weights can combine to make the weight room a dangerous place if proper precautions aren't taken. To help ensure your workouts are safe and productive, follow the guidelines in the box Safe Weight Training and the following suggestions.

Take CHARGE

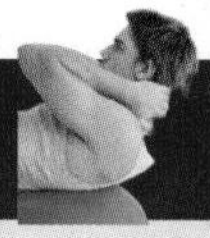

SAFE WEIGHT TRAINING

General Guidelines
- When beginning a program or trying new exercises or equipment, ask an instructor for help doing exercises safely and correctly.

- Lift weights from a stabilized body position; keep weights as close to your body as possible.
- Protect your back by maintaining control of your spine and avoiding dangerous positions. Don't twist your body while lifting.
- Observe proper lifting techniques and good form at all times. Don't lift beyond the limits of your strength.
- Don't hold your breath while doing weight training exercises. Doing so causes a decrease in blood returning to the heart and can make you become dizzy and faint. It can also increase blood pressure to dangerous levels. Exhale when exerting the greatest force, and inhale when moving the weight into position for the active phase of the lift. Breathe smoothly and steadily.
- Don't use defective equipment. Be aware of broken collars or bolts, frayed cables, broken chains, or loose cushions.
- Don't exercise if you're ill, injured, or overtrained. Do not try to work through the pain.

Free Weights

- Make sure the bar is loaded evenly on both sides and weights are secured with collars or spring clips.
- When you pick a weight up from the ground, keep your back straight and your head level. Don't bend at the waist with straight legs.
- Lift weights smoothly; don't jerk them. Control the weight through the entire range of motion.
- Do most of your lifting with your legs. Keep your hips and buttocks tucked in. When doing standing lifts, maintain a good posture to protect your back. Bend at the hips, not with the spine. Feet should be shoulder-width apart, heels and balls of the feet in contact with the floor, and knees slightly bent.
- Don't bounce weights against your body during an exercise.

Spotting

- Use spotters for free-weight exercises in which the bar crosses the face or head (e.g., the bench press), is placed on the back (e.g., squats), or is racked in front of the chest (e.g., overhead press from the rack).
- If one spotter is used (photo a), the spotter should stand behind the lifter; if two spotters are used (photo b), one spotter should stand at each end of the barbell.

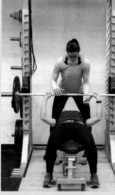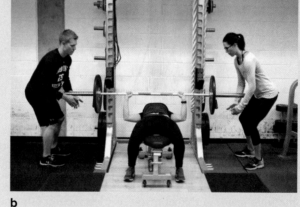

a   b

Courtesy of Paula J Gorman

- For squats with heavy resistance, use at least three spotters—one behind the lifter (hands near lifter's hips, waist, or torso) and one on each side of the bar. Squatting in a power rack will increase safety during this exercise. A power rack consists of four vertical posts with two movable horizontal bar catchers on each side.
- Spot dumbbell exercises as close to the wrists as possible to control the load.
- For over-the-face and over-the-head lifts, the spotter should hold the bar with an alternate grip (one palm up and one palm down) inside the lifter's grip.
- Spotter and lifter should ensure good communication by agreeing on verbal signals before the exercise.

Use Proper Lifting Technique

Every exercise has a proper technique that is important for obtaining maximum benefits and preventing injury. Your instructor or weight room attendant can help explain the specific techniques for different exercises and weight machines.

Perform exercises smoothly and with good form. Lift or push the weight forcefully during the active phase of the lift and then lower it slowly with control. Perform all lifts through the full range of motion and strive to maintain a neutral spine position during each exercise.

Fitness Tip

Doing three sets of resistance exercise is more anabolic than one set, meaning that doing multiple sets enhances muscle protein synthesis. If you're serious about strength training, do multiple sets of exercises to maximize muscle protein synthesis and muscle growth.

Use Spotters and Collars with Free Weights

Spotters are necessary when an exercise has potential for danger; a weight that is out of control or falls can cause a serious injury. A spotter can assist you if you cannot complete a lift or if the weight tilts. A spotter can also help you move a weight into position before a lift and provide help or additional resistance during a lift. Spotting requires practice and coordination between the lifter and the spotter(s).

Collars are devices that secure weights to a barbell or dumbbell. Although people lift weights without collars, doing so is dangerous. It is easy to lose your balance or to raise one side of the weight faster than the other. Without collars, the weights on one side of the bar will slip off and crash to the floor. If you use spring clip collars, make sure they fit the bar tightly. Worn spring collars can easily slide off the bar.

Be Alert for Injuries

Report any obvious muscle or joint injuries to your instructor or physician, and stop exercising the affected area. Training with an injured joint or muscle can lead to a more serious injury. Make sure you get the necessary first aid. Even minor injuries heal faster if you use the R-I-C-E principle for treating injuries described in Chapter 3.

Consult a physician if you have any unusual symptoms during exercise or if you're uncertain whether weight training is a proper activity for you. Weight training can aggravate conditions such as heart disease and high blood pressure. Immediately report symptoms such as headaches; dizziness; laboured breathing; numbness; vision disturbances; and chest, neck, or arm pains. As discussed in Chapter 3, pushing muscles to failure can sometimes result in rhabdomyolysis (destruction of muscle cells), which can cause serious illness or even death.

LO5 A Caution about Natural Health Products and Drugs

Many active people use a wide variety of **natural health products (NHPs)** and drugs in the quest for improved performance and appearance.

natural health products (NHPs)   Any products set out by the Natural Health Products Regulations in the Food and Drug Act governed by Health Canada. These products are considered to be safe as over-the-counter products and do not require a prescription to be sold.

Wellness Tip

Health Canada has issued several consumer warnings about dietary supplements—particularly the kinds that are marketed to people who want to build muscle and lose fat. A number of products have been pulled off store shelves after Health Canada found they were not safe. Talk to your doctor before considering any dietary supplement.

Natural Health Product and Drug Use by Active People

The variety and combinations of NHPs and drugs used by physically active people make it extremely difficult to determine the efficacy of these products or to predict their side effects. Many medical studies describe catastrophic side effects from use of unsafe drugs and NHPs. Most NHPs simply don't work.

Keep in mind that no NHP or drug will change a weak, untrained person into a strong, fit person. Those changes require regular training that stresses the muscles, heart, lungs, and metabolism, and causes the body to adapt. They also require a healthy, balanced diet, as described in Chapter 7. The next section describes weight training exercises that can help you reach your goals. See the box Natural Health Products: A Consumer Dilemma for more information on the safety of NHPs.

Critical CONSUMER

NATURAL HEALTH PRODUCTS: A CONSUMER DILEMMA

In January 2004, Canada's Department of Justice registered the Natural Health Products Regulations (NHPRs) under its *Food and Drugs Act*. The NHPRs are a regulatory framework from which consumers can gain a sense of confidence in the safety and quality of natural health products (NHPs) sold in Canada. The NHPRs include regulations stating the following:

- To classify as an NHP, substances cannot be classified as controlled drugs and substances by the *Food and Drug Act*. The Government of Canada provides a list of these drugs on its website at https://www.canada.ca/en/health-canada/services/drugs-health-products/natural-non-prescription.html
- All NHPs must be licensed by the Department of Justice before they can be sold in Canada. Licensing is by paper application and the NHP is not physically tested for its effects or potential benefits, whereas controlled drugs and substances are physically tested.
- Manufacturers/distributors of licensed NHPs can make health claims about their products. The efficacy of these claims is the responsibility of the manufacturer/distributor.

Given that manufacturers/distributors of licensed NHPs can advertise their products by using health claims, it can be difficult to wade through the advertising hype when choosing an NHP. It's

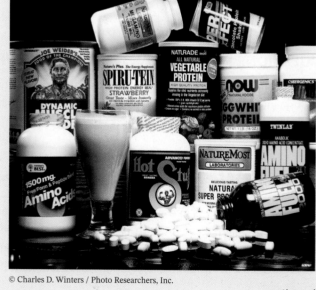

© Charles D. Winters / Photo Researchers, Inc.

continued

only human nature to want to feel, perform, and look as good as possible, but there is no guarantee that advertising claims about NHPs are true.

When faced with the decision about which NHP might be helpful to you, consider the following questions:

- **Do you really need an NHP at all?** Nutritional authorities agree that most athletes and young adults can obtain all the necessary ingredients for health and top athletic performance by eating a well-balanced diet and training appropriately. There is no NHP that outperforms wholesome real food and a good training regimen. Remember, too, that athletic performance and appearance are not life and death issues. It's one thing to take a cancer chemotherapy drug with many known adverse effects if there is a reasonable chance that it will save your life; it's another to take a potentially dangerous dietary supplement that may not even work for you when your goal is to increase your sports performance.
- **Is the product safe and effective?** The fact that an NHP is available in your local store is no guarantee of safety. As mentioned, the Department of Justice doesn't regulate NHPs in the same way as drugs. The only way to determine if an NHP really works is to perform carefully controlled research on human subjects. Testimonials from individuals who claim to have benefited from the product don't count. Few NHPs have undergone careful human testing, so it is difficult to tell which of them may actually work.
- **Can you be sure that the specific product is of high quality?** In 1999, the Government of Canada created the Natural and Non-prescription Health Products Directorate whose "role is to ensure that Canadians have ready access to natural health products that are safe, effective and of high quality while respecting freedom of choice and philosophical and cultural diversity" (https://www.canada.ca /en/health-canada/corporate/about-health-canada/branches-agencies/health-products-food-branch /natural-non-prescription-health-products-directorate.html).

Fitness Tip

As you create a personalized weight training program, focus on specificity and eliminate training methods that do not help you achieve your goal. Follow a well-designed training program that builds strength gradually and progressively. Don't adopt the program of the week just because it's popular.

Ask Yourself

QUESTIONS FOR CRITICAL THINKING AND REFLECTION

Do you think athletes should be allowed to use drugs and supplements to improve their sports performance? Would you be tempted to use a banned performance-enhancing drug if you thought you could get away with it? Why or why not?

LO6 4.4 Weight Training Exercises

A general book on fitness and wellness cannot include a detailed description of all weight training exercises. The following pages present a basic program for developing muscular strength and endurance for general fitness using body weight (no equipment), free weights, and weight machines. Photographs and a list of the muscles being trained accompany instructions for each exercise. (Figure 4.4 is a diagram of the muscular system.)

FIGURE 4.4

The muscular system. The muscle names enclosed in brackets refer to deep muscles.

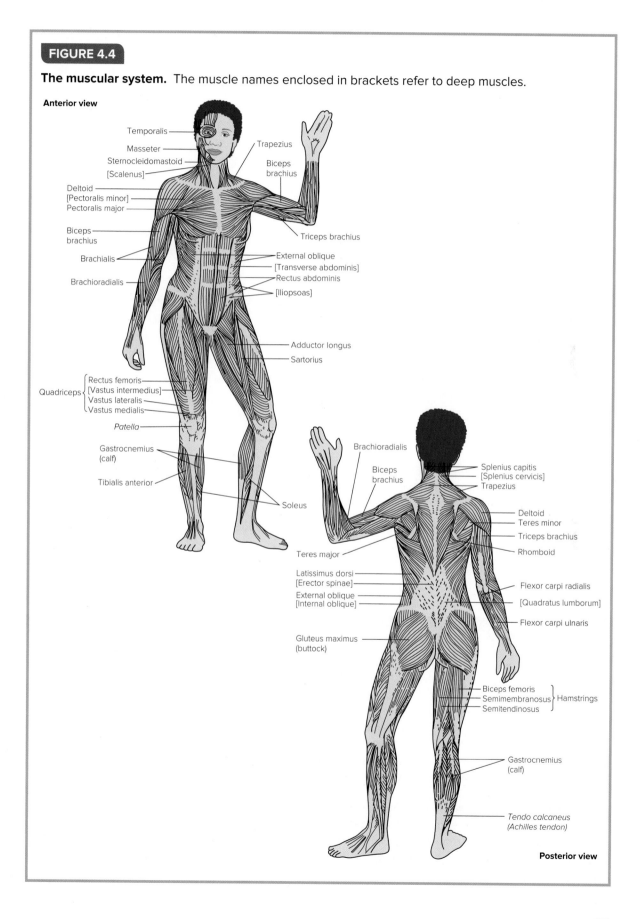

Anterior view

Temporalis
Masseter
Sternocleidomastoid
[Scalenus]
Deltoid
[Pectoralis minor]
Pectoralis major
Biceps brachius
Brachialis
Brachioradialis

Trapezius
Biceps brachius
Triceps brachius
External oblique
[Transverse abdominis]
Rectus abdominis
[Iliopsoas]
Adductor longus
Sartorius

Quadriceps {
Rectus femoris
[Vastus intermedius]
Vastus lateralis
Vastus medialis

Patella
Gastrocnemius (calf)
Tibialis anterior
Soleus

Brachioradialis
Biceps brachius
Teres major
Latissimus dorsi
[Erector spinae]
External oblique
[Internal oblique]
Gluteus maximus (buttock)

Splenius capitis
[Splenius cervicis]
Trapezius
Deltoid
Teres minor
Triceps brachius
Rhomboid
Flexor carpi radialis
[Quadratus lumborum]
Flexor carpi ulnaris

Biceps femoris
Semimembranosus
Semitendinosus
} Hamstrings

Gastrocnemius (calf)

Tendo calcaneus (Achilles tendon)

Posterior view

163

Labs 4.2 and 4.3 will help you assess your current level of muscular endurance and design your own weight training program. If you want to develop strength for a particular activity, your program should contain exercises for general fitness, exercises for the muscle groups most important for the activity, and exercises for muscle groups most often injured. Regardless of the goals of your program or the type of equipment you use, your program should be structured so that you obtain maximum results without risking injury.

Tips for Today and the Future

You don't need a complicated or heavy training program to improve strength: Just one set of 8 to 12 repetitions of 8 to 10 exercises, done 2 to 4 days per week, is enough for general fitness.

RIGHT NOW YOU CAN

- Do a set of static (isometric) exercises. If you're sitting, try tightening your abdominal muscles as you press your lower back into the seat or work your arms by placing the palms of your hands on top of your thighs and pressing down. Hold the contraction for 6 seconds and do 5 to 10 repetitions; don't hold your breath.

- Think of three things you've done in the past 24 hours that would have been easier or more enjoyable if you increased your level of muscular strength and endurance. Visualize improvements in your quality of life that could come from increased muscular strength and endurance.

IN THE FUTURE YOU CAN

- Make an appointment with a trainer at your campus or neighbourhood fitness facility. A trainer can help you put together an appropriate weight training program and introduce you to the equipment at the facility.

- Invest in an inexpensive set of free weights, kettlebells, a stability ball, or a resistance band. Then make a regular appointment with yourself to use your new equipment.

Common Questions ANSWERED

Q Will I gain weight if I do resistance exercises?

A Your weight probably will not change significantly as a result of a general fitness program consisting of one set of 8 to 12 repetitions of 8 to 10 exercises, performed on at least two nonconsecutive days per week. You will lose body fat, so your weight will stay about the same. You may notice a change in how your clothes fit, however, because muscle is more dense than fat. Increased muscle mass will help you control body fat. Muscle increases your metabolism, which means you burn more calories every day. If you combine resistance exercises with cardiovascular (endurance) exercises, you will be on your way to developing a healthier body composition. Concentrate on fat loss rather than weight loss.

Q Do I need more protein in my diet when I train with weights?

A No. Although there is some evidence that power athletes involved in heavy training have a higher-than-normal protein requirement, there is no reason for most people to consume extra protein.

Most Canadians take in more protein than they need, so even if there is an increased protein need during heavy training, it is probably supplied by the average diet. Consuming a protein-rich snack before or after training may promote muscle hypertrophy. (See Chapter 7 for more on dietary needs of athletes and specific recommendations for protein intake.)

Q What causes muscle soreness the day or two following a weight training workout?

A The muscle pain you feel a day or two after a heavy weight training workout is caused by injury to the muscle fibres and surrounding connective tissue. Contrary to popular belief, delayed-onset muscle soreness is not caused by lactic acid buildup. Scientists believe that injury to muscle fibres causes inflammation, which in turn causes the release of chemicals that break down part of the muscle tissue and cause pain. After a bout of intense exercise that causes muscle injury and delayed-onset muscle soreness, the muscles produce protective proteins that prevent soreness during future workouts. If you don't work out regularly, you lose these protective proteins and become susceptible to muscle soreness again.

Q Will strength training improve my sports performance?

A Strength developed in the weight room does not automatically increase your power in sports such as skiing, tennis, or cycling. Hitting a forehand in tennis and making a turn on skis are precise skills that require coordination between your nervous system and muscles. For skilled people, movements become reflex; you don't think about them when you do them. Increasing strength can disturb this coordination. Only by simultaneously practising a sport and improving fitness can you expect to become more powerful in the skill. Practice helps you integrate your new strength with your skills, which makes you more powerful. Consequently, you can hit the ball harder in tennis or make more graceful turns on the ski slopes. (Refer to Chapter 2 for more on the concept of specificity of physical training.)

Q Will I improve faster if I train every day?

A No. Your muscles need time to recover between training sessions. Doing resistance exercises every day will cause you to become overtrained, which will increase your chance of injury and impede your progress. If your strength training program has reached a plateau, try one of these strategies:

- Vary the number of sets. If you have been performing one set of each exercise, add sets.
- Train less frequently. If you are currently training the same muscle groups three or more times per week, you may not be allowing your muscles to fully recover from intense workouts.
- Change exercises. Using different exercises for a particular muscle group may stimulate further strength development.
- Vary the load and number of repetitions. Try increasing or decreasing the loads you are using and changing the number of repetitions accordingly.
- If you are training alone, find a motivated training partner. A partner can encourage you and assist you with difficult lifts, forcing you to work harder.

Q If I stop weight training, will my muscles turn to fat?

A No. Fat and muscle are two different kinds of tissue, and one cannot turn into the other. Muscles that aren't used become smaller (atrophy), and body fat may increase if caloric intake exceeds calories burned. Although the result of inactivity may be smaller muscles and more fat, the change is caused by two separate processes.

Q Should I wear a weight belt when I lift?

A Until recently, most experts advised people to wear weight belts. However, several studies have shown that weight belts do not prevent back injuries and may, in fact, increase the risk of injury by encouraging people to lift more weight than they are capable of lifting with good form. Although wearing a belt may allow you to lift more weight in some lifts, you may not get the full benefit of your program because use of a weight belt reduces the effectiveness of the workout on the muscles that help support your spine.

Weight Training Exercises: Body Weight

connect

Exercise 1

Air Squats

Instructions:

(photo a) Keep your back straight and head level; stand with feet slightly more than shoulder-width apart and toes pointed slightly outward.

(photo b) Hold your hands out in front of you. Squat down until your thighs are below parallel with the floor. Let your thighs move laterally (outward) so that you "squat between your legs." Hinge at your hips and don't let your back sag. This will help keep your back straight and your heels on the floor. Drive upward toward the starting position, hinging at the hips and keeping your back in a fixed position throughout the exercise.

Muscles developed: Quadriceps, gluteus maximus, hamstrings, gastrocnemius

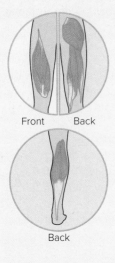

Front   Back

Back

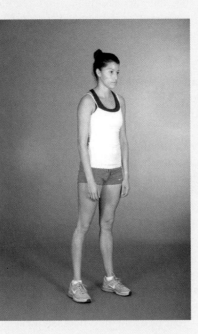

a

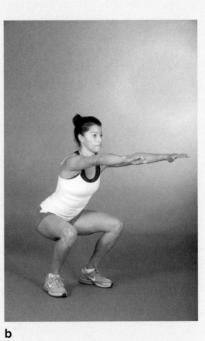

b

© Taylor Robertson Photography

Exercise 2

Lunges

Instructions:

(photo a) Stand with one foot about 60 cm in front of the other.

(photo b) Lunge forward with the front leg, bending it until the thigh is parallel to the floor. The heel of the lead leg should stay on the ground. Do not shift your weight so far forward that the knee moves out past the toes. Repeat the exercise using the other leg. Keep your back and head as straight as possible and maintain control while performing the exercise.

Muscles developed: Quadriceps, gluteus maximus, hamstrings, gastrocnemius

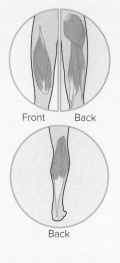

Front   Back

Back

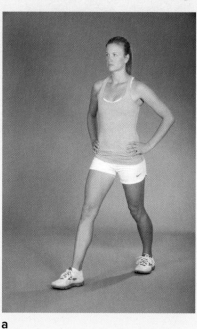

a

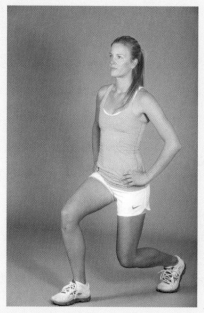

b

© Taylor Robertson Photography

Exercise 3

Burpees with a Push-Up

Instructions:

(photo a) From a standing position, squat down and place your hands on the floor; then kick your legs behind you and land in the "up" push-up position. Do a push-up.

(photo b) Then move your knees forward until you are in a squat position;

(photo c) spring up as high as you can into a full jump. Repeat.

Muscles developed: Quadriceps, gluteus maximus, hamstrings, gastrocnemius, deltoids, pectoralis major, triceps

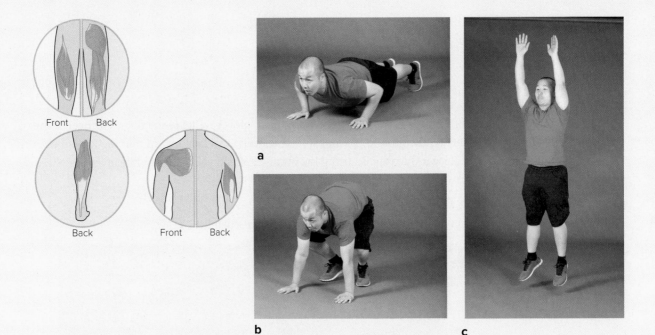

Front   Back

Back

Front   Back

a

b

c

© Taylor Robertson Photography

Exercise 4

Curl-Up or Crunch

Instructions:

(photo a) Lie on your back on the floor with your arms folded across your chest and your feet on the floor or on a bench.

(photo b) Curl your trunk up, minimizing your head and shoulder movement. Lower to the starting position. Focus on using your abdominal muscles rather than the muscles in your shoulders, chest, and neck.

Muscles developed: Rectus abdominis, obliques

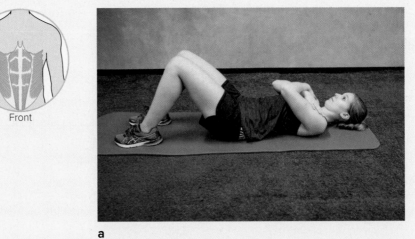

Front

a

Courtesy of Paula J Gorman

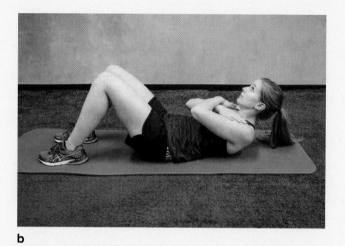

b

Courtesy of Paula J Gorman

Exercise 5

Spine Extension ("Bird Dog") (Isometric Exercise)

Instructions: Begin on all fours with your knees below your hips and your hands below your shoulders.

Unilateral spine extension:

(photo a)   Extend your right leg to the rear and reach forward with your right arm. Keep your spine neutral and your raised arm and leg in line with your torso. Don't arch your back or let your hip or shoulder sag. Hold this position for 10 to 30 seconds. Repeat with your left leg and left arm.

Bilateral spine extension:

Extend your left leg to the rear and reach forward with your right arm. Keep your spine neutral and your raised arm and leg in line with your torso. Don't arch your back or let your hip or shoulder sag. Hold this position for 10 to 30 seconds. Repeat with your right leg and left arm.

Muscles developed: Erector spinae, gluteus maximus, hamstrings, deltoids

Variation: Make this exercise more difficult by making box patterns with your arms and legs.

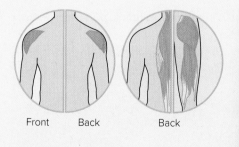

Front   Back   Back

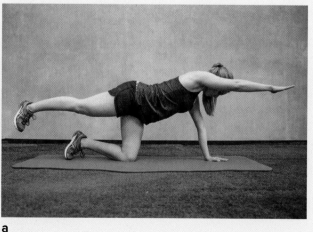

a

Courtesy of Paula J Gorman

169

Exercise 6

Isometric Side Bridge

Instructions: Lie on the floor on your side with your knees bent and your top arm lying alongside your body. Lift and drive your hips forward so your weight is supported by your forearm and knee. Hold this position for 3 to 10 seconds, breathing normally. Repeat on the other side. Perform 3 to 10 repetitions on each side.

Muscles developed: Obliques, quadratus lumborum

Variation: Make the exercise more difficult by keeping your legs straight and supporting yourself with your feet and forearm (see Lab 5.3) or with your feet and hand (with elbow straight). An advanced version of this exercise that builds the core and shoulder muscles is to do a side bridge on the right side, rotate to a front plank, and then rotate to a side bridge on the left side. Hold each position for three seconds.

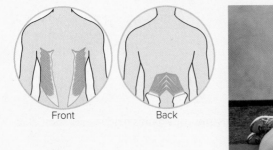

Front Back

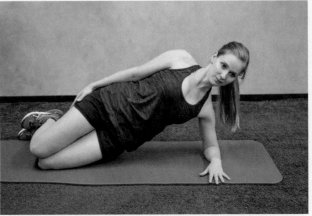

Courtesy of Paula J Gorman

Exercise 7

Front Plank

Instructions: Lying on your front with body straight, raise your body upward, supporting your weight on forearms and toes. Hold the position. Begin with 10-second holds and progress until you can hold the plank for at least 2 minutes. Breathe normally. Tighten your abs, glutes, and quads as you do this exercise.

Muscles developed: Rectus abdominis, erector spinae, trapezius, rhomboids, deltoids, pectorals, gluteals

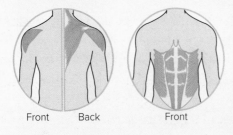

Front Back Front

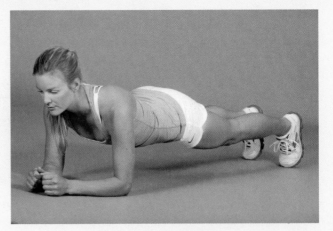

© Taylor Robertson Photography

170

Exercise 8

Push-Ups

Instructions: Start in the push-up position with your body weight supported by your hands and feet. Your arms and back should be straight and your fingers pointed forward. Lower your chest to the floor with your back straight, and then return to the starting position.

Muscles developed: Pectoralis muscles, triceps, deltoids

Variation: Do modified push-ups if you can't do at least 10 regular push-ups. Start with your body weight supported by your hands and knees. Your arms and back should be straight and your fingers pointed forward. Lower your chest to the floor with your back straight, and then return to the starting position.

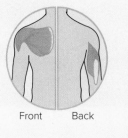

Front   Back

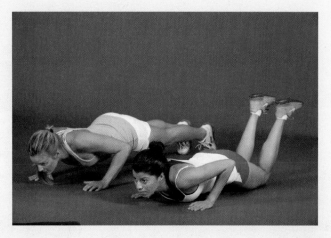

© Taylor Robertson Photography

Exercise 9

Pull-Up

Instructions:

(photo a)   Begin by grasping the pull-up bar with both hands, palms facing forward and elbows extended fully.

(photo b)   Pull yourself upward until your chin goes above the bar. Then return to the starting position.

Assisted pull-up:

(photo c)   This is done as described for a pull-up, except that a spotter assists by pushing upward at the waist, hips, or legs during the exercise.

Muscles developed: Latissimus dorsi, biceps

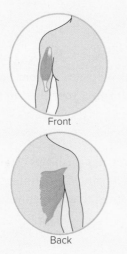

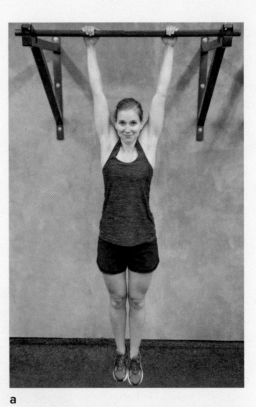

a

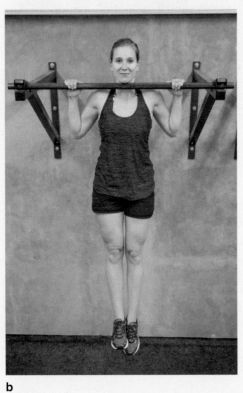

b

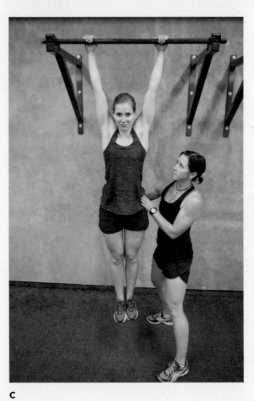

c

Courtesy of Paula J Gorman

Weight Training Exercises: Free Weights

connect

Exercise 1

Bench Press

Instructions:

(photo a)   Lying on a bench on your back with your feet on the floor, grasp the bar with palms upward and hands shoulder-width apart. If the weight is on a rack, move the bar carefully from the supports to a point over the middle of your chest or slightly above it (at the lower part of the sternum).

(photo b)   Lower the bar to your chest. Then press it in a straight line to the starting position. Don't arch your back or bounce the bar off your chest. You can also do this exercise with dumbbells or one arm at a time (unilateral training).

Muscles developed: Pectoralis major, triceps, deltoids

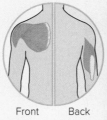

Front   Back

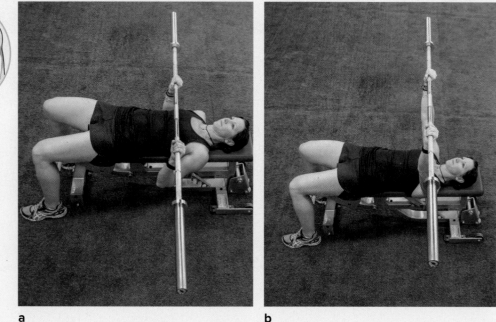

a   b

Courtesy of Paula J Gorman

Note: *To allow an optimal view of exercise technique, a spotter does not appear in these demonstration photographs; however, spotters should be used for most exercises with free weights.*

Exercise 2

Shoulder Press (Overhead or Military Press)

Instructions: This exercise can be done standing or seated, with dumbbells or a barbell. The shoulder press begins with the weight at your chest, preferably on a rack.

(photo a)   Grasp the weight with your palms facing away from you.

(photo b) Push the weight overhead until your arms are extended. Then return to the starting position (weight at chest). Be careful not to arch your back excessively.

If you are a more advanced weight trainer, you can "clean" the weight (lift it from the floor to your chest). The clean should be attempted only after instruction from a knowledgeable coach; otherwise, it can lead to injury.

Muscles developed: Deltoids, triceps, trapezius

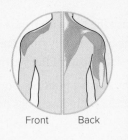

Front   Back

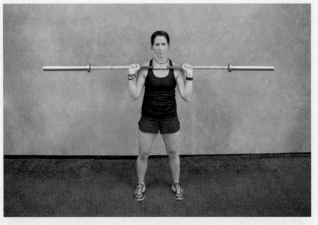

a

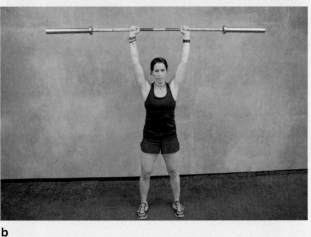

b

Courtesy of Paula J Gorman

Exercise 3

Upright Rowing

Instructions: This exercise can be done using dumbbells, a weighted bar (shown), or a barbell.

(photo a) From a standing position with arms extended fully, grasp a barbell with a close grip (hands about 15–30 cm apart) and palms toward the body.

(photo b)   Raise the bar to about the level of your collarbone, keeping your elbows above bar level at all times. Return to the starting position.

Muscles developed: Trapezius, deltoids, biceps

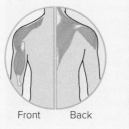

Front   Back

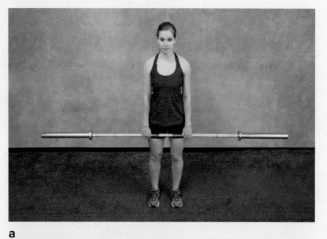

a

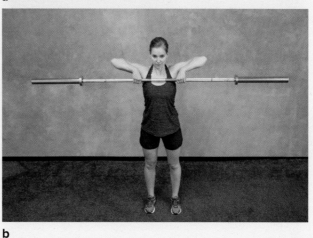

b

Courtesy of Paula J Gorman

Exercise 4

Biceps Curl

Instructions: This exercise can be done using dumbbells, a curl or weighted bar (shown), or a barbell; some people find that using a curl bar places less stress on the wrists.

(photo a)   From a standing position, grasp the bar with palms upward and hands shoulder-width apart.

(photo b)   Keeping your upper body rigid, flex (bend) your elbows until the bar reaches a level slightly below the collarbone. Return the bar to the starting position.

Muscles developed: Biceps, brachialis

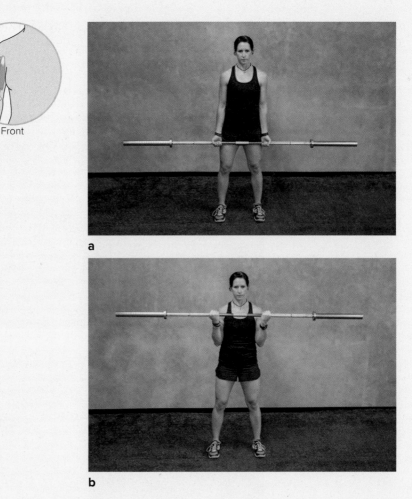

Front

a

b

Courtesy of Paula J Gorman

Exercise 5

Lateral Raise

Instructions:

(photo a) Stand with feet shoulder-width apart and a dumbbell in each hand. Hold the dumbbells parallel to each other.

(photo b) With elbows slightly bent, slowly lift both weights until they reach shoulder level. Keep your wrists in a neutral position, in line with your forearms. Return to the starting position.

Muscles developed: Deltoids

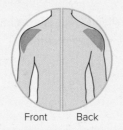

Front   Back

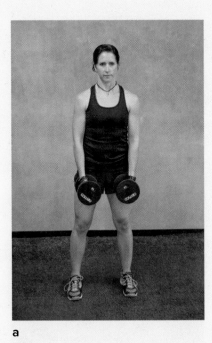

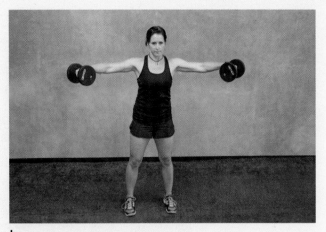

Courtesy of Paula J Gorman

Exercise 6

Squat

Instructions: If the bar is racked, place the bar on the fleshy part of your upper back and grasp the bar at shoulder width. Keeping your back neutral and head level, remove the bar from the rack and take a step back. Stand with feet slightly more than shoulder-width apart and toes pointed slightly outward.

(photo a) Rest the bar on the back of your shoulders, holding it there with hands facing forward.

(photo b) Keeping your head level and lower back straight and pelvis back, squat down until your thighs are below parallel with the floor. Let your thighs move laterally (outward) so that you "squat between your legs." This will help keep your back straight and keep your heels on the floor. Drive upward toward the starting position, hinging at the hips and keeping your back in a fixed position throughout the exercise.

Muscles developed: Quadriceps, gluteus maximus, hamstrings, gastrocnemius

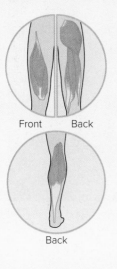

Front   Back

Back

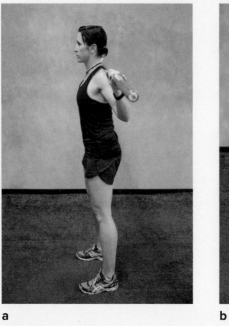

a

b

Courtesy of Paula J Gorman

Exercise 7

Thrusters

Instructions:

(photo a)   From a standing position, hold stones, soup cans, dumbbells, or barbells (or a single rock with both hands) at chest level with palms facing outward.

(photo b)   Squat down until your thighs are parallel with the floor.

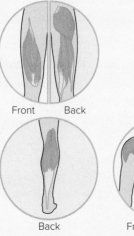

Front   Back

Back   Front   Back

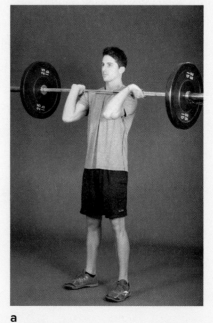

a

© Taylor Robertson Photography

(photo c)   Immediately stand and press the objects overhead in one continuous motion. Lower the objects to the starting position and immediately repeat the exercise.

Muscles developed: Quadriceps, gluteus maximus, hamstrings, gastrocnemius, deltoids, pectoralis major, triceps

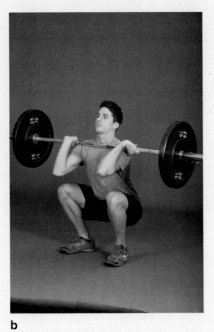

b

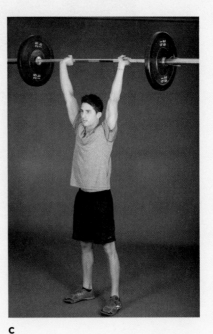

c

Exercise 8

Overhead Squats

Instructions:

(photo a)   Stand holding a broom handle, stones, barbell, or soup cans overhead with straight arms, feet placed slightly more than shoulder-width apart, toes pointed out slightly, head neutral, and back straight. Centre your weight over your arches or slightly behind.

(photo b)   Squat down, keeping your weight centred over your arches, and actively flex the hips (hinge at the hips with buttocks back) until your legs break parallel. During the movement, keep your back straight, shoulders back, and chest out, and let your thighs part to the side so that you are "squatting between your legs." Try to "spread the floor" with your feet. Push up to the starting position, maximizing the use of the posterior hip and thigh muscles, and maintaining a straight back and neutral head position.

Muscles developed: Quadriceps, gluteus maximus

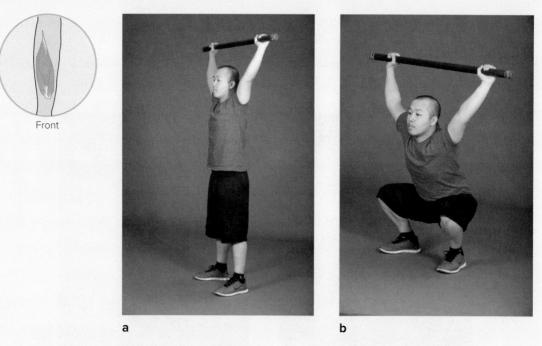

Front

a   b

© Taylor Robertson Photography

Exercise 9

Heel Raise

Instructions: Stand with feet shoulder-width apart and toes pointed straight ahead.

(photo a) Rest the bar on the back of your shoulders, holding it there with hands facing forward.

(photo b) Rest the bar on the back of your shoulders, holding it there with hands facing forward.

Muscles developed: Gastrocnemius, soleus

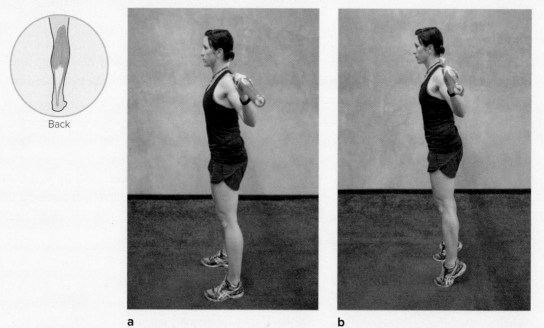

Back

a   b

Courtesy of Paula J Gorman

Exercise 10

Kettlebell Swing

Instructions:

(photo a) Begin by holding the kettlebell in both hands with palms facing toward you, in a standing position with knees bent, feet placed slightly more than shoulder-width apart, hips flexed, back straight, chest out, and head in a neutral position.

(photo b) Holding the kettlebell at knee level, swing the weight to a horizontal position by initiating the motion with the hips, thighs, and abs (tighten the quads, glutes, and ab muscles as hard as you can), keeping your arm straight and relaxed during the movement. Let the weight swing back between your legs in a "football hiking motion" and then repeat the exercise. During the movement, hinge at the hips and not at the spine.

Muscles developed: Quadriceps, gluteals, latissimus dorsi

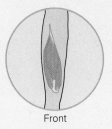

Front

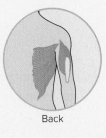

Back

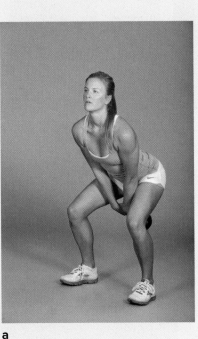

a

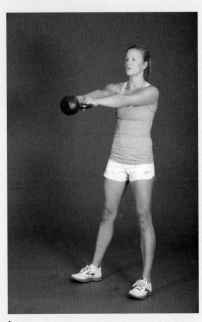

b

© Taylor Robertson Photography

Exercise 11

Kettlebell One-Arm Snatch

Instructions:

(photo a) Begin by holding the kettlebell in one hand with your palm facing toward you, in a standing position with knees bent, feet placed slightly more than shoulder-width apart, hips flexed, back straight, chest out, and head in a neutral position. Hold the kettlebell at knee level.

(photo b) Swing the weight to a horizontal position by initiating the motion with the hips, thighs, and abs (tighten the quads, glutes, and ab muscles as hard as you can), bending your arm as it approaches the chest and continuing the motion until straightening it overhead. The kettlebell should rotate from the front of your hand to the back during the motion. Use an upward punching motion at the top of the movement to prevent injuring your forearm.

(photo c) Let the weight swing back between your legs in a "football hiking motion" and then repeat the exercise. During the movement, hinge at the hips and not at the spine.

Muscles developed: Quadriceps, gluteals, latissimus dorsi, shoulder muscles

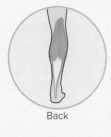
Back

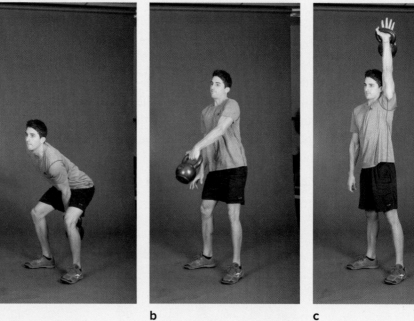
a   b   c

© Taylor Robertson Photography

Exercise 12

Kettlebell or Dumbbell Carry (Suitcase Carry)

Instructions: This is an excellent exercise for building the core muscles. Pick up a dumbbell or kettlebell in one or both hands. Maintaining good posture, walk 20 to 100 metres carrying the weight. Carry 5 kilograms or more, depending on your fitness.

Muscles developed: Core muscles, trapezius, leg and hip muscles

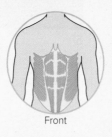
Front

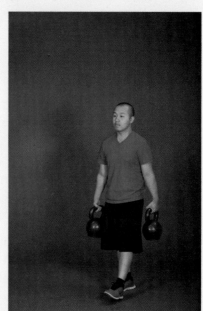

© Taylor Robertson Photography

Weight Training Exercises: Weight Machines

Mc Graw Hill Education **connect**

Exercise 1

Bench Press (Chest or Vertical Press)

Instructions: Sit or lie on the seat or bench, depending on the type of machine and the manufacturer's instructions. Your back, hips, and buttocks should be pressed against the machine pads. Place your feet on the floor or the foot supports.

(photo a)   Grasp the handles with your palms facing away from you; the handles should be aligned with your armpits.

(photo b)   Push the bars until your arms are fully extended, but don't lock your elbows. Return to the starting position.

Muscles developed: Pectoralis major, anterior deltoids, triceps

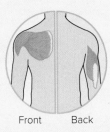

Front   Back

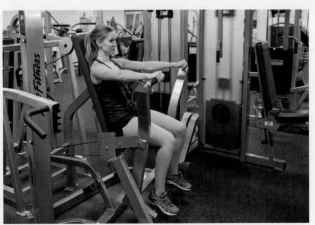

a

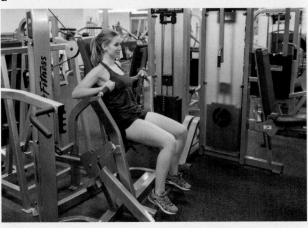

b

Courtesy of Paula J Gorman

Exercise 2

Lat Pull

Instructions: Begin in a seated or kneeling position, depending on the type of lat machine and the manufacturer's instructions.

(photo a)   Grasp the bar of the machine with arms fully extended.

(photo b)   Slowly pull the weight down until it reaches the top of your chest. Slowly return to the starting position.

Muscles developed: Latissimus dorsi, biceps

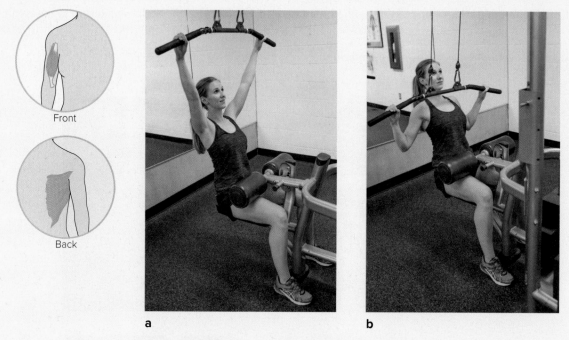

Front

Back

a   b

Courtesy of Paula J Gorman

Note: *This exercise focuses on the same major muscles as the assisted pull-up (Exercise 3); choose an appropriate exercise for your program based on your preferences and equipment availability.*

Exercise 3

Assisted Pull-Up

Instructions: Set the weight according to the amount of assistance you need to complete a set of pull-ups—the heavier the weight, the more assistance provided.

(photo a)   Stand or kneel on the assist platform, and grasp the pull-up bar with your elbows fully extended and your palms facing away.

(photo b)   Pull up until your chin goes above the bar and then return to the starting position.

Muscles developed: Latissimus dorsi, bicep

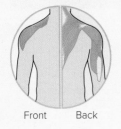

Front

Back

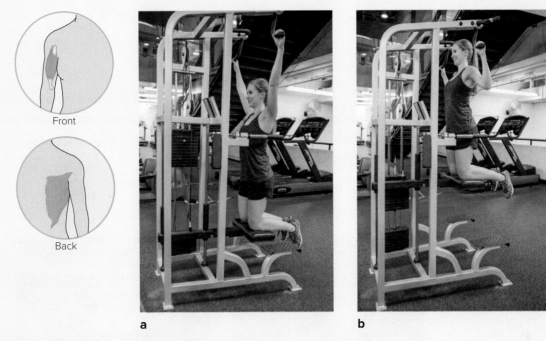

a   b

Courtesy of Paula J Gorman

Exercise 4

Overhead Press (Shoulder Press)

Instructions: Adjust the seat so that your feet are flat on the ground and the hand grips are slightly above your shoulders.

(photo a)   Sit down, facing away from the machine, and grasp the hand grips with your palms facing forward.

(photo b)   Press the weight upward until your arms are extended. Return to the starting position.

Muscles developed: Deltoids, trapezius, triceps

Front   Back

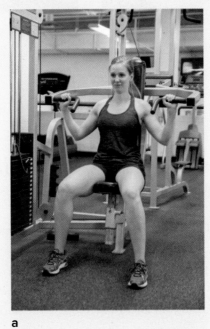

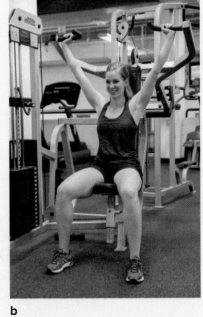

a   b

Courtesy of Paula J Gorman

Exercise 5

Biceps Curl

Instructions:

(photo a) Adjust the seat so your back is straight and your arms rest comfortably against the top and side pads. Place your arms on the support cushions and grasp the hand grips with your palms facing up.

(photo b) Keeping your upper body still, flex (bend) your elbows until the hand grips almost reach your collarbone. Return to the starting position.

Muscles developed: Biceps, brachialis

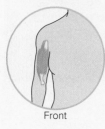

Front

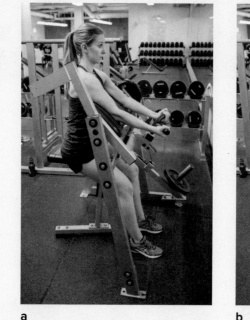

a

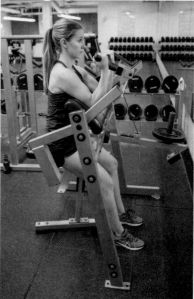

b

Courtesy of Paula J Gorman

Exercise 6

Leg Press

Instructions: Sit or lie on the seat or bench, depending on the type of machine and the manufacturer's instructions. Your head, back, hips, and buttocks should be pressed against the machine pads. Loosely grasp the handles at the side of the machine.

(photo a) Begin with your feet flat on the foot platform about shoulder-width apart. Extend your legs but do not forcefully lock your knees.

(photo b) Slowly lower the weight by bending your knees and flexing your hips until your knees are bent at about a 90-degree angle or your heels start to lift off the foot platform. Keep your lower back flat against the support pad. Then extend your knees and return to the starting position.

Muscles developed: Gluteus maximus, quadriceps, hamstrings

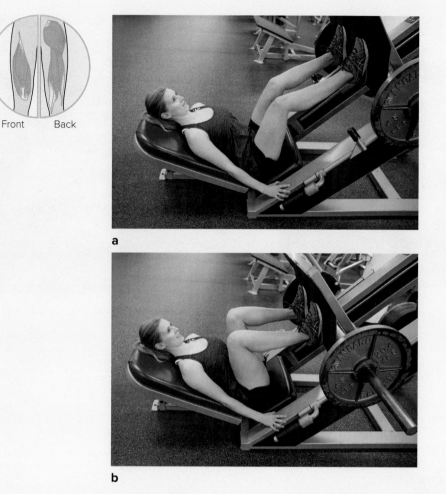

Front Back

a

b

Courtesy of Paula J Gorman

Exercise 7

Leg Extension (Knee Extension)

Instructions:

(photo a) Adjust the seat so that the pads rest comfortably on top of your lower shins. Loosely grasp the handles.

(photo b) Extend your knees until they are almost straight. Return to the starting position.

Note: *Knee extensions cause kneecap pain in some people. If you have kneecap pain during this exercise, check with an orthopedic specialist before repeating it.*

Muscles developed: Quadriceps

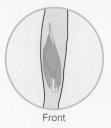

Front

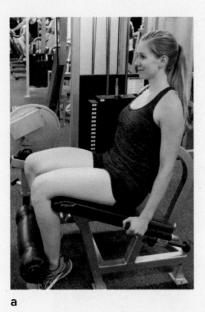

a

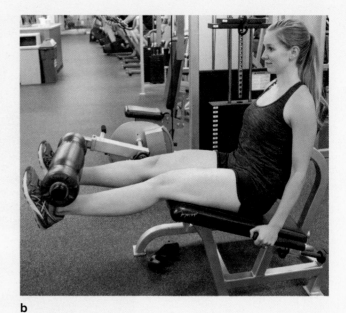

b

Courtesy of Paula J Gorman

Exercise 8

Seated Leg Curl

Instructions:

(photo a) Sit on the seat with your back against the back pad and the leg pad below your calf muscles.

(photo b) Flex your knees until your lower and upper legs form a 90 degree angle. Return to the starting position.

Muscles developed: Hamstrings, gastrocnemius

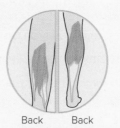

Back   Back

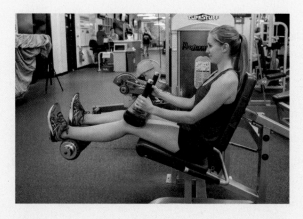

a

Courtesy of Paula J Gorman

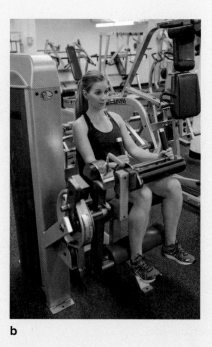

b

Note: *Abdominal machines and low-back machines are not recommended because of injury risk. Refer to the Free Weights exercise section for appropriate exercises to strengthen the abdominal and low-back muscles. For the rectus abdominus, obliques, and transvere abdominus, perform curl-ups (Exercise 4 in the Body Weight section), and for the erector spinae and quadratus lumborum, perform the spine extension and the isometric side bridge (Exercises 5 and 6 in the Body Weight section).*

SUMMARY

- Hypertrophy, or increased muscle fibre size, occurs when weight training causes the number of myofibrils to increase; total muscle size thereby increases. Strength also increases through muscle learning. Most women do not develop large muscles from weight training.

- Improvements in muscular strength and endurance lead to enhanced physical performance, protection against injury, improved body composition, better self-image, improved muscle and bone health with aging, reduced risk of chronic disease, and decreased risk of premature death.

- Muscular strength can be assessed by determining the amount of weight that can be lifted in one repetition of an exercise; muscular endurance can be assessed by determining the number of repetitions of a particular exercise that can be performed.

- Static (isometric) exercises involve contraction without movement. They are most useful when a person is recovering from an injury or surgery or needs to overcome weak points in a range of motion.

- Dynamic (isotonic) exercises involve contraction that results in movement. The two most common types are constant resistance (free weights) and variable resistance (many weight machines).

- Free weights and weight machines have pros and cons for developing fitness, although machines tend to be safer.

continued

- Lifting heavy weights for only a few repetitions helps develop strength. Lifting lighter weights for more repetitions helps develop muscular endurance.

- A strength training program for general fitness includes at least one set of 8 to 12 repetitions (enough to cause fatigue) of 8 to 10 exercises, along with warm-up and cool-down periods; the program should be carried out two to four nonconsecutive days a week.

- Safety guidelines for strength training include using proper technique, using spotters and collars when necessary, and taking care of injuries.

- Natural health products or drugs that are promoted as instant or quick "cures" usually don't work and are either dangerous or expensive or both.

FOR FURTHER EXPLORATION

Organizations and Websites

Canada's Physical Activity Guide. Offers many suggestions for incorporating physical activity into everyday life.

   http://www.phac-aspc.gc.ca/pau-uap/paguide/

American College of Sports Medicine Position Stand: Progression Models in Resistance Training for Healthy Adults. Provides an in-depth look at strategies for setting up a strength training program and making progress based on individual program goals.

   http://journals.lww.com/acsm-msse/Fulltext/2009/03000/-Progression_Models_in_Resistance _Training_for.26.aspx

Human Anatomy Online. Includes text, illustrations, and animation about the muscular system, nerve-muscle connections, muscular contraction, and other topics.

   http://www.innerbody.com/htm/body.html

National Strength and Conditioning Association. Offers information on strength development for fitness and athletic performance.

   http://www.nsca.com.

StrongFirst. Includes information about a school of strength, directed by kettlebell master Pavel Tsatsouline, which teaches men and women how to reach high levels of strength and fitness without interfering with work, school, family, or sport. The program offers clinics and web-based information.

   http://www.strongfirst.com

University of California, San Diego/Muscle Physiology Home Page. Contains an introduction to muscle physiology, including information about types of muscle fibres and energy cycles.

   http://muscle.ucsd.edu

University of Michigan/Muscles in Action. Provides interactive descriptions of muscle movements.

   http://www.med.umich.edu/lrc/Hypermuscle/Hyper.html

   See also the listings in Chapter 2.

Laboratory Activities

Name _____ Section _____ Date _____

Lab 4.1 Assessing Your Current Level of Muscular Strength

Mc Graw Hill Education **connect**

To assess your strength level and track the progress of your strength training program, you can use data from your weight training workouts to calculate 1 RM. On your workout card, record the amount of weight you lift and the number of repetitions you can complete using that weight. Perform as many repetitions as you can using correct form for each exercise. Use the table below to determine the 1 RM that corresponds to the amount of weight and number of repetitions you lifted. Fill in the following chart to use this method to track your strength gains in major muscle groups as your strength training program progresses. Fill in additional exercises as needed.

Exercise	Date_____ Weight	Reps	1-RM	Date_____ Weight	Reps	1-RM	Date_____ Weight	Reps	1-RM
Bench press									
Overhead press									
Lat pull									
Biceps curl									
Leg press									
Leg extension									

To use the following table to determine 1 RM, find the weight you lifted in the left column and move across the row until you reach the column for the number of repetitions you performed; the number in the corresponding row and column is your 1 RM for that exercise.

	Repetitions											
Wt (lb)	1	2	3	4	5	6	7	8	9	10	11	12
20	20	21	21	22	23	23	24	25	26	27	28	29
25	25	26	26	27	28	29	30	31	32	33	35	36
30	30	31	32	33	34	35	36	37	39	40	42	43
35	35	36	37	38	39	41	42	43	45	47	48	50
40	40	41	42	44	45	46	48	50	51	53	55	58
45	45	46	48	49	51	52	54	56	58	60	62	65
50	50	51	53	55	56	58	60	62	64	67	69	72
55	55	57	58	60	62	64	66	68	71	73	76	79
60	60	62	64	65	68	70	72	74	77	80	83	86
65	65	67	69	71	73	75	78	81	84	87	90	94
70	70	72	74	76	79	81	84	87	90	93	97	101
75	75	77	79	82	84	87	90	93	96	100	104	108
80	80	82	85	87	90	93	96	99	103	107	111	115

continued

85	85	87	90	93	96	99	102	106	109	113	118	122
90	90	93	95	98	101	105	108	112	116	120	125	130
100	95	98	101	104	107	110	114	118	122	127	132	137
100	100	103	106	109	113	116	120	124	129	133	139	144
105	105	108	111	115	118	122	126	130	135	140	145	151
110	110	113	116	120	124	128	132	137	141	147	152	158
115	115	118	122	125	129	134	138	143	148	153	159	166
120	120	123	127	131	135	139	144	149	154	160	166	173
125	125	129	132	136	141	145	150	155	161	167	173	180
130	130	134	138	142	146	151	156	161	167	173	180	187
135	135	139	143	147	152	157	162	168	174	180	187	194
140	140	144	148	153	158	163	168	174	180	187	194	202
145	145	149	154	158	163	168	174	180	186	193	201	209
150	150	154	159	164	169	174	180	186	193	200	208	216
155	155	159	164	169	174	180	186	192	199	207	215	223
160	160	165	169	175	180	186	192	199	206	213	222	230
165	165	170	175	180	186	192	198	205	212	220	229	238
170	170	175	180	185	191	197	204	211	219	227	235	245
175	175	180	185	191	197	203	210	217	225	233	242	252
180	180	185	191	196	203	209	216	223	231	240	249	259
185	185	190	196	202	208	215	222	230	238	247	256	266
190	190	195	201	207	214	221	228	236	244	253	263	274
195	195	201	206	213	219	226	234	242	251	260	270	281
200	200	206	212	218	225	232	240	248	257	267	277	288
205	205	211	217	224	231	238	246	255	264	273	284	295
210	210	216	222	229	236	244	252	261	270	280	291	303
215	215	221	228	235	242	250	258	267	276	287	298	310
220	220	226	233	240	248	256	264	273	283	293	305	317
225	225	231	238	245	253	261	270	279	289	300	312	324
230	230	237	244	251	259	267	276	286	296	307	319	331
235	235	242	249	256	264	273	282	292	302	313	325	339
240	240	247	254	262	270	279	288	298	309	320	332	346
245	245	252	259	267	276	285	294	304	315	327	339	353
250	250	257	265	273	281	290	300	310	322	333	346	360
255	255	262	270	278	287	296	306	317	328	340	353	367
260	260	267	275	284	293	302	312	323	334	347	360	375
265	265	273	281	289	298	308	318	329	341	353	367	382
270	270	278	286	295	304	314	324	335	347	360	374	389
275	275	283	291	300	309	319	330	341	354	367	381	396
280	280	288	296	305	315	325	336	348	360	373	388	403
285	285	293	302	311	321	331	342	354	367	380	395	411
290	290	298	307	316	326	337	348	360	373	387	402	418
295	295	303	312	322	332	343	354	366	379	393	409	425
300	300	309	318	327	338	348	360	372	386	400	416	432

Table generated using the Brzycki equation: $1 - RM = $ weight (kg)/(1.0278 − (0.0278 × repetitions)).

SOURCE: Adapted from Brzycki, M. 1993. Strength testing. Predicting a one-rep max from a reps-to-fatigue. *Journal of Physical Education, Recreation, and Dance* 64: 88–90, A publication of SHAPE America – Society of Health and Physical Educators, http://www.shapeamerica.org.

The Maximum Bench Press Test

Equipment

If you are using free weights, you will need the following equipment:

1. flat bench (with or without racks)
2. barbell
3. assorted weight plates, with collars to hold them in place
4. one or two spotters
5. weight scale

If you are using a weight machine, use the following equipment:

1. Universal Gym Dynamic Variable Resistance machine
2. weight scale

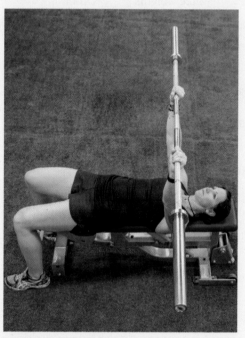

Courtesy of Paula J Gorman

Maximum bench press test.

Preparation

Try a few bench presses with a small amount of weight so you can practise your technique, warm up your muscles, and, if you use free weights, coordinate your movements with those of your spotters. Weigh yourself and record the results.

Body weight: _____ lb

Instructions

1. Use a weight that is lower than the amount you believe you can lift. For free weights, men should begin with a weight about 2/3 of their body weight; women should begin with the weight of just the bar (45 lb).
2. Lie on the bench with your feet firmly on the floor. If you are using a weight machine, grasp the handles with palms away from you; the tops of the handles should be aligned with the tops of your armpits.

If you are using free weights, grasp the bar slightly wider than shoulder width with your palms away from you. If you have one spotter, they should stand directly behind the bench; if you have two spotters, they should stand to the side, one at each end of the barbell. Signal to the spotter when you are ready to begin the test by saying "1, 2, 3." On "3," the spotter should help you lift the weight to a point over your midchest (nipple line).

3. Push the handles or barbell until your arms are fully extended. Exhale as you lift. If you are using free weights, the weight moves from a low point at the chest straight up. Keep your feet firmly on the floor, don't arch your back, and push the weight evenly with your right and left arms. Don't bounce the weight on your chest.

4. Rest for several minutes, then repeat the lift with a heavier weight. It will probably take several attempts to determine the maximum amount of weight you can lift (1 RM).

1 RM: _____ lb

Check one: _____ Universal _____ Free weights _____ Other

5. If you are using free weights, convert your free weights bench press score to an estimated value for 1 RM on the Universal bench press using the appropriate formula:

Males: Estimated Universal 1 RM = (1.016 × free weights 1 RM _____ lb) + 18.41 = _____ lb

Females: Estimated Universal 1 RM = (0.848 × free weights 1 RM _____ lb) + 21.37 = _____ lb

Rating Your Bench Press Result

1. Divide your Universal 1 RM value by your body weight.

1 RM _____ lb ÷ body weight _____ lb = _____

2. Find this ratio in the following table to determine your bench press strength rating. Record the rating here and in the chart at the end of this lab.

Bench press strength rating: _____

Strength Ratings for the Maximum Bench Press Test

				Pounds Lifted/Body Weight (lb)			
Men		*Very Poor*	*Poor*	*Fair*	*Good*	*Excellent*	*Superior*
Age:	Under 20	Below 0.89	0.89–1.05	1.06–1.18	1.19–1.33	1.34–1.75	Above 1.75
	20–29	Below 0.88	0.88–0.98	0.99–1.13	1.14–1.31	1.32–1.62	Above 1.62
	30–39	Below 0.78	0.78–0.87	0.88–0.97	0.98–1.11	1.12–1.34	Above 1.34
	40–49	Below 0.72	0.72–0.79	0.80–0.87	0.88–0.99	1.00–1.19	Above 1.19
	50–59	Below 0.63	0.63–0.70	0.71–0.78	0.79–0.89	0.90–1.04	Above 1.04
	60 and over	Below 0.57	0.57–0.65	0.66–0.71	0.72–0.81	0.82–0.93	Above 0.93
Women							
Age:	Under 20	Below 0.53	0.53–0.57	0.58–0.64	0.65–0.76	0.77–0.87	Above 0.87
	20–29	Below 0.51	0.51–0.58	0.59–0.69	0.70–0.79	0.80–1.00	Above 1.00
	30–39	Below 0.47	0.47–0.52	0.53–0.59	0.60–0.69	0.70–0.81	Above 0.81
	40–49	Below 0.43	0.43–0.49	0.50–0.53	0.54–0.61	0.62–0.76	Above 0.76
	50–59	Below 0.39	0.39–0.43	0.44–0.47	0.48–0.54	0.55–0.67	Above 0.67
	60 and over	Below 0.38	0.38–0.42	0.43–0.46	0.47–0.53	0.54–0.71	Above 0.71

SOURCE: Based on norms from the Cooper Institute for Aerobics Research, Dallas, Texas; from *The Physical Fitness Specialist Manual,* Revised 2005. Used with permission.

Functional Lower Body Strength Tests

The following tests assess functional leg movement skills using squats. Most people do squats improperly, increasing their risk of knee and back pain. Before you add weight-bearing squats to your weight training program, determine your functional leg strength, check your ability to squat properly, and give yourself a chance to master squatting movements. The following leg strength tests will help you in each of these areas.

These tests are progressively more difficult, so do not move to the next test until you have scored at least 3 on the current test. On each test, give yourself a rating of 0, 1, 3, or 5, as described in the instructions that follow the fifth test.

1. Chair Squat

Instructions

1. Sit up straight in a chair with your back resting against the backrest and your arms at your sides. Place your feet more than shoulder-width apart so you can get them under the body.

2. Begin the motion of rising out of the chair by flexing (bending) at the hips—not the back. Then squat up using a hip hinge movement (no spine movement). Stand without rocking forward, bending your back, or using external support, and keep your head in a neutral position.

3. Return to the sitting position while maintaining a straight back and keeping your weight centred over your feet. Your thighs should abduct (spread) as you sit back in the chair. Use your rear hip and thigh muscles as much as possible as you sit.

   Do five repetitions.

   Your rating: _____ (See rating instructions that follow.)

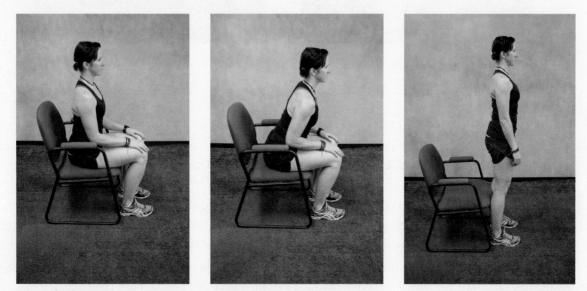

Courtesy of Paula J Gorman

2. Single-Leg Step-Up

Instructions

1. Stand facing a bench with your right foot placed on the middle of the bench, right knee bent at 90 degrees, and arms at your sides.

2. Step up on the bench until your right leg is straight, maximizing the use of the hip muscles.

3. Return to the starting position. Keep your hips stable, back straight, chest up, shoulders back, and head neutral during the entire movement.

Do five repetitions for each leg.

Your rating: _____ (See rating instructions that follow.)

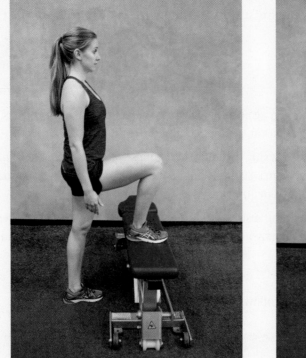 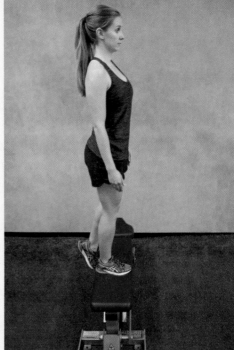

Courtesy of Paula J Gorman

3. Unweighted Squat

Instructions

1. Stand with your feet placed slightly more than shoulder-width apart, toes pointed out slightly, hands on hips or across your chest, head neutral, and back straight. Centre your weight over your arches or slightly behind.

2. Squat down, keeping your weight centred over your arches and actively flexing (bending) your hips until your legs break parallel. During the movement, keep your back straight, shoulders back, and chest out, and let your thighs part to the side so that you are "squatting between your legs."

3. Push back up to the starting position, hinging at the hips and not with the spine, maximizing the use of the rear hip and thigh muscles, and maintaining a straight back and neutral head position.

Do five repetitions.

Your rating: _____ (See rating instructions that follow.)

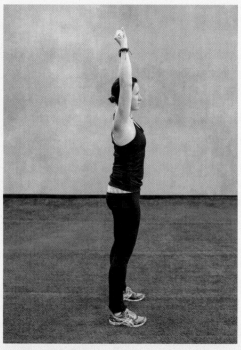
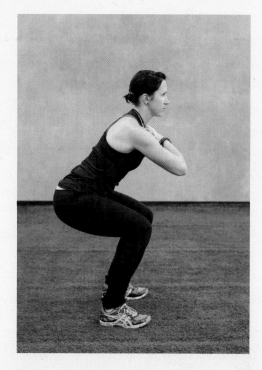

Courtesy of Paula J Gorman

4. Single-Leg Lunge-Squat with Rear-Foot Support

Instructions

1. Stand about 90 cm (3 feet) in front of a bench with your back to the bench.

2. Place the instep of your left foot on the bench, and put most of your weight on your right leg (your left leg should be bent), with your hands at your sides.

3. Squat on your right leg until your thigh is parallel with the floor. Keep your back straight, chest up, shoulders back, and head neutral.

4. Return to the starting position.

   Do three repetitions for each leg.

   Your rating: _____ (See rating instructions that follow.)

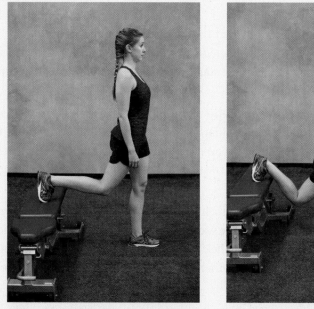

Courtesy of Paula J Gorman

5. Single-Leg Squat from a Bench Preparation

This exercise is the most difficult of the functional leg tests. Use spotters if you haven't done this exercise before or if you do not have the leg strength to perform three repetitions easily.

Instructions

1. Stand on the middle of a bench with your weight on your right leg and your arms extended in front of you. During the test, maintain a straight back and keep your weight over the arches of your feet.

2. Squat down on your right leg until your thigh is parallel with the ground, maximizing the use of your rear hip and thigh muscles. Do not rock forward on your toes or bend at the waist, and maintain a neutral head position.

3. Return to the starting position (stand up) by straightening your right hip and knee, maximizing the use of your rear hip and thigh muscles.

   Perform three repetitions for each leg.

   Your rating: _____ (See rating instructions that follow.)

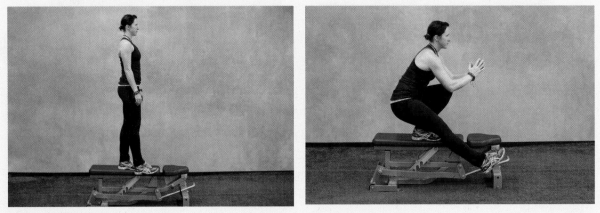

Courtesy of Paula J Gorman

Rating Your Functional Leg Strength Test Results

5 points: Performed the exercise properly with good back and thigh position, weight centred over the middle or rear of the foot, chest out, and shoulders back; good use of hip muscles on the way down and on the way up, with head in a neutral position throughout the movement; maintained good form during all repetitions; abducted (spread) the thighs on the way down during chair squats and double-leg squats; for single-leg exercises, showed good strength on both sides; for single-leg lunge-squat with rear-foot support, maintained straight back, and knees stayed behind toes.

3 points: Weight was forward on the toes, with some rounding of the back; used thigh muscles excessively, with little use of hip muscles; head and chest were too far forward; showed little abduction of the thighs during double-leg squats; when going down for single-leg exercises, one side was stronger than the other; form deteriorated with repetitions; for single-leg lunge-squat with rear-foot support and single-leg squat from a bench, could not reach parallel (thigh parallel with floor).

1 point: Had difficulty performing the movement, rocking forward and rounding back badly; used thigh muscles excessively, with little use of hip muscles on the way up or on the way down; chest and head were forward; on unweighted squats, had difficulty reaching parallel; and showed little abduction of the thighs; on single-leg exercises, one leg was markedly stronger than the other; could not perform multiple repetitions.

0 points: Could not perform the exercise.

Hand Grip Strength Test

Equipment

Grip strength dynamometer

Preparation

If necessary, adjust the hand grip size on the dynamometer into a position that is comfortable for you; then lock the grip in place. The second joint of your fingers should fit snugly under the handle of the dynamometer.

Instructions

1. Stand with the hand to be tested first at your side, away from your body. The dynamometer should be in line with your forearm and held at the level of your thigh. Squeeze the dynamometer as hard as possible without moving your arm; exhale as you squeeze. During the test, don't let the dynamometer touch your body or any other object.

2. Perform two trials with each hand, alternating trials between hands. Rest for about a minute between trials. Record the scores for each hand to the nearest kilogram.

Right hand: Trial 1: _____ kg   Trial 2: _____ kg   Right hand best trial _____ kg

Left hand: Trial 1: _____ kg   Trial 2: _____ kg   Left hand best trial _____ kg

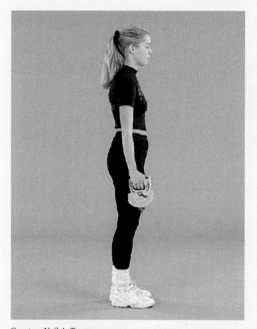

Courtesy Neil A. Tanner

Hand grip strength test.

Rating Your Hand Grip Strength

Refer to the following table for a rating of your grip strength. Record the rating below and in the chart at the end of this lab.

Total score (sum of the best trial for each hand) _____ Rating for hand grip strength: _____

Men		Grip Strength* (kg)				
		Poor	Fair	Good	Very Good	Excellent
Age:	15–19	≤ 78	79–89	90–97	98–107	≥ 108
	20–29	≤ 83	84–94	95–103	104–114	≥ 115
	30–39	≤ 83	84–94	95–103	104–114	≥ 115
	40–49	≤ 79	80–87	88–96	97–107	≥ 108
	50–59	≤ 75	76–83	84–91	92–100	≥ 101
	60–69	≤ 72	73–83	84–90	91–99	≥ 100
Women						
Age:	15–19	≤ 47	48–52	53–59	60–67	≥ 68
	20–29	≤ 51	52–57	58–62	63–69	≥ 70
	30–39	≤ 50	51–57	58–62	63–70	≥ 71
	40–49	≤ 48	49–53	54–60	61–68	≥ 69
	50–59	≤ 44	45–48	49–53	54–60	≥ 61
	60–69	≤ 40	41–44	45–47	48–53	≥ 54

*Combined right and left hand grip strength.

SOURCE: Table: Rating Your Hand Grip Strength (Males and Females). *Canadian Society for Exercise Physiology - Physical Activity training for Health* (CSEP-PATH®), © 2013. All rights reserved. Reprinted with permission.

Summary of Results

Maximum bench press test from either the 1 RM test or the multiple-repetition test:

Weight pressed: _____ lbs Rating: _____

Functional leg strength tests (0–5): Chair squat: _____ Single-leg step-up: _____ Unweighted squat: _____

Single-leg lunge-squat with rear-foot support: _____ Single-leg squat from a bench: _____

Hand grip strength test: Total score: _____ kg Rating: _____

Remember that muscular strength is specific; your ratings may vary considerably for different parts of your body.

Using Your Results

How did you score? Are you at all surprised by your rating for muscular strength? Are you satisfied with your current rating? When examining your ratings, CSEP suggests you consider the ratings to indicate the following:

- "Needs improvement" means health risks are present.
- "Fair" means some health benefits are obtained in addition to health risks being present.
- "Good" indicates that some health benefits are obtained.
- "Very good" means that considerable health benefits are seen.
- "Excellent" means optimal health benefits are obtained.

If you're not satisfied, set a realistic goal for improvement:

_____

_____

_____

Are you satisfied with your current level of muscular strength as evidenced in your daily life—for example, your ability to lift objects, climb stairs, and engage in sports and recreational activities? If you're not satisfied, set some realistic goals for improvement:

_____

_____

_____

What should you do next? Enter the results of this lab in the Preprogram Assessment column in Appendix B. If you've set goals for improvement, begin planning your strength training program by completing the plan in Lab 4.3. After several weeks of your program, complete this lab again and enter the results in the Postprogram Assessment column of Appendix B. How do the results compare?

_____

_____

_____

Name _____   **Section** _____   **Date** _____

Lab 4.2 Assessing Your Current Level of Muscular Endurance

![Mc Graw Hill Education] **connect**

For best results, don't do any strenuous weight training within 48 hours of any test. To assess endurance of the abdominal muscles, perform the partial curl-up test. To assess endurance of muscles in the upper body, perform the push-up test. To assess endurance of the muscles in the lower body, perform the squat endurance test.

The Partial Curl-Up Test

Equipment

1. four 15-cm strips of self-stick Velcro or heavy tape
2. ruler
3. metronome
4. partner
5. mat (optional)

Preparation

Affix the strips of Velcro or long strips of tape on the mat or testing surface. Place the strips 10 centimetres apart.

Instructions

1. Start by lying on your back on the floor or mat, arms straight and by your sides, shoulders relaxed, palms down and on the floor, and fingers straight. Adjust your position so that the longest fingertip of each hand touches the end of the near strip of Velcro or tape. Bend your knees about 90 degrees, with your feet about 30 to 45 centimetres from your buttocks.

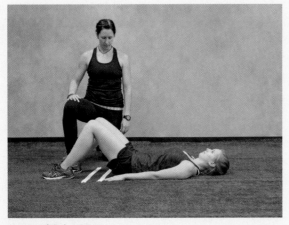
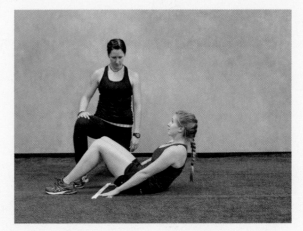

Courtesy of Paula J Gorman

Curl-up test: (a) Starting position.   (b) Curl-up.

2. To perform a curl-up, flex your spine while sliding your fingers across the floor until the fingertips of each hand reach the second strip of Velcro or tape. Then, return to the starting position; the shoulders must be returned to touch the mat between curl-ups, but the head need not touch. Shoulders must remain relaxed throughout the curl-up, and feet and buttocks must stay on the floor. Breathe easily, exhaling during the lift phase of the curl-up; do not hold your breath.

3. Make sure the palms of your hands and your heels remain in contact with the mat throughout the test. Do not anchor your feet during the test.

4. Once your partner says "go," perform as many partial curl-ups as you can at the metronome pace with correct form. Your partner counts the curl-ups you perform and calls a stop to the test if they notice any incorrect form or drop in your pace.

Number of partial curl-ups: _____

Rating Your Partial Curl-Up Test Result

Your score is the number of completed partial curl-ups. Refer to the appropriate portion of the following table for a rating of your abdominal muscular endurance. Record your rating below and in the chart at the end of this lab.

Rating: _____

Ratings for the Partial Curl-Up Test

	Number of Curl-Ups					
Men	*Very Poor*	*Poor*	*Average*	*Good*	*Excellent*	*Superior*
Age: 16–19	Below 48	48–57	58–64	65–74	75–93	Above 93
20–29	Below 46	46–54	55–63	64–74	75–93	Above 93
30–39	Below 40	40–47	48–55	56–64	65–81	Above 81
40–49	Below 38	38–45	46–53	54–62	63–79	Above 79
50–59	Below 36	36–43	44–51	52–60	61–77	Above 77
60–69	Below 33	33–40	41–48	49–57	58–74	Above 74
Women						
Age: 16–19	Below 42	42–50	51–58	59–67	68–84	Above 84
20–29	Below 41	41–51	52–57	58–66	67–83	Above 83
30–39	Below 38	38–47	48–56	57–66	67–85	Above 85
40–49	Below 36	36–45	46–54	55–64	65–83	Above 83
50–59	Below 34	34–43	44–52	53–62	63–81	Above 81
60–69	Below 31	31–40	41–49	50–59	60–78	Above 78

SOURCE: Ratings based on norms calculated from data collected by Robert Lualhati on 4545 college students, 16–80 years of age, at Skyline College, San Bruno, Calif. Used with permission.

The Push-Up Test

Equipment:

Mat or towel (optional)

Preparation

In this test, you will perform either standard push-ups or modified push-ups in which you support yourself with your knees. The modified technique reduces the need for upper-body strength in a test of muscular endurance. For an accurate assessment of upper-body endurance, men should perform standard push-ups and women should perform modified push-ups. (Note that when using push-ups as part of a strength training program, individuals should choose the technique most appropriate for increasing their level of strength and endurance—regardless of gender.)

Instructions

1. *For push-ups:* Start in the push-up position with your body supported by your hands and feet. *For modified push-ups:* Start in the modified push-up position with your body supported by your hands and knees. *For both positions,* your arms and your back should be straight and your fingers pointed forward.

2. Lower your chest to the floor with your back straight, and then return to the starting position.

3. Perform as many push-ups or modified push-ups as you can without stopping.

Number of push-ups: _____ or number of modified push-ups: _____

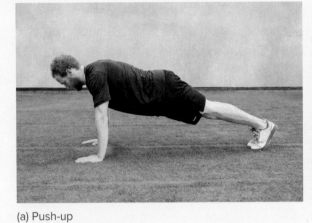

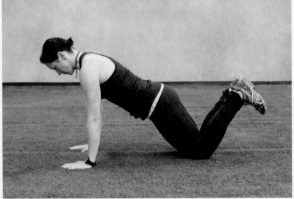

(a) Push-up

(b) Modified push-up

Courtesy of Paula J Gorman

Rating Your Push-Up Test Result

Your score is the number of completed push-ups or modified push-ups. Refer to the appropriate portion of the table below for a rating of your upper-body endurance. Record your rating below and in the chart at the end of this lab.

Rating: _____

Ratings for the Push-Up and Modified Push-Up Tests

				Number of Push-Ups		
Men		*Poor*	*Fair*	*Good*	*Very Good*	*Excellent*
Age:	15–19	≤ 17	18–22	23–28	29–38	≥ 39
	20–29	≤ 16	17–21	22–28	29–35	≥ 36
	30–39	≤ 11	12–16	17–21	22–29	≥ 30
	40–49	≤ 9	10–12	13–16	17–24	≥ 25
	50–59	≤ 6	7–9	10–12	13–20	≥ 21
	60–69	≤ 4	5–7	8–10	11–17	≥ 18
				Number of Modified Push-Ups		
Women		*Poor*	*Fair*	*Good*	*Very Good*	*Excellent*
Age:	15–19	≤ 11	12–17	18–24	25–32	≥ 33
	20–29	≤ 9	10–14	15–20	21–29	≥ 30
	30–39	≤ 7	8–12	13–19	20–26	≥ 27
	40–49	≤ 4	5–10	11–14	15–23	≥ 24
	50–59	≤ 1	2–6	7–10	11–20	≥ 21
	60–69	≤ 1	2–4	5–11	12–16	≥ 17

The Squat Endurance Test

Instructions

1. Stand with your feet placed slightly more than shoulder width apart, toes pointed out slightly, hands on hips or across your chest, head neutral, and back straight. Centre your weight over your arches or slightly behind.

2. Squat down, keeping your weight centred over your arches, until your thighs are parallel with the floor. Push back up to the starting position, maintaining a straight back and neutral head position.

3. Perform as many squats as you can without stopping.

   Number of squats: _____

Rating Your Squat Endurance Test Result

Your score is the number of completed squats. Refer to the appropriate portion of the table for a rating of your leg muscular endurance. Record your rating below and in the summary at the end of this lab.

   Rating: _____

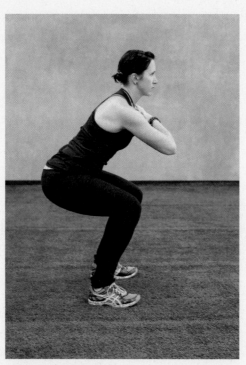

Courtesy of Paula J Gorman

Ratings for the Squat Endurance Test

Men		Very Poor	Poor	Below Average	Average	Above Average	Good	Excellent
				Number of Squats Performed				
Age:	18–25	< 25	25–30	31–34	35–38	39–43	44–49	> 49
	26–35	< 22	22–28	29–30	31–34	35–39	40–45	> 45
	36–45	< 17	17–22	23–26	27–29	30–34	35–41	> 41
	46–55	< 9	13–17	18–21	22–24	25–38	29–35	> 35
	56–65	< 9	9–12	13–16	17–20	21–24	25–31	> 31
	65 +	< 7	7–10	11–14	15–18	19–21	22–28	> 28

continued

Number of Squats Performed

		Very Poor	Poor	Below Average	Average	Above Average	Good	Excellent
Women								
Age:	18–25	< 18	18–24	25–28	29–32	33–36	37–43	> 43
	26–35	< 20	13–20	21–24	25–28	29–32	33–39	> 39
	36–45	< 7	7–14	15–18	19–22	23–26	27–33	> 33
	46–55	< 5	5–9	10–13	14–17	18–21	22–27	> 27
	56–65	< 3	3–6	7–9	10–12	13–17	18–24	> 24
	65 +	< 2	2–4	5–10	11–13	14–16	17–23	> 23

SOURCE: Topend Sports, http://www.topendsports.com/testing/tests/home-squat.htm.

Summary of Results

Curl-up test: Number of curl-ups: _____ Rating: _____

Push-up test: Number of push-ups/modifies push-ups: _____ Rating: _____

Squat endurance test: Number of squats: _____ Rating: _____

Remember that muscular endurance is specific: Your ratings may vary considerably for different parts of your body.

Using Your Results

How did you score? Are you at all surprised by your ratings for muscular endurance? Are you satisfied with your current ratings? If you're not satisfied, set realistic goals for improvement:

_____

_____

_____

Are you satisfied with your current level of muscular endurance as evidenced in your daily life—for example, your ability to carry groceries or your books, hike, and do yard work? If you're not satisfied, set some realistic goals for improvement:

_____

_____

_____

What should you do next? Enter the results of this lab in the Preprogram Assessment column in Appendix B. If you've set goals for improvement, begin planning your strength training program by completing the plan in Lab 4.3. After several weeks of your program, complete this lab again and enter the results in the Postprogram Assessment column of Appendix B. How do the results compare?

_____

_____

_____

Name _____ Section _____ Date _____

Lab 4.3 Designing and Monitoring a Strength Training Program

connect

1. **Set goals.** List goals for your strength training program. Your goals can be specific or general, short or long term. In the first section, include specific, measurable goals that you can use to track the progress of your fitness program. These goals might be things like raising your upper body muscular strength rating from fair to good or being able to complete 10 repetitions of a lat pull with 50 kilograms of resistance. In the second section, include long-term and more qualitative goals, such as improving self-confidence and reducing your risk for back pain.

Specific Goals: Current Status _____ **Final Goal** _____

_____   _____

_____   _____

_____   _____

Other goals: _____

_____

_____

2. **Choose exercises.** Based on your goals, choose 8 to 10 exercises to perform during each weight training session. If your goal is general training for wellness, use one of the sample programs in Figure 4.2. List your exercises and the muscles they develop in the program plan below.

3. **Frequency: Choose the number of training sessions per week.** Work out at least two nonconsecutive days per week. Indicate the days you will train on your program plan; be sure to include days of rest to allow your body to recover.

4. **Intensity: Choose starting weights.** Experiment with different amounts of weight until you settle on a good starting weight, one that you can lift easily for 10 to 12 repetitions. As you progress in your program, you can add more weight. Fill in the starting weight for each exercise on the program plan.

5. **Time: Choose a starting number of sets and repetitions.** Include at least one set of 8 to 12 repetitions of each exercise. (When you add weight, you may have to decrease the number of repetitions slightly until your muscles adapt to the heavier load.) If your program is focusing on strength alone, your sets can contain fewer repetitions using a heavier load. If you are over 50 to 60 years of age, your sets should contain more repetitions (10 to 15) using a lighter load. Fill in the starting number of sets and repetitions of each exercise on the program plan.

6. **Monitor your progress.** Use the workout card below to monitor your progress and keep track of exercises, weights, sets, and repetitions.

Program Plan for Weight Training											
Exercise	Muscle(s) Developed	Frequency (check √)							Intensity: Weight (kg)	Time	
		M	Tu	W	Th	F	Sa	Su		Repetitions	Sets

WORKOUT CARD FOR _____

Exercise/Date																														
	Wt																													
	Sets																													
	Reps																													
	Wt																													
	Sets																													
	Reps																													
	Wt																													
	Sets																													
	Reps																													
	Wt																													
	Sets																													
	Reps																													
	Wt																													
	Sets																													
	Reps																													
	Wt																													
	Sets																													
	Reps																													
	Wt																													
	Sets																													
	Reps																													
	Wt																													
	Sets																													
	Reps																													
	Wt																													
	Sets																													
	Reps																													
	Wt																													
	Sets																													
	Reps																													
	Wt																													
	Sets																													
	Reps																													
	Wt																													
	Sets																													
	Reps																													

Flexibility and Low-Back Health

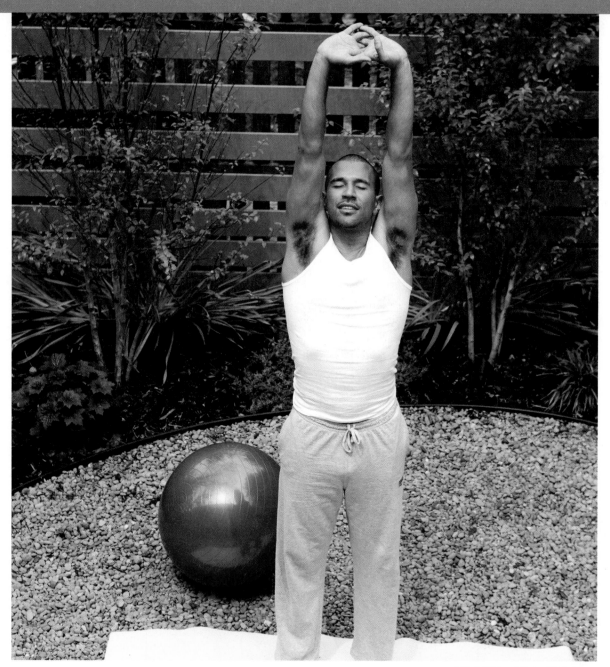

LEARNING OBJECTIVES

After reading this chapter, you should be able to

LO1 List the factors that affect a joint's flexibility

LO2 Identify the potential benefits of flexibility and stretching exercises

LO3 Describe the intensity, duration, and frequency of stretching exercises that will develop the most flexibility with the lowest risk of injury

LO4 Describe the different types of stretching exercises and how they affect muscles.

LO5 List safe stretching exercises for major joints

LO6 Explain how low-back pain can be prevented and managed

TEST YOUR KNOWLEDGE

1. **When should stretching exercises be performed?**
   a. at the start of a warm-up
   b. first thing in the morning
   c. after endurance exercise or strength training

2. **If you injure your back, it's usually best to rest in bed until the pain is completely gone.**

   True or false?

3. **It is better to hold a stretch for a short time than to "bounce" while stretching.**

   True or false?

ANSWERS

1. **C.** It's best to do stretching exercises when your muscles are warm. Intensely stretching muscles before exercise may reduce their explosive strength and interfere with neuromuscular control.

2. **FALSE.** Prolonged bed rest may actually worsen back pain. Limit bed rest to a day or less, treat pain and inflammation with cold and then heat, and begin moderate physical activity as soon as possible.

3. **TRUE.** "Bouncing" during stretching can damage your muscles. This type of stretching, called ballistic stretching, should be used only by well-conditioned athletes for specific purposes. A person of average fitness should stretch slowly, holding each stretch for 15 to 30 seconds.

Flexibility—the ability of a joint to move through its full **range of motion**—is important for general fitness and wellness. Flexibility is a highly adaptable physical fitness component. It increases in response to a regular program of stretching exercises and decreases with inactivity. Flexibility is also specific: Good flexibility in one joint doesn't necessarily mean good flexibility in another. You can increase your flexibility by doing regular stretching exercises for all major joints.

> **range of motion**   The full motion possible in a joint.

This chapter describes the factors that affect flexibility and the benefits of maintaining good flexibility. It provides guidelines for assessing your current level of flexibility and putting together a successful stretching program. It also examines the common problem of low-back pain.

LO1 5.1 What Determines Flexibility?

There are two basic types of flexibility:

- **Static flexibility** is the ability to hold an extended position at one end or point in a joint's range of motion. For example, static flexibility determines how far you can extend your arm across the front of your body or out to the side. Static flexibility depends on your ability to tolerate stretched muscles, the structure of your joints, and the elasticity of muscles.

- **Dynamic flexibility** is the ability to move a joint through its range of motion with little resistance. For example, it affects your ability to pitch a ball or swing a golf club. Dynamic flexibility depends on static flexibility, but it also involves strength, coordination, and resistance to movement.

Dynamic flexibility is important for daily activities and sports. Because static flexibility is easier to measure and better researched, however, most assessment tests and stretching programs target that type of flexibility.

The flexibility of a joint is affected by its structure, by muscle elasticity and length, and by nervous system regulation. Joint structure can't be changed, but other factors, such as the length of resting muscle fibres, can be changed through exercise; these factors should be the focus of a program to develop flexibility.

Joint Structure

How flexible a joint is depends partly on the nature and structure of the joint (Figure 5.1). *Hinge* joints such as those in your fingers and knees allow only limited forward and backward movement; they lock when fully extended. *Ball-and-socket* joints like the hip enable movement in many different directions and have a greater range of motion. **Joint capsules**, semi-elastic structures that give joints strength and stability but limit movement, surround the major joints. The bone surfaces within the joint are lined with cartilage and separated by synovial fluid, which cushions the bones and reduces friction as the joint moves. Ligaments, both inside and outside the joint capsule, strengthen and reinforce the joint.

> **joint capsules**   Semi-elastic structures, composed primarily of connective tissue, that surround major joints.

Heredity also plays a part in joint structure and flexibility; for example, although everyone has a broad range of motion in the ball-and-socket hip joint, not everyone can do a split. Gender may also play a role, with some studies finding that women on average have greater flexibility in certain joints.[1]

Muscle Elasticity and Length

Soft tissues, including skin, muscles, tendons, and ligaments, also affect the flexibility of a joint. Muscle tissue is the key to developing flexibility because regular stretching can lengthen it. The most important component of muscle tissue related to flexibility is the connective tissue that surrounds and envelops every part of muscle tissue, from

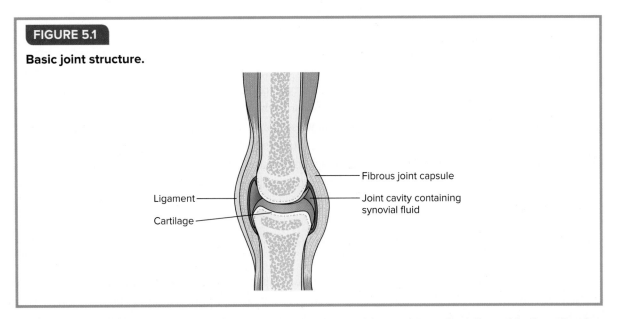

FIGURE 5.1

Basic joint structure.

Fibrous joint capsule

Joint cavity containing synovial fluid

Ligament

Cartilage

individual muscle fibres to entire muscles. Connective tissue provides structure, elasticity, and bulk and makes up about 30% of muscle mass. Two principal types of connective tissue are **collagen**, white fibres that provide structure and support, and **elastin**, yellow fibres that are elastic and flexible. The collagen and elastin are closely intertwined, so muscle tissue exhibits the properties of both types of fibres. A structural protein in muscles called *titin* also has elastic properties and contributes to flexibility.

soft tissues   Tissues of the human body that include skin, fat, linings of internal organs and blood vessels, connective tissues, tendons, ligaments, muscles, and nerves.
collagen   White fibres that provide structure and support in connective tissue.
elastin   Yellow fibres that make connective tissue flexible.

When a muscle is stretched, the wavelike elastin fibres straighten; when the stretch is relieved, they rapidly snap back to their resting position. This temporary lengthening is called **elastic elongation**. If stretched gently and regularly, connective tissues may lengthen and flexibility may improve. This long-term lengthening is called **plastic elongation**. Without regular stretching, the process reverses and these tissues shorten, resulting in decreased flexibility. Regular stretching may contribute to flexibility by lengthening muscle fibres through the addition of contractile units called *sarcomeres*.

elastic elongation   Temporary change in the length of muscles, tendons, and supporting connective tissues.
plastic elongation   Long-term change in the length of muscles, tendons, and supporting connective tissues.

A muscle can tolerate a limited amount of stretch. As the limits of its flexibility are reached, connective tissue becomes more brittle and may rupture if overstretched. A safe and effective program stretches muscles enough to slightly elongate the tissues but not so much that they are damaged. Research has shown that flexibility is improved best by stretching when muscles are warm[2] (following exercise or the application of heat) and the stretch is applied gradually and conservatively. Sudden, high-stress stretching is less effective and can lead to muscle damage.

Wellness Tip

Muscles shrink after injury or surgery. Rehabilitation exercises can help muscles grow again. One caution: Overuse of drugs like ibuprofen can slow the regrowth process. Use such drugs only as prescribed by your doctor.

Nervous System Regulation

Proprioceptors are nerves that send information about changes in the muscular and skeletal systems to the nervous system, which responds with signals to help control the speed, strength, and coordination of muscle contractions. When a muscle is stretched (lengthened), proprioceptors detect the amount and rate of the change in muscle length. The nerves send a signal to the spinal cord, which then sends a signal back to the muscle, triggering a muscle contraction that resists the change in muscle length. Another signal is sent to the antagonistic, or opposing, muscle, causing it to relax and facilitate contraction of the stretched muscle. These reflexes occur frequently in active muscles and allow for fine control of muscle length and movement. Muscle flexibility is linked to strength. Practising lower-body eccentric exercise (lengthening contractions) increases strength and flexibility and might decrease the risk of lower body muscle injury.

proprioceptors Nerves that send information about the muscular and skeletal systems to the nervous system.

Small movements that only slightly stimulate these receptors cause small reflex actions. Rapid, powerful, and sudden movements that strongly stimulate the receptors cause large, powerful reflex muscle contractions. Thus stretches that involve rapid, bouncy movements can be dangerous and cause injury. Each bounce causes a reflex contraction, which means a muscle might be stretching at the same time it is contracting. Performing a gradual stretch and then holding it allows the proprioceptors to adjust to the new muscle length and to reduce the signals it sends to the spinal cord, thereby allowing muscles to lengthen and, over time, improving flexibility.

The stretching technique called *proprioceptive neuro-muscular facilitation (PNF)* takes advantage of nerve activity to improve flexibility. For example, contracting a muscle prior to stretching it can help allow the muscle to stretch farther. The advanced strength training technique called *plyometrics* (see Chapter 4) also takes advantage of the nervous system action in stretching and contracting muscles.

Modifying nervous control through movement and specific exercises is the best way to improve the functional range of motion. Regular stretching trains the proprioceptors to allow the muscles to lengthen. Proprioceptors adapt very quickly to stretching (or lack of stretching), so frequent training helps develop flexibility. Stretching before exercising, however, can disturb proprioceptors and interfere with motor control during exercise. This is another good reason to stretch after exercising.

LO2 5.2 Benefits of Flexibility

Good flexibility provides benefits for the entire musculoskeletal system. Flexibility training increases range of motion and may prevent muscle strains. As long as you don't overstretch, flexibility training will increase strength and the quality of movement, which might decrease the risk of some sports injuries. Most studies, however, show that stretching does not prevent overuse injuries.

Joint Health

Good flexibility is essential to good joint health. When the muscles and other tissues that support a joint are tight, the joint is subject to abnormal stresses that can cause joint deterioration. For example, tight thigh muscles cause excessive pressure on the kneecap, leading to pain in the knee joint. Poor joint flexibility can also cause abnormalities in joint lubrication, leading to deterioration of the sensitive cartilage cells lining the joint; pain and further joint injury can result.

Improved flexibility can greatly improve your quality of life, particularly as you get older. People tend to exercise less as they age, leading to loss of joint mobility and increased incidence of joint pain. Aging also decreases the natural elasticity of muscles, tendons, and joints, resulting in stiffness. The problem is often compounded by arthritis (see the box Does Physical Activity Increase or Decrease the Risk of Bone and Joint Disease?). Good joint flexibility may prevent arthritis, and stretching may lessen pain in people who have the condition. Another benefit of good flexibility for older adults is that it increases balance and stability.

The Evidence *for* EXERCISE

DOES PHYSICAL ACTIVITY INCREASE OR DECREASE THE RISK OF BONE AND JOINT DISEASE?

Most college and university students don't worry much about developing fall-related fractures or chronic bone-related illnesses such as osteoporosis (loss of bone mass) or osteoarthritis (degeneration of the cartilage lining the bones inside joints). Even so, bone health should be a concern throughout life: Girls amass 85% of their adult bone mass by age 18 and boys build the same amount by age 20, and most people begin losing bone mass around age 30. For many, bone loss is accelerated by poor diet and lack of exercise. According to Osteoporosis Canada, at least one in three women and one in five men will break a bone due to osteoporosis. It is estimated that 2 million Canadians are affected by osteoporosis.

Getting enough nutrients is important for bone health (see Chapter 8), but there is mounting evidence that exercise can preserve or improve bone health. For example, several studies have shown an inverse relationship between physical activity and the risk for bone fractures. That is, the more you exercise, the less likely you are to suffer fractures, especially of the upper leg and hip. Research has not determined conclusively how much exercise is required to reduce fracture risk, but reduced risk seems to become apparent when people walk at least four hours per week and devote at least one hour per week to other forms of physical activity. These findings seem to be consistent for women and men, but some studies disagree on this point, so further research is needed.

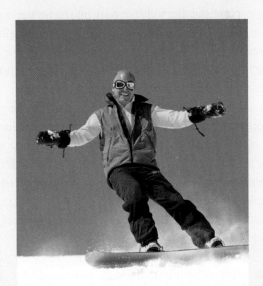

Ingram Publishing

One way in which exercise helps both men and women is by increasing the mineral density of bones, or at least by decreasing the loss of mineral density over time. Several one-year-long studies found that exercise can increase bone mineral density by 1–2% per year, which is significant—especially considering that older people can lose the same amount of bone mineral density every one to four years. Currently, Heath Canada and the Canadian Society for Exercise Physiology recommend that adults perform weight-bearing physical activities (such as walking) three to five days per week and strength training exercises two to four days per week to increase bone mass or avoid loss of mineral density.

The evidence is less conclusive for the effect of exercise on osteoarthritis, but it is still fairly positive. All experts agree that regular, moderate-intensity exercise is necessary for joint health. However, they also warn that vigorous or too-frequent exercise may contribute to joint damage and encourage the onset of osteoarthritis. For this reason, experts try to strike a balance in their exercise recommendations, especially for people with a family history of osteoarthritis. Research seems to support this

continued

cautionary approach. Some studies have found that regular physical activity (as recommended for general health) does not increase osteoarthritis risk; other studies show that moderate activity may provide some protection against the disease, but this evidence is limited.

A few studies also reveal that the type of exercise you do may increase your risk. For example, competitive or strenuous sports such as ballet, orienteering, football, basketball, soccer, and tennis have been associated with the disease, whereas sports such as cross-country skiing, running, swimming, biking, and walking have not.

The bottom line is that the earlier in life you become physically active, the greater your protection against bone loss and bone-related diseases. However, if you have a family history of osteoporosis or osteoarthritis, or if you have already developed symptoms of one of these ailments, be sure to talk to your physician before beginning an exercise program.

SOURCES: American College of Sports Medicine. 2013. *ACSM's Guidelines for Exercise Testing and Prescription,* 9th ed. Philadelphia: Wolters Kluwer/Lippincott Williams & Wilkins Health; Giangregorio, L. M., et al. 2015. Too fit to fracture: Outcomes of a Delphi consensus process on physical activity and exercise recommendations for adults with osteoporosis with or without vertebral fractures. *Osteoporosis International* 26(3): 891–910; Osteoporosis Canada. 2017. *About the Disease* (https://osteoporosis.ca/about-the-disease/; retrieved November 07, 2017); Canadian Society for Exercise Physiology 2013. *CSEP—Physical Activity Training for Health*, Ontario, Canada: CSEP.

Prevention of Low-Back Pain and Injuries

Poor spinal stability puts pressure on the nerves leading out from the spinal column and can lead to low-back pain. It is estimated that over 80% of Canadians will suffer from low-back pain at some point in their lifespan.[3] Strength and flexibility in the back, pelvis, and thighs may help prevent this type of back pain, but may or may not improve back health or reduce the risk of injury. Good hip and knee flexibility do protect the spine from excessive motion during the tasks of daily living.

Although scientific evidence is limited, people with either high or low flexibility seem to have an increased risk for injury.[4] Extreme flexibility reduces joint stability, and poor flexibility limits a joint's range of motion. People with an average level of fitness should try to attain normal flexibility in joints throughout the body, meaning each joint can move through its normal range of motion with no difficulty. Stretching programs are particularly important for older adults, people involved in high-power sports that include rapid changes in direction (such as football and tennis), workers involved in brief bouts of intense exertion (such as police officers and firefighters), and people who sit for prolonged periods (such as office workers and students).

However, stretching before a high-intensity activity (such as sprinting or basketball) may increase the risk of injury by interfering with neuromuscular control and reducing the muscles' natural ability to stretch and contract. When injuries occur, flexibility exercises can reduce symptoms and help restore normal range of motion in affected joints.

Additional Potential Benefits

- **Relief of aches and pains.** Studying or working in one place for a long time can make your muscles tense. Stretching helps relieve tension so you can go back to work refreshed and effective. Stretching reduces the symptoms of exercise-induced muscle damage, and flexible muscles are less susceptible to the damage.

- **Relief of muscle cramps.** Recent research suggests that exercise-related muscle cramps are caused by increased electrical activity within the affected muscle. The best treatment for muscle cramps is gentle stretching, which reduces the electrical activity and allows the muscle to relax.

- **Improved body position and strength for sports (and life).** Good flexibility lets you assume more efficient body positions and exert force through a greater range of motion. For example, swimmers with more flexible shoulders have stronger strokes because they can pull their arms through the water in the optimal position. Some studies suggest that flexibility training enhances strength development.

- **Maintenance of good posture and balance.** Good flexibility also contributes to body symmetry and good posture. Bad posture can gradually change your body structures. Sitting in a slumped position, for example, can lead to tightness in the muscles in the front of your chest and overstretching and looseness in the upper spine, causing a rounding of the upper back. This condition, called *kyphosis,* is common in older people. Stretching regularly may prevent it.

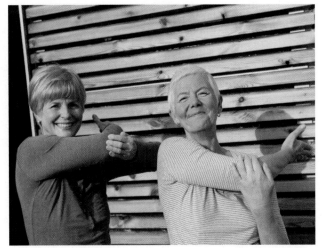
© Image Source / Alamy

Flexibility training helps maintain pain-free joints as you age.

- **Relaxation.** Flexibility exercises, particularly when practised in combination with yoga or tai chi, reduce mental tension, slow your breathing rate, and reduce blood pressure.

- **Improving impaired mobility.** Stretching often decreases pain and improves functional capacity in people with arthritis, stroke, or muscle and nerve diseases, and in people who are recovering from surgery or injury.

Assessing Flexibility

Because flexibility is specific to each joint, there are no tests of general flexibility. The most commonly used flexibility test is the sit-and-reach test, which rates the flexibility of the muscles in the lower back and hamstrings. To assess your flexibility and identify inflexible joints, complete Lab 5.1.

LO3 5.3 Creating a Successful Program to Develop Flexibility

A successful program for developing flexibility includes safe exercises executed with the most effective techniques. Your goal should be to at least attain normal flexibility in the major joints. Balanced flexibility (not too much or too little) provides joint stability and facilitates smooth, economical movement patterns. You can achieve balanced flexibility by performing stretching exercises regularly and by using a variety of stretches and stretching techniques.

Applying the FITT Principle

As with other programs, the acronym FITT can be used to remember key components of a stretching program: Frequency, Intensity, Time, and Type of exercise.

Frequency

Health Canada recommends that individuals perform stretching exercises a minimum of two to three days a week, and ideally four to seven days a week. To prevent injury and improve flexibility, it's best to stretch when your muscles are warm, either after cardiorespiratory endurance exercise or weight training.

217

As described earlier, static stretching can adversely affect muscle performance in the short term. So, if you are planning a workout for which high-performance is important, it is best to perform static stretches after your workout but while your muscles are still warm and your joints are lubricated. Stretching isn't the same thing as a cool-down, so be sure to do the cardiorespiratory cool-down first so you can transition to a lower level of intensity before stretching. If the plan for your workout includes a moderate activity like walking, then static stretching prior to your workout isn't likely to impact performance in a significant way.

Dynamic stretching, described in the next section, may have less of an impact on muscle performance and so is sometimes included as part of an active warm-up. However, dynamic stretching is more challenging to learn and perform.

Intensity and Time (Duration)

For each exercise, slowly stretch your muscles to the point of slight tension or mild discomfort—but not to the point of pain. Hold the stretch for 15 to 30 seconds. As you hold the stretch, the feeling of slight tension should slowly subside; at that point, try to stretch a bit farther. Throughout the stretch, try to relax and breathe easily. Rest for about 30 to 60 seconds between each stretch, and do two to four repetitions of each stretch. A complete flexibility workout usually takes about 10 to 30 minutes (Figure 5.2).

FIGURE 5.2

A flexibility workout.

Warm-up 5–10 minutes or following an endurance or strength training workout	Stretching exercises for major joints	
	Sample program	
	Exercise	*Areas stretched*
	Head turns and tilts	Neck
	Towel stretch	Triceps, shoulders, chest
	Across-the-body and overhead stretches	Shoulders, upper back, back of arm
	Upper-back stretch	Upper back
	Lateral stretch	Trunk muscles
	Step stretch	Hip, front of thigh
	Side lunge	Inner thigh, hip, calf
	Inner-thigh stretch	Inner thigh, hip
	Hip and trunk stretch	Trunk, outer thigh, hip, buttocks, lower back
	Modified hurdler stretch	Back of thigh, lower back
	Alternate leg stretcher	Back of thigh, hip, knee, ankle, buttocks
	Lower-leg stretch	Calf, soleus, Achilles tendon

Frequency: 2–3 days per week (minimum); 4–7 days per week (ideal)

Intensity: Stretch to the point of mild discomfort, not pain

Time (duration): All stretches should be held for 15–30 seconds and performed 2–4 times

Type of activity: Stretching exercises that focus on major joints

LO4   Types of Stretching Techniques

Stretching techniques vary from simply stretching the muscles during the course of normal activities to sophisticated methods based on patterns of muscle reflexes. Improper stretching can do more harm than good, so it's important to understand the different types of stretching exercises and how they affect the muscles. Four common techniques are static stretches, ballistic stretches, dynamic stretches, and PNF.

Static Stretching

In **static stretching**, each muscle is gradually stretched and the stretch is held for 15 to 30 seconds. A slow stretch prompts less reaction from proprioceptors, and the muscles can safely stretch farther than usual. Static stretching is the type most often recommended by fitness experts because it is safe and effective.

> **static stretching** A technique in which a muscle is slowly and gently stretched and then held in the stretched position.

The key to this technique is to stretch the muscles and joints to the point where a pull is felt, but not to the point of pain. (One note of caution: Excess static stretching can decrease joint stability and increase the risk of injury. This may be a particular concern for women, who naturally have joints that are less stable and more flexible than men.) The sample stretching program presented later in this chapter features static stretching exercises.

Ballistic Stretching

In **ballistic stretching**, the muscles are stretched suddenly in a forceful bouncing movement. For example, touching the toes repeatedly in rapid succession is a ballistic stretch for the hamstrings. A problem with this technique is that the heightened activity of proprioceptors caused by the rapid stretches can continue for some time, possibly causing injuries during any physical activities that follow. Another concern is that triggering strong responses from the nerves can cause a reflex muscle contraction that makes it harder to stretch. For these reasons, ballistic stretching is usually not recommended for people of average fitness.

> **ballistic stretching** A technique in which muscles are stretched by the force generated as a body part is repeatedly bounced, swung, or jerked.

Ballistic stretching trains the muscle dynamically, so it can be an appropriate stretching technique for some well-trained athletes. For example, tennis players stretch their hamstrings and quadriceps ballistically when they lunge for a ball during a tennis match. Because this movement is part of their sport, they might benefit from ballistic training of these muscle groups.

Dynamic (Functional) Stretching

The emphasis in **dynamic stretching** is on functional movements. Dynamic stretching is similar to ballistic stretching in that it includes movement, but it differs in that it does not involve rapid bouncing. Instead, dynamic stretching involves moving the joints through the range of motion used in a specific exercise or sport in an exaggerated but slow and controlled manner; movements are fluid rather than jerky. An example of a dynamic stretch is the lunge walk, in which a person takes slow steps with an exaggerated stride length and reaches a lunge stretch position with each step.

> **dynamic stretching** A technique in which muscles are stretched by moving joints slowly and fluidly through their range of motion in a controlled manner; also called functional stretching.

Slow dynamic stretches can lengthen the muscles in many directions without developing high tension in the tissues. These stretches elongate the tissues and train the neuromuscular system. Because dynamic stretches are based on sports movements or movements used in daily life, they develop functional flexibility that translates well into activities.

Dynamic stretches are more challenging than static stretches because they require balance and coordination and may carry a greater risk of muscle soreness and injury. People just beginning a flexibility program might want to start off with static stretches and try dynamic stretches only after they are comfortable with static stretching techniques and have improved their flexibility. It is also a good idea to seek expert advice on dynamic stretching technique and program development.

Functional flexibility training can also be combined with functional strength training. For example, lunge curls, which combine dynamic lunges with free weights biceps curls, stretch the hip, thigh, and calf muscles; stabilize the core muscles in the trunk; and build strength in the arm muscles. Many activities build functional flexibility and strength at the same time, including yoga, Pilates, tai chi, Olympic weight lifting, plyometrics, stability training (including Swiss and Bosu ball exercises), medicine ball exercises, and functional training machines (for example, Life Fitness and Cybex).

Proprioceptive Neuromuscular Facilitation (PNF)

PNF techniques use reflexes initiated by both muscle and joint receptors to cause greater training effects. The most popular PNF stretching technique is the *contract-relax* stretching method, in which a muscle is contracted before it is stretched. The contraction activates proprioceptors, causing relaxation in the muscle about to be stretched. For example, in a seated stretch of calf muscles, the first step in PNF is to contract the calf muscles. The individual or a partner can provide resistance for an isometric contraction. Following a brief period of relaxation, the next step is to stretch the calf muscles by pulling the tops of the feet toward the body. A duration of 6 seconds for the contraction at 20–75% of maximum effort and 10 to 30 seconds for the stretch is recommended. PNF appears to be most effective if the individual pushes hard during the isometric contraction.

Another example of a PNF stretch is the *contract-relax-contract pattern.* In this technique, begin by contracting the muscle to be stretched and then relaxing it. Next, contract the opposing muscle (the antagonist). Finally, stretch the first muscle. For example, using this technique to stretch the hamstrings (the muscles in the back of the thigh) would require the following steps: contract the hamstrings, relax the hamstrings, contract the quadriceps (the muscles in the front of the thigh), stretch the hamstrings.

PNF appears to allow more effective stretching, and greater immediate increases in flexibility than static stretching.[5] It also usually requires a partner and takes more time.

Passive versus Active Stretching

Stretches can be done either passively or actively. In **passive stretching**, an outside force or resistance provided by yourself, a partner, gravity, or a weight helps your joints move through their range of motion. For example, a seated stretch of the hamstring and back muscles can be done by reaching the hands toward the feet until a pull is felt in those muscles. You can achieve a greater range of motion (a more intense stretch) using passive stretching. However, because the stretch is not controlled by the muscles themselves, there is a greater risk of injury. Communication between partners in passive stretching is very important to ensure that joints aren't forced outside their normal functional range of motion.

passive stretching   A technique in which muscles are stretched by force applied by an outside force.

Wellness Tip

You don't have to be at the gym to stretch. There are lots of simple, small-movement stretches you can do anywhere—even at your desk. For some examples, visit a good health website such as MayoClinic.com and search for "stretching exercises."

In **active stretching**, a muscle is stretched by a contraction of the opposing muscle (the muscle on the opposite side of the limb). For example, an active seated stretch of the calf muscles occurs when a person actively contracts the muscles on the top of the shin. The contraction of this opposing muscle produces a reflex that relaxes the muscles to be stretched. The muscle can be stretched farther with a low risk of injury.

active stretching A technique in which muscles are stretched by the contraction of the opposing muscles.

The only disadvantage of active stretching is that a person may not be able to produce enough stress (enough stretch) to increase flexibility using only the contraction of opposing muscle groups. The safest and most convenient technique is active static stretching, with an occasional passive assist. For example, you might stretch your calves both by contracting the muscles on the top of your shin and by pulling your feet toward you. This way you combine the advantages of active stretching—safety and the relaxation reflex—with those of passive stretching—greater range of motion. People who are just beginning flexibility training may be better off doing active rather than passive stretches. For PNF techniques, it is particularly important to have a knowledgeable partner.

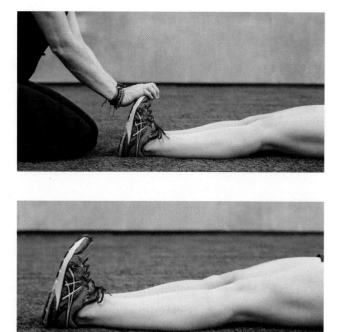

(top and bottom), Courtesy of Paula J Gorman

In passive stretching (top), an outside force—such as pressure exerted by another person—helps move the joint and stretch the muscles. In active stretching (bottom), the force to move the joint and stretch the muscles is provided by a contraction of the opposing muscles.

CAREER OPTIONS IN...

FLEXIBILITY

Instructing: yoga, tai chi, sport-related coaching

Rehabilitation: therapeutic assistant, kinesiologist, recreation therapy

Self-Employed: flexibility workshop presenter, life balance trainer

SOURCE: Physical and Health Education Canada (http://www.phecanada.ca).

Making Progress

As with any type of training, you will make progress and improve your flexibility if you stick with your program. Judge your progress by simply noting your body position while stretching. For example, note how far you can lean forward during a modified hurdler stretch. Repeat the assessment tests that appear in Lab 5.1 periodically and be sure to take the test at the same time of day each time. You will likely notice some improvement after only two to three weeks of stretching, but you may need at least two months to attain significant improvements. By then, you can expect flexibility increases of about 10–20% in many joints.

LO5 Exercises to Improve Flexibility: A Sample Program

There are hundreds of exercises that can improve flexibility. Your program should include exercises that work all the major joints of the body by stretching their associated muscles (refer back to Figure 5.2). The exercises illustrated in the next section are simple to do and pose a minimum risk of injury. Use these exercises to create a well-rounded program for developing flexibility. Be sure to perform each stretch using the proper technique. Hold each position for 15 to 30 seconds and perform two to four repetitions of each exercise. Complete Lab 5.2 when you are ready to start your program.

Fitness Tip

Many people have stopped stretching after hearing mixed results from research studies. This may be a mistake. Stretching after an intense workout can relieve soreness, in addition to providing all the other benefits listed here.

Flexibility Exercises

Mc Graw Hill Education **connect**

Exercise 1

Head Turns and Tilts

Area stretched: Neck

Instructions: *Head turns:* Turn your head to the right and hold the stretch. Repeat to the left. *Head tilts:* Tilt your head to the left and hold the stretch. Repeat to the right.

Variation: Place your right palm on your right cheek; try to turn your head to the right as you resist with your hand. Repeat on the left side.

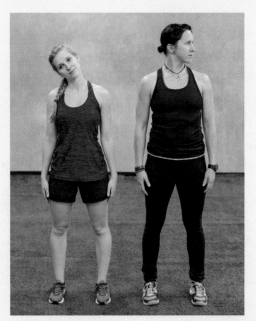

Courtesy of Paula J Gorman

Exercise 2

Towel Stretch

Areas stretched: Triceps, shoulders and chest

Instructions: Roll up a towel and grasp it with both hands, palms down. With your arms straight, slowly lift it back over your head as far as possible. The closer together your hands are, the greater the stretch.

Variation: Repeat the stretch with your arms down and the towel behind your back. Grasp the towel with your palms forward and thumbs pointing out. Gently raise your arms behind your back. This exercise can also be done without a towel.

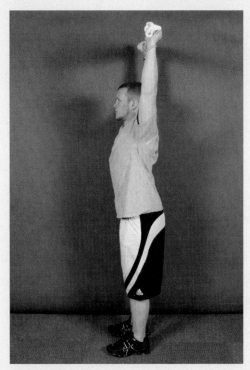

© Wayne Glusker

Exercise 3

Across-the-Body and Overhead Stretches

Areas stretched: Shoulders, upper back, back of the arm (triceps)

Instructions:

(photo a) Keeping your back straight, cross your right arm in front of your body and grasp it with your left hand. Stretch your arm, shoulders, and back by gently pulling your arm as close to your body as possible. Hold.

(photo b) Bend your right arm over your head, placing your right elbow as close to your right ear as possible. Grasp your right elbow with your left hand over your head. Stretch the back of your arm by gently pulling your right elbow back and toward your head. Hold. Repeat both stretches on your left side.

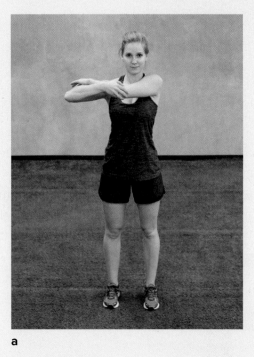
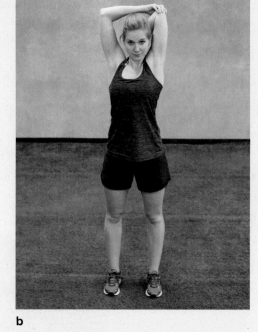

a   b

Courtesy of Paula J Gorman

Exercise 4

Upper-Back Stretch

Areas stretched: Upper back

Instructions: Stand with your feet shoulder-width apart, knees slightly bent, and pelvis tucked under. Lace your fingers in front of your body and press your palms forward.

Variation: In the same position, wrap your arms around your body as if you were giving yourself a hug.

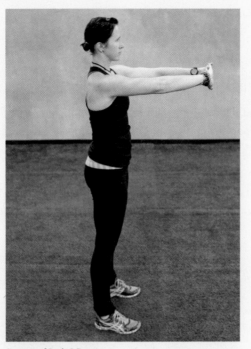

Courtesy of Paula J Gorman

Exercise 5

Lateral Stretch

Areas stretched: Trunk muscles

Instructions: Stand with your feet shoulder-width apart, knees slightly bent, and pelvis tucked under. Raise one arm over your head and bend sideways from the waist. Support your trunk by placing the hand or forearm of your other arm on your thigh or hip for support. Be sure you bend directly sideways and don't move your body below the waist. Repeat on the other side.

Variation: Perform the same exercise in a seated position.

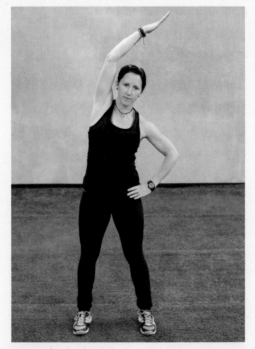

Courtesy of Paula J Gorman

Exercise 6

Step Stretch

Areas stretched: Hip, front of thigh (quadriceps)

Instructions: Step forward and flex your forward knee, keeping your knee directly above your ankle. Stretch your other leg back so that it is parallel to the floor. Press your hips forward and down to stretch. Your arms can be at your sides, on top of your knee, or on the ground for balance. Repeat on the other side.

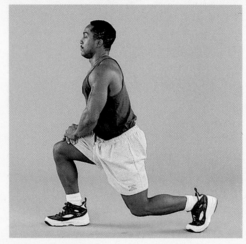

Courtesy Neil A. Tanner

Exercise 7

Side Lunge

Areas stretched: Inner thigh, hip, calf

Instructions: Stand in a wide straddle with your legs turned out from your hip joints and your hands on your thighs. Lunge to one side by bending one knee and keeping the other leg straight. Keep your knee directly over your ankle; do not bend it more than 90 degrees. Repeat on the other side.

Variation: In the same position, lift the heel of the bent knee to provide additional stretch. The exercise may also be performed with your hands on the floor for balance.

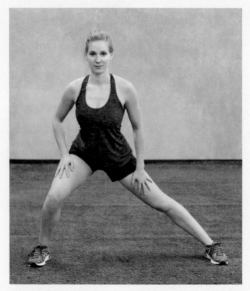

Courtesy of Paula J Gorman

Exercise 8

Inner Thigh Stretch

Areas stretched: Inner thigh, hip

Instructions: Sit with the soles of your feet together. Push your knees toward the floor using your hands or forearms.

Variation: When you first begin to push your knees toward the floor, use your legs to resist the movement. Then, relax and press your knees down as far as they will go.

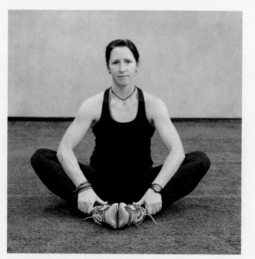

Courtesy of Paula J Gorman

Exercise 9

Hip and Trunk Stretch

Areas stretched: Trunk, outer thigh and hip, buttocks, lower back

Instructions: Sit with your left leg straight, right leg bent and crossed over the left knee, and right hand on the floor next to your right hip. Turn your trunk as far as possible to the right by pushing against your right leg with your left forearm or elbow. Keep your right foot on the floor. Repeat on the other side.

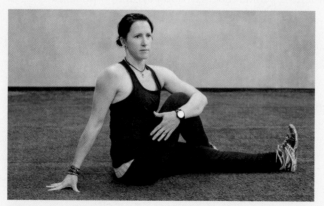

Courtesy of Paula J Gorman

Exercise 10

Modified Hurdler Stretch (Seated Single-Leg Hamstring)

Areas stretched: Back of the thigh (hamstring), lower back

Instructions: Sit with your left leg straight and your right leg tucked close to your body. Reach toward your left foot as far as possible. Repeat for the other leg.

Variation: As you stretch forward, alternately flex and point the foot of your extended leg.

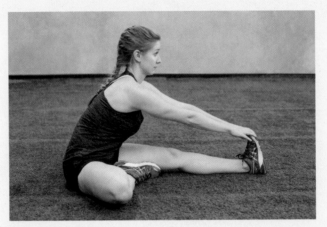

Courtesy of Paula J Gorman

Exercise 11

Alternate Leg Stretcher

Areas stretched: Back of the thigh (hamstring), hip, knee, ankle, buttocks

Instructions: Lie flat on your back with both legs straight.

> **(photo a)** Grasp your left leg behind the thigh and pull in to your chest.

> **(photo b)** Hold this position, and then extend your left leg toward the ceiling.

> **(photo c)** Hold this position, and then bring your left knee back to your chest and pull your toes toward your shin with your left hand. Stretch the back of the leg by attempting to straighten your knee. Repeat for the other leg.

Variation: Perform the stretch on both legs at the same time.

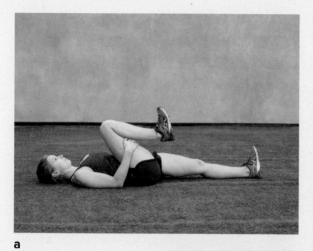

a

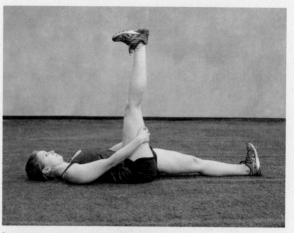

b

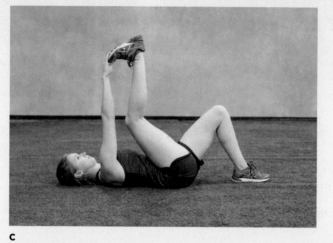

c

Courtesy of Paula J Gorman

Exercise 12

Lower-Leg Stretch

Areas stretched: Back of the lower leg (calf, soleus, Achilles tendon)

Instructions: Stand with one foot about 30 to 50 cm in front of the other, with both feet pointing forward.

    (photo a) Keeping your back leg straight, lunge forward by bending your front knee and pushing your rear heel backward. Hold.

    (photo b) Then, pull your back foot in slightly, and bend your back knee. Shift your weight to your back leg. Hold. Repeat on the other side.

Variation: Place your hands on a wall and extend one foot back, pressing your heel down to stretch; or stand with the balls of your feet on a step or bench and allow your heels to drop below the level of your toes.

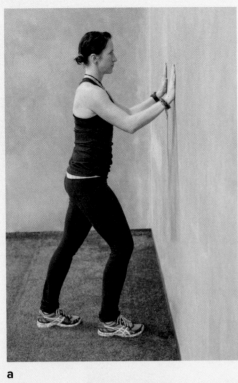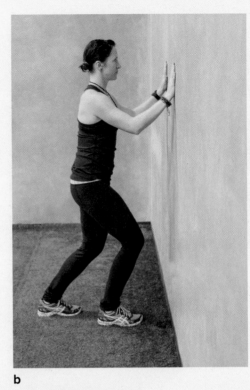

a   b

Courtesy of Paula J Gorman

Exercise 13

Single-Leg Deadlift

Areas stretched: Stretches and loads the hamstrings and glute muscles both eccentrically and concentrically (lengthening and shortening contractions)

Instructions: Start with a dumbbell or kettlebell placed slightly outside the foot of one leg. Bend down to the weight by hinging at the hips and bending at the knee. Your other leg should be bent and relaxed. Pick up the weight and tighten your body and extend the hip and knee as you stand straight, locking out your hip and contracting your glute. Repeat with the other leg.

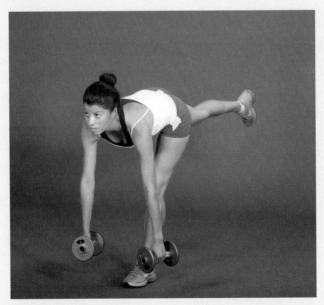

© Taylor Robertson Photography

LO6 5.4 Preventing and Managing Low-Back Pain

Approximately two-thirds of Canadians experience back pain in a given year and of those who are working, about 15% take time off work as a result of their back pain. Low-back pain is estimated to cost as much as $12 billion a year in Canada in direct costs such as treatment and rehabilitation alone.[6]

Back pain can result from sudden traumatic injuries, but it is more often the long-term result of weak and inflexible muscles, poor posture, or poor body mechanics during activities like lifting and carrying. Any abnormal strain on the back can result in pain. Most cases of low-back pain clear up within a few weeks or months, but some people have recurrences or suffer from chronic pain.

Function and Structure of the Spine

The spinal column performs many important functions in the body, including the following:

- Provides structural support for the body, especially the thorax (upper-body cavity).
- Surrounds and protects the spinal cord.
- Supports much of the body's weight and transmits it to the lower body.
- Serves as an attachment site for a large number of muscles, tendons, and ligaments.
- Allows movement of the neck and back in all directions.

The spinal column is made up of bones called **vertebrae** that provide structural support to the body and protect the spinal cord (Figure 5.3 on the next page). The spine consists of 7 cervical vertebrae in the neck, 12 thoracic vertebrae in the upper back, and 5 lumbar vertebrae in the lower back. The nine vertebrae at the base of the spine are fused into two sections and form the sacrum and the coccyx (tailbone). The spine has four curves: the cervical, thoracic, lumbar, and sacral curves. These curves help bring the body weight supported by the spine in line with the axis of the body.

> **vertebrae** Bony segments composing the spinal column that provide structural support for the body and protect the spinal cord.

Although the structure of vertebrae depends on their location on the spine, the different types of vertebrae share common characteristics. Each consists of a body, an arch, and several bony processes (Figure 5.4 on the next page). The vertebral body is cylindrical, with flattened surfaces where **intervertebral disks** are attached. The vertebral body is designed to carry the stress of body weight and physical activity. The vertebral arch surrounds and protects the spinal cord. The bony processes serve as joints for adjacent vertebrae and attachment sites for muscles and ligaments. **Nerve roots** from the spinal cord pass through notches in the vertebral arch.

> **intervertebral disks** Elastic disks located between adjoining vertebrae, consisting of a gel- and water-filled nucleus surrounded by fibrous rings; they serve as a shock absorbers for the spinal column.
>
> **nerve roots** The bases of each of the 31 pairs of spinal nerves that branch off the spinal cord through spaces between vertebrae.

Intervertebral disks, which absorb and disperse the stresses placed on the spine, separate vertebrae from each other. Disks are made up of a gel- and water-filled nucleus surrounded by a series of fibrous rings. The liquid nucleus can change shape when it is compressed, allowing the disk to absorb shock. The intervertebral disks also help maintain the spaces between vertebrae where the spinal nerve roots are located.

FIGURE 5.3

The spinal column. The spine is made up of five separate regions and has four distinct curves. An intervertebral disk is located between adjoining vertebrae.

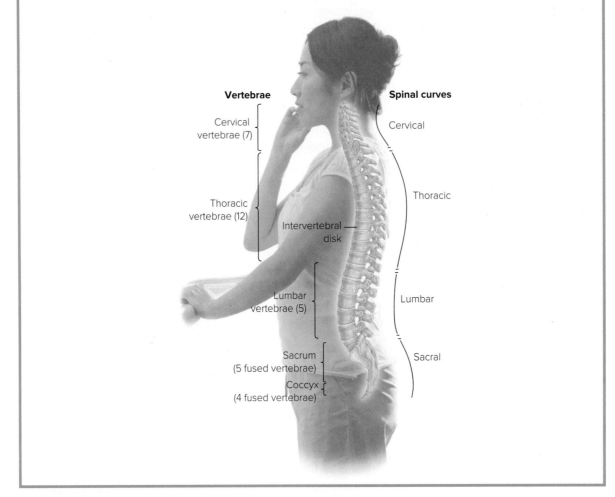

FIGURE 5.4

Vertebrae and an intervertebral disk.

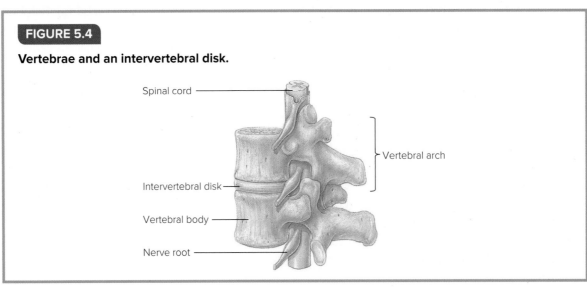

Core Muscle Fitness

The **core muscles** are the trunk muscles extending from the hips to the upper back, including those in the abdomen, pelvic floor, sides of the trunk, back, buttocks, hip, and pelvis (Figure 5.5). There muscles are attached to the ribs, hips, spinal column, and other bones in the trunk of the body. The core muscles stabilize the spine and help transfer force between the upper body and lower body. They also stabilize the midsection when you sit, stand, reach, walk, jump, twist, squat, throw, or bend. The muscles on the front, back, and sides of your trunk support your spine when you sit in a chair and they fix your midsection as you use your legs to stand up. When hitting a forehand in tennis or batting a softball, most of the force is transferred from the legs and hips, across the core muscles, to the arms. Strong core muscles make movements more forceful and help prevent back pain.

core muscles   The trunk muscles extending from the hips to the upper back.

Major core muscles.

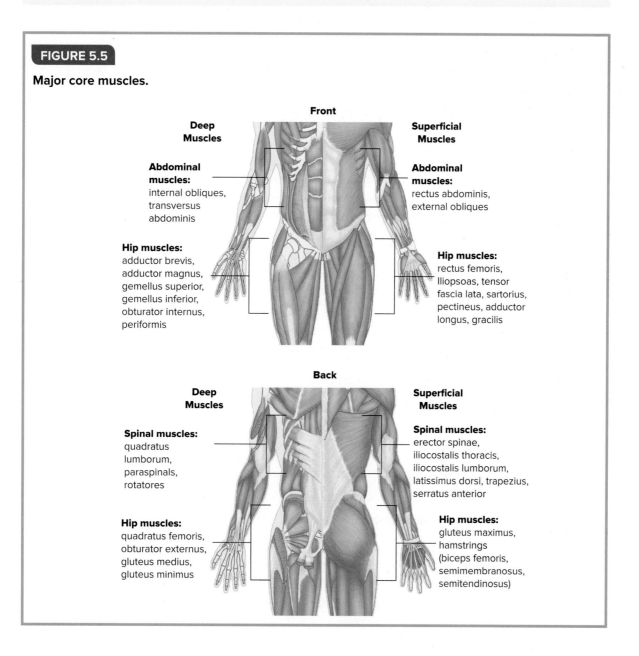

Front

Deep Muscles

Abdominal muscles:
internal obliques, transversus abdominis

Hip muscles:
adductor brevis, adductor magnus, gemellus superior, gemellus inferior, obturator internus, periformis

Superficial Muscles

Abdominal muscles:
rectus abdominis, external obliques

Hip muscles:
rectus femoris, Iliopsoas, tensor fascia lata, sartorius, pectineus, adductor longus, gracilis

Back

Deep Muscles

Spinal muscles:
quadratus lumborum, paraspinals, rotatores

Hip muscles:
quadratus femoris, obturator externus, gluteus medius, gluteus minimus

Superficial Muscles

Spinal muscles:
erector spinae, iliocostalis thoracis, iliocostalis lumborum, latissimus dorsi, trapezius, serratus anterior

Hip muscles:
gluteus maximus, hamstrings (biceps femoris, semimembranosus, semitendinosus)

During any dynamic movement, the core muscles work together; some shorten to cause movement, while others contract and hold to provide stability, lengthen to brake the movement, or send signals to the brain about the movements and positions of the muscles and bones (proprioception). When specific core muscles are weak or tired, the nervous system steps in and uses other muscles. This substitution causes abnormal stresses on the joints, decreases power, and increases the risk of injury.

The best exercises for low-back health are whole-body exercises that force the core muscles to stabilize the spine in many different directions. The low-back exercises presented later in this chapter include several exercises that focus on the core muscles, including the step stretch (lunge), side bridges, and spine extensions. These exercises are generally safe for beginning exercisers and, with physician approval, people with some back pain. More challenging core exercises use stability balls or free weights. Stability ball exercises require the core muscles to stabilize the ball (and the body) while performing nearly any type of exercise. Many traditional exercises with free weights can strengthen the core muscles if done in a standing position. Weight machines train muscles in isolation, while exercises with free weights done while standing help train the body for real-world movements—an essential principle of core training.

Fitness Tip

Swiss ball exercises are great for building core muscles. Swiss ball training increases trunk flexion and extension, strength, abdominal endurance, lower back flexibility, and balance.

Causes of Back Pain

Back pain can occur at any point along your spine. The lumbar area, because it bears the majority of your weight, is the most common site. Any movement that causes excessive stress on the spinal column can result in injury and pain. The spine is well equipped to bear body weight and the force or stress of body movements along its long axis. However, it is less capable of bearing loads at an angle to its long axis or when the trunk is flexed (bent). You do not have to carry a heavy load or participate in a vigorous contact sport to injure your back. Picking a pencil up from the floor using poor body mechanics—reaching too far out in front of you or bending over with your knees straight, for example—can also result in back pain. Risk factors associated with low-back pain include:

- age greater than 34 years
- degenerative diseases such as arthritis or osteoporosis
- a family or personal history of back pain or trauma
- a sedentary lifestyle
- low job satisfaction
- low socioeconomic status[7]
- smoking, which increases risk because it appears to increase degenerative changes in the spine
- excess body weight, which increases strain on the back
- psychological stress or depression, which can cause muscle tension and back pain
- occupations and activities that involve physically hard work, such as frequent lifting, twisting, bending, standing up, or straining in forced positions; those requiring high concentration demands (such as computer programming); and those involving vibrations affecting the entire body (such as truck driving)

Underlying causes of back pain include poor muscle endurance and strength in the muscles of the abdomen, back, hips, and legs; excess body weight; poor posture or body position when standing, sitting, or sleeping; and poor body mechanics when performing actions like lifting and carrying, or sports movements. Strained muscles, tendons, or ligaments can cause pain and can, over time, lead to injuries to vertebrae or the intervertebral disks.

Physical stress can cause disks to break down and lose some of their ability to absorb shock. A damaged disk may bulge out between vertebrae and put pressure on a nerve root, a condition commonly referred to as a *slipped* or *herniated disk.* Painful pressure on nerves can also occur if damage to a disk narrows the space between two vertebrae. With age, you lose fluid from the disks, making them more likely to bulge and put pressure on nerve roots. Depending on the amount of pressure on a nerve, symptoms may include numbness in the back, hip, leg, or foot; radiating pain; loss of muscle function; depressed reflexes; and muscle spasm. If the pressure is severe enough, loss of function can be permanent.

Preventing Low-Back Pain

Incorrect posture is responsible for many back injuries. Strategies for maintaining good posture during daily activities are presented in the box Good Posture and Low-Back Health. You can follow the same guidelines for posture and movement when you engage in sports or recreational activities. Make sure to control your movements and warm up thoroughly before you exercise, and take special care when lifting weights.

The role of exercise in preventing and treating back pain is still being investigated. However, many experts do recommend exercise, especially for people who have already experienced an episode of low-back pain. Regular exercise aimed at increasing muscle endurance and strength in the back and abdomen is often recommended to prevent back pain, as is lifestyle physical activity such as walking. Movement helps lubricate your spinal disks and increases muscle fitness in your trunk and legs. Other lifestyle recommendations for preventing back pain include the following:

- Maintain a healthy weight. Excess fat contributes to poor posture, which can place harmful stress on the spine.
- Stop smoking.
- Reduce stress.
- Avoid sitting, standing, or working in the same position for too long. Stand up every hour or half-hour and move around.
- Use a supportive seat and a medium-firm mattress.
- Use lumbar support when driving, particularly for long distances, to prevent back muscle fatigue and pain.
- Warm up thoroughly before exercising.
- Progress gradually when attempting to improve strength or fitness.

Take CHARGE

GOOD POSTURE AND LOW-BACK HEALTH

Changes in everyday posture and behaviour can help prevent and alleviate low-back pain.

- **Lying down.** When resting or sleeping, lie on your side with your knees and hips bent. If you lie on your back, place a pillow under your knees. Don't lie on your stomach. Use a medium-firm mattress.

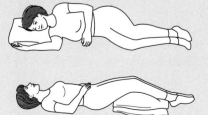

continued

- **Sitting at a computer.** Sit in a slightly reclined position of 100 to 110 degrees, not an upright 90-degree position. Adjust your chair so your knees are slightly lower than your hips. If your back flattens as you sit, try using a lumbar roll to maintain your back's natural curvature. Place your feet flat on the floor or on a footrest. Place the monitor directly in front of you and adjust it so your eyes are level with the top of the screen; you should be looking slightly downward at the middle of the screen. Adjust the keyboard and mouse so your forearms and wrists are in a neutral position, parallel with the floor.

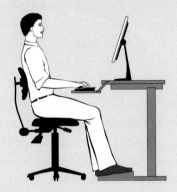

- **Lifting.** If you need to lower yourself to grasp an object, bend at the knees and hips rather than at the waist. Your feet should be about shoulder-width apart. Lift gradually, keeping your arms straight, by standing up or by pushing with your leg muscles. Keep the object close to your body. Don't twist; change the position of your feet so that you pivot your body as a whole rather than twisting at your waist or shoulders.

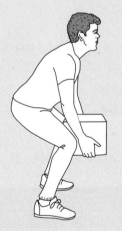

- **Standing**. When you are standing, a straight line should run from the top of your ear through the centre of your shoulder, the centre of your hip, the back of your kneecap, and the front of your ankle bone. Support your weight mainly on your heels, with one or both knees slightly bent. Don't let your pelvis tip forward or your back arch. Shift your weight back and forth from foot to foot. Avoid prolonged standing.

    To check your posture, stand in a normal way with your back to a wall. Your upper back and buttocks should touch the wall; your heels may be a several centimetres away. Slide one hand into the space between your lower back and the wall. It should slide in easily but should almost touch both your back and the wall. Adjust your posture as needed, and try to hold this position as you walk away from the wall.

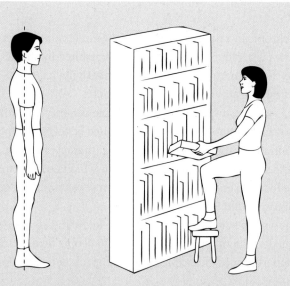

- **Walking.** Walk with your toes pointed straight ahead. Keep your back flat, head up and centred over your body, and chin in. Swing your arms freely. Don't wear tight or high-heeled shoes. Walking briskly is better for back health than walking slowly.

Managing Acute Back Pain

Sudden (acute) back pain usually involves tissue injury. Symptoms may include pain, muscles spasms, stiffness, and inflammation. Many cases of acute back pain go away by themselves within a few days or weeks. However, in some cases you may have to actively treat the symptoms with one or more of the following recommendations:

- You may be able to reduce pain and inflammation by applying cold and then heat. Begin with a cold treatment and apply ice several times a day. Once inflammation and spasms subside, apply heat using a heating pad or a warm bath.

- If the pain is bothersome, an over-the-counter, nonsteroidal anti-inflammatory medication such as ibuprofen or naproxen may be helpful; stronger pain medications and muscle relaxants are available by prescription.

- Bed rest immediately following the onset of back pain may make you feel better, but it should be of very short duration. Prolonged bed rest—five days or more—was once thought to be an effective treatment for back pain, but most physicians now advise against it because it may weaken muscles and actually worsen pain. Limit bed rest to one day and begin moderate physical activity as soon as possible.

- Exercise can increase muscular endurance and flexibility and protect your disks from loss of fluid. Three of the back exercises discussed later in the chapter may be particularly helpful following an episode of acute back pain: curl-ups, side bridges, and back extensions.

See your physician if acute back pain doesn't resolve within a short time. Other warning signals of a more severe problem that requires a professional evaluation include severe pain, numbness, pain that radiates down one or both legs, problems with bladder or bowel control, fever, or rapid weight loss.

Managing Chronic Back Pain

Low-back pain is considered chronic if it persists for more than three months. Symptoms vary—some people experience stabbing or shooting pain, others a steady ache accompanied by stiffness. Sometimes pain is localized; in other cases, it radiates to another part of the body. Underlying causes of chronic back pain include injuries, infection, muscle or ligament strains, and disk herniations.

Because symptoms and causes are so varied, different people benefit from different treatment strategies, and researchers have found that many treatments have only limited benefits. Potential treatments may include over-the-counter or prescription medications; exercise; physical therapy, massage, or chiropractic care; acupuncture; percutaneous electrical nerve stimulation (PENS), in which acupuncture-like needles are used to deliver an electrical current; education and advice about posture, exercise, and body mechanics; and surgery (see the box Yoga for Relaxation and Pain Relief).

Psychological therapy may also be beneficial in some cases. Reducing emotional stress that causes muscle tension can provide direct benefits, and other therapies can help people deal better with chronic pain and its effects on their daily lives. Support groups and expressive writing are beneficial for people with chronic pain and other conditions.

In FOCUS

YOGA FOR RELAXATION AND PAIN RELIEF

Exercise, such as yoga and tai chi, can provide relief from back pain, depending on the pain's underlying cause. Effective exercises stretch the muscles and connective tissue in the hips, stabilize the spine, and strengthen and build endurance in the core muscles of the back and abdomen.

Yoga may be an option for many back pain sufferers because it offers a variety of exercises that target the spine and the core muscles. Yoga is an ancient practice involving slow, gentle movements performed with controlled breathing and focused attention. Yoga practitioners slowly move into a specific posture (called an asana) and hold the posture for up to 60 seconds. There are hundreds of asanas, many of which are easy to do and provide good stretches.

Yoga also involves simple breathing exercises that gently stretch the muscles of the upper back while helping the practitioner focus. Yoga experts say that breathing exercises not only encourage relaxation, but also clear the mind and can help relieve mild to moderate pain. Yoga enthusiasts end their workouts energized and refreshed, but also calm and relaxed.

Many medical professionals now recommend yoga for patients with back pain, particularly postures that involve arching and gently stretching the back, such as the cat pose (similar to the cat stretch shown in the "Low-Back Exercises" section of this chapter). These are basic asanas that most people can perform repeatedly and hold for a relatively long time.

Because asanas must be performed correctly to be beneficial, qualified instruction is recommended. For those with back pain, physicians advise choosing an instructor who is not only accomplished in yoga, but also knowledgeable about back pain and its causes. Such instructors can steer students away from exercises that do more harm than good. It is especially important to choose postures that will benefit the back without worsening the underlying problem. Some asanas can aggravate an injured or painful back if they are performed incorrectly or too aggressively. In fact, a few yoga postures should not be done at all by people with back pain.

If you have back pain, see your physician to determine its cause before beginning any type of exercise program. Even gentle exercise or stretching can be bad for an already injured back, especially if the spinal disks or nerves are involved. For some back conditions, rest or therapy may be better options than exercise, at least in the short term.

Wellness Tip

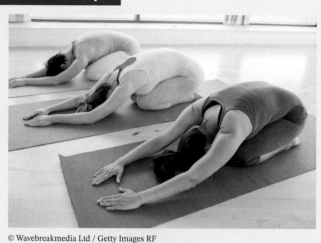

Wellness Tip When practising yoga, it is important to choose postures, such as this child pose, that will benefit the back without worsening the underlying problem. Some asanas can aggravate an injured or painful back if they are performed incorrectly or too aggressively. In fact, people with back pain should avoid a few yoga postures, such as a standing forward bend.

© Wavebreakmedia Ltd / Getty Images RF

Exercises for the Prevention and Management of Low-Back Pain

The tests in Labs 5.3 and 5.4 can help you assess low-back muscular endurance. The exercises in the following section are designed to help you maintain a healthy back by stretching and strengthening the major muscle groups that affect the back—the abdominal muscles, the muscles along your spine and sides, and the muscles of your hips and thighs. If you have back problems, check with your physician before beginning any exercise program. Perform the exercises slowly and progress very gradually. Stop and consult your physician if any exercise causes back pain. General guidelines for back exercise programs include the following:

- Do low-back exercises at least three days per week. Most experts recommend daily back exercises.
- Emphasize muscular endurance rather than muscular strength—endurance is more protective.
- Don't do spine exercises involving a full range of motion early in the morning. Because your disks have a high fluid content early in the day, injuries may result.
- Engage in regular endurance exercise such as cycling or walking in addition to performing exercises that specifically build muscular endurance and flexibility. Brisk walking with a vigorous arm swing may help relieve back pain. Start with fast walking if your core muscles are weak or you have back pain.
- Be patient and stick with your program. Increased back fitness and pain relief may require as long as three months of regular exercise.
- Always use good form and stop if you feel pain. The adage "no pain, no gain" does not apply to back exercises.
- Build core stiffness through stabilization exercises; they strengthen muscles, improve muscular endurance, reduce low back pain, and boost sports performance. Greater core stiffness also transfers strength and speed to the limbs, increases the load bearing capacity of the spine, and protects the internal organs during sports movements. When working on abdominal muscles, emphasize stabilization exercises, such as side-bridges, carry exercises, planks, bird-dogs, and the "stir-the-pot" exercise rather than spinal flexion exercises such as sit-ups. Poor performance on the spinal endurance activities (see Lab 5.3) means that you are not training your abdominal muscles correctly.

Low-Back Exercises

connect

Exercise 1

Cat Stretch

Target: Improved flexibility, relaxation, and reduced stiffness in the spine

Instructions: Begin on all fours with your knees below your hips and your hands below your shoulders. Slowly and deliberately move through a cycle of extension and flexion of your spine.

- Begin by slowly pushing your back up and dropping your head slightly until your spine is extended (rounded).

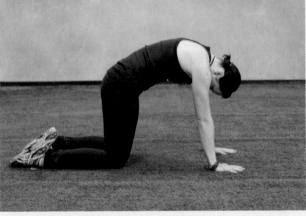

Courtesy of Paula J Gorman

- Then, slowly lower your back and lift your chin slightly until your spine is flexed (relaxed and slightly arched). *Do not press at the ends of the range of motion.* Stop if you feel pain. Do 10 slow, continuous cycles of the movement.

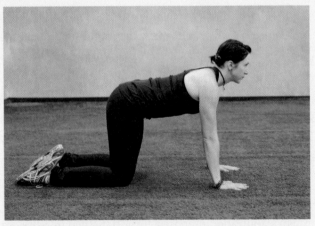

Courtesy of Paula J Gorman

Exercise 2

Step Stretch

(see Exercise 6 in Flexibility Exercises)

Target: Improved flexibility, strength, and endurance in the muscles of the hip and the front of the thigh

Instructions: Hold each stretch for 10 to 30 seconds and do 2 to 4 repetitions on each side.

Exercise 3

Alternate Leg Stretcher

(see Exercise 11 in Flexibility Exercises)

Target: Improved flexibility in the back of the thigh, hip, knee, and buttocks

Instructions: Hold each stretch for 10 to 30 seconds and do 2 to 4 repetitions on each side.

Exercise 4

Trunk Twist

Target: Improved flexibility in the lower back and sides

Instructions: Lie on your side with top knee bent, lower leg straight, lower arm extended out in front of you on the floor, and upper arm at your side. Push down with your upper knee while you twist your trunk backward. Try to get your shoulders and upper body flat on the floor, turning your head as well. Return to the starting position, and then repeat on the other side. Hold the stretch for 10 to 30 seconds and do 2 to 4 repetitions on each side.

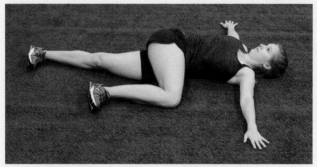

Courtesy of Paula J Gorman

Exercise 5

Curl-Up

(see Exercise 4 in the Body Weight section in Chapter 4)

Target: Improved strength and endurance in the abdomen

Variation: Add a twist to develop other abdominal muscles. When you have curled up so that your shoulder blades are off the floor, twist your upper body so that one shoulder is higher than the other; reach past your knee with your upper arm. Hold and then return to the starting position. Repeat on the opposite side. Curl-ups can also be done using an exercise ball.

Exercise 6

Isometric Side Bridge

(see Exercise 6 in the Body Weight sectionin Chapter 4)

Target: Increased strength and endurance in the muscles along the sides of the abdomen

Instructions: Hold the bridge position for 10 seconds, breathing normally. Work up to a 60-second hold. Perform one or more repetitions on each side.

Variation: You can make the exercise more difficult by keeping your legs straight and supporting yourself with your feet and forearm (see Lab 5.3) or with your feet and hand (with elbow straight).

Exercise 7

Spine Extensions

(see Exercise 5 in the Body Weight section in Chapter 4)

Target: Increased strength and endurance in the back, buttocks, and back of the thighs

Instructions: Hold each position for 10 to 30 seconds. Begin with one repetition on each side and work up to several repetitions.

Variation: If you have experienced back pain in the past or if this exercise is very difficult for you, do the exercise with both hands on the ground rather than with one arm lifted. You can make this exercise more difficult by doing it while balancing on an exercise ball. Find a balance point on your chest while lying face down on the ball with one arm and the opposite leg on the ground. Tense your abdominal muscles while reaching and extending with one arm and reaching and extending with the opposite leg. Repeat this exercise using the other arm and leg.

Exercise 8

Wall Squat (Phantom Chair)

Target: Increased strength and endurance in the lower back, thighs, and abdomen

Instructions: Lean against a wall and bend your knees as though you are sitting in a chair. Support your weight with your legs. Begin by holding the position for 5 to 10 seconds. Build up to 1 minute or more. Perform one or more repetitions.

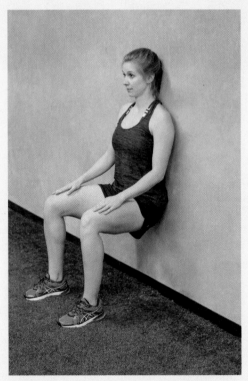

Courtesy Neil A. Tanner

Exercise 9

Pelvic Tilt

Target: Increased strength and endurance in the abdomen and buttocks

Instructions: Lie on your back with knees bent and arms extended to the side. Tilt your pelvis under and try to flatten your lower back against the floor. Tighten your buttock and abdominal muscles while you hold this position for 5 to 10 seconds. Don't hold your breath. Work up to 10 repetitions of the exercise. Pelvic tilts can also be done standing or leaning against a wall.

Note: *Although this is a popular exercise with many therapists, some experts question the safety of pelvic tilts. Stop if you feel pain in your back at any time during the exercise.*

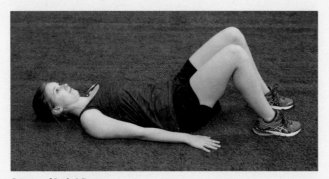

Courtesy of Paula J Gorman

Exercise 10

Back Bridge

Target: Increased strength and endurance in the hips and buttocks

Instructions: Lie on your back with knees bent and arms extended to the side. Tuck your pelvis under, and then lift your tailbone, buttocks, and lower back from the floor. Hold this position for 5 to 10 seconds with your weight resting on your feet, arms, and shoulders, and then return to the starting position. Work up to 10 repetitions of the exercise.

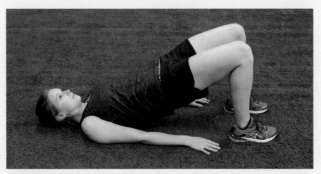

Courtesy of Paula J Gorman

Exercise 11

Stir the Pot

Target: Increased strength and endurance in the core muscles and shoulders.

Instructions: Assume a plank position on an exercise ball, with forearms on the ball and legs extended to the rear. Maintaining a stiff torso and neutral spine, rotate on the ball in a clockwise direction for 10 repetitions, and then repeat in a counterclockwise direction for 10 repetitions.

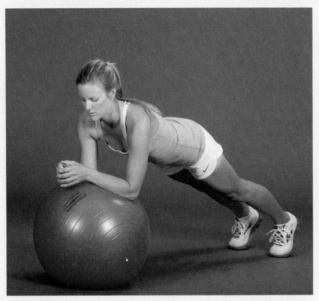

© Taylor Robertson Photography

Exercise 12

Kettlebell or Dumbbell Carry (Suitcase Carry)

Target: Core muscles, trapezius, leg and hip muscles

Instructions: This is an excellent exercise for building the core muscles. Pick up a dumbbell or kettlebell in one or both hands. Maintaining good posture, walk 20 to 100 metres carrying the weights. Carry 5 to a few hundred kilograms, depending on your fitness.

Tips for Today and the Future ✓

To improve and maintain your flexibility, perform stretches that work the major joints at least twice a week.

RIGHT NOW YOU CAN

- Stand up and stretch—do either the upper-back stretch or the across-the-body stretch shown in the chapter.

- Practise the recommended sitting and standing postures suggested in the chapter. If needed, adjust your chair or find something to use as a footrest.

IN THE FUTURE YOU CAN

- Build up your flexibility by incorporating more sophisticated stretching exercises into your routine.

- Increase the frequency of your flexibility workouts to five or more days per week.

- Increase the efficiency of your workouts by adding stretching exercises to the cool-down period of your endurance or strength workouts.

Common Questions ANSWERED

Q Is stretching the same as warming up?

A No. They are two distinct activities. A warm-up involves moving the joints through the same motions used during the activity; it increases body temperature so your metabolism works better when you're exercising at high intensity. Stretching increases the movement capability of your joints so you can move more easily with less risk of injury. It is best to stretch at the end of your aerobic or weight training workout, when your muscles are warm. Warmed muscles stretch better than cold ones and are less prone to injury.

Q How much flexibility do I need?

A This question is not always easy to answer. If you're involved in a sport such as gymnastics, figure skating, or ballet, you are often required to reach extreme joint motions to achieve success. However, nonathletes do not need to reach these extreme joint positions. In fact, too much flexibility may, in some cases, increase your risk of injury. As with other types of fitness, moderation is the key. You should regularly stretch your major joints and muscle groups but not aspire to reach extreme flexibility.

Q Can I stretch too far?

A Yes. As muscle tissue is progressively stretched, it reaches a point where it becomes damaged and may rupture. The greatest danger occurs during passive stretching when a partner is doing the stretching for you. It is critical that your stretching partner not force your joint outside its normal functional range of motion.

Q Can physical training limit flexibility?

A When done properly, weight training increases flexibility. However, because of the limited range of motion used during the running stride, jogging tends to compromise flexibility. It is important for runners to practise flexibility exercises for the hamstrings and quadriceps regularly.

Q Does stretching affect muscular strength?

A Flexibility training increases muscle strength over time, but several recent studies have found that stretching causes short-term decreases in strength, power, and motor control. This is one reason some experts suggest that people not stretch as part of their exercise warm-up, particularly if they plan to engage in a high-performance activity. It is important to warm up before any workout by engaging in 5 to 10 minutes of light exercise, such as walking or slow jogging.

SUMMARY

- Flexibility, the ability of joints to move through their full range of motion, is highly adaptable and specific to each joint.

- Range of motion can be limited by joint structure, muscle inelasticity, and stretch receptor activity.

continued

- The spinal column consists of vertebrae separated by intervertebral disks. It provides structure and support for the body and protects the spinal cord. The core muscles stabilize the spine and transfer force between the upper and lower body.

- Developing flexibility depends on stretching the elastic tissues within muscles regularly and gently until they lengthen. Overstretching can make connective tissue brittle and lead to rupture.

- Signals sent between muscle and tendon nerves and the spinal cord can enhance flexibility.

- The benefits of flexibility include preventing abnormal stresses that lead to joint deterioration and possibly reducing the risk of injuries and low-back pain.

- Stretches should be held for 10 to 30 seconds; perform two to four repetitions. Flexibility training should be done a minimum of two or three days a week (ideally, four to seven days per week), preferably following activity, when muscles are warm.

- Static stretching is done slowly and held to the point of mild tension. Ballistic stretching consists of bouncing stretches and can lead to injury. Dynamic stretching moves joints slowly and fluidly through their range of motions. Proprioceptive neuromuscular facilitation uses muscle receptors in contracting and relaxing a muscle.

- Passive stretching, using an outside force in moving muscles and joints, achieves a greater range of motion (and has a higher injury risk) than active stretching, which uses opposing muscles to initiate a stretch.

- Acute back pain can be treated as a soft tissue injury, with cold treatment followed by application of heat (once swelling subsides); prolonged bed rest is not recommended. A variety of treatments have been suggested for chronic back pain, including regular exercise, physical therapy, acupuncture, education, and psychological therapy.

- In addition to good posture, proper body mechanics, and regular physical activity, a program for preventing low-back pain includes exercises that stretch and strengthen major muscle groups that affect the lower back.

FOR FURTHER EXPLORATION

Organizations and Websites

The Arthritis Society. Includes general information about the role of exercise for those with various forms of arthritis. Also contains an open forum to ask questions of physicians.

http://www.arthritis.ca

Back Fit Pro. Provides evidence-based information on preventing and treating back pain. website is maintained by Dr. Stuart McGill, a professor of spine biomechanics at the University of Waterloo.

http://www.backfitpro.com

Bone and Joint Canada. Promotes the preservation of bone and joint health to improve the health-related quality of life for those with musculo-skeletal disorders.

http://boneandjointcanada.com/

The Canadian Academy of Sports Medicine. Promotes the practice of medicine as it applies to all areas of physical activity.

http://casem-acmse.org/

Canadian Chiropractic Association. Includes information to create awareness about back pain and the role of chiropractors in its treatment. Also provides a questionnaire to assess your risk for suffering low back pain.

http://ccachiro.org

The Canadian Orthopaedic Foundation. Offers information on research, education, and care of those with bone and joint disorders.

http://whenithurtstomove.org/

Canadian Physiotherapy Association. Outlines SMART stretching tips for a variety of activities.

http://www.physiotherapy.ca/

International Yoga Federation. Includes information and resources for yoga organizations around the world.

http://www.internationalyogafederation.net

Mayo Clinic: Focus on Flexibility. Offers an easy-to-use program of basic stretching exercises for beginners, with a focus on the benefits of greater flexibility.

https://www.mayoclinic.org/healthy-lifestyle/fitness/in-depth/stretching/art-20047931

International Fitness Association. Provides information about the physiology of stretching and different types of stretching exercises.

http://www.ifafitness.com/stretch/index.html

See also the listings for Chapter 2 and Chapter 4.

Laboratory Activities

Name _____ Section _____ Date _____

Lab 5.1 Assessing Your Current Level of Flexibility

![McGraw Hill Education] connect®

Part I Sit-and-Reach Test

Equipment

Use a modified Wells and Dillon flexometer or construct your own measuring device using a firm box or two pieces of wood about 30 cm high attached at right angles to each other. Attach a metric ruler to measure the extent of reach. With the low numbers of the ruler toward the person being tested, set the 26-cm mark of the ruler at the footline of the box. (Individuals who cannot reach as far as the footline will have scores below 26 cm; those who can reach past their feet will have scores above 26 cm.) Most studies show no relationship between performance on the sit-and-reach test and the incidence of back pain.

Preparation

Warm up your muscles with a low-intensity activity such as walking or easy jogging. Then perform slow stretching movements.

Instructions

1. Remove your shoes and sit facing the flexibility measuring device with your knees fully extended and your feet flat against the device about 10 cm apart.

2. Reach as far forward as you can, with palms down, arms evenly stretched, and knees fully extended; hold the position of maximum reach for about two seconds.

3. Perform the stretch two times, recording the distance of maximum reach to the nearest 0.5 cm: _____ cm

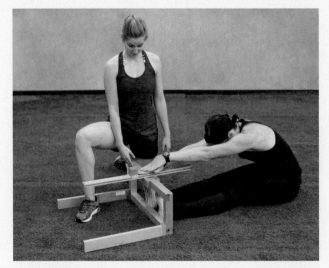

Courtesy of Paula J Gorman

Rating Your Flexibility

Find the score in the following table to determine your flexibility rating. Record it here and at the end of this lab.

Rating: _____

Ratings for Sit-and-Reach Test

		Rating/Score (cm)*				
Men		*Poor*	*Fair*	*Good*	*Very Good*	*Excellent*
Age:	15–19	≤23	24–28	29–33	34–38	≤39
	20–29	≤24	25–29	30–33	34–39	≤40
	30–39	≤22	23–27	28–32	33–37	≤38
	40–49	≤17	18–23	24–28	29–34	≤35
	50–59	≤15	16–23	24–27	28–34	≤35
	60–69	≤14	15–19	20–24	25–32	≤33
Women						
Age:	15–19	≤28	29–33	34–37	38–42	≤43
	20–29	≤27	28–32	33–36	37–40	≤41
	30–39	≤26	27–31	32–35	36–40	≤41
	40–49	≤24	25–29	30–33	34–37	≤38
	50–59	≤24	25–29	30–32	33–38	≤39
	60–69	≤22	23–26	27–30	31–34	≤35

*Footline is set at 26 cm.

Part II Range-of-Motion Assessment

This portion of the lab can be completed by doing visual comparisons or by measuring joint range of motion with a goniometer or other instrument.

Equipment

1. A partner to do visual comparisons or to measure the range of motion of your joints or a mirror to perform your own visual comparisons

2. A goniometer, flexometer, or other instrument to measure range of motion

Preparation

Warm up your muscles with some low-intensity activity such as walking or easy jogging.

Instructions

The average range of motion for some of the major joints is illustrated and listed below. Visually assess the range of motion in your joints and compare it to that shown in the illustrations. For each joint, note (with a check mark) whether your range of motion is above average, average, or below average and in need of improvement. Average values for range of motion are given in degrees for each joint in the assessment. You can also complete the assessment by measuring your range of motion with a goniometer, flexometer, or other instrument. If you are using this measurement method, identify your rating (above average, average, or below average) and record your range of motion in degrees next to the appropriate category. Although the measurement method is more time-consuming, it allows you to track the progress of your stretching program more precisely and to note changes within the broader ratings categories (below average, above average).

Record your ratings below and on the chart at the end of this lab. (Ratings were derived from several published sources.)

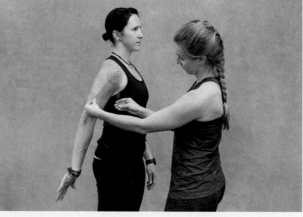

Courtesy of Paula J Gorman

Assessment of range of motion using a goniometer.

1. Shoulder Abduction and Adduction

For each position and arm, check one of the following; also fill in degrees if using the measurement method.

Shoulder abduction—raise arm up to the side

Right	Left	
_____	_____	Below average/needs improvement
_____	_____	Average (92–95°)
_____	_____	Above average

Shoulder adduction—move arm down and in front of body

Right	Left	
_____	_____	Below average/needs improvement
_____	_____	Average (124–127°)
_____	_____	Above average

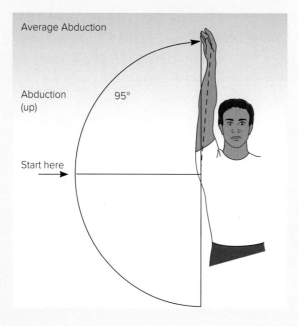

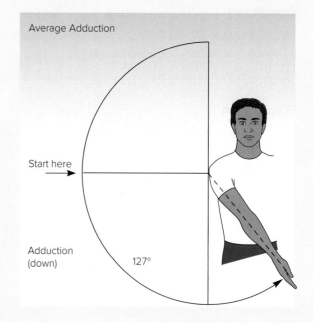

2. Shoulder Flexion and Extension

For each position and arm, check one of the following; also fill in degrees if using the measurement method.

Shoulder flexion—raise arm up in front of the body

Right   Left

_____   _____   Below average/needs improvement

_____   _____   Average (92–95°)

_____   _____   Above average

Shoulder extension—move arm down and behind the body

Right   Left

_____   _____   Below average/needs improvement

_____   _____   Average (145–150°)

_____   _____   Above average

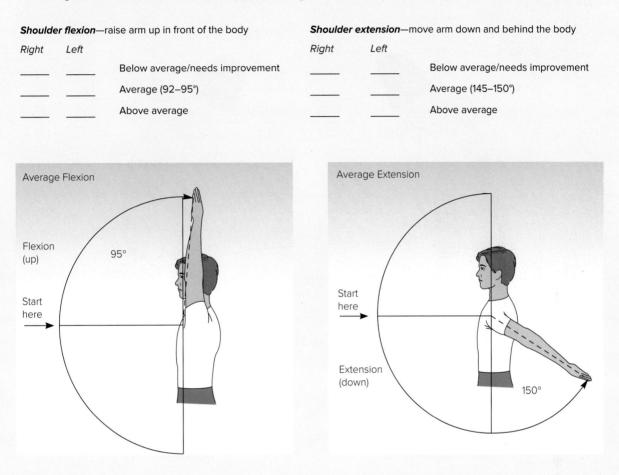

3. Trunk/Low Back Lateral Flexion

Bend directly sideways at your waist. To prevent injury, keep your knees slightly bent and support your trunk by placing your hand or forearm on your thigh. Check one of the following for each side; also fill in degrees if using the measurement method.

Right   Left

_____   _____   Below average/needs improvement

_____   _____   Average (36–40°)

_____   _____   Above average

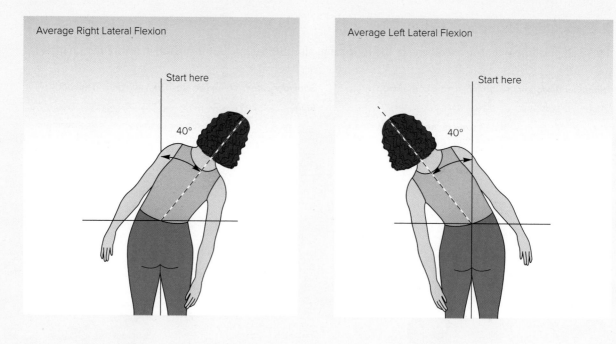

Average Right Lateral Flexion

Start here

40°

Average Left Lateral Flexion

Start here

40°

4. Hip Abduction

Raise your leg to the side at the hip. Check one of the following for each leg; also fill in degrees if using the measurement method.

Right	*Left*	
_____	_____	Below average/needs improvement
_____	_____	Average (40–45°)
_____	_____	Above average

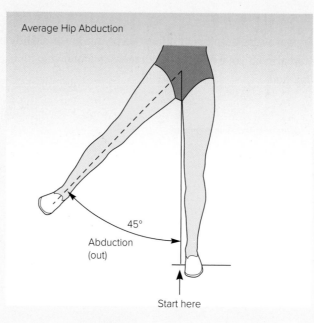

Average Hip Abduction

45°

Abduction
(out)

Start here

5. Hip Flexion (Bent Knee)

With one leg flat on the floor, bend the other knee and lift the leg up at the hip. Check one of the following for each leg; also fill in degrees if using the measurement method.

Right   *Left*

_____   _____   Below average/needs improvement

_____   _____   Average (121–125°)

_____   _____   Above average

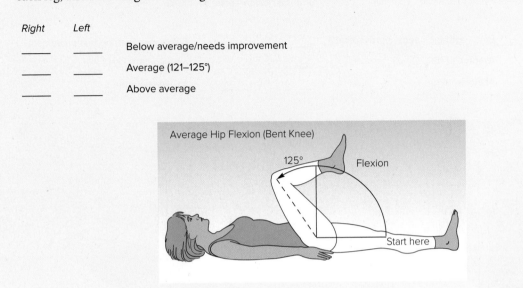

6. Hip Flexion (Straight Leg)

With one leg flat on the floor, raise the other leg at the hip, keeping both legs straight. Take care not to put excess strain on your back. Check one of the following for each leg; also fill in degrees if using the measurement method.

Right   *Left*

_____   _____   Below average/needs improvement

_____   _____   Average (79–81°)

_____   _____   Above average

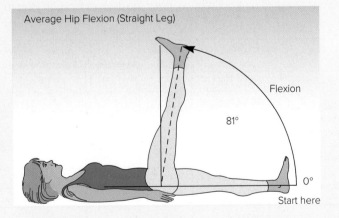

7. Ankle Dorsiflexion and Plantar Flexion

For each position and foot, check one of the following; also fill in degrees if using the measurement method.

Ankle dorsiflexion—pull your toes toward your shin

Right   Left

_____   _____   Below average/needs improvement

_____   _____   Average (9–13°)

_____   _____   Above average

Plantar flexion—point your toes

Right   Left

_____   _____   Below average/needs improvement

_____   _____   Average (50–55°)

_____   _____   Above average

Average Ankle Dorsiflexion
Start here
Dorsiflexion   13°

Average Ankle Plantar Flexion
Start here
55° Plantar flexion

Rating Your Flexibility

Sit-and-Reach Test: Score: _____ cm. Rating: _____

Range-of-Motion Assessment

Identify your rating for each joint on each side of the body. If you used the comparison method, put check marks in the appropriate categories; if you measured range of motion, enter the degrees for each joint in the appropriate category.

Joint/Assessment		Right Below Average	Right Average	Right Above Average	Left Below Average	Left Average	Left Above Average
1. Shoulder abduction and adduction	Abduction						
	Adduction						
2. Shoulder flexion and extension	Flexion						
	Extension						
3. Trunk/low-back lateral flexion	Flexion						
4. Hip abduction	Abduction						
5. Hip flexion (bent knee)	Flexion						
6. Hip flexion (straight leg)	Flexion						
7. Ankle dorsiflexion and plantar flexion	Dorsiflexion						
	Plantar flexion						

Using Your Results

How did you score? Do your scores for the flexibility tests surprise you? Are you satisfied with your current ratings? If you're not satisfied, set a realistic goal for improvement:

_____

_____

_____

Are you satisfied with your current level of flexibility as expressed in your daily life—for example, your ability to maintain good posture and move easily and without pain?

If you're not satisfied, set some realistic goals for improvement:

_____

_____

_____

What should you do next? Enter the results of this lab in the Preprogram Assessment column in Appendix B. If you've set goals for improvement, begin planning your flexibility program by completing the plan in Lab 5.2. After several weeks of your program, complete this lab again and enter the results in the Postprogram Assessment column of Appendix B. How do the results compare?

_____

_____

_____

Name _____ Section _____ Date _____

Lab 5.2 Creating a Personalized Program for Developing Flexibility

![connect logo] Mc Graw Hill Education **connect**

Goals: List goals for your flexibility program. On the left, include specific, measurable goals that you can use to track the progress of your fitness program. These goals might be things like raising your sit-and-reach score from fair to good or your bent-leg hip flexion rating from below average to average. On the right, include long-term and more qualitative goals, such as reducing your risk for back pain.

Specific Goals: Current Status   *Final Goals*

_____   _____

_____   _____

_____   _____

Other goals:

_____

_____

Exercises: The exercises in the program plan below are from the general stretching program presented in Chapter 5. You can add or delete exercises depending on your needs, goals, and preferences. For any exercises you add, fill in the areas of the body affected.

Frequency: A minimum frequency of two to three days per week is recommended; four to seven days per week is ideal. You may want to do your stretching exercises the same days you plan to do cardio-respiratory endurance exercise or weight training because muscles stretch better following exercise, when they are warm.

Intensity: All stretches should be done to the point of mild discomfort, not pain.

Program Plan for Flexibility								
Exercise	**Areas Stretched**	**Frequency (check ✓)**						
		M	T	W	Th	F	Sa	Su
Head turns and tilts	Neck							
Towel stretch	Triceps, shoulders, chest							
Across-the-body and overhead stretches	Shoulders, upper back, back of the arm							
Upper-back stretch	Upper back							
Lateral stretch	Trunk muscles							
Step stretch	Hip, front of thigh							
Side lunge	Inner thigh, hip, calf							
Inner-thigh stretch	Inner thigh, hip							
Hip and trunk stretch	Trunk, outer thigh and hip, lower back							
Modified hurdler stretch	Back of the thigh, lower back							
Leg stretcher	Back of the thigh, hip, knee, ankle, buttocks							
Lower-leg stretch	Back of the lower leg							
Single-leg deadlift	Hamstrings and gluteal muscles							

Time/duration: All stretches should be held for 10 to 30 seconds. (PNF techniques should include a 6-second contraction followed by a 10- to 30-second assisted stretch.) All stretches should be performed 2 to 4 times. You can monitor your program using a chart like the following flexibility program chart.

Flexibility Program Chart

Fill in the dates (Frequency) you perform each stretch (Type), the number of seconds (Time) you hold each stretch (should be 15–30 seconds), and the number of repetitions of each (should be 2–4). For an easy check on the duration of your stretches, count "one thousand one, one thousand two," and so on. You will probably find that over time you'll be able to hold each stretch longer (in addition to being able to stretch farther). Recall that your intensity is based on stretching to the point of mild discomfort, not pain.

Exercise/Date																				
	Duration																			
	Reps																			
	Duration																			
	Reps																			
	Duration																			
	Reps																			
	Duration																			
	Reps																			
	Duration																			
	Reps																			
	Duration																			
	Reps																			
	Duration																			
	Reps																			
	Duration																			
	Reps																			
	Duration																			
	Reps																			
	Duration																			
	Reps																			
	Duration																			
	Reps																			
	Duration																			
	Reps																			
	Duration																			
	Reps																			
	Duration																			
	Reps																			
	Duration																			
	Reps																			
	Duration																			
	Reps																			
	Duration																			
	Reps																			

Name _____ Section _____ Date _____

Lab 5.3 Assessing Muscular Endurance for Low-Back Health
connect

The three tests in this lab evaluate the muscular endurance of major spine stabilizing muscles.

Side Bridge Endurance Test

Equipment

1. stopwatch or clock with a second hand
2. exercise mat
3. partner

Preparation

Warm up your muscles with some low-intensity activity such as walking or easy jogging. Practise assuming the side bridge position described below.

Instructions

1. Lie on the mat on your side with your legs extended. Place your top foot in front of your lower foot for support. Lift your hips off the mat so that you are supporting yourself on one elbow and your feet. Your body should maintain a straight line. Breathe normally; don't hold your breath.

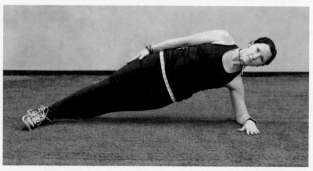

Courtesy of Paula J Gorman

2. Hold the position as long as possible. Your partner should keep track of the time and make sure that you maintain the correct position. Your final score is the total time you are able to hold the side bridge with correct form—from the time you lift your hips until your hips return to the mat.

3. Rest for 5 minutes and then repeat the test on the other side. Record your times here and on the chart at the end of the lab.

Right side bridge time: _____ sec.   Left side bridge time: _____ sec.

Trunk Flexors Endurance Test

(also called the V-sit Flexor Endurance Test)

Equipment

1. stopwatch or clock with a second hand
2. exercise mat or padded exercise table

3. two helpers

4. a wedge angled at 55° from the floor or padded bench (optional)

Preparation

Warm up with some low-intensity activity such as walking or easy jogging.

Instructions

1. To start, assume a sit-up posture with your back supported at an angle of 60° from the floor; support can be provided by a jig, a padded bench, or a spotter. Your knees and hips should both be flexed at 90°, and your arms should be folded across your chest with your hands placed on the opposite shoulders. Your toes should be secured under a toe strap or held by a partner.

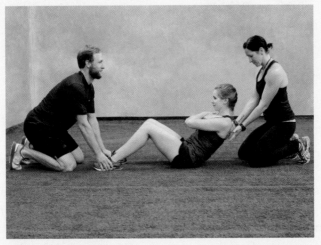

Courtesy of Paula J Gorman

2. Your goal is to hold the starting position (isometric contraction) as long as possible after the support is pulled away. To begin the test, a helper pulls the jig or other support back about 10 centimetres. A helper keeps track of the time; if a spotter is acting as your support, they should be ready to support your weight as soon as your torso begins to move back. Your final score is the total time you are able to hold the contraction—from the time the support is removed until any part of your back touches the support. Remember to breathe normally throughout the test.

3. Record your time here and on the chart at the end of the lab.

Trunk flexors endurance time: _____ sec.

Back Extensors Endurance Test

Equipment

1. stopwatch or clock with a second hand

2. extension bench with padded ankle support or any padded bench

3. partner

Preparation

Warm up with some low-intensity activity such as walking or easy jogging.

Instructions

1. Lie face down on the test bench with the upper body extending out over the end of the bench and the pelvis, hips, and knees flat on the bench. Your arms should be folded across your chest with your hands placed on the opposite shoulders. Your feet should be secured under a padded strap or held by a partner.

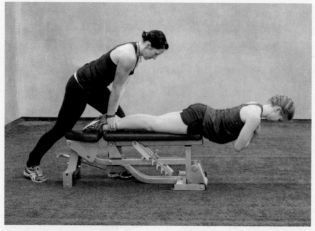

Courtesy of Paula J Gorman

2. Your goal is to hold your upper body in a straight horizontal line with your lower body as long as possible. Keep your neck straight and neutral; don't raise your head and don't arch your back. Breathe normally. Your partner keeps track of the time and watches your form. Your final score is the total time you are able to hold the horizontal position—from the time you assume the position until your upper body drops from the horizontal position.

3. Record your time here and on the chart below.

Back extensors endurance time: _____ sec.

Front Plank Test

Equipment

1. stopwatch or clock with a second hand
2. exercise mat
3. partner

Preparation

Warm up your muscles with some low-intensity activity such as walking or easy jogging. Practise assuming the front plank position described below.

Instructions

1. Assume a front plank position by lying on your front and then lifting your hips, supporting your weight on your forearms and toes and keeping the torso rigid. Your body should maintain a straight line; keep your hands together and elbows directly under your shoulders. Breathe normally and don't hold your breath.

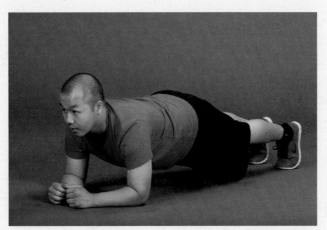

© Taylor Robertson Photography

2. Hold the position as long as possible. Your partner keeps track of the time and makes sure you maintain the correct position. Your final score is the total time you are able to hold the front plank with correct form—from the time you lift your hips until your hips return to the mat.

3. Record your time here and on the chart at the end of the lab.

Front plank time:_____sec

Rating Your Test Results for Muscular Endurance for Low-Back Health

The table below shows mean endurance test times for healthy young college/university students ages 17 to 25, based on a study of 181 university students. Compare your scores with the times shown in the table. Your percentile on each test tells you the percent of the students in the study scored at or below your score.

Percentiles Ranks for Torso Muscle Endurance Tests for College-Age Men and Women (age 17–25)

Percentiles	Trunk flexor test (sec)		Back extensor test (sec)		Side bridge test, right (sec)		Side bridge test, left (sec)		Front plank test (sec)	
	Men	Women	Men	Women	Men	Women	Men	Women	Men	Women
99%	276	246	246	265	193	130	187	133	400	213
95%	234	208	215	232	164	112	160	114	336	181
90%	211	188	199	215	149	102	146	104	302	165
85%	196	174	188	204	140	96	137	97	280	154
80%	184	163	179	194	131	91	129	92	261	145
75%	174	154	171	186	124	86	122	87	245	137
70%	164	145	164	179	118	83	116	83	231	130
65%	156	138	159	173	113	79	111	79	219	124
60%	148	130	152	167	107	76	106	75	206	118
55%	140	123	147	161	102	72	101	72	195	112
50%	132	116	141	155	97	69	96	68	183	106
45%	124	109	135	149	92	66	91	64	171	100
40%	117	102	130	143	87	63	86	61	160	95

continued

Percentiles	Trunk flexor test (sec)		Back extensor test (sec)		Side bridge test, right (sec)		Side bridge test, left (sec)		Front plank test (sec)	
	Men	Women	Men	Women	Men	Women	Men	Women	Men	Women
35%	108	94	123	137	81	59	81	57	147	88
30%	100	87	118	131	76	55	76	53	135	82
25%	90	78	111	124	70	52	70	49	121	75
20%	80	69	103	116	63	47	63	44	105	67
15%	68	58	94	106	54	42	55	39	86	58
10%	53	44	83	95	45	36	46	32	64	47
5%	30	24	67	78	30	26	32	22	30	31
1%	0	0	36	45	1	8	5	3	0	0

NOTE: The percentiles are based on data collected on 181 university kinesiology students ages 17–25. The results might not be representative of other populations.

SOURCE: Percentile charts calculated from the data of McGill, S., M. Belore, I. Crosby, and C. Russell. 2010. Clinical tools to quantify torso flexion endurance: Normative data from student and firefighter populations. Occupational Ergonomics 9(1): 55–61.

Record Your Scores

Test	Time	Percentile
Right Side Bridge		
Left Side Bridge		
Trunk Flexors		
Back Extensions		
Front Plank		

Using Your Results

How did you score? Are you at all surprised by your scores for the low-back tests? Are you satisfied with your current ratings?

If you're not satisfied, set a realistic goal for improvement. The norms in this lab are based on healthy young adults, so a score above the mean may or may not be realistic for you. Instead, you may want to set a specific goal based on time rather than rating; for example, set a goal of improving your time by 10%. Imbalances in muscular endurance have been linked with back problems, so if your rating is significantly lower for one of the three tests, you should focus particular attention on that area of the body.

Goal:

_____

_____

_____

What should you do next? Enter the results of this lab in the Preprogram Assessment column in Appendix B. If you've set a goal for improvement, begin a program of low-back exercises such as that suggested in this chapter. After several weeks of your program, complete this lab again and enter the results in the Postprogram Assessment column of Appendix B. How do the results compare?

_____

_____

_____

Body Composition

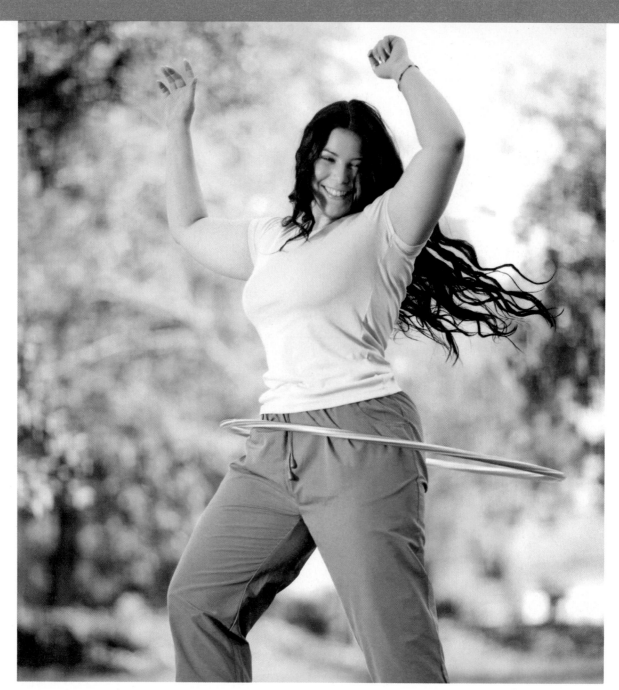

LEARNING OBJECTIVES

After reading this chapter, you should be able to

LO1   Define fat-free mass and body fat and describe their functions in the body

LO2   Explain how body composition affects overall health and wellness

LO3   Describe how body mass index, body composition, and body fat distribution are measured and assessed

LO4   Explain how to set goals based on recommended body weight and body fat distribution

TEST YOUR KNOWLEDGE

1. **Exercise helps reduce the risks associated with overweight and obesity even if it doesn't result in improvements in body composition.**

   True or false?

2. **Which of the following is the most significant risk factor for type 2 diabetes (the most common type of diabetes)?**
   a. smoking
   b. low-fibre diet
   c. overweight or obesity
   d. inactivity

3. **In women, excessive exercise and low energy (calorie) intake can cause which of the following?**
   a. unhealthy reduction in body fat levels
   b. amenorrhea (absent menstruation)
   c. bone density loss and osteoporosis
   d. muscle wasting and fatigue

ANSWERS

1. **TRUE.** Regular physical activity provides protection against the health risks of overweight and obesity. People who are fit and obese live longer, healthier lives than normal weight people who are sedentary. However, it is best to both be active and maintain a healthy weight.

2. **C.** All four are risk factors for diabetes, but overweight/obesity is the most significant. It's estimated that 90% of cases of type 2 diabetes could be prevented if people adopted healthy lifestyle behaviours.

3. **ALL FOUR.** Very low levels of body fat, and the behaviours used to achieve them, have serious health consequences for both men and women.

Body composition, the body's relative amount of fat and fat-free mass, is an important component of fitness for health and wellness. People whose body composition is optimal tend to be healthier, move more efficiently, and feel better about themselves. They also have a lower risk of many chronic diseases.

Many people, however, don't succeed in their efforts to obtain a fit and healthy body because they set unrealistic goals and emphasize short-term weight loss rather than the permanent changes in lifestyle that lead to fat loss and a healthy body composition. Successful management of body composition requires the long-term, consistent coordination of many aspects of a wellness program. Even in the absence of changes in body composition, an active lifestyle improves wellness and decreases the risk of disease and premature death (see the box Why Is Physical Activity Important Even If Body Composition Doesn't Change?).

The Evidence *for* EXERCISE

WHY IS PHYSICAL ACTIVITY IMPORTANT EVEN IF BODY COMPOSITION DOESN'T CHANGE?

Physical activity is important for health even if it produces no changes in body composition—that is, even if a person remains overweight or obese. Physical activity confers benefits no matter how much you weigh; conversely, physical inactivity operates independently of body composition as a risk factor for health problems.

Regular physical activity and exercise block many of the destructive effects of obesity. For example, physical activity improves blood pressure, blood glucose levels, cholesterol levels, and body fat distribution. It also lowers the risk of cardiovascular disease, diabetes, and premature death. Although physical activity and exercise produce these improvements quickly in some people and slowly in others due to genetic differences, the improvements do occur. Physical activity is particularly important for the many people who have metabolic syndrome or prediabetes, both of which are characterized by insulin resistance. Exercise encourages the body's cells to take up and use insulin efficiently for converting nutrients into usable energy. Being physically inactive for just one day decreases the capacity of the cells to take up and use blood sugar. Exercise makes fat cells fit by improving the function of their mitochondria (powerhouses of the cell) and decreasing inflammation.

Although being physically active and not being sedentary may sound identical, experts describe them as different dimensions of the same health issue. Data suggest that it is important not only to be physically active, but also to avoid prolonged sitting. In one study, people who watched TV or used

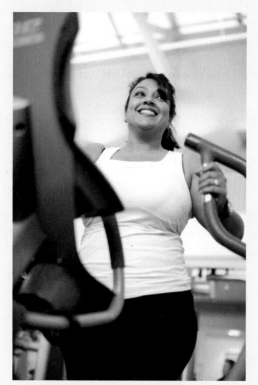
© yellowdog / age fotostock

a computer four or more hours a day had twice the risk of having metabolic syndrome as those who spent less than one hour a day in these activities; other studies reported similar results. Thus, in addition to increasing physical activity, avoiding or reducing sedentary behaviour is an important—and challenging—health goal.

Physical activity, then, is important even if it doesn't change body composition. But at a certain level, physical activity and exercise do improve body composition (meaning less fat and more lean muscle mass). Evidence supports a *dose-response* relation between exercise and fat loss: The more you exercise, the more fat you will lose. This includes both total body fat and abdominal fat. Additionally, the more body fat a person has, the greater is the loss of abdominal fat with exercise. Studies show that, even without calorie reduction, walking 150 minutes per week at a pace of 6.5 kilometres per hour, or jogging 75 minutes a week at 9.5 kilometres per hour, produces a decrease in total fat and abdominal fat that is associated with improved metabolic health.

Studies also show, however, that combining exercise with an appropriate reduction in calories is an even better way to reduce levels of body fat and increase lean muscle mass. The results of combining exercise and calorie reduction may not show up as expected on the scale because the weight of body fat lost is partially offset by the weight of muscle mass gained. Still, body composition, physical fitness, and overall health have improved.

The question is sometimes asked, Which is more important in combating the adverse health effects of obesity—physical activity or physical fitness? Many studies suggest that both are important; the more active and fit you are, the lower your risk of having health problems and dying prematurely. Of the two, however, physical activity appears to be more important than physical fitness for health.

SOURCES: Earnest, C. P., et al. 2013. Cardiometabolic risk factors and metabolic syndrome in the Aerobics Center Longitudinal Study. *Mayo Clinics Proceedings* 88(3): 259–270; Loprinzi, P., et al. 2014. The "fit but fat" paradigm addressed using accelerometer-determined physical activity data. *North American Journal of Medical Sciences* 6(7): 295–301; Vieira-Potter, V. J., et al. 2015. Exercise (and estrogen) make fat cells "fit." *Exercise Sport Sciences Reviews,* 43(3):172–178.

This chapter focuses on defining and measuring body composition. The aspects of lifestyle that affect body composition are discussed in detail in other chapters: physical activity and exercise in Chapters 2, Chapter 3, Chapter 4, and Chapter 5, sound nutritional habits in Chapter 7, specific strategies for weight management in Chapter 8, and healthy techniques for managing stress in Chapter 12.

LO1 6.1 What Is Body Composition, and Why Is It Important?

The human body can be divided into fat-free mass and body fat. As defined in Chapter 2, fat-free mass is composed of all the body's nonfat tissues: bone, water, muscle, connective tissue, organ tissues, and teeth.

Body fat is incorporated into the nerves, brain, heart, lungs, liver, mammary glands, and other body organs and tissues. A certain amount of body fat is necessary for the body to function. It is the main source of stored energy in the body; it also cushions body organs and helps regulate body temperature. This **essential fat**

essential fat   Fat incorporated in various tissues of the body; critical for normal body functioning.

makes up about 3–5% of total body weight in men and 8–12% in women (see Figure 6.1). The percentage is higher in women due to fat deposits in the breasts, uterus, and other gender-specific sites.

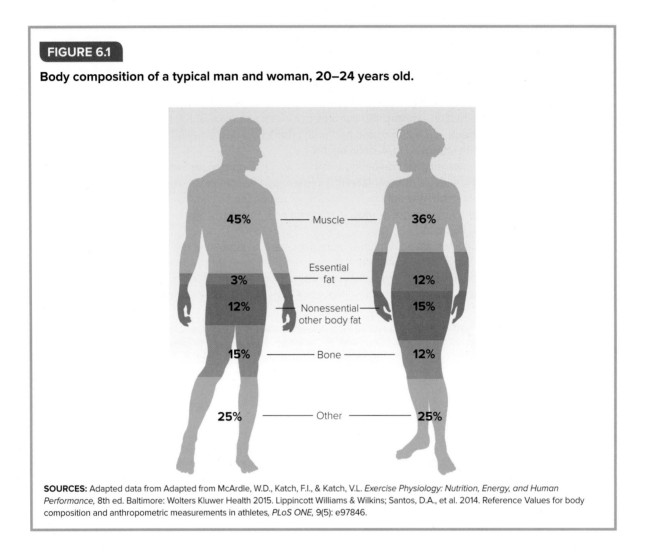

FIGURE 6.1

Body composition of a typical man and woman, 20–24 years old.

	Man		Woman
Muscle	45%		36%
Essential fat	3%		12%
Nonessential other body fat	12%		15%
Bone	15%		12%
Other	25%		25%

SOURCES: Adapted data from Adapted from McArdle, W.D., Katch, F.I., & Katch, V.L. *Exercise Physiology: Nutrition, Energy, and Human Performance,* 8th ed. Baltimore: Wolters Kluwer Health 2015. Lippincott Williams & Wilkins; Santos, D.A., et al. 2014. Reference Values for body composition and anthropometric measurements in athletes, *PLoS ONE,* 9(5): e97846.

Most of the fat in the body is stored in fat cells, or **adipose tissue**, located under the skin **(subcutaneous fat)** and around major organs **(visceral** or **intra-abdominal fat)**. People have a genetically determined number of fat cells, but these cells can increase or decrease in size depending on how much fat is being stored. The amount of stored fat depends on several factors, including age, sex, metabolism, diet, and activity level. The primary source of excess body fat is excess calories consumed in the diet—that is, calories consumed beyond what is expended in metabolism, physical activity, and exercise. A kilogram of body fat is equal to 7700 calories, so an intake of just 100 calories a day in excess of calories expended will result in a 4.5 kilogram weight gain over the course of a year. Excess stored body fat is associated with increased risk of chronic diseases like diabetes and cardiovascular disease, as described later in this chapter.

adipose tissue   Connective tissue in which fat is stored.
subcutaneous fat   Fat located under the skin.
visceral (intra-abdominal) fat   Fat located around major organs.

Overweight and Obesity Defined

When looking at body composition, the most important consideration is the proportion of the body's total weight that is fat—the **percent body fat**. For example, two women may both be 165 centimetres tall and weigh 60 kilograms, but one woman, a runner, may have only 20% of her body weight as fat, whereas the second, sedentary woman could have 34% body fat. Although neither woman is overweight by most standards, the second woman is overfat, meaning she has more than a healthy amount of body fat. Too much body fat (not total weight) has a negative effect on health and well-being. Just as the amount of body fat is important, so is its location on your body. For example, visceral fat (around major organs) is more harmful to health than subcutaneous fat (under the skin).

percent body fat   The percentage of total body weight that is composed of fat.

Overweight is usually defined as total body weight above the recommended range for good health (as determined by large-scale population surveys). **Obesity** is defined as a more serious degree of overweight that carries multiple major health risks. The cut-off point for obesity may be set in terms of percent body fat or in terms of some measure of total body weight.

overweight   Body weight above the recommended range for good health; sometimes defined as a body mass index between 25 and 29.9, a measure of the proportion of weight to height.
obesity   Severely overweight, characterized by an excessive accumulation of body fat; may also be defined in terms of some measure of total body weight or a body mass index of 30 or more.

Wellness Tip

Sleep problems increase the risk of obesity, especially in children and young adults. Sleep loss increases production of the hormone ghrelin, which boosts appetite and slows metabolic rate. Fatigue can also make it hard to live a healthy lifestyle and maintain a healthy weight.

Prevalence of Overweight and Obesity among Canadians

By any measure, North Americans are getting fatter. In Canada, the prevalence of obesity increased from 13.8% in 1978/79 to almost 19% in 2013.[1] The number of Canadians who report themselves as either overweight or obese has also risen to 62% for males and 45% for females—a significant increase from 2012 for males, but a stable number since 2009 for females. Digging a little deeper, it should be noted that although rates appear steady for females, the number of Canadian women reporting as obese has steadily increased since 2003; conversely, rates of obesity in men have shown no statistical difference since 2007.[2]

Comparatively, approximately 34% of Americans are obese and about 67% are considered overweight.[3] Possible explanations for the increasing numbers of overweight and obese North Americans include more time spent in sedentary work and leisure activities, fewer short trips on foot and more by automobile, fewer daily gym classes for students, more meals eaten outside the home, greater consumption of fast food, increased portion sizes, and increased consumption of soft drinks and convenience foods. In addition, fewer than half of North Americans meet the minimum recommendation of 30 minutes per day of moderate physical activity.

LO2 Excess Body Fat and Wellness

As rates of overweight and obesity increase, so do the problems associated with them. The direct financial cost of obesity in Canada alone is reported to be close to $2 billion[4] ($117 billion in the United States[5]), and obesity is now the second-leading preventable cause of death after cigarette smoking. Excess body fat can also impact overall wellness through its effects on chronic disease risk, ability to perform physical activities, and body image.

Metabolic Syndrome and Premature Death

Many overweight and obese people—especially those who are sedentary and eat a poor diet—suffer from a group of symptoms called **metabolic syndrome** (or insulin resistance syndrome). Metabolic syndrome is diagnosed if a person has at least three out of five of these key factors: large waistline (fat deposits in the abdominal region), high blood pressure, high fasting blood sugar, high triglycerides, and low HDL ("good" cholesterol). Associated conditions include **chronic inflammation**, erectile dysfunction, and **fatty liver** disease. Metabolic syndrome increases the risk of heart disease by up to three times in men and six times in women.[6] According to the Canadian Health Measures Survey (2009–2011), about 22% of adult Canadians have metabolic syndrome.

> **metabolic syndrome** A cluster of symptoms present in many overweight and obese people that greatly increases their risk of heart disease, diabetes, and other chronic illnesses; symptoms include insulin resistance, abnormal blood fats, abdominal fat deposition, type 2 diabetes, high blood pressure, and chronic inflammation.
> **chronic inflammation** A response of blood vessels to harmful substances, such as germs, damaged cells, or irritants; can lead to heart disease, cancer, allergies, and muscle degeneration.
> **fatty liver** Increased fat storage in the liver that can lead to liver inflammation and failure.

Obesity is also associated with an increased risk of death from many types of cancer (e.g., breast, colorectal, endometrial). Other health problems associated with obesity include impaired immune function, gallbladder and kidney disease, skin problems, sleep and breathing disorders, erectile dysfunction, back pain, arthritis, and other bone and joint disorders.

Being obese in itself does not imply that the risk for chronic disease and premature death will be equal. In fact, Statistics Canada has identified differing levels of risk depending upon the status or level of obesity that Canadians suffer from. As obese Canadians move from Class I obesity (BMI = 30) to Class II obesity (BMI = 35) to Class III obesity (BMI = 40), there is an escalation in their health risk. In 2011, 16.2% of obese Canadians were in Class I, 6.3% were in Class II, and 3.6% were in Class III.

Strengthening Mental Wellness

Researchers have found strong associations between obesity and mental disorders (depression in particular); and these associations become stronger as people become more obese. Be sure to consider all your risk factors for mental wellness and stay active and eat a healthy diet in an effort to minimize your risk for obesity.

Body Fat Distribution and Health

The distribution of body fat (the locations of fat on the body) is also an important indicator of health. Men and postmenopausal women tend to store fat in the upper regions of their bodies, particularly in the abdominal area (the "apple shape"). Premenopausal women usually store fat in the hips, buttocks, and thighs (the "pear shape"). Excess fat in the abdominal area increases risk of several diseases, including high blood pressure, diabetes, early-onset heart disease, stroke, certain cancers, and mortality. The reason for this increased risk is not entirely clear, but it appears that fat in the abdomen is more easily mobilized and sent into the bloodstream, increasing disease-related blood fat levels.

A measure of waist circumference helps assess the risks of unhealthy body fat distribution. A total waist measurement of more than 102 centimetres (40 inches) for men and more than 88 centimetres (35 inches) for women is associated with a significantly increased risk of disease. Because waist circumference tends to be higher in taller people, waist-to-height ratio is a more accurate measure than waist circumference alone. Your waist measurement should be less than half your height. Using this index, a person who is 173 centimetres (5 feet 8 inches) tall should have a waist circumference of less than 86.5 centimetres (34 inches). A person who is 193 centimetres (6 feet 4 inches) tall should have a waist circumferences of less than 96.5 centimetres (38 inches).

Performance of Physical Activities

Too much body fat makes physical activity difficult because moving the body through everyday activities entails working harder and using more energy. In general, overfat people are less fit than others and don't have the muscular strength, endurance, and flexibility that make normal activity easy. Because exercise is more difficult they might do less of it, depriving themselves of an effective way to improve body composition.

Emotional Wellness and Self-Image

Obesity can affect psychological as well as physical wellness. Being perceived as fat can be a source of judgment, ostracism, and sometimes discrimination by others. It can also contribute to psychological problems such as depression, anxiety, and low self-esteem.

The popular image of the "ideal" body has changed greatly in the past 50 years, evolving from slightly plump to unhealthily thin. The ideal body—as presented by the media—is an unrealistic goal for most Canadians. This is because a person's ability to change body composition depends on heredity as well as diet and exercise. (Body image, problems with body image, and unhealthy ways of dealing with a negative body image are all discussed in Chapter 8.)

Diabetes and Excess Body Fat

Even mild to moderate overweight is associated with a substantial increase in the risk of type 2 diabetes. Obese people are more than three times as likely as nonobese people to develop type 2 diabetes, and the incidence of this disease among Canadians has increased dramatically as the rate of obesity has climbed.

Diabetes mellitus is a disease that disrupts normal metabolism. The pancreas normally secretes the hormone insulin, which stimulates cells to take up glucose (blood sugar) to produce energy. Diabetes interferes with this process, causing a buildup of glucose in the bloodstream. Diabetes is associated with kidney failure; nerve damage; circulation problems; retinal damage and blindness; and increased rates of heart attack, stroke, and hypertension. Diabetes is currently the sixth leading cause of death in Canada

More than 9.1 million Canadians live with either diabetes or prediabetes. There are two major forms of diabetes. About 10% of people with diabetes have the more serious form, known as *type 1 diabetes*. In this type of diabetes, the pancreas produces little or no insulin, which means a person can lapse into a coma. Daily doses of insulin are required, and other medications to control blood sugar levels and other complications of the disease may also be necessary. Type 1 diabetes usually strikes before age 30.

The remaining 90% of Canadians with diabetes have *type 2 diabetes*. This condition can develop slowly, and about 25% of affected individuals are unaware of their condition. In type 2 diabetes, the pancreas doesn't produce enough insulin, cells are resistant to insulin, or both. This condition is usually diagnosed in people over age 40, although there has been a tenfold increase in type 2 diabetes in children in the past two decades. About one-third of people with type 2 diabetes must take insulin; others may take medications that increase insulin production or stimulate cells to take up glucose.

A third type of diabetes occurs in 2% to 10% of women during pregnancy. *Gestational diabetes* usually disappears after pregnancy, but 5–10% of women with gestational diabetes go on to have type 2 diabetes immediately after pregnancy. Women who had gestational diabetes during pregnancy have up to a 60% chance of developing diabetes within 10 to 20 years.

The term *prediabetes* describes blood glucose levels that are higher than normal but not high enough for a diagnosis of full-blown diabetes. The Public Health Agency of Canada estimates that prediabetes affects roughly 5 million Canadians over the age of 20; experts warn that most people with the condition will develop type 2 diabetes unless they adopt preventive lifestyle measures.

The major factors involved in the development of diabetes are age, obesity, physical inactivity, a family history of diabetes, and lifestyle. Excess body fat reduces cell sensitivity to insulin, and insulin resistance is usually a precursor of type 2 diabetes. Ethnicity also plays a role. According to the Canadian Diabetes Association, Canadians who are of Aboriginal, Hispanic, Asian, South Asian, or African descent are at greater risk of being diagnosed with type 2 diabetes.

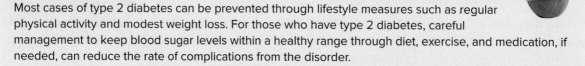

Wellness Tip

Most cases of type 2 diabetes can be prevented through lifestyle measures such as regular physical activity and modest weight loss. For those who have type 2 diabetes, careful management to keep blood sugar levels within a healthy range through diet, exercise, and medication, if needed, can reduce the rate of complications from the disorder.

Treatment

There is no cure for diabetes, but it can be managed successfully by keeping blood sugar levels within safe limits through diet, exercise, and, if necessary, medication. Individuals can monitor blood sugar levels with a home test, and close control of glucose levels can significantly reduce the rate of serious complications.

The majority of people with type 2 diabetes are overweight when diagnosed, including 55% who are obese. An important step in treatment is to lose weight. Even a small amount of exercise and weight loss can be beneficial. The Canadian Diabetes Association reports that in one study, people at risk of type 2 diabetes were able to reduce their risk by 58% by exercising moderately for 30 minutes a day and by losing 5–7% of their body weight. In people age 60 and older, the risk was cut by almost 71%. Regular exercise and a healthy diet are often sufficient to control type 2 diabetes.

Prevention

It is estimated that 90% of cases of type 2 diabetes could be prevented if people adopted healthy lifestyle behaviours, including regular physical activity, a moderate diet, and modest weight loss. For people with prediabetes, lifestyle measures are more effective than medication for delaying or preventing the development of diabetes. Exercise (endurance and/or strength training) makes cells more sensitive to insulin and helps stabilize blood glucose levels; it also helps keep body fat at healthy levels.

A moderate diet to control body fat is perhaps the most important dietary recommendation for the prevention of diabetes. However, the composition of the diet may also be important. Studies have linked diets low in fibre and high in sugar, refined carbohydrates, saturated fat, red meat, and high-fat dairy products to increased risk of diabetes. Specific foods linked to higher diabetes risk include soft drinks, white bread, white rice, French fries, processed meats, and sugary desserts. Diets rich in whole grains, fruits, vegetables, legumes, fish, and poultry may be protective.

Warning Signs and Testing

Be alert for the following warning signs of diabetes:

- frequent urination
- extreme hunger or thirst
- unexplained weight loss
- extreme fatigue
- blurred vision
- frequent infections
- cuts and bruises that are slow to heal
- tingling or numbness in the hands or feet
- generalized itching with no rash

The best way to avoid complications is to recognize these symptoms and get early diagnosis and treatment. Because type 2 diabetes is often asymptomatic in the early stages, major health organizations now recommend routine screening for people over age 45 and anyone younger who is at high risk, including those who are obese. Screening involves a blood test to check glucose levels after either a period of fasting or the administration of a set dose of glucose. A fasting glucose level of 7 mmol/L or higher indicates diabetes; a level of 5.6 mmol/L indicates prediabetes. If you are concerned about your risk for diabetes, talk with your physician about being tested.

Strengthening Mental Wellness

While physical activity increases self-confidence and self-worth, being overweight, obese, or underweight can lead to a decrease in self-perception. In fact, those who are obese are more likely to perceive themselves to be less athletically capable and to have a lower overall self-worth. To change your self-perception, reach out to organizations such as the Canadian Women's Foundation or the Canadian Women's Health Network.

Problems Associated with Very Low Levels of Body Fat

Though not as prevalent a problem as overweight or obesity, having too little body fat is also dangerous. Essential fat is necessary for the functioning of the body, and health experts generally view too little body fat—less than about 8–12% for women and 3–5% for men—as a threat to health. Extreme leanness is linked with reproductive, circulatory, and immune system disorders and with premature death. Extremely lean people may experience muscle wasting and fatigue. They are also more likely to suffer from dangerous eating disorders, which are described in more detail in Chapter 8. For women, an extremely low percentage of body fat is associated with **amenorrhea** and loss of bone mass (see the box The Female Athlete Triad on the next page).

amenorrhea   Absent or infrequent menstruation, sometimes related to low levels of body fat and excessive quantity or intensity of exercise.

DIVERSITY Matters

THE FEMALE ATHLETE TRIAD

Even while obesity is at epidemic levels in North America, many girls and women strive for unrealistic thinness in response to pressure from peers and a society obsessed with appearance. This quest for thinness has led to an increasingly common, underreported condition called the **female athlete triad**.

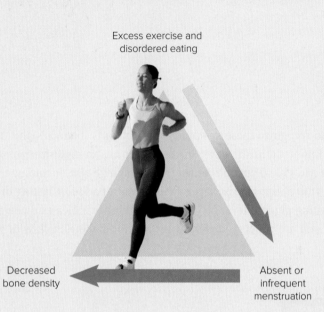

Excess exercise and disordered eating

Decreased bone density

Absent or infrequent menstruation

The triad consists of three inter-related disorders: abnormal eating patterns (and excessive exercising), followed by lack of menstrual periods (amenorrhea), followed by decreased bone density (premature osteoporosis). Left untreated, the triad can lead to decreased physical performance, increased incidence of bone fractures, disturbances of heart rhythm and metabolism, and even death.

Abnormal eating is the event from which the other two components of the triad flow. Abnormal eating ranges from moderately restricting food intake, to binge eating and purging (bulimia), to severely restricting food intake (anorexia nervosa). Whether serious or relatively mild, eating disorders prevent women from consuming enough calories to meet their bodies' needs.

Disordered eating, combined with intense exercise and emotional stress, can suppress the hormones that control the menstrual cycle. If the menstrual cycle stops for three consecutive months, the condition is called amenorrhea. Prolonged amenorrhea can lead to osteoporosis; bone density may erode to the point that a woman in her 20s will have the bone density of a woman in her 60s. Women with osteoporosis have fragile, easily fractured bones. Some researchers have found that even a few missed menstrual periods can decrease bone density.

All physically active women and girls have the potential to develop one or more components of the female athlete triad; for example, it is estimated that 5–20% of women who exercise regularly and vigorously may develop amenorrhea. But the triad is most prevalent among athletes who participate in certain sports: those in which appearance is highly important, that emphasize a prepubertal body shape, that require contour-revealing clothing for competition, that require endurance, and that use weight categories for participation. Such sports include gymnastics, figure skating, swimming, distance running, cycling, cross-country skiing, track, volleyball, rowing, horse racing, and cheerleading.

The female athlete triad can be life-threatening, and health professionals are taking it seriously. Typical signs of the eating disorders that trigger the condition are extreme weight loss, dry skin, loss of hair, brittle fingernails, cold hands and feet, low blood pressure and heart rate, swelling around the ankles and hands, and weakening of the bones. Female athletes who have repeated stress fractures may be suffering from the condition.

female athlete triad A condition consisting of three interrelated disorders: abnormal eating patterns (and excessive exercising) followed by lack of menstrual periods (amenorrhea) and decreased bone density (premature osteoporosis).

Early intervention is the key to stopping this series of interrelated conditions. Unfortunately, once the condition has progressed, long-term consequences, especially bone loss, are unavoidable. Teen-agers may need only to learn about good eating habits; university-age women with a long-standing problem may require psychological counselling.

SOURCES: Joy, E., et al. 2014. Female Athlete Triad coalition consensus statement on treatment and return to play of the Female Athlete Triad. *Current Sports Medicine Reports* 13(4): 219–232; Mallinson, R. J., and M. J. De Souza. 2014. Current perspectives on the etiology and manifestation of the "silent" component of the Female Athlete Triad. *International Journal Women's Health* 6: 451–467; Mountjoy, M., et al. 2014. The IOC consensus statement: Beyond the Female Athlete Triad–Relative Energy Deficiency in Sport (RED-S). *British Journal Sports Medicine* 48(7):491–497.

LO3 6.2 Assessing Body Mass Index, Body Composition, and Body Fat Distribution

Although a scale can tell your total weight, it can't reveal whether a fluctuation in weight is due to a change in muscle, body water, or fat. Most importantly, a scale can't differentiate between overweight and overfat. Some methods of assessing and classifying body composition are based on body fat, while others are based on total body weight. Although methods based on total body weight are less accurate, they are commonly used because body weight is easier to measure than body fat. Various methods of assessing body composition are described later in the chapter.

In the past, many people relied on height/weight tables (which were based on insurance company mortality statistics) to determine whether they were at a healthy weight. Such tables, however, can be highly inaccurate for some people. Because muscle tissue is denser and heavier than fat, a fit person can easily weigh more than the recommended weight on a height/weight table. For the same reason, an unfit person may weigh less than the table's recommended weight.

There are a number of simple, inexpensive ways to estimate healthy body weight and healthy body composition that are more accurate than the bathroom scale. These assessments can provide you with information about the health risks associated with your current body weight and body composition. They can also help you establish reasonable goals and set a starting point for current and future decisions about weight loss and weight gain.

Calculating Body Mass Index

Body mass index (BMI) is a measure of body weight that is useful for classifying the health risks of body weight if you don't have access to more sophisticated methods. Though more accurate than height-weight tables, body mass index is also based on the concept that weight should be proportional to height. BMI is easy to calculate and rate. Researchers frequently use BMI in studies that examine the health risks associated with body weight.

body mass index (BMI)   A measure of relative body weight correlating highly with more direct measures of body fat, calculated by dividing total body weight (in kilograms) by the square of body height (in metres).

BMI is calculated as follows:

1. Multiply your height in metres by itself to obtain the square of the height measurement.

2. Divide your weight in kilograms by the result of step 1.

The following example is for a person who is 5 feet, 3 inches tall (63 inches) and weighs 130 pounds:

1. Divide body weight in pounds by 2.2 to convert weight to kilograms: $130 \div 2.2 = 59.1$

2. Multiply height in inches by 0.0254 to convert height to metres: $63 \times 0.0254 = 1.6$

3. Multiply the result of step 2 by itself to get the square of the height measurement: $1.6 \times 1.6 = 2.56$

4. Divide the result of step 1 by the result of step 3 to determine BMI: $59.1 \div 2.56 = 23$

An alternative equation, based on pounds and inches, is

$$BMI = [weight/(height \times height)] \times 703$$

Space for your own calculations can be found in Lab 6.1, and a complete BMI chart appears in Lab 6.2.

Under federal guidelines from Health Canada, a BMI between 18.5 and 24.9 is considered healthy. A person is classified as overweight if they have a BMI of 25 or above and obese if they have a BMI of 30 or above (see Table 6.1). A person with a BMI below 18.5 is classified as underweight, although low BMI values may be healthy in some cases if they are not the result of smoking, an eating disorder, or an underlying disease. A BMI of 17.5 or less is sometimes used as a diagnostic criterion for the eating disorder anorexia nervosa (see Chapter 8).

TABLE 6.1

Body Mass Index (BMI) Classification and Disease Risk

BMI Category	BMI (kg/m²)	Obesity Class	Disease Risk Relative to Normal Weight and Waist Circumference[a]
			BMI Risk
Underweight[b]	<18.5		Increased
Normal	18.5–24.9		Least
Overweight	25.0–29.9		Increased
Obesity	30.0–34.9	I	High
	35.0–39.9	II	Very high
	≥40.0	III	Extremely high

[a] Disease risk for type 2 diabetes, hypertension, and cardiovascular disease. The waist circumference cut-off points for increased risk are 90 cm for men and 80 cm for women.
[b] Research suggests that a low BMI can be healthy in some cases, as long as it is not the result of smoking, an eating disorder, or an underlying disease process. A BMI of 17.5 or less is sometimes used as a diagnostic criterion for the eating disorder anorexia nervosa.

SOURCE: Table: Rating your BMI. Health Risk for BMI, *Canadian Society for Exercise Physiology - Physical Activity training for Health* (CSEP-PATH®), © 2013. All rights reserved. Reprinted with permission.

In classifying the health risks associated with overweight and obesity, the Health Canada and the World Health Organization (WHO) guidelines consider body fat distribution and other disease risk factors in addition to BMI. As described earlier, excess fat in the abdomen is of greater concern than excess fat in other areas. Measurement of waist circumference (see Table 6.2) is one method of assessing body fat distribution, as discussed later in the chapter. At a given level of overweight, people with a large waist circumference and/or additional disease risk factors are at greater risk for health problems. For example, a man with a BMI of 27, a waist circumference of more than 94 centimetres, and high blood pressure is at greater risk for health problems than another man who has a BMI of 27 but has a smaller waist circumference and no other risk factors. In Lab 6.1 you will evaluate your health risk from a combined BMI-WC score.

TABLE 6.2

Waist Circumference Classifications

Classification	Waist Circumference in Centimetres (Inches)	
	Women	Men
Normal	<80 cm (32 in.)	<94 cm (37 in.)
Increased	≥80 cm (32 in.)	≥94 cm (37 in.)
Substantially increased	≥88 cm (35 in.)	≥102 cm (40 in.)

SOURCE: Adapted from World Health Organization. 2008. *Waist Circumference and Waist-to-Hip Ratio. Report of a WHO Expert Consultation.* Geneva: WHO.

Optimal BMI for good health depends on many factors. If your BMI is 25 or above, consult a physician for help in determining a healthy BMI for you. (Weight loss recommendations based on Canadian Society for Exercise Physiology [CSEP] guidelines are discussed further in Chapter 8.)

Because BMI doesn't distinguish between fat weight and fat-free weight, it is inaccurate for some groups. For example, athletes who weight train have more muscle mass—and thus weigh more—than average people and may be classified as overweight by the BMI scale. Because their "excess" weight is in the form of muscle, however, it is healthy. Further, BMI is not particularly useful for tracking changes in body composition—gains in muscle mass and losses of fat. BMI also does not take into account differences in gender; women are likely to have more body fat for a given BMI than men. In addition, BMI measurements have over- and underestimated the prevalence of obesity in several ethnic groups, such as Hispanics and blacks, because of racial and ethnic differences in muscle mass and muscle density. Finally, BMI is a poor predictor of health in people short in stature, whose gene function may have been altered by environmental factors early in life. If you are an athlete, a serious weight trainer, or a person of short stature, do not use BMI as your primary means of assessing whether your current weight is healthy. Instead, try one of the methods described in the next section for estimating percent body fat.

Estimating Percent Body Fat

Estimating percent body fat can be one method of tracking changes in body composition over time. Unfortunately, an autopsy—the dissection and chemical analysis of the body—is the only method for directly measuring the percentage of body weight that is fat. However, there are other indirect techniques that can provide an estimate of percent body fat. One of the most accurate is underwater weighing. Other techniques include skinfold measurements, the Bod Pod, bioelectrical impedance analysis, and dual-energy X-ray absorptiometry.

All of these methods have a margin of error, so it is important not to focus too much on precise values. For example, underwater weighing has an error of about ±3%, meaning that if a person's percent body fat is actually 17%, the test result may be between 14% and 20%; skinfold measurements have an error rate of about ±6%. The results of different methods may also vary, so if you plan to track changes in body composition over time, be sure to use the same method each time to perform the assessment. Table 6.3 (on the next page) provides estimated ranges for healthy percent body fat. As with BMI, the percent body fat ratings indicate cut-off points for health risks associated with underweight and obesity.

TABLE 6.3

Percent Body Fat Classification

	Percent Body Fat (%)				Percent Body Fat (%)		
	20–39 Years	*40–59 Years*	*60–79 Years*		*20–39 Years*	*40–59 Years*	*60–79 Years*
Women				**Men**			
Essential[a]	8–12	8–12	8–12	Essential[a]	3–5	3–5	3–5
Low/athletic[b]	13–20	13–22	13–23	Low/athletic[b]	6–7	6–10	6–12
Recommended	21–32	23–33	24–35	Recommended	8–19	11–21	13–24
Overfat[c]	33–38	34–39	36–41	Overfat[c]	20–24	22–27	25–29
Obese[c]	≥39	≥40	≥42	Obese[c]	≥25	≥28	≥30

NOTE: The cutoffs for recommended, overfat, and obese ranges in this table are based on a study that linked body mass index classifications from the National Institutes of Health with predicted percent body fat (measured using dual-energy X-ray absorptiometry).

[a] Essential body fat is necessary for the basic functioning of the body.
[b] Percent body fat in the low/athletic range may be appropriate for some people as long as it is not the result of illness or disordered eating habits.
[c] Health risks increase as percent body fat exceeds the recommended range.

SOURCES: Gallagher, D., et al. 2009. Healthy percentage body fat ranges: An approach for developing guidelines based on body mass index. *American Journal of Clinical Nutrition* 72: 694–701; Swain, D. P. 2013. *ACSM's Resource Manual for Guidelines for Exercise Testing and Prescription,* 7th ed. Philadelphia: Wolters Kluwer/Lippincott Williams & Wilkins Health.

Underwater Weighing

In hydrostatic (underwater) weighing, an individual is weighed under water and on land. The percentages of fat and fat-free weight are then calculated from body density. Muscle has a higher density and fat has a lower density than water. Therefore, people with more body fat tend to float and weigh less under water, and lean people tend to sink and weigh more under water. Most university exercise physiology departments or sports medicine laboratories have an underwater weighing facility. If you want an accurate assessment of your body composition, find a place that does underwater weighing or has a Bod Pod (described in the next section).

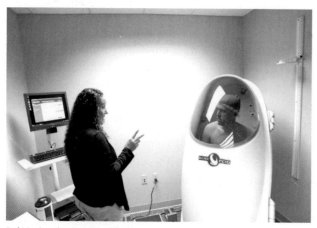

Joel Martinez / United States Air Force

The Bod Pod

The Bod Pod

The Bod Pod is a small chamber containing computerized sensors that measures body composition by air displacement. The technique's technical name is *plethysmography*. It determines the percentage of fat by calculating how much air is displaced by the person sitting inside the chamber. The Bod Pod has an error rate of ±2–4% in determining percent body fat.

Skinfold Measurements

Skinfold measurement is a simple, inexpensive, and practical way to assess body composition. Skinfold measurements can be used to assess body composition because equations can link the thickness of skinfolds at various sites to percent body fat calculations from more precise laboratory techniques.

Skinfold assessment typically involves measuring the thickness of skinfolds at several different places on the body. You can sum up the skinfold values as an indirect measure of body fatness. For example, to create a fitness (and dietary change) program to improve body composition, compare the sum of skinfold values over time as an indicator of your program's progress and of improvements in body composition. You can also plug your skinfold values into equations like those in Lab 6.1 that predict percent body fat. When using these equations, however, it is important to remember that they have a fairly substantial margin of error—($\pm$4% if performed by a skilled technician)—so don't focus too much on specific values. The sum represents only a relative measure of body fatness.

Skinfolds are measured with a device called a **caliper**, which consists of a pair of spring-loaded, calibrated jaws. High-quality calipers are made of metal and have parallel jaw surfaces and constant spring tension. Inexpensive plastic calipers are also available, but you need to make sure they are spring-loaded and have metal jaws to ensure accuracy. Refer to Lab 6.1 for instructions on how to take skinfold measurements.

caliper   A pressure-sensitive measuring instrument with two jaws that can be adjusted to determine thickness.

Taking accurate measurements with calipers requires patience, experience, and considerable practice. It's best to take several measurements at each site (or have several different people take each measurement). Be sure to take the measurements in the exact location called for in the procedure. Because the amount of water in your body changes during the day, skinfold measurements taken in the morning and evening often differ. If you repeat the measurements in the future to track changes in your body composition, measure skinfolds at approximately the same time of day.

Bioelectrical Impedance Analysis (BIA)

The BIA technique works by sending a small electrical current through the body and measuring the body's resistance to it (see the box Using BIA at Home on the next page). Fat-free tissues, where most body water is located, are good conductors of electrical current, whereas fat is not. Thus, the amount of resistance to electrical current is related to the amount of fat-free tissue in the body (the lower the resistance, the greater the fat-free mass) and can be used to estimate percent body fat.

Bioelectrical impedance analysis has an error rate of $\pm$4–5%. To reduce error, follow the manufacturer's instructions carefully and avoid overhydration or underhydration (more or less body water than normal). Because measurement varies with the type of BIA analyzer, use the same instrument to compare measurements over time.

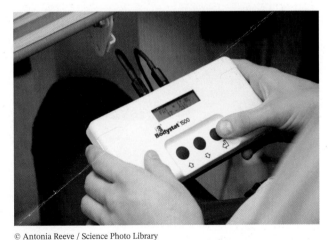

© Antonia Reeve / Science Photo Library

Using bioelectrical impedance analysis to estimate percent body fat.

Wellness *in the* DIGITAL AGE

USING BIA AT HOME

As described in this chapter, scientists can use several techniques to accurately measure body composition, including underwater weighing, air displacement, and dual-energy X-ray absorptiometry (DEXA). These methods are costly, however, and require technical expertise.

You can estimate your body fat and fat-free weight simply and accurately, at home, without the help of a technician. All you need is a digital home scale with a built-in bioelectrical impedance analyzer (BIA) or a hand-held BIA unit. BIA works by measuring the resistance in the body to a small electric current. Electricity flows more slowly through fat tissue than through muscle, so the more fat you have, the more slowly such a current will flow through your body. Conversely, a current will pass through your body more quickly if you have more fat-free (muscle) weight.

Before using a BIA, be sure to read and follow the fluid intake and exercise instructions that are included with your unit. If no such instructions are included, be sure to seek professional advice from a fitness professional before relying on the measures you receive from a BIA unit. When the body is dehydrated, fat estimations can be incorrect.

To use a BIA scale, stand on the scale with bare feet. As it checks your weight, the BIA sends a low-voltage electrical current through your body and analyzes the speed at which the current travels. Checking your weight and body composition takes no longer than checking your weight alone. Most BIA units can remember your last weight and body composition measurement, making it easy to compare the measurements from day to day or week to week. Some scales can remember measurements for multiple people, as well.

A study of 22 weight-trained men showed that BIA compared favourably to underwater weighing for measuring body composition. Measurements of fat and lean mass are most valuable for measuring changes in body composition during diet and exercise programs.

Popular BIA scales are manufactured by Taylor, Whynter, Omron, RemedyT, and Tanita. These scales are available in most department stores and online, and cost between $50 and $200, depending on features.

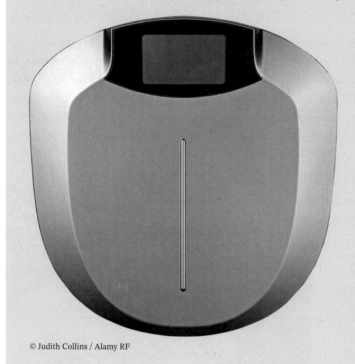

© Judith Collins / Alamy RF

Advanced Techniques: DEXA and TOBEC

Dual-energy X-ray absorptiometry (DEXA) works by measuring the tissue absorption of high- and low-energy X-ray beams. The procedure has an error rate of $\pm 2\%$. Total body electrical conductivity (TOBEC) estimates lean body mass by passing a body through a magnetic field. These methods are often used in sophisticated research projects but are seldom available to the average person. We mention them because they are often used for comparison with some of the field tests described in this chapter.

Assessing Body Fat Distribution

Researchers have studied many different methods for determining the risk associated with body fat distribution. Two of the simplest to perform are waist circumference measurement and waist-to-hip ratio calculation. In the first method, you measure your waist circumference; in the second, you divide your waist circumference by your hip circumference. Waist circumference has been found to be a better indicator of abdominal fat than waist-to-hip ratio. More research is needed to determine the precise degree of risk associated with specific values for these two assessments of body fat distribution. However, as noted earlier, a total waist measurement of more than 102 centimetres for men and 88 centimetres for women and a waist-to-hip ratio above 0.94 for young men and 0.82 for young women are associated with a significantly increased risk of heart disease and diabetes. Lab 6.1 shows you how to measure your body fat distribution.

Somatotype

As discussed in Chapter 2, somatotype describes your basic body build. The three somatotypes are endomorph, mesomorph, and ectomorph.

Endomorphs are round and pear shaped, with wide hips and shoulders. They gain weight easily and will typically regain weight rapidly if they resume their normal lifestyle after losing weight. Endomorphs often excel at weight lifting and might enjoy weight-supported aerobic exercises such as swimming or cycling. Conversely, they might find distance running difficult and painful.

Mesomorphs are lean and muscular and respond well to exercise. They have wedged-shaped bodies, broad shoulders, narrow hips, and little body fat. They gain fitness easily and usually excel at almost any kind of physical activity or sport.

Ectomorphs are thin and linear, with narrow hips and shoulders. They typically have little muscle or fat. Their light frame helps make them successful in activities such as distance running and gymnastics.

Few people have extreme body types—most of us are a mixture of all three. People with every body type can benefit from some form of physical activity.

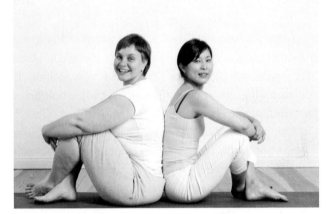

© Fred Froese / Getty Images RF

Wellness Tip

Many body shapes and sizes are associated with good health. Focus on positive lifestyle behaviours rather than on unrealistic goals related to body weight or shape.

LO4 6.3 Setting Body Composition Goals

If assessment tests indicate that fat loss would be beneficial for your health, your first step is to establish a goal. You can use the ratings in Table 6.1 or Table 6.3 to choose a target value for BMI or percent body fat, depending on which assessment you completed.

Set a realistic goal that will ensure good health. Heredity limits your capacity to change your body composition, and few people can expect to develop the body of a fashion model or competitive bodybuilder.

However, you can improve your body composition through a program of regular exercise and a healthy diet. If your body composition is in or close to the recommended range, you may want to set a lifestyle goal rather than a specific percent body fat or BMI goal. For example, you might set a goal of increasing your daily physical activity from 20 to 60 minutes or beginning a program of weight training, and then let any improvements in body composition occur as a secondary result of your primary target (physical activity). Remember, a lifestyle that includes regular exercise may be more important for health than trying to reach any ideal weight.

If you are significantly overfat or if you have known risk factors for disease (such as high blood pressure or high cholesterol), consult your physician to determine a body composition goal for your individual risk profile. For people who are obese, small losses of body weight (5–15%) over a 6 to 12 month period can result in significant health improvements.

Strengthening Mental Wellness

Research suggests that the type of goals you set for yourself can also help to motivate you to continue exercising. Choose goals that are not only specific and detailed, but that also focus on the process that you are engaging in. For example, what will you do to change your body composition? Will you raise your heart rate to 70% of your maximum heart rate for 20 minutes? Can you strive to push to 15 repetitions on each exercise for the upper body muscles? By using these types of goals, you will be better prepared to stick with your program by focusing your mental energy on aspects of the program that will contribute to your goals.

After you've established a body composition goal, you can then set a target range for body weight. Although body weight is not an accurate method of assessing body composition, it's a useful method for tracking progress in a program to change body composition. If you're losing a small or moderate amount of weight and exercising, you're probably losing fat while building muscle mass. Lab 6.2 will help you determine a range for recommended body weight.

Using percent body fat or BMI will generate a fairly accurate target body weight for most people. However, it's best not to stick rigidly to a recommended body weight calculated from any formula; individual genetic, cultural, and lifestyle factors are also important. Decide whether the body weight that the formulas generate for you is realistic, meets all your goals, is healthy, *and* is reasonable for you to maintain.

6.4 Making Changes in Body Composition

In general, your focus should be on lifestyle—regular physical activity, endurance exercise, strength training, and a moderate energy intake. Making significant cuts in food intake in order to lose weight and body fat is a difficult strategy to maintain; focusing on increased physical activity is a better approach for many people. In studies of people who have lost weight and maintained the loss, physical activity was the key to long-term success. (Chapter 8 includes specific strategies for losing or gaining weight and improving body composition.)

You can track your progress toward your target body composition by checking your body weight regularly. You can also monitor how much energy you have and how your clothes fit. To get a more accurate idea of your progress, you should directly reassess your body composition occasionally during your program. Body composition changes as weight changes. Losing a lot of weight usually includes losing some muscle mass no matter how hard you exercise, partly because carrying less weight requires the muscular system to bear a smaller burden. Conversely, a large gain in weight without exercise still causes some gain in muscle mass because muscles are working harder to carry the extra weight.

Tips for Today and the Future

A wellness lifestyle can lead naturally to a body composition that is healthy and appropriate for you.

RIGHT NOW YOU CAN

- Find out what types of body composition assessment techniques are available at facilities on your campus or in your community.
- Do 30 minutes of physical activity five days per week—walk, jog, bike, swim, or climb stairs.
- Drink a glass of water instead of a carbonated beverage, and include a high-fibre food such as whole-grain bread or cereal, popcorn, apples, berries, or beans in your next snack or meal.

IN THE FUTURE YOU CAN

- Think about your image of the ideal body type for your sex. Consider where your idea comes from, whether you use this image to judge your own body, and whether it is a realistic goal for you.
- Be aware of media messages (especially visual images) that make you feel embarrassed or insecure about your body. Remind yourself that these messages are usually designed to sell a product; they should not form the basis of your body image.

Common Questions ANSWERED

Q Is spot reducing effective?

A Spot reducing refers to attempts to lose body fat in specific parts of the body by doing exercises for those parts. Danish researchers have shown that fat use increases in adipose tissue surrounding active muscle, but it is not known if short-term fat use helps reduce fat in specific sites. Most studies show that spot-reducing exercises contribute to fat loss only to the extent that they burn calories. The best way to reduce fat in any specific area is to create an overall negative energy balance: Take in less energy (food) than you use up through exercise and metabolism.

Q How does exercise affect body composition?

A Cardiorespiratory endurance exercise burns calories, thereby helping create a negative energy balance. Weight training does not use many calories and therefore is of little use in creating a negative energy balance. However, weight training increases muscle mass, which maintains a high metabolic rate (the body's energy level) and helps improve body composition. To minimize body fat and increase muscle mass, thereby improving body composition, combine cardiorespiratory endurance exercise and weight training (see figure below).

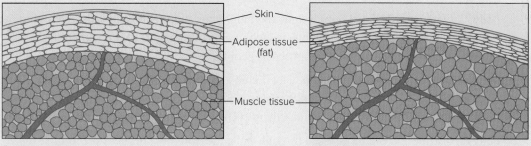

Before training   **After training**

Effects of exercise on body composition. Endurance exercise and strength training both reduce body fat and increase muscle mass.

continued

Q   Are people who have a desirable body composition physically fit?

A   Having a healthy body composition is not necessarily associated with overall fitness. For example, many bodybuilders have very little body fat but have poor cardiorespiratory capacity and flexibility. Some athletes, such as football players, weigh 150 kilograms or more; they have to lose the weight when they retire if they don't want to jeopardize their health. To be fit, you must rate high on all the components of fitness.

Q   What is liposuction, and will it help me lose body fat?

A   Suction lipectomy, popularly known as liposuction, is not performed as often in Canada as it is in the United States, where it has become the most commonly performed cosmetic procedure. The procedure involves removing limited amounts of fat from specific areas. Typically, no more than 2.5 kilograms of adipose tissue is removed at a time. The procedure is usually successful if the amount of excess fat is limited and skin elasticity is good. The procedure is most effective if integrated into a program of dietary restriction and exercise. Side effects include infection, dimpling, and wavy skin contours. Liposuction has a death rate of 1 in 5000 patients, primarily from pulmonary thromboembolism (a blood clot in the lungs) or fat embolism (circulatory blockage caused by a dislodged piece of fat). Other serious complications include shock, bleeding, and impaired blood flow to vital organs.

Q   What is cellulite, and how do I get rid of it?

A   Cellulite is the name commonly given to ripply, wavy fat deposits that collect just under the skin. The "cottage cheese" appearance stems from the breakdown of tissues supporting the fat. These rippling fat deposits are really the same as fat deposited anywhere else in the body. The only way to control them is to create a negative energy balance—burn up more calories than are taken in. There are no creams or lotions that will rub away surface (subcutaneous) fat deposits, and spot reducing is also ineffective. The solution is sensible eating habits and exercise.

SUMMARY

- The human body is composed of fat-free mass (which includes bone, muscle, organ tissues, and connective tissues) and body fat (essential and nonessential).

- Having too much body fat has negative health consequences, especially in terms of cardiovascular disease and diabetes. Distribution of fat is also a significant factor in health.

- A fit and healthy-looking body, with the right body composition for a particular person, develops from habits of proper nutrition and exercise.

- Measuring body weight is not an accurate way to assess body composition because it does not differentiate between muscle weight and fat weight.

- Body mass index (calculated from weight and height measurements) and waist circumference can help classify the health risks associated with being overweight. BMI is sometimes inaccurate, however, particularly in muscular people.

- Techniques for estimating percent body fat include underwater weighing, the Bod Pod, skinfold measurements, bioelectrical impedance analysis (BIA), dual-energy X-ray absorptiometry (DEXA), and total body electrical conductivity (TOBEC).

- Body fat distribution can be assessed through waist measurement or the waist-to-hip ratio.

- Somatotype—endomorph (round), mesomorph (muscular), or ectomorph (linear)—is a useful tool for describing basic body characteristics.

- To determine a recommended body composition and weight, choose a target BMI or target body fat percentage. Keep heredity in mind when setting a goal, and focus on positive changes in lifestyle.

FOR FURTHER EXPLORATION

Organizations and Websites

Canadian Diabetes Association. Provides numerous resources on diabetes including local resources.

http://www.diabetes.ca/

Canadian Obesity Network. Includes research information on obesity.

http://www.obesitynetwork.ca/

Health Canada. Offers information on Canada's Food Guide and making healthy food choices.

http://www.hc-sc.gc.ca/ahc-asc/branch-dirgen/hpfb-dgpsa/onpp-bppn/index-eng.php

Heart and Stroke Foundation of Canada. Includes a BMI calculator and other information on healthy living.

http://www.heartandstroke.ca/

Methods of Body Composition Analysis Tutorials. Contains information about body composition assessment techniques, such as underwater weighing, BIA, and DEXA.

http://nutrition.uvm.edu/bodycomp

Public Health Agency of Canada. Includes comprehensive information about the population of Canada and the trends in body composition across ages, ethnicities, and regions.

http://www.phac-aspc.gc.ca/chn-rcs/index-eng.php

See also the listings for Chapters 2, Chapter 7, and Chapter 8.

Laboratory Activities

Name _____ Section _____ Date _____

Lab 6.1 Assessing Anthropometric Health Risk

Mc Graw Hill Education connect

In this lab, you will gather two anthropometric measures (body mass index and waist circumference) that will help predict your health risk. In addition, skinfold measurements will be used to calculate your estimated body fat percentage.

Body Mass Index (BMI)
Equipment

1. Weight scale

2. Tape measure or other means of measuring height
   Instructions
   Measure your height and weight, and record the results. Be sure to record the unit of measurement.
   Height: _____
   Weight: _____

Calculating BMI (see also the shortcut chart of BMI values in Lab 6.2)

1. Square your height measurement.

   Height _____ m × height _____ m = height _____ m²

2. BMI equals body weight in kilograms divided by height in metres squared (kg/m²).

   Body weight _____ kg ÷ height _____ m² = BMI _____ kg/m²

   (from step 1)

Rating Your BMI

Refer to this table for a rating of your BMI. Record the results below and at the end of this section.

BMI Category	BMI (kg/m²)
Underweight	<18.5
Normal	18.5–24.9
Overweight	25.0–29.9
Obesity (I)	30.0–34.9
Obesity (II)	35.0–39.9
Extreme obesity (III)	≥40.0

(Refer to Table 6.1 for additional information.)

BMI _____ kg/m²

BMI Category (from table) _____

Waist Circumference (WC)

Equipment

1. Tape measure

2. Partner to take measurements

Preparation

Wear clothes that will not add significantly to your measurements.

Instructions

Stand with your feet together and your arms at your sides. Raise your arms only high enough to allow you to take the measurements. Your partner should ensure the tape is horizontal around the entire circumference and pulled snugly against your skin. The tape shouldn't be pulled so tight that it causes indentations in your skin. At the end of a normal expiration, record the measurement to the nearest half-centimetre.

Waist. Measure just above the superior (top) aspect of the iliac crest. To find your iliac crest, feel for the top edge of the supraillium (see Skinfold Measurement below).

WC _____ cm

Assessing Your Health Risk

Record your results and refer to the chart below to discover your combined BMI-WC health risk.

Measurements

Body Mass Index: _____ kg/m²

Waist circumference: _____ cm

Health Risk: _____

BMI & WC Scoring for Adults 20-65 yrs

BMI	BMI Category	BMI Risk	WC for Men (cm)	WC for Women (cm)	BMI-WC Risk
<18.5	Underweight	Increased	—	—	—
18.5–24.9	Normal Weight	Least	≥90	≥80	High
25.0–29.9	Overweight	Increased	≥100	≥90	Very High
30.0–34.9	Obese Class I	High	≥110	≥105	Extremely High
35.0–39.9	Obese Class II	Very High	≥125	≥115	Extremely High
≥40	Obese Class III	Extremely High	≥125	≥125	Extremely High

SOURCE: Table: Rating your BMI. Health Risk for BMI and for Combined BMI-Waist Circumference (WC), *Canadian Society for Exercise Physiology - Physical Activity training for Health* (CSEP-PATH®), © 2013. All rights reserved. Reprinted with permission.

Skinfold Measurements—Estimated Body Fat Percentage

Equipment

1. Skinfold calipers

2. Partner to take measurements

3. Marking pen (optional)

Instructions

1. Select and locate the correct sites for measurement. All measurements should be taken on the right side of the body with the subject standing. Skinfolds are normally measured on the natural fold line of the skin, either vertically or at a slight angle. The skinfold measurement sites for males are chest, abdomen, and thigh; for females, triceps, suprailium, and thigh. If the person taking skinfold measurements is inexperienced, it may be helpful to mark the correct sites with a marking pen.

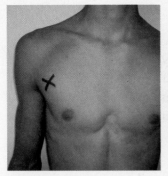 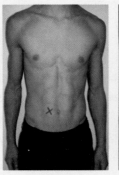 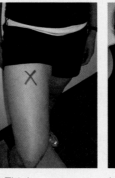 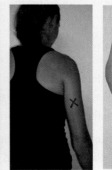 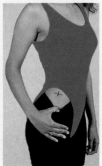

(a) Chest   (b) Abdomen   (c) Thigh   (d) Triceps   (e) Suprailium

Courtesy of Ilsa Wong

(a) Chest. Pinch a diagonal fold halfway between the nipple and the shoulder crease.

(b) Abdomen. Pinch a vertical fold about 2 centimetres to the right of the umbilicus (navel).

(c) Thigh. Pinch a vertical fold midway between the top of the hipbone and the kneecap.

(d) Triceps. Pinch a vertical skinfold on the back of the right arm midway between the shoulder and elbow. The arm should be straight and should hang naturally.

(e) Suprailium. Pinch a fold at the top front of the right hipbone. The skinfold here is taken slightly diagonally according to the natural fold tendency of the skin.

2. **Measure the appropriate skinfolds**. Pinch a fold of skin between your thumb and forefinger. Pull the fold up so that no muscular tissue is included; don't pinch the skinfold too hard. Hold the calipers perpendicular to the fold and measure the skinfold about 0.5 centimetres away from your fingers. Allow the tips of the calipers to close on the skinfold and let the reading settle before marking it down. Take readings to the nearest half-millimetre. Continue to repeat the measurements until two consecutive measurements match, releasing and repinching the skinfold between each measurement. Make a note of the final measurement for each site.

Time of day of measurements: _____

Men		*Women*	
Chest: _____ mm		Triceps: _____ mm	
Abdomen: _____ mm		Suprailium: _____ mm	
Thigh: _____ mm		Thigh: _____ mm	

Determining Percent Body Fat

Add the measurements of your three skinfolds. Use this sum as a point of comparison for future assessments and/or find the percent body fat that corresponds to your total in the appropriate table. For example, a 19-year-old female with measurements of 16 mm, 19 mm, and 22 mm would have a skinfold sum of 57 mm; according to the table below, her percent body fat is 22.7.

Sum of three skinfolds: _____ mm

Percent body fat: _____ %

Percent Body Fat Estimate for Women: Sum of Triceps, Suprailium, and Thigh Skinfolds

Sum of Skinfolds (mm)	Age								
	Under 22	23–27	28–32	33–37	38–42	43–47	48–52	53–57	Over 57
23–25	9.7	9.9	10.2	10.4	10.7	10.9	11.2	11.4	11.7
26–28	11.0	11.2	11.5	11.7	12.0	12.3	12.5	12.7	13.0
29–31	12.3	12.5	12.8	13.0	13.3	13.5	13.8	14.0	14.3
32–34	13.6	13.8	14.0	14.3	14.5	14.8	15.0	15.3	15.5
35–37	14.8	15.0	15.3	15.5	15.8	16.0	16.3	16.5	16.8
38–40	16.0	16.3	16.5	16.7	17.0	17.2	17.5	17.7	18.0
41–43	17.2	17.4	17.7	17.9	18.2	18.4	18.7	18.9	19.2
44–46	18.3	18.6	18.8	19.1	19.3	19.6	1 9.8	20.1	20.3
47–49	19.5	19.7	20.0	20.2	20.5	20.7	21.0	21.2	21.5
50–52	20.6	20.8	21.1	21.3	21.6	21.8	22.1	22.3	22.6
53–55	21.7	21.9	22.1	22.4	22.6	22.9	23.1	23.4	23.6
56–58	22.7	23.0	23.2	23.4	23.7	23.9	24.2	24.4	24.7
59–61	23.7	24.0	24.2	24.5	24.7	25.0	25.2	25.5	25.7
62–64	24.7	25.0	25.2	25.5	25.7	26.0	26.7	26.4	26.7
65–67	25.7	25.9	26.2	26.4	26.7	26.9	27.2	27.4	27.7
68–70	26.6	26.9	27.1	27.4	27.6	27.9	28.1	28.4	28.6
71–73	27.5	27.8	28.0	28.3	28.5	28.8	29.0	29.3	29.5
74–76	28.4	28.7	28.9	29.2	29.4	29.7	29.9	30.2	30.4
77–79	29.3	29.5	29.8	30.0	30.3	30.5	30.8	31.0	31.3
80–82	30.1	30.4	30.6	30.9	31.1	31.4	31.6	31.9	32.1
83–85	30.9	31.2	31.4	31.7	31.9	32.2	32.4	32.7	32.9
86–88	31.7	32.0	32.2	32.5	32.7	32.9	33.2	33.4	33.7
89–91	32.5	32.7	33.0	33.2	33.5	33.7	33.9	34.2	34.4
92–94	33.2	33.4	33.7	33.9	34.2	34.4	34.7	34.9	35.2
95–97	33.9	34.1	34.4	34.6	34.9	35.1	35.4	35.6	35.9
98–100	34.6	34.8	35.1	35.3	35.5	35.8	36.0	36.3	36.5
101–103	35.3	35.4	35.7	35.9	36.2	36.4	36.7	36.9	37.2
104–106	35.8	36.1	36.3	36.6	36.8	37.1	37.3	37.5	37.8
107–109	36.4	36.7	36.9	37.1	37.4	37.6	37.9	38.1	38.4
110–112	37.0	37.2	37.5	37.7	38.0	38.2	38.5	38.7	38.9
113–115	37.5	37.8	38.0	38.2	38.5	38.7	39.0	39.2	39.5
116–118	38.0	38.3	38.5	38.8	39.0	39.3	39.5	39.7	40.0
119–121	38.5	38.7	39.0	39.2	39.5	39.7	40.0	40.2	40.5
122–124	39.0	39.2	39.4	39.7	39.9	40.2	40.4	40.7	40.9
125–127	39.4	39.6	39.9	40.1	40.4	40.6	40.9	41.1	41.4
128–130	39.8	40.0	40.3	40.5	40.8	41.0	41.3	41.5	41.8

SOURCE: Jackson, A.S., and M.L. Pollock. 1985. Practical assessment of body composition. *Physician and Sportsmedicine* 13(5): 76–90. Table 5. Reprinted by permission of the publisher Taylor & Francis Ltd, http://www.tandfonline.com.

Percent Body Fat Estimate for Men: Sum of Chest, Abdomen, and Thigh Skinfolds

Sum of Skinfolds (mm)	Age								
	Under 22	23–27	28–32	33–37	38–42	43–47	48–52	53–57	Over 57
8–10	1.3	1.8	2.3	2.9	3.4	3.9	4.5	5.0	5.5
11–13	2.2	2.8	3.3	3.9	4.4	4.9	5.5	6.0	6.5
14–16	3.2	3.8	4.3	4.8	5.4	5.9	6.4	7.0	7.5
17–19	4.2	4.7	5.3	5.8	6.3	6.9	7.4	8.0	8.5
20–22	5.1	5.7	6.2	6.8	7.3	7.9	8.4	8.9	9.5
23–25	6.1	6.6	7.2	7.7	8.3	8.8	9.4	9.9	10.5
26–28	7.0	7.6	8.1	8.7	9.2	9.8	10.3	10.9	11.4
29–31	8.0	8.5	9.1	9.6	10.2	10.7	11.3	11.8	12.4
32–34	8.9	9.4	10.0	10.5	11.1	11.6	12.2	12.8	13.3
35–37	9.8	10.4	10.9	11.5	12.0	12.6	13.1	13.7	14.3
38–40	10.7	11.3	11.8	12.4	12.9	13.5	14.1	14.6	15.2
41–43	11.6	12.2	12.7	13.3	13.8	14.4	15.0	15.5	16.1
44–46	12.5	13.1	13.6	14.2	14.7	15.3	15.9	16.4	17.0
47–49	13.4	13.9	14.5	15.1	15.6	16.2	16.8	17.3	17.9
50–52	14.3	14.8	15.4	15.9	16.5	17.1	17.6	18.2	18.8
53–55	15.1	15.7	16.2	16.8	17.4	17.9	18.5	19.1	19.7
56–58	16.0	16.5	17.1	17.7	18.2	18.8	19.4	20.0	20.5
59–61	16.9	17.4	17.9	18.5	19.1	19.7	20.2	20.8	21.4
62–64	17.6	18.2	18.8	19.4	19.9	20.5	21.1	21.7	22.2
65–67	18.5	19.0	19.6	20.2	20.8	21.3	21.9	22.5	23.1
68–70	19.3	19.9	20.4	21.0	21.6	22.2	22.7	23.3	23.9
71–73	20.1	20.7	21.2	21.8	22.4	23.0	23.6	24.1	24.7
74–76	20.9	21.5	22.0	22.6	23.2	23.8	24.4	25.0	25.5
77–79	21.7	22.2	22.8	23.4	24.0	24.6	25.2	25.8	26.3
80–82	22.4	23.0	23.6	24.2	24.8	25.4	25.9	26.5	27.1
83–85	23.2	23.8	24.4	25.0	25.5	26.1	26.7	27.3	27.9
86–88	24.0	24.5	25.1	25.7	26.3	26.9	27.5	28.1	28.7
89–91	24.7	25.3	25.9	26.5	27.1	27.6	28.2	28.8	29.4
92–94	25.4	26.0	26.6	27.2	27.8	28.4	29.0	29.6	30.2
95–97	26.1	26.7	27.3	27.9	28.5	29.1	29.7	30.3	30.9
98–100	26.9	27.4	28.0	28.6	29.2	29.8	30.4	31.0	31.6
101–103	27.5	28.1	28.7	29.3	29.9	30.5	31.1	31.7	32.3
104–106	28.2	28.8	29.4	30.0	30.6	31.2	31.8	32.4	33.0
107–109	28.9	29.5	30.1	30.7	31.3	31.9	32.5	33.1	33.7
110–112	29.6	30.2	30.8	31.4	32.0	32.6	33.2	33.8	34.4
113–115	30.2	30.8	31.4	32.0	32.6	33.2	33.8	34.5	35.1
116–118	30.9	31.5	32.1	32.7	33.3	33.9	34.5	35.1	35.7
119–121	31.5	32.1	32.7	33.3	33.9	34.5	35.1	35.7	36.4
122–124	32.1	32.7	33.3	33.9	34.5	35.1	35.8	36.4	37.0
125–127	32.7	33.3	33.9	34.5	35.1	35.8	36.4	37.0	37.6

SOURCE: Jackson, A.S., and M.L. Pollock. 1985. Practical assessment of body composition. *Physician and Sportsmedicine* 13(5): 76–90. Table 8. Reprinted by permission of the publisher Taylor & Francis Ltd, http://www.tandfonline.com

Rating Your Body Composition

Refer to Table 6.3 to rate your percent body fat. Record it below:

Rating: _____

Using Your Results

How did you score? Are you at all surprised by your ratings for health risk? Are your current ratings in the range for good health? Are you satisfied with your current body composition? Why or why not?

_____

_____

_____

If you're not satisfied, set a realistic goal for improvement:

_____

_____

_____

What should you do next? Enter the results of this lab in the Preprogram Assessment column in Appendix B. If you've determined that you need to change your body composition, plan your program using the labs in Chapters 7 and Chapter 9 and the weight management section of the Daily Fitness and Nutrition Journal. After several weeks or months of an exercise and/or dietary change program, complete this lab again and enter the results in the Postprogram Assessment column of Appendix B.

Name _____ **Section** _____ **Date** _____

Lab 6.2 Setting Goals for Target Body Weight

![Mc Graw Hill Education] **connect**

This lab is designed to help you set body weight goals based on a target BMI or percent body fat. If the results of Lab 6.1 indicate that a change in body composition would be beneficial for your health, you may want to complete this lab to help you set goals.

Remember that a wellness lifestyle—including a balanced diet and regular exercise—is more important for your health than achieving any specific body weight, BMI, or percent body fat. You may want to set goals for improving your diet and increasing physical activity and let your body composition change as a result. If so, use the labs in Chapter 3, Chapter 4, Chapter 7, and Chapter 8 as your guides.

Equipment

Calculator (or pencil and paper for calculations).

Preparation

Determine percent body fat and/or calculate BMI as described in Lab 6.1. Keep track of height and weight as measured for these calculations.

Height: _____ Weight: _____

Instructions: Target Body Weight from Target BMI

Use the diagram below to find the target body weight that corresponds to your target BMI. Find your height on the y-axis, and then move across the appropriate row until you enter the BMI zone that you would like to

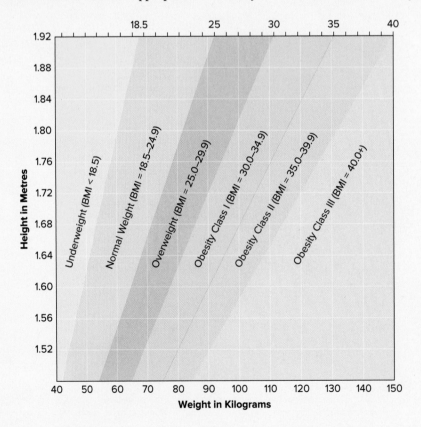

achieve. Follow that zone down to the x-axis to discover the range in weight that corresponds to your target BMI zone. Remember, BMI is only an indirect measurement of body composition. It is possible to improve body composition without any significant change in weight. For example, a weight training program may result in increased muscle mass and decreased fat mass without any change in overall weight. For this reason, you may want to set alternative or additional goals, such as improving the fit of your clothes or decreasing your waist measurement.

Current BMI: _____ Target BMI zone: _____ Target body weight range (from chart): _____

Alternative/additional goals:

_____

_____

_____

Note: You can calculate target body weight from target BMI more precisely by using the following formula: (1) convert your height measurement to metres; (2) square your height measurement; (3) multiply this number by your target BMI to get your target weight in kilograms:

1. Height _____ in. $\times$ 0.0254 m/in. = height _____ m

2. Height _____ m $\times$ height _____ m = _____ m^2

3. Target BMI _____ $\times$ height _____ m^2 = target weight _____ kg

Note: If you are more comfortable referring to your weight in pounds, multiply your weight in kg by 2.2 to estimate your weight in pounds.

Setting a Goal

Based on these calculations and other factors (including heredity, individual preference, and current health status), select a target weight or range of weights for yourself.

Target body weight: _____

Nutrition

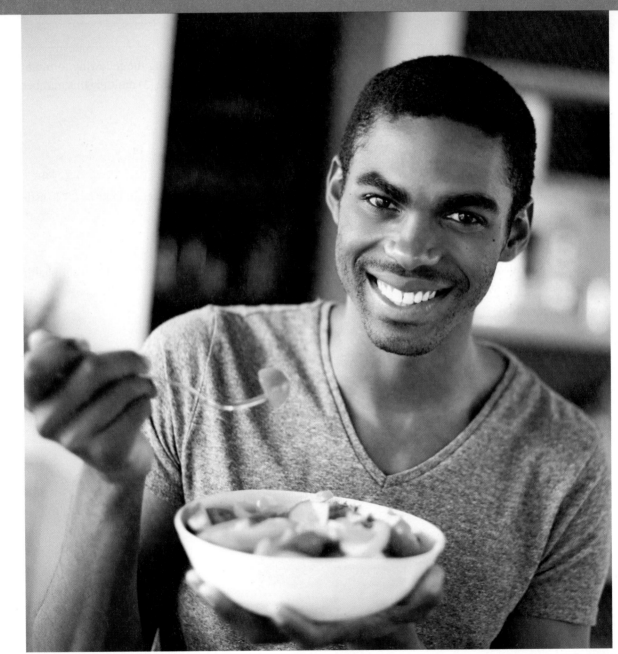

LEARNING OBJECTIVES

After reading this chapter, you should be able to

LO1 List the essential nutrients and describe the functions they perform in the body

LO2 Describe the guidelines that have been developed to help people choose a healthy diet, avoid nutritional deficiencies, and reduce their risk of diet-related chronic diseases

LO3 Describe nutritional guidelines for vegetarians and for special population groups

LO4 Explain how to use food labels and other consumer tools to make informed choices about foods

LO5 Create a personal nutrition plan based on affordable foods that you enjoy and that will promote wellness today and in the future

TEST YOUR KNOWLEDGE

1. **It is recommended that all adults consume one serving each of fruits and vegetables every day.**
   True or false?

2. **Candy is the leading source of added sugars in the North American diet.**
   True or false?

3. **Which of the following is NOT a whole grain?**
   a. brown rice
   b. wheat flour
   c. popcorn

ANSWERS

1. **FALSE.** For someone consuming 2000 calories per day, 2½ cups of vegetables and 2 cups of fruit are recommended daily.

2. **FALSE.** Regular (nondiet) carbonated beverages are the leading source of added sugars, with an average of 99.7 litres consumed per person per year in Canada. Each 360 mL beverage supplies about 10 teaspoons of sugar, the total recommended daily limit for a 2000-calorie diet.

3. **B.** Unless labelled "whole wheat," wheat flour is processed to remove the bran and germ and is not a whole grain.

In your lifetime, you'll spend about six years eating—about 70 000 meals and 60 tonnes of food. What you eat affects your energy level, well-being, and overall health. Your nutritional habits help determine your risk of major chronic diseases, including heart disease, cancer, stroke, and diabetes. Choosing foods that provide adequate amounts of the nutrients you need while limiting the substances linked to disease should be an important part of your daily life.

Choosing a healthy diet is a two-part project. First, you have to know which nutrients are necessary and in what amounts. Second, you have to translate those requirements into a diet consisting of foods you like to eat that are both available and affordable, and that fit into your lifestyle. After you have an idea of what constitutes a healthy diet for you, you can adjust your current diet to bring it into line with your goals.

This chapter provides the basic principles of **nutrition**. It introduces the six classes of essential nutrients, explaining their role in the functioning of the body. It also provides guidelines that you can use to design a healthy eating plan. Finally, it offers practical tools and advice to help you apply the guidelines to your life.

> **nutrition**   The science of food and how the body uses it in health and disease.

LO1 7.1 Nutritional Requirements: Components of a Healthy Diet

You probably think about your diet in terms of the foods you like to eat. More important for your health, though, are the nutrients contained in those foods. Your body requires proteins, fats, carbohydrates, vitamins, minerals, and water—about 45 **essential nutrients**. The word *essential* in this context means that you must get these substances from food because your body is unable to manufacture them at all, or at least not fast enough or in sufficient amounts to meet your physiological needs. The six classes of nutrients, along with their functions and major sources, are listed in Table 7.1.

> **essential nutrients**   Substances the body must get from food because it cannot manufacture them at all or fast enough to meet its needs. These nutrients include proteins, fats, carbohydrates, vitamins, minerals, and water.

The body needs some essential nutrients in relatively large amounts. These **macronutrients** include protein, fat, carbohydrate, and water. **Micronutrients**, such as vitamins and minerals, are required in much smaller amounts. Your body obtains nutrients through the process of **digestion**, which breaks down food into compounds that the gastrointestinal tract can absorb and the body can use (see Figure 7.1). A diet that provides enough essential nutrients is vital because they provide energy, help build and maintain body tissues, and help regulate body functions.

> **macronutrients**   Essential nutrients required by the body in relatively large amounts.
> **micronutrients**   Essential nutrients required by the body in minute amounts.
> **digestion**   The process of breaking down foods in the gastrointestinal tract into compounds the body can absorb.

Food is partially broken down by being chewed and mixed with saliva in the mouth. After travelling to the stomach via the esophagus, food is broken down further by stomach acids and other secretions. As food moves through the digestive tract, it is mixed by muscular contractions and broken down by chemicals. Most absorption of nutrients occurs in the small intestine, aided by secretions from the pancreas, gallbladder, and intestinal lining. The large intestine reabsorbs excess water; the remaining solid wastes are collected in the rectum and excreted through the anus.

TABLE 7.1

The Six Classes of Essential Nutrients

Nutrient	Function	Major Sources
Proteins (4 calories/gram)	Form important parts of muscles, bone, blood, enzymes, some hormones, and cell membranes; repair tissue; regulate water and acid-base balance; help in growth; supply energy	Meat, fish, poultry, eggs, milk products, legumes, nuts
Carbohydrates (4 calories/gram)	Supply energy to cells in brain, nervous system, and blood; supply energy to muscles during exercise	Grains (breads and cereals), fruits, vegetables, milk
Fats (9 calories/gram)	Supply energy; insulate, support, and cushion organs; provide medium for absorption of fat-soluble vitamins	Animal foods, grains, nuts, seeds, fish, vegetables
Vitamins	Promote (initiate or speed up) specific chemical reactions within cells	Abundant in fruits, vegetables, and grains; also found in meat and dairy products
Minerals	Help regulate body functions; aid in the growth and maintenance of body tissues; act as catalysts for the release of energy	Found in most food groups
Water	Makes up 50–60% of body weight; provides a medium for chemical reactions; transports chemicals; regulates temperature; removes waste products	Fruits, vegetables, and liquids

FIGURE 7.1

The Digestive System

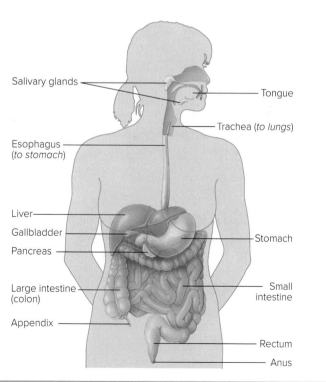

Calories

The energy in foods is expressed as **kilocalories**. One kilocalorie represents the amount of heat it takes to raise the temperature of 1 litre of water 1°C. A person needs about 2000 kilocalories a day to meet energy needs. In common usage, people usually refer to kilocalories as calories, which is a much smaller energy unit: 1 kilocalorie contains 1000 calories. This text uses the familiar word *calorie* to stand for the larger energy unit; you'll also find *calorie* used on food labels.

> **kilocalorie**   A measure of energy content in food; 1 kilocalorie represents the amount of heat needed to raise the temperature of 1 litre of water 1°C; commonly referred to as a *calorie*.

Of the six classes of essential nutrients, three supply energy:

- fat = 9 calories per gram
- protein = 4 calories per gram
- carbohydrate = 4 calories per gram

Alcohol, although it is not an essential nutrient, also supplies energy, providing 7 calories per gram.

Just meeting energy needs is not enough; our bodies need enough of all the essential nutrients to function properly. Practically all foods contain mixtures of nutrients, although foods are commonly classified according to their predominant nutrients. For example, spaghetti is considered a carbohydrate food although it contains small amounts of other nutrients. The following sections discuss the functions and sources of each class of nutrients.

> **Fitness Tip**
>
> A kilogram of body fat is equal to 7700 calories. If you eat 100 calories more than you expend every day, you will gain more than 4.5 kilograms in a year.

Proteins—The Basis of Body Structure

Proteins form important parts of the body's main structural components, muscles and bones. Proteins also form important parts of blood, enzymes, cell membranes, and some hormones.

> **protein**   An essential nutrient that forms important parts of the body's main structures (muscle and bones) as well as blood, enzymes, hormones, and cell membranes; also provides energy.

Amino Acids

The building blocks of proteins are called **amino acids**. Twenty common amino acids are found in food, and nine of these are essential (or indispensable). As long as foods supply certain nutrients, the body can produce the other 11 amino acids.

> **amino acids**   The building blocks of proteins.

Complete and Incomplete Proteins

Individual protein sources are considered "complete" if they supply all the essential amino acids in adequate amounts and "incomplete" if they do not. Meat, fish, poultry, eggs, milk, cheese, and soy provide complete proteins. Incomplete proteins, which come from plant sources such as nuts and **legumes** (dried beans and peas), are good sources of most essential amino acids, but are usually low in one or more.

legumes   Vegetables such as peas and beans that are high in fibre and are also important sources of protein.

Combining two vegetable proteins, such as wheat and peanuts in a peanut butter sandwich, allows each vegetable protein to make up for the amino acids missing in the other protein. The combination yields a complete protein. It was once believed that vegetarians had to complement their proteins at each meal in order to receive the benefit of a complete protein. We now know that proteins consumed throughout the course of the day can complement each other to form a pool of amino acids from which the body can draw to produce proteins. Vegetarians should include a variety of vegetable protein sources in their diets to make sure they get all the essential amino acids in adequate amounts. (Healthy vegetarian diets are discussed later in the chapter.)

Strengthening Mental Wellness

Research shows that some protein-rich foods can give you a quick mental boost, which can be helpful before an exam. The theory is that proteins contain the amino acid tyrosine, which is used by the body to manufacture the neurotransmitters dopamine and norepinephrine. Some researchers postulate that eating protein-containing foods could increase the synthesis of these neurotransmitters, which can speed reaction time and increase alertness. Whether this really works, especially in well-nourished individuals who have not been lacking these nutrients to begin with, remains to be seen. In the meantime, it wouldn't hurt—and it might even help—to include some protein in the meal you eat prior to your next big exam.

Recommended Protein Intake

Adequate daily intake of protein for adults is 0.8 gram per kilogram of body weight, or about 50 grams of protein per day for someone who weighs 64 kilograms (140 pounds) and 65 grams of protein for someone who weighs 82 kilograms (180 pounds). Table 7.2 lists some popular food items and the amount of protein each provides.

TABLE 7.2

Protein Content of Common Food Items

Item	Protein (grams)
90 g lean meat, poultry, or fish	20–27
¼ block (90 g) tofu	7
1 cup cooked beans	15–19
1 cup yogourt	8–13
30 g cheese	6–8
1 cup cottage or ricotta cheese	23–28

The majority of Canadians consume acceptable levels of protein required for adequate nutrition.[1] Protein consumed beyond what the body needs is synthesized into fat for energy storage or burned for energy requirements. A little extra protein is not harmful, but it can contribute fat to the diet because protein-rich foods can be high in fat, especially saturated fat.

A fairly broad range of protein intake is associated with good health. Health Canada recommends that the amount of protein adults eat should fall within the range of 10–30% of the total daily calorie intake. The average Canadian adult diet includes about 16% of total daily calories as protein.[2] (See Chapter 8 for more information about high-protein diets advocated for weight loss.)

Fats—Essential in Small Amounts

Fats, also known as *lipids*, are the most concentrated source of energy, at 9 calories per gram. The fats stored in your body represent usable energy, help insulate your body, and support and cushion your organs. Fats in the diet help your body absorb fat-soluble vitamins and add flavour and texture to foods. Fats are the major fuel for the body during periods of rest and light activity.

Two fats, linoleic acid and alpha-linolenic acid—the essential fatty acids—are necessary components of the diet. They are used to make compounds that are key regulators of such body functions as the maintenance of blood pressure and the progress of a healthy pregnancy.

Types and Sources of Fats

Food fats are usually composed of both **saturated** and **unsaturated** fatty acids (Table 7.3). The dominant type of fatty acid determines the fat's characteristics. Saturated fats come mostly from animal products—red meats (e.g., hamburger, steak, roasts), whole milk, cheese, hot dogs, and lunch meats—but are also found in tropic oils, such as coconut and palm oils. They are usually solid at room temperature. Most unsaturated fats in

TABLE 7.3

Types of Fatty Acids

Type of Fatty Acid	Found In[a]
Saturated	• Animal fats (especially fatty meats and poultry fat and skin) • Butter, cheese, and other high-fat dairy products • Palm and coconut oils
Trans	• Some frozen pizza • Some types of popcorn • Deep-fried fast foods • Stick margarine and shortening • Packaged cookies and crackers • Processed snacks and sweets
Monounsaturated	• Olive, canola, and safflower oils • Avocados, olives • Peanut butter (without added fat) • Many nuts, including almonds, cashews, pecans, and pistachios
Polyunsaturated—Omega-3[b]	• Fatty fish, including salmon, white albacore tuna, mackerel, anchovies, and sardines • Compared to fish, lesser amounts are found in walnut, flaxseed, canola, and soybean oils; tofu; walnuts; flaxseeds; and dark green leafy vegetables
Polyunsaturated—Omega-6[b]	• Corn, soybean, and cottonseed oils (often used in margarine, mayonnaise, and salad dressings)

[a] Food fats contain a combination of types of fatty acids in various proportions. For example, canola oil is composed mainly of monounsaturated fatty acids (62%) but also contains polyunsaturated (32%) and saturated (6%) fatty acids.
[b] The essential fatty acids are polyunsaturated; linoleic acid is an omega-6 fatty acid and alpha-linolenic acid is an omega-3 fatty acid.

foods come from plant sources and are liquid at room temperature. Most of the fats in food are fairly similar in composition, generally including a molecule of glycerol (an alcohol) plus three fatty acid chains attached to it. The resulting structure is called a triglyceride. Animal fat, for example, is primarily made of triglycerides.

> **saturated**   Fatty acids found mostly in animal products and tropical oils; usually solid at room temperature.
> **unsaturated**   Fatty acids usually found in plant foods; usually liquid at room temperature.

Depending on their structure, unsaturated fatty acids can be further divided into *monounsaturated* and *polyunsaturated* fats. Olive, canola, safflower, and peanut oils contain mostly monounsaturated fatty acids. Soybean, corn, and cottonseed oils contain mostly polyunsaturated fatty acids. You may sometimes also see polyunsaturated fats described more specifically by chemical structure as either omega-3 or omega-6 fats.

Hydrogenation

When unsaturated vegetable oils undergo the process of **hydrogenation**, a mixture of saturated and unsaturated fatty acids is produced, creating a more solid fat from a liquid oil. Hydrogenation also changes some unsaturated fatty acids into **trans fatty acids (trans fats)**, unsaturated fatty acids with an atypical shape that affects their behaviour in the body.

> **hydrogenation**   A process by which hydrogens are added to unsaturated fats, increasing the degree of saturation and turning liquid oils into solid fats. Hydrogenation produces a mixture of saturated fatty acids and standard and trans forms of unsaturated fatty acids.
> **trans fatty acids (trans fats)**   A type of unsaturated fatty acid produced during the process of hydrogenation; trans fats have an atypical shape that affects their chemical activity.

Trans fats can be found in many foods. Some occur naturally in animal fat, particularly beef, lamb, and dairy products, but the majority of trans fat in the Canadian diet are artificial, from partially hydrogenated oils. Many baked and fried foods are prepared with hydrogenated vegetable oils, which means they can be relatively high in saturated and trans fatty acids. Food manufacturers use hydrogenation to increase the stability of an oil so it can be reused for deep frying; to improve the texture of certain foods (to make pastries and pie crusts flakier, for example); and to extend the shelf life of foods made with oil. Hydrogenation is also used to transform liquid oil into margarine or vegetable shortening.

In general, the more solid a hydrogenated oil is, the more saturated and trans fats it contains. For example, stick margarines typically contain more saturated and trans fats than do tub or squeeze margarines.

Hydrogenated vegetable oils are not the only plant fats that contain saturated fats. Palm and coconut oils, although derived from plants, are also highly saturated. Yet fish oils, derived from an animal source, are rich in polyunsaturated fats.

Fats and Health

Scientists are still unravelling the complex effects that individual types of fats and overall dietary patterns have on health and the risk for specific diseases. Recently, most health experts have agreed on the dangers of artificial trans fats because of their double-negative effect on heart health—they raise levels of **low-density lipoprotein (LDL)**—"bad" cholesterol—and they also lower **high-density lipoprotein (HDL)**—"good" cholesterol. Consuming trans fats appears to increase the risk of both cardiovascular disease and type 2 diabetes.

> **low-density lipoprotein (LDL)**   Blood fat that transports cholesterol to organs and tissues; excess amounts result in the accumulation of fatty deposits on artery walls.
> **high-density lipoprotein (HDL)**   Blood fat that helps transport cholesterol out of the arteries, thereby protecting against heart disease.

Canadians were once the largest consumers of trans fats in the world. Fortunately, Canadian consumption of trans fats has declined by about 40% over the last decade (8.3–4.9 g per day).[3] In January 2003, Canada became the first country to require the inclusion of trans fatty acid content on food labels. In 2017, as part of its Healthy Eating Strategy, Health Canada banned industrial trans fats in all food sold in Canada.

What about other types of fats? Many studies have examined the effects of dietary fat intake on blood **cholesterol** levels and the risk of heart disease. Although there are numerous conflicting thoughts about fat consumption, the general consensus is that we are still strongly advised to lower saturated fat intake to reduce cardiovascular risk, especially those people with risk factors for heart disease. Continued research on the health risks and benefits of individual fats is ongoing. For example, do saturated fats in beef, butter, milk, and chocolate all have the same effect on heart disease risk? And what are the health effects of shifts in the intake of particular fats within the overall context of the diet?

> **cholesterol** A waxy substance found in the blood and cells and needed for cell membranes, vitamin D, and hormone synthesis.

Dietary fat affects health in other ways besides heart disease risk. Diets high in fatty red meat are associated with an increased risk of certain forms of cancer, especially colon cancer. A high-fat diet can also make weight management more difficult because fat is a concentrated source of calories. If you are trying to limit overall energy intake, consuming a high-fat diet can make it more difficult to consume all essential nutrients at your target calorie level.

What does all this mean for you? Although more research is needed on the precise effects of different types and amounts of fat on overall health, evidence suggests that most people benefit from keeping their overall fat and saturated fat intake at recommended levels. Dietary patterns are more important for health than a focus on a single nutrient. The fats in your diet are found in foods that contain other nutrients, and the foods you consume are in the context of your overall diet. Increased body weight, aging, and gender are more important for predicting negative health events than eating one kind of dietary fat rather than another.

Health Canada recommends that Canadians limit their intake of saturated fat to less than 10% of total calories per day—but that they do so in the context of a healthy dietary pattern that emphasizes vegetables, fruits, whole grains, low- or non-fat dairy, seafood, legumes, and nuts; is lower in red and processed meat; and is low in sugar-sweetened foods and drinks and refined grains. Don't replace one less-than-healthy choice with another. Healthy dietary patterns are described in detail later in this chapter.

Wellness Tip

An isolated focus on reducing dietary fat intake contributed to an explosion in the availability of processed foods promoted as being low in fat. Many of these choices, however, are high in refined grains and added sugars and are not healthy choices. Focus on your overall dietary pattern and limit your intake of both saturated fats and added sugars. Choose unsaturated fats, whole grains, and fruits and vegetables.

Recommended Fat Intake

To meet the body's need for essential fats, adult men need about 17 grams per day of linoleic acid and 1.6 grams per day of alpha-linolenic acid. Women need 12 grams of linoleic acid and 1.1 grams of alpha-linolenic acid per day. It only takes about 3 to 4 teaspoons (15–20 grams) of vegetable oil per day incorporated into your diet to supply the essential fats. Most Canadians get enough essential fats; limiting unhealthy fats is a much greater health concern.

Limits for total, saturated, and trans fat intake have been set by a number of government and research organizations. In 2002, the Food and Nutrition Board, in conjunction with Health Canada, released recommendations for the balance of energy sources in a healthful diet. These recommendations, called Acceptable Macronutrient Distribution Ranges (AMDRs), are based on ensuring adequate intake of essential nutrients while also reducing the risk of chronic diseases like heart disease and cancer. As with protein, a range of levels of fat intake is associated with good health; the AMDR for total fat is 20–35% of total calories. Although more difficult for consumers to monitor, AMDRs have also been set for omega-6 fatty acids (5–10%) and omega-3 fatty acids (0.6–1.2%) as part of total fat intake. Because any amount of saturated and trans fat increases the risk of heart disease, saturated and trans fat intake should be kept as low as possible and most fat in a healthy diet should be unsaturated. Canadian adults currently consume about 31% of total calories as fat.

For advice on setting individual intake goals, see the box, Setting Intake Goals for Protein, Fat, and Carbohydrates. To determine how close you are to meeting these intake goals for fat, keep a running total over the course of the day. For prepared foods, food labels list the number of grams of fat, protein, and carbohydrates. Nutrition information is also available in many grocery stores, in published nutrition guides, and online (see For Further Exploration at the end of the chapter). By checking these resources, you can keep track of the total grams of fat, protein, and carbohydrates you eat and assess your current diet.

In reducing fat intake to recommended levels, the emphasis should be on lowering saturated and trans fats. You can still eat high-fat foods, but it makes good sense to limit the size of your portions and to balance your intake with low-fat foods. For example, peanut butter is high in fat, with 8 grams (72 calories) of fat in each 90-calorie tablespoon. Two tablespoons of peanut butter eaten on whole-wheat bread and served with a banana, carrot sticks, and a glass of nonfat milk makes a nutritious lunch—high in protein and carbohydrates, and relatively low in total and saturated fat (500 calories, 18 grams of total fat, 4 grams of saturated fat). By comparison, 4 tablespoons of peanut butter on high-fat crackers with potato chips, cookies, and whole milk is a less healthy combination (1000 calories, 62 grams of total fat, 15 grams of saturated fat). So although it's important to evaluate individual food items for their fat content, it is more important to look at them in the context of your overall diet.

Take CHARGE

SETTING INTAKE GOALS FOR PROTEIN, FAT, AND CARBOHYDRATES

The Food and Nutrition Board and Health Canada have established goals to help ensure adequate intake of the essential amino acids, fatty acids, and carbohydrates. The daily goals for adequate intake for adults are as follows:

	Men	Women
Protein	56 grams	46 grams
Fat: Linoleic acid	17 grams	12 grams
Alpha-linolenic acid	1.6 gram	1.1 grams
Carbohydrates	130 grams	130 grams

Protein intake goals can be calculated more specifically by multiplying your body weight in kilograms by 0.8. (Refer to the Nutrition Resources section at the end of the chapter for information for specific age groups and life stages.)

To meet your daily energy needs, you need to consume more than the minimally adequate amounts of the energy-providing nutrients listed above, which alone supply only about 800 to 900 calories. The

continued

Food and Nutrition Board provides additional guidance in the form of Acceptable Macronutrient Distribution Ranges (AMDRs). The ranges can help you balance your intake of the energy-providing nutrients in ways that ensure adequate intake, while reducing the risk of chronic disease. The AMDRs for protein, total fat, and carbohydrates are as follows:

Protein	10–30% of total daily calories
Total fat	20–35% of total daily calories
Carbohydrates	45–65% of total daily calories

To set individual goals, begin by estimating your total daily energy (calorie) needs; if your weight is stable, your current energy intake is the number of calories you need to maintain your weight at your current activity level. Next, select percentage goals for protein, fat, and carbohydrates. You can allocate your total daily calories among the three classes of macronutrients to suit your preferences; just make sure that the three percentage values you select total 100% and that you meet the minimum intake goals listed. Two samples reflecting different total energy intake and nutrient intake goals are shown below.

To translate your own percentage goals into daily intake goals expressed in calories and grams, multiply the appropriate percentages by total calorie intake and then divide the results by the corresponding calories per gram. For example, a fat limit of 35% applied to a 2200-calorie diet would be calculated as follows: $0.35 \times 2200 = 770$ calories of total fat; $770 \div 9$ calories per gram = 86 grams of total fat. (Remember that fat has 9 calories per gram and that protein and carbohydrates have 4 calories per gram.)

Two Sample Macronutrient Distributions

Nutrient	AMDR	Sample 1 Individual Goals	Sample 1 Amounts for a 1600-calorie diet	Sample 2 Individual Goals	Sample 2 Amounts for a 2800-calorie diet
Protein	10–30%	15%	240 calories = 60 grams	30%	840 calories = 210 grams
Fat	20–35%	30%	480 calories = 53 grams	25%	700 calories = 78 grams
Carbohydrates	45–65%	55%	880 calories = 220 grams	45%	1260 calories = 315 grams

SOURCE: Food and Nutrition Board, Institute of Medicine, National Academies. 2002. *Dietary Reference Intakes: Energy, Carbohydrate, Fibre, Fat, Fatty Acids, Cholesterol, Protein, and Amino Acids.* Washington, DC: National Academy Press. Reprinted with permission from *Dietary Reference Intakes: Applications in Dietary Planning.* Copyright © 2003 by the National Academy of Sciences. Courtesy of the National Academies Press, Washington, DC.

Carbohydrates—An Ideal Source of Energy

Carbohydrates or "carbs" supply energy to body cells. Some cells, such as those in the brain and other parts of the nervous system and in the blood, use only carbohydrate glucose for fuel. During high-intensity exercise, muscles use carbohydrates for fuel.

carbohydrate An essential nutrient; sugars, starches, and dietary fibre are all carbohydrates.

Simple and Complex Carbohydrates

Carbohydrates are classified into two groups: simple and complex. *Simple carbohydrates* are the single sugar molecules (monosaccharides) and the double sugars (disaccharides). Three monosaccharides are glucose, fructose, and galactose. Glucose, the most common of the sugars, is used by both animals and plants for energy. Fructose is a very sweet sugar that is found in fruits, and galactose is the sugar in milk.

The disaccharides, pairs of single sugars, include sucrose (table sugar: fructose + glucose), maltose (malt sugar: glucose + glucose), and lactose (milk sugar: galactose + glucose). Simple carbohydrates add sweetness to foods. They are found naturally in fruits and milk and are added to soft drinks, fruit drinks, candy, and desserts. There is no evidence that any type of simple carbohydrate is more nutritious than others.

Complex carbohydrates include starches and most types of dietary fibre. Starches are found in a variety of plants, especially grains (e.g., wheat, rye, rice, oats, barley, millet), legumes, and tubers (e.g., potatoes, yams). Most other vegetables contain a mix of starches and simple carbohydrates. Fibre, which is discussed later in this chapter, is found in fruits, vegetables, and grains.

During digestion, your body breaks down carbohydrates into simple sugar molecules, such as **glucose**, for absorption. Once the glucose is in the bloodstream, the pancreas releases the hormone insulin, which allows cells to take up glucose and use it for energy. The liver and muscles also take up glucose and store it in the form of a starch called **glycogen**. The muscles use glucose from glycogen as fuel during endurance events or long workouts.

> **glucose** A simple sugar that is the body's basic fuel.
> **glycogen** An animal starch stored in the liver and muscles.

Refined Carbohydrates versus Whole Grains

Complex carbohydrates can be further divided between refined, or processed, carbohydrates and unrefined carbohydrates, or whole grains. Before they are processed, all grains are **whole grains**, consisting of an inner layer of germ, a middle layer called the endosperm, and an outer layer of bran (Figure 7.2). During processing, the germ and bran are often removed, leaving just the starchy endosperm. The refinement of whole grains transforms whole-wheat flour to white flour, brown rice to white rice, and so on.

> **whole grain** The entire edible portion of a grain such as wheat, rice, or oats, including the germ, endosperm, and bran. During milling or processing, parts of the grain are removed, often leaving just the endosperm.

FIGURE 7.2

The parts of a whole grain kernel.

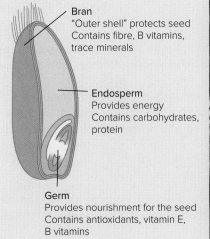
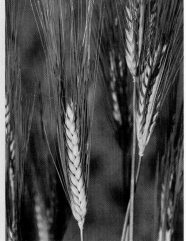

Bran
"Outer shell" protects seed
Contains fibre, B vitamins, trace minerals

Endosperm
Provides energy
Contains carbohydrates, protein

Germ
Provides nourishment for the seed
Contains antioxidants, vitamin E, B vitamins

Refined carbohydrates usually retain all the calories of their unrefined counterparts, but they tend to be much lower in fibre, vitamins, minerals, and other beneficial compounds. Refined grain products are often enriched or fortified with vitamins and minerals, but many of the nutrients lost in processing are not replaced.

Unrefined carbohydrates tend to take longer to chew and digest than refined ones; they also enter the bloodstream more slowly. This slower digestive pace tends to make people feel full sooner and for a longer period. In addition, a slower rise in blood glucose levels following consumption of complex carbohydrates may help in the prevention and management of diabetes. Whole grains are also high in dietary fibre (discussed later in this chapter).

Consumption of whole grains has been linked to reduced risk for heart disease, diabetes, and cancer, and plays an important role in gastrointestinal health and body weight management. For all these reasons, whole grains are recommended over those that have been refined. See the box Choosing More Whole-Grain Foods for tips on increasing your intake of whole grains.

Wellness Tip

Recent evidence suggests that people who eat more whole grains, especially those high in dietary fibre, tend to have a lower body weight than people who eat fewer whole grains.

Take CHARGE

CHOOSING MORE WHOLE-GRAIN FOODS

What Are Whole Grains?

The first step in increasing your intake of whole grains is to correctly identify them. The following are whole grains:

whole wheat	whole-grain corn
whole rye	popcorn
whole oats	brown rice
oatmeal	barley

Other choices include bulgur (cracked wheat), millet, kasha (roasted buckwheat kernels), quinoa, teff, wheat and rye berries, amaranth, graham flour, whole-grain kamut, whole-grain spelt, and whole-grain triticale.

Wheat flour, unbleached flour, enriched flour, and degerminated corn meal are not whole grains. Wheat germ and wheat bran are also not whole grains, but they are the constituents of wheat typically left out when wheat is processed and so are healthier choices than regular wheat flour, which typically contains just the endosperm.

Checking Packages for Whole Grains

To find packaged foods—such as bread or pasta—that are rich in whole grains, read the list of ingredients and check for special health claims related to whole grains. The first item on the list of ingredients should be one of the whole grains listed above. In addition, Health Canada has recently suggested that Canadian manufacturers follow US Food and Drug Administration guidelines, which allow manufacturers to include special health claims for foods that contain 51% or more whole-grain ingredients. Such products may contain a statement such as the following on their packaging:

- "Rich in whole grain."
- "Made with 100% whole grain."
- "Diets rich in whole-grain foods may help reduce the risk of heart disease and certain cancers."

However, many whole-grain products do not carry such claims. This is one more reason to check the ingredient list to make sure you're buying a product made from one or more whole grains.

Glycemic Index and Glycemic Response

Insulin and glucose levels rise and fall following a meal or snack containing any type of carbohydrate. Some foods cause a quick and dramatic rise in glucose and insulin levels, while others have a slower, more moderate effect. A food that has a strong effect on blood glucose levels is said to have a high **glycemic index**. The glycemic index of a food indicates the type of carbohydrate in that food. Unrefined complex carbohydrates, high-fibre foods, and high-fat foods tend to have a lower glycemic index.

glycemic index (GI)   A measure of how high and how fast a particular food raises blood glucose levels.

Attempting to base food choices on glycemic index is a difficult task, however. For people with particular health concerns, such as diabetes, glycemic index may be an important consideration in choosing foods. In addition to the type of carbohydrate in the food, the total amount of carbohydrates in the diet is important for diabetes management. Your best bet, therefore, is to choose a variety of vegetables daily and limit refined grains as well as foods that are high in added sugars and low in other nutrients.

Strengthening Mental Wellness

Certain carbohydrate-rich foods, such as a bagel or a plain baked potato, can have a temporary calming effect on some people during stressful situations.

Recommended Carbohydrate Intake

On average, Canadians consume 358 grams of carbohydrate per day, well above the 130 grams needed to meet the body's requirement for essential carbohydrate.[4] A range of intakes is associated with good health, and experts recommend that adults consume 45–65% of total daily calories as carbohydrate, about 225 to 325 grams of carbohydrate for someone consuming 2000 calories per day. The focus should be on consuming a variety of foods rich in complex carbohydrates, especially whole grains.

Health experts offer separate guidelines for intake of added sugars as part of total carbohydrate consumption. The Food and Nutrition Board and Health Canada set an AMDR for added sugars of 25% or less of total daily calories, but many health experts recommend a substantially lower intake—as low as 5–10%. Foods high in added sugar are generally high in calories and low in nutrients and fibre, thus providing "empty" calories. To reduce your intake of added sugars, limit soft drinks, candy, sweet desserts, and sweetened fruit drinks.

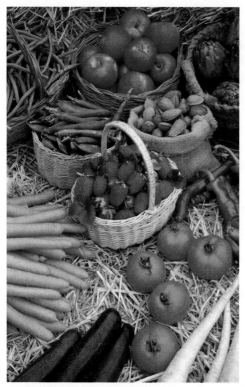

© Pixtal / AGE Fotostock

Fruits, vegetables, and whole grains are excellent sources of carbohydrates and fibre.

The simple carbohydrates in your diet should come from food sources in which they are found naturally, including fruits, which are excellent sources of vitamins and minerals, and from milk, which is high in protein and calcium.

Athletes in training can especially benefit from high carbohydrate diets (60–70% of total daily calories), which enhance the amount of carbohydrates stored in their muscles as glycogen and therefore provide more carbohydrate fuel for use during endurance events or long workouts. Carbohydrates consumed during prolonged athletic events (e.g., sport beverages and gels) can provide fluid, electrolytes, and glucose to help fuel muscles and extend the availability of the glycogen stored in muscles.

Fibre—A Closer Look

Fibre is the term given to nondigestible carbohydrates provided mainly by plants. Instead of being digested, like starch, fibre passes through the intestinal tract and provides bulk for feces in the large intestine, which in turn facilitates elimination. In the large intestine, some types of fibre are broken down by bacteria into acids and gases, which explains why eating too much fibre can lead to intestinal gas. Even though humans don't digest fibre, it is necessary for good health.

Types of Fibre

The Food and Nutrition Board and Health Canada have defined two types of fibre:

- **Dietary fibre** is the nondigestible carbohydrates (and the noncarbohydrate substance lignin) that are present naturally in plants such as grains, legumes, and vegetables.

- **Functional fibre** is any nondigestible carbohydrates that have been either isolated from natural sources or synthesized in a lab and then added to a food product or supplement.

dietary fibre Nondigestible carbohydrates and lignin that are intact in plants.
functional fibre Nondigestible carbohydrates either isolated from natural sources or synthesized; these may be added to foods and dietary supplements.

Total fibre is the sum of dietary and functional fibre in a person's diet.

total fibre The total amount of dietary fibre and functional fibre in the diet.

Fibres have different properties that lead to different physiological effects in the body. **Soluble (viscous) fibre**, such as that found in oat bran or legumes, can delay stomach emptying, slow the movement of glucose into the blood after eating, and reduce absorption of cholesterol. **Insoluble fibre**, such as that found in wheat bran or psyllium seed, increases fecal bulk and helps prevent constipation, hemorrhoids, and other digestive disorders.

soluble (viscous) fibre Fibre that dissolves in water or is broken down by bacteria in the large intestine.
insoluble fibre Fibre that does not dissolve in water and is not broken down by bacteria in the large intestine.

A high-fibre diet can help reduce the risk of type 2 diabetes, heart disease, and pulmonary disease, as well as improve gastrointestinal health and aid in the management of metabolic syndrome and body weight. Some studies have linked high-fibre diets with a reduced risk of colon and rectal cancer.

Sources of Fibre

All plant foods contain some dietary fibre. Fruits, legumes, oats (especially oat bran), and barley all contain the viscous types of fibre that help lower blood glucose and cholesterol levels. Wheat (especially wheat bran), cereals, grains, and vegetables are all good sources of cellulose and other fibres that help prevent constipation. Psyllium, which is often added to cereals or used in fibre supplements and laxatives, improves intestinal health and also helps control glucose and cholesterol levels. The processing of packaged foods can remove fibre, so it's important to depend on fresh fruits and vegetables and foods made from whole grains as sources of dietary fibre.

Recommended Intake of Dietary Fibre

To reduce the risk of chronic disease and maintain intestinal health, the Food and Nutrition Board and Health Canada recommend a daily fibre intake of 38 grams for adult men and 25 grams for adult women. Canadians currently consume about 14 grams of fibre per day.[5] Fibre should come from foods, not supplements, which should be used only under medical supervision. Drink plenty of water, at least eight cups daily, to get the most health benefits from the fibre you consume.

Wellness Tip

To avoid intestinal discomfort, add fibre to your diet slowly so you can build a tolerance to it.

Vitamins—Organic Micronutrients

Vitamins are organic (carbon-containing) substances required in very small amounts to regulate various processes within living cells (see Table 7.4 on the next page). Humans need 13 vitamins. Four are fat-soluble (A, D, E, and K), and nine are water-soluble (C and the eight B-complex vitamins: thiamin, riboflavin, niacin, vitamin B-6, folate, vitamin B-12, biotin, and pantothenic acid).

vitamins Organic substances needed in small amounts to help promote and regulate chemical reactions and processes in the body.

Solubility affects how a vitamin is absorbed, transported, and stored in the body. The water-soluble vitamins are absorbed directly into the bloodstream, where they travel freely. Excess water-soluble vitamins are removed by the kidneys and excreted in urine. Fat-soluble vitamins require a more complex absorptive process. They are usually carried in the blood by special proteins and are stored in the body in fat tissues rather than excreted.

Functions of Vitamins

Many vitamins help chemical reactions take place. They provide no energy to the body directly but help unleash the energy stored in carbohydrates, proteins, and fats. Vitamins are critical in the production of red blood cells and the maintenance of the nervous, skeletal, and immune systems. Some vitamins act as **antioxidants**, which help preserve healthy cells in the body. Key vitamin antioxidants include vitamin E, vitamin C, and the vitamin A precursor beta-carotene. (Antioxidants are described later in the chapter.)

antioxidant A substance that protects against the breakdown of body constituents by free radicals; actions include binding oxygen, donating electrons to free radicals, and repairing damage to molecules.

TABLE 7.4

Facts about Vitamins

Vitamin	Important Dietary Sources	Major Functions	Signs of Prolonged Deficiency	Toxic Effects of Megadoses
Fat-Soluble				
Vitamin A	Liver, milk, butter, cheese, and fortified margarine; carrots, spinach, and other orange and deep-green vegetables and fruits	Maintenance of vision, skin, linings of the nose, mouth, digestive and urinary tracts, immune function	Night blindness; dry, scaling skin; increased susceptibility to infection; loss of appetite; anemia; kidney stones	Liver damage, miscarriage and birth defects, headache, vomiting and diarrhea, vertigo, double vision, bone abnormalities
Vitamin D	Fortified milk and margarine, fish oils, butter, egg yolks (sunlight on skin also produces vitamin D)	Development and maintenance of bones and teeth, promotion of calcium absorption	Rickets (bone deformities) in children; bone softening, loss, and fractures in adults	Kidney damage, calcium deposits in soft tissues, depression, death
Vitamin E	Vegetable oils, whole grains, nuts and seeds, green leafy vegetables, asparagus, peaches	Protection and maintenance of cellular membranes	Red blood cell breakage and anemia, weakness, neurological problems, muscle cramps	Relatively nontoxic, but may cause excess bleeding or formation of blood clots
Vitamin K	Green leafy vegetables; smaller amounts widespread in other foods	Production of proteins essential for blood clotting and bone metabolism	Hemorrhaging	None reported
Water-Soluble				
Biotin	Cereals, yeast, egg yolks, soy flour, liver; widespread in foods	Synthesis of fat, glycogen, and amino acids	Rash, nausea, vomiting, weight loss, depression, fatigue, hair loss	None reported
Folate	Green leafy vegetables, yeast, oranges, whole grains, legumes, liver	Amino acid metabolism, synthesis of RNA and DNA, new cell synthesis	Anemia, weakness, fatigue, irritability, shortness of breath, swollen tongue	Masking of vitamin B-12 deficiency
Niacin	Eggs, poultry, fish, milk, whole grains, nuts, enriched breads and cereals, meats, legumes	Conversion of carbohydrates, fats, and protein into usable forms of energy	Pellagra (symptoms include diarrhea, dermatitis, inflammation of mucous membranes, dementia)	Flushing of the skin, nausea, vomiting, diarrhea, liver dysfunction, glucose intolerance
Pantothenic acid	Animal foods, whole grains, broccoli, potatoes; widespread in foods	Metabolism of fats, carbohydrates, and proteins	Fatigue, numbness and tingling of hands and feet, gastrointestinal disturbances	None reported

Vitamin	Important Dietary Sources	Major Functions	Signs of Prolonged Deficiency	Toxic Effects of Megadoses
Riboflavin	Dairy products, enriched breads and cereals, lean meats, poultry, fish, green vegetables	Energy metabolism; maintenance of skin, mucous membranes, and nervous system structures	Cracks at corners of mouth, sore throat, skin rash, hypersensitivity to light, purple tongue	None reported
Thiamine	Whole-grain and enriched breads and cereals, organ meats, lean pork, nuts, legumes	Conversion of carbohydrates into usable forms of energy, maintenance of appetite and nervous system function	Beriberi (symptoms include muscle wasting, mental confusion, anorexia, enlarged heart, nerve changes)	None reported
Vitamin B6	Eggs, poultry, fish, whole grains, nuts, soybeans, liver, kidney, pork	Metabolism of amino acids and glycogen	Anemia, convulsions, cracks at corners of mouth, dermatitis, nausea, confusion	Neurological abnormalities and damage
Vitamin B12	Meat, fish, poultry, fortified cereals	Synthesis of blood cells; other metabolic reactions	Anemia, fatigue, nervous system damage, sore tongue	None reported
Vitamin C	Peppers, broccoli, Brussels sprouts, spinach, citrus fruits, strawberries, tomatoes, potatoes, cabbage, other fruits and vegetables	Maintenance and repair of connective tissue, bones, teeth, and cartilage; promotion of healing; aid in iron absorption	Scurvy, anemia, reduced resistance to infection, loosened teeth, joint pain, poor wound healing, hair loss, poor iron absorption	Urinary stones in some people, acid stomach from ingesting supplements in pill form, nausea, diarrhea, headache, fatigue

Sources: Food and Nutrition Board, Institute of Medicine. 2006. *Dietary Reference Intakes: The Essential Guide to Nutrient Requirements.* Washington, DC: National Academies Press. The complete Dietary Reference Intake reports are available from the National Academies Press (http://www.nap.edu). Shils, M.E., et al., eds. 2005. *Modern Nutrition in Health and Disease,* 10th ed. Baltimore: Lippincott Williams and Wilkins.

Sources of Vitamins

The human body must obtain vitamins from foods, and they are abundant in fruits, vegetables, and grains. In addition, many processed foods, such as flour and breakfast cereals, contain added vitamins. A few vitamins are made in certain parts of the body: The skin makes vitamin D when it is exposed to sunlight, and intestinal bacteria make vitamin K. Nonetheless, you still need to obtain vitamin D and vitamin K from foods (see Table 7.4).

Vitamin Deficiencies and Excesses

If your diet lacks sufficient amounts of a particular vitamin, characteristic symptoms of deficiency develop (see Table 7.4). For example, vitamin A deficiency can cause blindness, and people whose diets lack vitamin B12 can develop anemia. Vitamin deficiency diseases are most often seen in developing countries; they are relatively rare in Canada because vitamins are readily available from our food supply. However, many Canadians consume lower-than-recommended amounts of several vitamins.

Nutrient intake that is consistently below recommended levels can have adverse effects on health even if it is not low enough to cause a deficiency disease. For example, low intake of folate increases a woman's chance of giving birth to a baby with a neural tube defect (a congenital malformation of the central nervous system). Low intake of folate and vitamins B6 and B12 has been linked to increased heart disease risk. Recent research suggests that vitamin D supplementation can reduce the risk of cardiovascular disease and of several cancers. As important as vitamins are, many Canadians consume less-than-recommended amounts of vitamins A, C, B6, and E.

Extra vitamins in the diet can be harmful, especially when taken as supplements. Megadoses of fat-soluble vitamins are particularly dangerous because the excess will be stored in the body rather than excreted, increasing the risk of toxicity. Even when supplements are not taken in excess, relying on them for an adequate intake of vitamins can problematic. There are many substances in foods other than vitamins and minerals that have important health effects. Later in this chapter we discuss specific recommendations for vitamin intake and when a supplement is advisable. For now, keep in mind that it's best to obtain most of your vitamins from foods rather than supplements.

The vitamins and minerals in foods can be easily lost or destroyed during storage or cooking. To retain their value, you should eat or process vegetables immediately after buying them. If you can't do this, then store them in a cool place, covered to retain moisture—either in the refrigerator (for a few days) or in the freezer (for a longer term). To reduce nutrient losses during food preparation, minimize the amount of water used and the total cooking time. Develop a taste for a crunchier texture in cooked vegetables. Baking, steaming, broiling, grilling, and microwaving are all good methods of preparing vegetables.

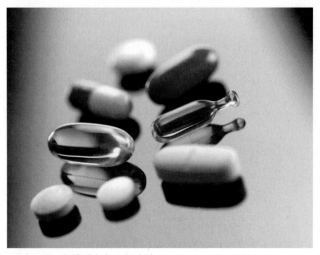

© Cultura Creative (RF) / Alamy Stock Photo

Vitamin and mineral supplements are popular, but they are not usually necessary for healthy people who eat a balanced diet.

CAREER OPTIONS IN...

NUTRITION

Health Care: dietitian/nutritionist, professor, doctor

Community: life sciences or home economics teacher, wellness coordinator

Industry: food scientist, product health claims researcher, food and nutrition administration

SOURCES: Physical and Health Education Canada (http://www.phecanada.ca); Mount Saint Vincent University. Nutrition Related Career Options (http://www.msvu.ca/en/home/programsdepartments/professionalstudies/appliedhumannutrition /becomingadietitiannutritionprofessional/nutritioncareers.aspx).

Minerals—Inorganic Micronutrients

Minerals are inorganic (non-carbon-containing) elements that you need in small amounts to help regulate body functions, aid in the growth and maintenance of body tissues, and help release energy (Table 7.5).

minerals Inorganic compounds needed in small amounts for regulation, growth, and maintenance of body tissues and functions.

TABLE 7.5

Facts about Selected Minerals

Mineral	Important Dietary Sources	Major Functions	Signs of Prolonged Deficiency	Toxic Effects of Megadoses
Calcium	Milk and milk products, tofu, fortified orange juice and bread, green leafy vegetables, bones in fish	Formation of bones and teeth; control of nerve impulses, muscle contraction, blood clotting	Stunted growth in children, bone mineral loss in adults; urinary stones	Kidney stones, calcium deposits in soft tissues, inhibition of mineral absorption, constipation
Fluoride	Fluoridated water, tea, marine fish eaten with bones	Maintenance of tooth and bone structure	Higher frequency of tooth decay	Increased bone density, mottling of teeth, impaired kidney function
Iodine	Iodized salt, seafood, processed foods	Essential part of thyroid hormones, regulation of body metabolism	Goitre (enlarged thyroid), cretinism (birth defect)	Depression of thyroid activity, hyperthyroidism in susceptible people
Iron	Meat and poultry, fortified grain products, dark-green vegetables, dried fruit	Component of hemoglobin, myoglobin, and enzymes	Iron-deficiency anemia, weakness, impaired immune function, gastrointestinal distress	Nausea, diarrhea, liver and kidney damage, joint pains, sterility, disruption of cardiac function, death
Magnesium	Widespread in foods and water (except soft water); especially found in grains, legumes, nuts, seeds, green vegetables, milk	Transmission of nerve impulses, energy transfer, activation of many enzymes	Neurological disturbances, cardiovascular problems, kidney disorders, nausea, growth failure in children	Nausea, vomiting, diarrhea, central nervous system depression, coma; death in people with impaired kidney function
Phosphorus	Present in nearly all foods, especially milk, cereal, peas, eggs, meat	Bone growth and maintenance, energy transfer in cells	Impaired growth, weakness, kidney disorders, cardiorespiratory and nervous system dysfunction	Drop in blood calcium levels, calcium deposits in soft tissues, bone loss
Potassium	Meats, milk, fruits, vegetables, grains, legumes	Nerve function and body water balance	Muscular weakness, nausea, drowsiness, paralysis, confusion, disruption of cardiac rhythm	Cardiac arrest
Selenium	Seafood, meat, eggs, whole grains	Defence against oxidative stress and regulation of thyroid hormone action	Muscle pain and weakness, heart disorders	Hair and nail brittleness and loss, nausea and vomiting, weakness, irritability

Mineral	Important Dietary Sources	Major Functions	Signs of Prolonged Deficiency	Toxic Effects of Megadoses
Sodium	Salt, soy sauce, fast food, and processed foods, especially lunch meats, canned soups and vegetables, salty snacks, and processed cheese	Body water balance, acid-base balance, nerve function	Muscle weakness, loss of appetite, nausea, vomiting; deficiency is rarely seen	Edema, hypertension in sensitive people
Zinc	Whole grains, meat, eggs, liver, seafood (especially oysters)	Synthesis of proteins, RNA, and DNA; wound healing; immune response; ability to taste	Growth failure, loss of appetite, impaired taste acuity, skin rash, impaired immune function, poor wound healing	Vomiting, impaired immune function, decline in blood HDL levels, impaired copper absorption

Sources: Food and Nutrition Board, Institute of Medicine. 2006. *Dietary Reference Intakes: The Essential Guide to Nutrient Requirements.* Washington, DC: National Academies Press. The complete Dietary Reference Intake reports are available from the National Academies Press (http://www.nap.edu). Shils, M.E., et al., eds. 2005. *Modern Nutrition in Health and Disease,* 10th ed. Baltimore: Lippincott Williams and Wilkins.

There are about 17 essential minerals. The major minerals, those that the body needs in amounts exceeding 100 milligrams per day, include calcium, phosphorus, magnesium, sodium, potassium, and chloride. The essential trace minerals, those that you need in minute amounts, include copper, fluoride, iodine, iron, selenium, and zinc.

Characteristic symptoms develop if an essential mineral is consumed in a quantity too small or too large for good health. The minerals most commonly lacking in the Canadian diet are iron, calcium, magnesium, and potassium.[6] Focus on good food choices for these nutrients (see Table 7.5). Iron-deficiency **anemia** is a problem in some age groups, and researchers fear poor calcium intakes are sowing the seeds for future **osteoporosis**, especially in women. See the box Eating for Healthy Bones to learn more.

anemia   A deficiency in the oxygen-carrying material in the red blood cells.
osteoporosis   A condition in which the bones become thin and brittle and break easily.

Take CHARGE

EATING FOR HEALTHY BONES

Osteoporosis is a condition in which the bones become dangerously thin and fragile over time. It currently afflicts as many as 2 million Canadians, with women over the age of 50 being twice as likely to suffer from it as males over the age of 50.

Most bone mass is built by age 18. After bone density peaks between the ages of 25 and 35, bone mass is lost over time. To prevent osteoporosis, the best strategy is to build as much bone as possible during your youth and do everything you can to maintain it as you age. Up to 50% of bone loss is determined by controllable lifestyle factors such as diet and exercise. Key nutrients for bone health include the following.

Calcium   Getting enough calcium is important throughout the life span to build and maintain bone mass. Health Canada recommends that most adults consume 1000 to 2000 mg of calcium per day. Milk, yogourt, canned salmon and sardines with the bones, and calcium-fortified orange juice, bread, and cereals are all good sources.

Vitamin D   Vitamin D is necessary for bones to absorb calcium; 600 IU (15 mcg) a day is recommended for children and adults aged 9 to 70 years. Vitamin D can be obtained from foods and is manufactured by the skin when exposed to sunlight. Because the sun is weaker in northern latitudes, most Canadians are good candidates for vitamin D supplements. People who don't eat many foods rich in vitamin D, such as milk, eggs, and oily fish, and those who don't expose their face, arms, and hands to the sun (without sunscreen) for 5 to 15 minutes a few times each week, are at risk.

Vitamin K   Vitamin K promotes the synthesis of proteins that help keep bones strong. Broccoli and leafy green vegetables are rich in vitamin K.

Other nutrients   Other nutrients that may play an important role in bone health include vitamin C, magnesium, potassium, manganese, zinc, copper, and boron.

On the flip side, several dietary substances that may have a negative effect on bone health, especially if consumed in excess. These include alcohol, sodium, caffeine, and retinol (a form of vitamin A). Drinking lots of carbonated beverages, which often replace milk in the diet and which are high in phosphorus (a mineral that may interfere with calcium absorption), has been shown to increase the risk of bone fracture in teenage girls.

The effect of protein intake on bone mass depends on other nutrients. Protein helps build bone as long as calcium and vitamin D intake are adequate. However, if intake of calcium and vitamin D is low, high protein intake can lead to bone loss.

Weight-bearing aerobic activities help maintain bone mass throughout life. In fact, just jumping in place or skipping rope for two minutes a day can help maintain bone density. Normal weight-bearing activities of daily living (such as carrying a load of laundry up a flight of stairs) also go a long way to keeping your bones strong. Walking is a great way keep bones strong. Strength training improves bone density, muscle mass, strength, and balance.

SOURCE: Osteoporosis Canada (http://www.osteoporosis.ca) and Health Canada. 2010. *Food and Nutrition: Vitamin D and Calcium: Updated Dietary Reference Intakes* (http://www.hc-sc.gc.ca/fn-an/nutrition/vitamin/vita-d-eng.php#t5; retrieved December 10, 2011).

Wellness Tip

If you take a supplement, *never* take more than the recommended dosage unless your doctor tells you to.

Water—Vital but Often Ignored

Water is the major component in both foods and the human body: You are composed of about 50–60% water. Your need for other nutrients, in terms of weight, is much less than your need for water. In fact, you can live up to 50 days without food, but only a few days without water.

Water is distributed all over the body, among lean and other tissues and in urine and other body fluids. Water is used in the digestion and absorption of food and is the medium in which most of the chemical reactions take place within the body. Some water-based fluids like blood transport substances around the body; other fluids serve as lubricants or cushions. Water also helps regulate body temperature.

Water is contained in almost all foods, particularly in liquids, fruits, and vegetables. The foods and fluids you consume provide 80–90% of your daily water intake; the remainder is generated through metabolism. You lose water each day in urine, feces, and sweat, and through evaporation in your lungs.

Most people maintain a healthy water balance by consuming beverages at meals and drinking fluids in response to thirst. In 2004, the Food and Nutrition Board and Health Canada set levels of adequate water intake to maintain hydration (Table 7.6); all fluids, including those containing caffeine, can count toward your total daily fluid intake. Men need to consume about 3.7 total litres of water, with 3.0 litres (about 13 cups) coming from beverages; women need 2.7 total litres, with 2.2 litres (about 9 cups) coming from beverages. (See Table 1 in the Nutrition Resources section at the end of the chapter for recommendations for specific age groups.) If you exercise vigorously or live in a hot climate, you need to consume additional fluids to maintain a balance between water consumed and water lost. Severe dehydration causes weakness and can lead to death. See the Do Athletes Need a Different Diet? box later in the chapter for more on the fluid needs of athletes and active people.

TABLE 7.6

Adequate Daily Water Intake

Life Stage		Total Water Intake from Fluids and Food	Fluid Intake (Water and Beverages) as Part of Total Water Intake
Children	1–3 years	1.3 litres	0.9 litres (about 4 cups)
	4–8 years	1.7 litres	1.2 litres (about 5 cups)
Males	9–13 years	2.4 litres	1.8 litres (about 8 cups)
	14–18 years	3.3 litres	2.6 litres (about 11 cups)
	19 years and older	3.7 litres	3.0 litres (about 13 cups)
Females	9–13 years	2.1 litres	1.6 litres (about 7 cups)
	14–18 years	2.3 litres	1.8 litres (about 8 cups)
	19 years and older	2.7 litres	2.2 litres (about 9 cups)

Infant fluid intake (0.7–0.8 litres/day) is assumed to be from human milk and, for infants 7–12 months, from complementary foods and beverages.

SOURCE: Reprinted with permission from the National Academy of Science. "Dietary Reference Intake: Water, Potassium, Sodium, Chloride, and Sulfate." 2004. Institute of Medicine, National Academies.

Fitness Tip

Drink plenty of water before, during, and after workouts, especially when the weather is warm. Proper hydration helps you avoid cramps and heat-related problems such as heat stroke.

Other Substances in Food

Many substances in food are not essential nutrients but they may influence health.

Antioxidants

When the body uses oxygen or breaks down certain fats or proteins as a normal part of metabolism, substances called **free radicals** are produced. A free radical is a chemically unstable molecule that reacts with fats, proteins, and DNA, damaging cell membranes and mutating genes. Free radicals have been implicated in aging, cancer, cardiovascular disease, and other degenerative diseases like arthritis. Environmental factors such as cigarette smoke, exhaust fumes, radiation, excessive sunlight, certain drugs, and stress can increase free radical production.

> **free radical** An electron-seeking compound that can react with fats, proteins, and DNA, damaging cell membranes and mutating genes in its search for electrons; produced through chemical reactions in the body and by exposure to environmental factors such as sunlight and tobacco smoke.

Antioxidants found in foods can help protect the body by blocking the formation and action of free radicals and repairing the damage they cause. Some antioxidants, such as vitamin C, vitamin E, and selenium, are also essential nutrients. Others, such as carotenoids, found in yellow, orange, and dark-green leafy vegetables, are not. Research has identified herbs, spices, berries, nuts, and chocolate as some of the top antioxidant ingredients and foods. Also high in antioxidants are Brussels sprouts, kale, cauliflower, and pomegranates.

Phytochemicals

Antioxidants fall into the broader category of **phytochemicals**, substances found in plant foods that may help prevent chronic disease. For example, certain substances found in soy foods may help lower cholesterol levels. Sulforaphane, a compound isolated from broccoli and other **cruciferous vegetables**, may render some carcinogenic compounds harmless. Allyl sulfides, a group of chemicals found in garlic and onions, appear to boost the activity of cancer-fighting immune cells. Phytochemicals found in whole grains are associated with a reduced risk of cardiovascular disease, diabetes, and cancer. Carotenoids found in green vegetables may help preserve eyesight with age. Further research on phytochemicals may extend the role of nutrition to the prevention and treatment of many chronic diseases.

> **phytochemicals** Naturally occurring substances found in plant foods that may help prevent and treat chronic diseases such as heart disease and cancer; *phyto* means plant.
> **cruciferous vegetables** Vegetables of the cabbage family, including cabbage, broccoli, Brussels sprouts, kale, and cauliflower; the flower petals of these plants form the shape of a cross, hence the name.

To increase your intake of phytochemicals, eat a variety of fruits and vegetables rather than relying on supplements. Like many vitamins and minerals, isolated phytochemicals may be harmful if taken in high doses. In many cases, their health benefits may be the result of chemical substances working in combination. The role of phytochemicals in disease prevention is discussed further in Chapter 11 and Chapter 12.

LO2 7.2 Nutritional Guidelines: Planning Your Diet

Various tools have been created by scientific and government groups to help people design healthy diets. The **Dietary Reference Intakes (DRIs)** are standards for nutrient intake designed to prevent nutritional deficiencies and reduce the risk of chronic disease. **Canada's Food Guide** translates these nutrient recommendations into a balanced food-group plan that includes all essential nutrients. Together, the DRIs and the Food Guide make up a complete set of resources for dietary planning.

> **Dietary Reference Intakes (DRIs)** An umbrella term for four types of nutrient standards: Adequate Intake (AI), Estimated Average Requirement (EAR), and Recommended Dietary Allowance (RDA) set levels of intake considered adequate to prevent nutrient deficiencies and reduce the risk of chronic disease; Tolerable Upper Intake Level (UL) sets the maximum daily intake that is unlikely to cause health problems.
> **Canada's Food Guide** A food-group plan that provides practical advice to ensure a balanced intake of the essential nutrients.

Dietary Reference Intakes (DRIs)

How much vitamin C, iron, calcium, and other nutrients do you need to stay healthy? The Food and Nutrition Board of the National Academy of Sciences and Health Canada have partnered to establish dietary standards, or recommended intake levels, for North Americans of all ages. The current set of standards, called Dietary Reference Intakes (DRIs), were introduced in 1997. An earlier set of standards, called the **Recommended Dietary Allowances (RDAs)**, focused on preventing nutritional deficiency diseases such as anemia; the RDAs were established in 1941 and updated periodically, most recently in 1989. The newer DRIs have a broader focus because recent research has looked not just at the prevention of nutrient deficiencies, but also at the role of nutrients in promoting optimal health and preventing chronic diseases such as cancer, osteoporosis, and heart disease.

> **Recommended Dietary Allowances (RDAs)**   Amounts of certain nutrients considered adequate to prevent deficiencies in most healthy people; will eventually be replaced by the Dietary Reference Intakes (DRIs).

The DRIs include standards for both recommended intakes and maximum safe intakes. The recommended intake of each nutrient is expressed as either a *Recommended Dietary Allowance (RDA)* or an *Adequate Intake (AI)*. An AI is set when there is not enough information available to set an RDA value; regardless of the type of standard used, however, the DRI represents the best available estimate of intake for optimal health. The *Tolerable Upper Intake Level (UL)* sets the maximum daily intake by a healthy person that is unlikely to cause health problems. For example, the RDA for calcium for an 18-year-old female is 1300 mg per day; the UL is 3000 mg per day.

Because of lack of data, ULs have not been set for all nutrients. This does not mean that people can tolerate long-term intakes of these vitamins and minerals above recommended levels. Like all chemical agents, nutrients can produce adverse effects if intakes are excessive. There is no established benefit from consuming nutrients at levels above the RDA or AI. The DRIs can be found in the Nutrition Resources section. For more information, visit the website of the National Academies' Food and Nutrition Board (see For Further Exploration at the end of the chapter.)

Daily Values

Because the DRIs are far too cumbersome to use as a basis for food labels, the US Food and Drug Administration developed another set of dietary standards, the **Daily Values**. The Daily Values are based on several different sets of guidelines and include standards for fat, cholesterol, carbohydrates, dietary fibre, and selected vitamins and minerals. The Daily Values represent appropriate intake levels for a 2000-calorie diet. The percent Daily Value shown on a food label indicates how well that food contributes to your recommended daily intake. Food labels are described in detail later in this chapter.

> **Daily Values**   A simplified version of the RDAs used on food labels; also included are values for nutrients with no established RDA.

Should You Take Supplements?

The aim of the DRIs is to guide you in meeting your nutritional needs primarily with food, rather than with vitamin and mineral supplements. Supplements lack the potentially beneficial synergistic balance of nutrients, phytochemicals, and fibre that are found only in whole foods. Although many Canadians can get the vitamins and minerals they need by eating a varied, nutritionally balanced diet like the one recommended by Canada's Food Guide, many also choose to supplement. The 2015 Canadian Community Health Survey reported that almost 46% of Canadians use at least one nutritional supplement.

Over the past two decades, high-dose supplement use has been promoted as a way to prevent or delay the onset of many diseases, including heart disease and several forms of cancer. These claims remain controversial. According to the latest research, a balanced diet of whole foods—not high-dose supplementation—is the best way to promote health and prevent disease.

In setting the DRIs, the Food and Nutrition Board recommends supplements of particular nutrients for the following groups:

- Women who are capable of becoming pregnant should take 400 μg per day of folic acid (the synthetic form of the vitamin folate) from fortified foods and/or supplements in addition to folate from a varied diet. Research indicates that this level of folate intake will reduce the risk of neural tube defects. Enriched breads, flours, corn meals, rice, noodles, and other grain products have been fortified with small amounts of folic acid. Folate is found naturally in leafy green vegetables, legumes, oranges and orange juice, and strawberries.

- People over age 50 should consume foods fortified with vitamin B12, B12 supplements, or both to meet the majority of the DRI of 2.4 mg of B12 daily. Up to 30% of people over age 50 have problems absorbing protein-bound B12 in foods.

- Because of the oxidative stress caused by smoking, smokers should get 35 mg *more* vitamin C per day than the RDA set for their age and sex (for adults, the recommended daily vitamin C intake for nonsmokers is 90 mg for men and 75 mg for women). However, supplements are not usually needed because this extra vitamin C can easily be found in foods. For example, a 250-millilitre (8 ounce) glass of orange juice has about 100 mg of vitamin C.

Supplements may also be recommended in other cases. For instance, women with heavy menstrual flows may need extra iron. Older people, people with dark skin, and people exposed to little sunlight may need extra vitamin D. Some vegetarians may need supplemental calcium, iron, zinc, and vitamin B12, depending on their food choices. Other people may benefit from supplementation based on their lifestyle, physical condition, medicines, or dietary habits.

Although dietary supplements are sold over the counter, the question of whether to take supplements is a serious one. Some vitamins and minerals are dangerous when ingested in excess, as described previously in Tables 7.4 and 7.5. Large doses of particular nutrients can also cause health problems by affecting the absorption of other vitamins and minerals or interacting with medications. For all these reasons, think carefully about whether to take high-dose supplements and consult a physician or registered dietitian.

Canada's Food Guide

Canada's Food Guide (see Figure 7.3 on the next page) outlines what to eat each day. It is not a rigid prescription, but rather a general guide that lets you choose a healthful diet that's right for you. It calls for eating a variety of foods to get the nutrients you need and at the same time the right amount of calories to maintain a healthy weight. To access the online version of Canada's Food Guide, go to http://www.hc-sc.gc.ca/fn-an/food-guide-aliment/index-eng.php and click on "My Food Guide" to create your own personal food guide based on your daily requirements. Your personal food guide will identify how many servings of each food group that you should be consuming on a daily basis.

Food Guide Servings and Their Sizes

The number of servings (see Figure 7.3) recommended for each group in Canada's Food Guide is based on specific serving sizes that may differ from your own typical portion sizes and the serving sizes listed on food labels. For example, one serving of pasta is about 125 millilitres (½ cup); if your portion at a meal is

FIGURE 7.3

Canada's Food Guide and recommended servings.

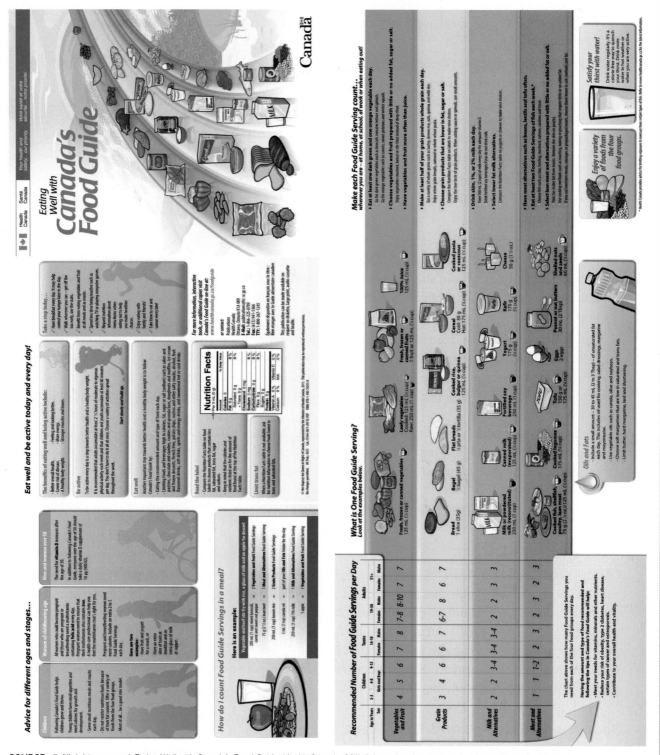

350 millilitres (1½ cups) of pasta, it would count as three servings toward your daily total from the Grain Products food group. When evaluating your current diet or planning dietary changes, it is very important to consider the serving sizes given in the Food Guide. If you are one of the many people who have trouble identifying 30 grams of cereal or a half-cup of rice, see the strategies in the box Judging Serving Sizes.

Take CHARGE

JUDGING SERVING SIZES

Studies have shown that most people underestimate the size of their food portions, in many cases by as much as 50%. If you need to retrain your eye, try using measuring cups and spoons and an inexpensive kitchen scale when you eat at home. With a little practice, you'll learn the difference between different serving sizes of chicken or meat and what a half-cup of rice really looks like. For quick estimates, use these equivalents:

- 1 teaspoon of margarine = one dice
- 30 grams of cheese = your thumb, four dice stacked together
- 60 grams of chicken or meat = a deck of cards
- ½ cup of rice, pasta, or potato = ½ a baseball
- 2 tablespoons of peanut butter = a ping-pong ball
- 1 60-gram bagel = a hockey puck
- 1 60-gram muffin or roll = a large egg
- 1 medium fruit (apple or orange) = a baseball
- ¼ cup nuts = a golf ball
- small cookie or cracker = a poker chip

Grain Products (3 to 8 Servings)

Foods from this group are usually low in fat and rich in complex carbohydrates, dietary fibre (if grains are unrefined), and many vitamins and minerals, including thiamine, riboflavin, iron, niacin, folate, and zinc. Although three to eight servings may seem like a large amount of food, many people eat several servings at a time. A single serving is the equivalent of the following:

- 1 slice of bread or half a hamburger bun, English muffin, or bagel
- 1 small roll, biscuit, or muffin
- 30 grams of ready-to-eat cereal
- ½ cup cooked cereal, rice, or pasta
- 5–6 small or 2–3 large crackers
- 1 18-cm corn or flour tortilla

Choose foods that are typically made with little fat or sugar (e.g., bread, rice, pasta) over those that are high in fat and sugar (e.g., croissants, chips, cookies, doughnuts). The key message is to *make at least half your grains whole grains.*

Fruit and Vegetables (4 to 10 Servings)

Fruit and vegetables are rich in carbohydrates, dietary fibre, vitamin A, vitamin C, folate, magnesium, and other nutrients. They are also naturally low in fat (both) and sodium (fruits). A serving of vegetables is equivalent to the following:

- 1 cup raw leafy vegetables
- 1 medium sized fruit or vegetable

- ½ cup tomato sauce
- ½ cup fruit or vegetable juice
- ½ cup cooked dry beans (legumes)
- 1 cup bean or vegetable soup

Because fruits and vegetables vary in the nutrients they provide, it is important to consume a variety of types to obtain maximum nutrition. Many Canadians consume only a few different types of vegetables, with white potatoes (baked or served as french fries) being the most popular. A suggestion would be to try to consume at least one serving from each of the following vegetable groups on most days of the week:

- dark-green vegetables like spinach, chard, collards, broccoli, romaine, and turnip and mustard greens
- deep-yellow and orange vegetables like carrots, winter squash, sweet potatoes, and pumpkin
- legumes like pinto beans, kidney beans, black beans, lentils, chickpeas, and tofu; legumes can be counted as servings of vegetables or as alternatives to meat
- starchy vegetables like corn, green peas, and white potatoes
- other vegetables such as tomatoes, bell peppers (red, orange, yellow, or green), green beans, and cruciferous vegetables like cauliflower

Choose whole fruits often—they are higher in fibre and often lower in calories than fruit juices. Fruit juices typically contain more nutrients and less added sugar than fruit drinks. The key message is to *fill half your plate with fruits and vegetables.*

Milk and Alternatives (2 to 4 Servings)

Foods from this group are high in protein, carbohydrates, calcium, riboflavin, and vitamin D. To limit the fat in your diet, choose servings of low-fat or nonfat items from this group:

- 1 cup milk
- 50 grams of block cheese
- 2 slices of processed cheese
- 175 grams of yogourt

Cottage cheese is lower in calcium than most other cheeses, and one cup of cottage cheese counts as only half a serving for this food group. Ice cream is also lower in calcium than many other dairy products (½ cup is equivalent to ⅓ serving); in addition, it is high in sugar and fat. The number of servings you should consume each day will depend on your age and health status (see Figure 7.4). The key message is to *switch to fat-free or low-fat (1%) milk and dairy products.*

Meat and Alternatives (2 to 3 Servings)

This food group provides protein, niacin, iron, vitamin B6, zinc, and thiamine; the animal foods in the group also provide vitamin B12. Canada's Food Guide recommends two to three servings each day of foods from this group. The total amount of these servings should be the equivalent of 150 to 300 grams of cooked lean meat, poultry, or fish a day. Many people misjudge what makes up a single serving for this food group:

- An average hamburger or a medium chicken breast half is about 100 grams; ½ cup of drained canned tuna counts as about 75 grams.
- The following portions of nonmeat foods are equivalent to 30 grams of lean meat: ½ cup cooked dry beans (if not counted as a vegetable), 1 egg, 2 tablespoons peanut butter, ⅓ cup nuts, ¼ cup seeds, and ⅓ cup tofu.

One egg at breakfast, a cup of pinto beans at lunch, and a hamburger at dinner would add up to the equivalent of 225 grams of lean meat for the day. To limit your intake of fat and saturated fat, choose lean cuts of meat and skinless poultry, eat nuts and seeds in moderation, and watch your serving sizes carefully. Additionally, you may choose to eat fish such as salmon twice a week to increase your consumption of healthier fats. Choose at least one serving of plant proteins such as black beans, lentils, or tofu every day.

Canada's Food Guide also includes a category for Oils and Fats, which gives advice on foods such as oils and sugars that are not found in the Food Guide. Health Canada suggests that you consume products found in this group in moderation. Foods in this group tend to be higher in fat and calorie content. See the box Reducing the Saturated and Trans Fats in Your Diet for ways to reduce their intake. In addition, a new Beverages section helps to identify healthier selections of beverages that may even count toward other food groups in the guide.

Take CHARGE

REDUCING THE SATURATED AND TRANS FATS IN YOUR DIET

Your overall goal is to limit total fat intake to no more than 35% of total calories. Choose unsaturated fats over saturated and trans fats. Here are some steps that can help reduce these types of fat in your diet:

- Be moderate in your consumption of foods high in fat, including fast food, commercially prepared baked goods and desserts, deep-fried foods, meat, poultry (with skin), nuts and seeds, and regular dairy products.
- When you do eat high-fat foods, limit your portion sizes and balance your intake with foods low in fat.
- Choose lean cuts of meat, and trim any visible fat from meat before and after cooking. Remove skin from poultry before or after cooking.
- Drink fat-free or low-fat milk instead of whole milk, and use lower-fat varieties when cooking or baking. Substitute plain low-fat yogourt, low-fat cottage cheese, or buttermilk for sour cream.
- Use vegetable oil instead of butter or margarine. Use tub or squeeze margarine instead of stick margarine. Look for margarines that are free of trans fats. Minimize intake of coconut or palm oil.
- Season vegetables, seafood, and meats with herbs and spices rather than with creamy sauces, butter, or margarine.
- Use olive oil or lemon juice on salad, or use a yogourt-based salad dressing instead of mayonnaise or sour cream dressings.
- Steam, boil, bake, or microwave vegetables, or stir-fry them in a small amount of canola or vegetable oil.
- Roast, bake, or broil meat, poultry, or fish so that fat drains away as the food cooks.
- Use a nonstick pan for cooking so that added fat will be unnecessary; use a vegetable spray for frying.
- Substitute egg whites for whole eggs when baking; limit the number of egg yolks when scrambling eggs.
- Choose fruits as desserts most often.
- Eat a low-fat vegetarian main dish at least once a week.

Canada's Food Guide to Healthy Eating provides a general guide to what you should eat every day. By eating a balanced variety of foods from each of the four food groups and including some plant proteins, you can ensure that your daily diet is adequate in all nutrients. A diet using low-fat food choices contains only about 1800 calories but meets all known nutritional needs, except possibly for iron in some women who have heavy menstrual periods. For these women, foods fortified in iron, such as breakfast cereals, can make up the deficit.

Complementing Canada's Food Guide

Health Canada recognizes that people may consume diets that include foods not found in the Food Guide, or include foods required in different ratios. In 2007, *Eating Well with Canada's Food Guide—First Nations, Inuit, and Métis* (see Figure 7.4) was published in three languages (Cree, Ojibwe, and Inuktitut). In addition, the following section details the use of a guide that enables many vegetarians to consume foods that will assist in meeting daily intake values.

LO3 The Vegetarian Alternative

Vegetarians choose a diet with one essential difference from the diets described previously—they eliminate or restrict foods of animal origin (i.e., meat, poultry, fish, eggs, milk). Many people choose such diets for health reasons; vegetarian diets tend to be lower in total calories and calories from fat, saturated fat, cholesterol, and animal protein, and higher in complex carbohydrates, dietary fibre, folate, vitamins C and E, carotenoids, and phytochemicals. Some people adopt a vegetarian diet out of concern for the environment, for financial considerations, or for reasons related to ethics or religion.

vegetarian Someone who follows a diet that restricts or eliminates foods of animal origin.

Types of Vegetarian Diets

There are various vegetarian styles. The wider the variety of the diet eaten, the easier it is to meet nutritional needs.

- **Vegans** eat only plant foods.
- **Lacto-vegetarians** eat plant foods and dairy products.
- **Lacto-ovo-vegetarians** eat plant foods, dairy products, and eggs.

vegan A vegetarian who eats no animal products at all.
lacto-vegetarian A vegetarian who includes milk and cheese products in the diet.
lacto-ovo-vegetarian A vegetarian who eats no meat, poultry, or fish, but does eat eggs and milk products.

Others can be categorized as **partial vegetarians**, **semivegetarians**, or **pescovegetarians**. These people eat plant foods, dairy products, eggs, and usually a small selection of poultry, fish, and other seafood. Many other people frequently choose vegetarian meals but are not strictly vegetarian. Including some animal protein (such as dairy products) in a vegetarian diet makes planning easier, but it is not necessary.

partial vegetarians, semivegetarians, or pescovegetarians Vegetarians who include eggs, dairy products, and small amounts of poultry and seafood in their diet.

A Food Guide for Vegetarians

Health Canada's latest version of Canada's Food Guide is considered to be more "friendly" to vegetarians in that its Meat and Alternatives group places a greater emphasis on the consumption of vegetarian options instead of meat-only products. Although a vegetarian-only version of Canada's Food Guide has not been created, the Dietitians of Canada have produced a Vegetarian Food Guide Rainbow (see Figure 7.5 on p. 326) that can be a good resource.

FIGURE 7.4

Eating Well with Canada's Food Guide—First Nations, Métis, and Inuit.

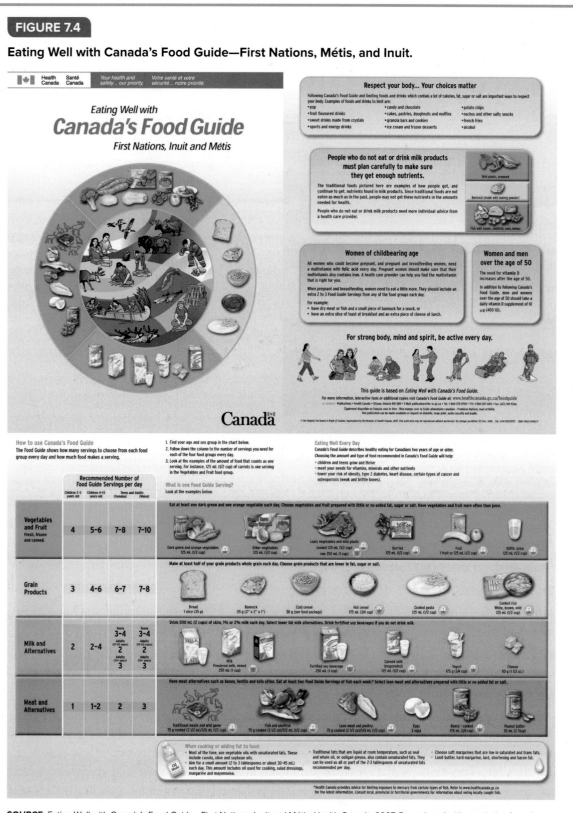

SOURCE: Eating Well with Canada's Food Guide—First Nations, Inuit and Métis. Health Canada, 2007. Reproduced with permission from the Minister of Health, 2015.

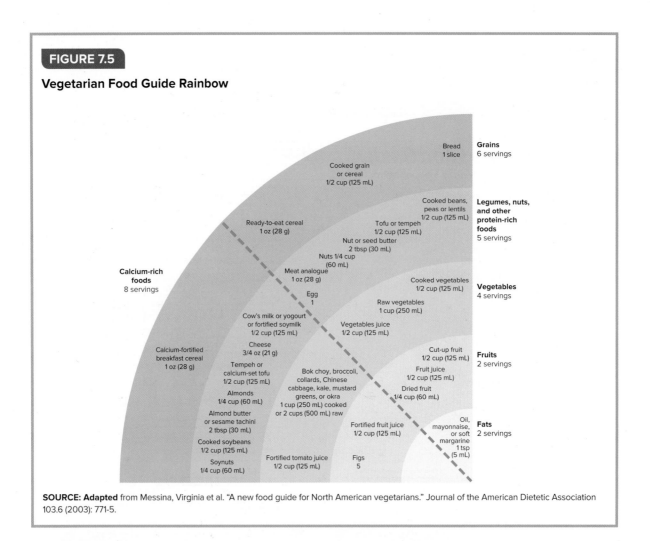

FIGURE 7.5

Vegetarian Food Guide Rainbow

Grains
6 servings

Bread
1 slice

Cooked grain
or cereal
1/2 cup (125 mL)

Cooked beans,
peas or lentils
1/2 cup (125 mL)

Legumes, nuts,
and other
protein-rich
foods
5 servings

Ready-to-eat cereal
1 oz (28 g)

Tofu or tempeh
1/2 cup (125 mL)

Nut or seed butter
2 tbsp (30 mL)

Nuts 1/4 cup
(60 mL)

Calcium-rich
foods
8 servings

Meat analogue
1 oz (28 g)

Cooked vegetables
1/2 cup (125 mL)

Vegetables
4 servings

Egg
1

Raw vegetables
1 cup (250 mL)

Cow's milk or yogourt
or fortified soymilk
1/2 cup (125 mL)

Vegetables juice
1/2 cup (125 mL)

Calcium-fortified
breakfast cereal
1 oz (28 g)

Cheese
3/4 oz (21 g)

Cut-up fruit
1/2 cup (125 mL)

Fruits
2 servings

Tempeh or
calcium-set tofu
1/2 cup (125 mL)

Bok choy, broccoli,
collards, Chinese
cabbage, kale, mustard
greens, or okra
1 cup (250 mL) cooked
or 2 cups (500 mL) raw

Fruit juice
1/2 cup (125 mL)

Almonds
1/4 cup (60 mL)

Dried fruit
1/4 cup (60 mL)

Almond butter
or sesame tachini
2 tbsp (30 mL)

Fortified fruit juice
1/2 cup (125 mL)

Oil,
mayonnaise,
or soft
margarine
1 tsp
(5 mL)

Fats
2 servings

Cooked soybeans
1/2 cup (125 mL)

Soynuts
1/4 cup (60 mL)

Fortified tomato juice
1/2 cup (125 mL)

Figs
5

SOURCE: Adapted from Messina, Virginia et al. "A new food guide for North American vegetarians." Journal of the American Dietetic Association 103.6 (2003): 771-5.

Vegetarians can adapt the basic Food Guide with only a few key modifications (see Table 1 in the Nutrition Resources section at the end of the chapter):

- Grain Products group (5–12 servings per day)

- Fruit and Vegetables group (5–10 servings per day)

- Milk and Alternatives group (0–4 servings per day); vegans and other vegetarians who do not consume any dairy products must find other rich sources of calcium (see below)

- Dry Beans, Nuts, Seeds, Eggs, and Meat Substitutes group (2–3 servings per day); this group includes such foods as soy milk, legumes, eggs or egg whites, nuts, seeds, tofu (soybean curd), tempeh (a cultured soy product), and peanut butter

A healthy vegetarian diet emphasizes a wide variety of plant foods. Although plant proteins are generally of a lower quality than animal proteins, choosing a variety of plant foods will supply all of the essential amino acids. Choosing minimally processed and unrefined foods will maximize nutrient value and provide ample dietary fibre. Daily consumption of a variety of plant foods in amounts that meet total energy needs can provide all needed nutrients, except vitamin B12 and possibly vitamin D. Strategies for obtaining these and other nutrients of concern include the following:

- Vitamin B12 is found naturally only in animal foods; if dairy products and eggs are limited or avoided, B12 can be obtained from fortified foods such as ready-to-eat cereals, soy beverages, meat substitutes, and special yeast products or from supplements.

- Vitamin D can be obtained by spending 5 to 15 minutes a day out in the sun, by consuming vitamin D-fortified products like ready-to-eat cereals and soy or rice milk, or by taking a supplement.

- Calcium is found in legumes, tofu processed with calcium, dark-green leafy vegetables, nuts, tortillas made from lime-processed corn, and fortified orange juice, soy milk, bread, and other foods.

- Iron is found in whole grains, fortified bread and breakfast cereals, dried fruits, green leafy vegetables, nuts and seeds,

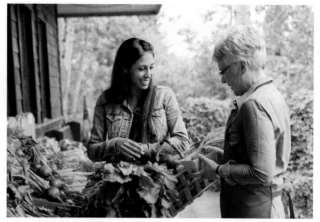

© Hero Images / Getty Images

Variety is the key to maintaining a healthy, balanced vegetarian diet.

legumes, and soy foods. The iron in plant foods is more difficult for the body to absorb than the iron from animal sources. Eating or drinking a good source of vitamin C with most meals is helpful because vitamin C improves iron absorption.

- Zinc is found in whole grains, nuts, legumes, and soy foods.

If you are a vegetarian, remember it's especially important to eat as wide a variety of foods as possible to ensure that all your nutritional needs are satisfied. Consulting with a registered dietitian will make your planning easier. Vegetarian diets for children, teens, and pregnant and lactating women warrant professional guidance.

Fitness Tip

Consumption of red meats, sweets, eggs, and butter is greatly reduced or eliminated entirely in most forms of the Mediterranean diet.

Dietary Challenges for Various Population Groups

Canada's Food Guide to Healthy Eating provides a basis that everyone can use to create a healthy diet. However, different population groups should be aware of special dietary challenges.

Children and Teenagers

The best approach for parents with younger children is to provide a variety of foods. For example, parents can add vegetables to casseroles and fruit to cereal, or they can offer fruit and vegetable juices or homemade yogourt or fruit shakes instead of sugary drinks. Many children and teenagers enjoy eating at fast-food restaurants, but they should be encouraged to select the healthiest menu choices and to balance the day's diet with low-fat, nutrient-rich foods. Allowing children to help prepare meals is another good way to encourage good eating habits.

University/College Students

Foods that are convenient for university and college students are not always the healthiest choices. Students who eat in buffet-style dining halls, cafeterias, and snack bars can easily overeat, and the foods offered are not necessarily high in nutrients or low in fat. The same is true of meals at fast-food restaurants. However, it is possible to make healthy eating both convenient and affordable. See the tips in the box Eating Strategies for University/College Students.

Take CHARGE

EATING STRATEGIES FOR UNIVERSITY/COLLEGE STUDENTS

Eating Wherever

- Eat a colourful, varied diet. The more colourful your diet is, the more varied and rich in fruits and vegetables it will be. Fruits and vegetables are typically inexpensive, delicious, rich in nutrients, and low in fat and calories.
- Eat breakfast. You'll have more energy in the morning and be less likely to grab an unhealthy snack later on.
- Choose healthy snacks—fruits, vegetables, grains, and cereals.
- Drink nonfat milk, water, mineral water, or 100% fruit juice more often than soft drinks or other sweetened beverages.
- Pay attention to portion sizes.
- Combine physical activity with healthy eating.

Eating on Campus

- Choose a meal plan that includes breakfast.
- Decide what you want to eat before you get in line, and stick to your choices.
- Build your meals around whole grains and vegetables. Ask for small servings of meat and high-fat main dishes.
- Choose leaner poultry, fish, or bean dishes rather than high-fat meats and fried entrées.
- Ask that gravies and sauces be served on the side; limit your intake.
- Choose broth-based or vegetable soups rather than cream soups.
- At the salad bar, load up on leafy greens, beans, and fresh vegetables. Avoid mayonnaise-coated salads (macaroni salad, potato salad), bacon, croutons, and high-fat dressings. Put dressing on the side; dip your fork into it rather than pouring it over the salad.
- Choose fruit for dessert rather than pastries, cookies, or cakes.

Eating in Fast-Food Restaurants

- Most fast-food chains provide a brochure with a nutritional breakdown of the foods on the menu. Ask for it, or check the restaurant's website for nutritional information. (See also the information in Appendix A.)
- Order small single burgers with no cheese instead of double burgers with many toppings.
- Ask for items to be prepared without mayonnaise, tartar sauce, sour cream, or other high-fat sauces. Ketchup, mustard, and fat-free mayonnaise or sour cream are better choices and are available at many fast-food restaurants.
- Choose whole-grain buns or bread for sandwiches.
- Choose chicken items made from chicken breast, not processed chicken.
- Order vegetable pizzas without extra cheese.
- If you order french fries or onion rings, get the smallest size and/or share them with a friend. Better yet, get a salad or fruit cup instead.

Eating on the Run

- When you need to eat in a hurry, remember that you can carry healthy foods in your backpack or a small insulated lunch sack (with a frozen gel pack to keep fresh food from spoiling).

- Carry items that are small and convenient but nutritious, such as fresh fruits or vegetables, whole-wheat buns or muffins, snack-size cereal boxes, and water.
- Make healthy choices at vending machines such as water or 100% fruit juice for beverages and whole grain crackers or pretzels, nuts, seeds, baked chips, low-fat popcorn, and low-fat granola bars as snacks.

Pregnant and Breastfeeding Women

Good nutrition is essential to a healthy pregnancy. Nutrition counselling before conception can help women establish a balanced eating plan and healthy body weight for a healthy pregnancy. Women have special nutritional needs during pregnancy and while breastfeeding. Pregnant or breastfeeding women are often advised to take a nutrient supplement in addition to following a special diet, as recommended by Canada's Food Guide. To reduce the risk of neural tube defects in the fetus, it is also recommended that all women of childbearing age get 400 μg of folic acid daily from fortified foods or supplements.

Older Adults

Nutrient needs do not change much as people age, but because older adults tend to become less active, they don't need as many calories to maintain body weight. At the same time, the absorption of nutrients tends to be lower in older adults because of age-related changes in the digestive tract. For these reasons, older adults should focus on eating nutrient-dense foods. For example, foods fortified with vitamin B12 and/or B12 supplements are recommended for people over age 50. Calcium and vitamin D intake can be inadequate; therefore, physicians may suggest supplementation to reduce bone loss and risk of osteoporosis. Antioxidants from fruits and vegetables are important in older adults to reduce age-related changes in vision and cognitive functioning. Because constipation is a common problem, consuming foods high in dietary fibre and drinking enough liquids are important goals.

Athletes

Key dietary concerns for athletes include meeting increased energy and fluid requirements for training and making healthy food choices throughout the day. For more on this topic, see the box Do Athletes Need a Different Diet?.

The Evidence *for* EXERCISE

DO ATHLETES NEED A DIFFERENT DIET?

If you exercise vigorously and frequently, or if you are an athlete in training, you likely have increased energy and fluid requirements. Research supports the following recommendations for athletes:

- **Energy intake.** Those engaged in a vigorous training program may have energy needs as high as 6000 calories per day—far greater than the energy needs of a moderately active person. It is recommended that athletes consume a diet with 60–65% of calories coming from carbohydrates, 10–15% from protein, and no more than 30% from fat.

  Athletes who need to maintain low body weight and fat (such as gymnasts, skaters, and wrestlers) need to get enough calories and nutrients while avoiding unhealthy eating patterns such as bulimia. The combination of low body fat, high physical activity, disordered eating habits—and, in women,

continued

amenorrhea—is associated with osteoporosis, stress fractures, and other injuries. If keeping your weight and body fat low for athletic reasons is important to you, seek dietary advice from a qualified dietitian and make sure your physician is aware of your eating habits.

- **Carbohydrates.** Endurance athletes involved in competitive events lasting longer than 90 minutes may benefit from increasing carbohydrate intake to 65–70% of their total calories. Specifically, the American College of Sports Medicine (ACSM) recommends that athletes consume 6 to 10 grams per kilogram of body weight daily, depending on their weight, sport, and other nutritional needs. This increase should come in the form of complex carbohydrates.

  High carbohydrate intake builds and maintains glycogen stores in the muscles, resulting in greater endurance and delayed fatigue during competitive events. The ACSM recommends that before exercise, an active adult or athlete eat a meal or snack that is relatively high in carbohydrates, moderate in protein, and low in fat and fibre. Eating carbohydrates 30 minutes, two hours, and four hours after exercise can help replenish glycogen stores in the liver and muscles.

- **Fat.** It is recommended that all athletes get 20–35% of calories from fat in their diets. This is in line with the daily intake suggested by Health Canada. Reducing fat intake to less than 20% of daily calories can negatively affect performance and be harmful to health.

- **Protein.** For endurance and strength-trained athletes, the ACSM and the Dietitians of Canada recommend eating 1.2 to 1.7 grams of protein per kilogram of body weight each day, which is considerably higher than the standard DRI of 0.8 gram per kilogram. This level of protein is easily obtainable from foods; in fact, most Canadians eat more protein than they need every day. A balanced, moderate-protein diet can provide the protein most athletes need.

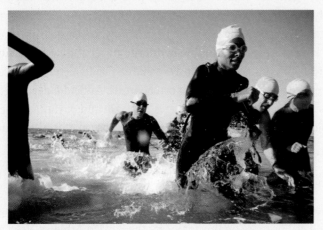

© Fuse / Corbis / Getty Images

  There is no evidence that consuming supplements containing vitamins, minerals, protein, or specific amino acids builds muscle or improves sports performance. Strength and muscle are built with exercise, not extra protein, and carbohydrates provide the fuel needed for muscle-building exercise.

- **Fluids.** If you exercise heavily or live in a hot climate, you should drink extra fluids to maximize performance and prevent heat illness. For a strenuous endurance event, prepare yourself the day before by drinking plenty of fluids. The ACSM and Dietitians of Canada recommend drinking 4 to 6 millilitres of fluid per kilogram of body weight about four hours before the event. During the event, take in enough fluids to compensate for fluid loss due to sweating; the amount required depends on the individual and their sweat rate. Afterwards, drink enough to replace lost fluids—about 1040 to 1560 mL for every kilogram of weight lost.

  Water is a good choice for fluid replacement for events lasting 60 to 90 minutes. For longer workouts or events, a sports drink can be a good choice. These contain water, electrolytes, and carbohydrates and can provide some extra energy, as well as replace electrolytes like sodium lost in sweat.

SOURCE: ADAPTED FROM "Nutrition and Athletic Performance." *Medicine & Science in Sports & Exercise*: March 2009 (Volume 41, Issue 3): p 709-731. doi: 10.1249/MSS.0b013e31890eb86. SPECIAL COMMUNICATIONS: Position Stands (http://journals.lww.com/acsm -msse/Fulltext/2009/03000/Nutrition_and_Athletic_Performance.27.aspx).

People with Special Health Concerns

Many Canadians have special health concerns that affect their dietary needs. For example, people with diabetes benefit from a well-balanced diet that is low in simple sugars, high in complex carbohydrates, and relatively rich in monounsaturated fats. People with high blood pressure need to limit their sodium consumption and control their weight. If you have a health problem or concern that may require a special diet, discuss your situation with a physician or registered dietitian.

LO4 7.3 Nutritional Planning: Making Informed Choices about Food

Knowing about nutrition is a good start to making sound choices about food. It also helps if you can interpret food labels, understand food additives, and avoid foodborne illnesses.

Reading Food Labels

Consumers can get help in applying the principles of the Food Guide and the DRIs from nutrition labels. Since 2003, nutrition labelling on all pre-packaged foods in Canada has been mandatory. Every nutrition label shows a variety of information such as serving sizes and the amount of fat, saturated fat, cholesterol, protein, dietary fibre, and sodium in each serving. To make intelligent choices about food, learn to read and understand nutrition labels (see the box Using Nutrition Labels). Research has shown that people who read nutrition labels eat less fat.

Critical CONSUMER

USING NUTRITION LABELS

Nutrition labels are designed to help consumers make food choices based on the nutrients that are most important to good health. In addition to listing nutrient content by weight, the label puts the information in the context of a daily diet of 2000 calories that includes no more than 65 grams of fat (approximately 30% of total calories). For example, if a serving of a particular product has 13 grams of fat, the label will show that the serving represents 20% of the daily fat allowance. If your daily diet contains fewer or more than 2000 calories, you need to adjust these calculations accordingly.

Nutrition labels contain uniform serving sizes. This means that if you look at different brands of salad dressing, for example, you can compare calories and fat content based on the serving amount. (Note that nutrition label serving sizes may be larger or smaller than Food Guide serving sizes, however.) Regulations also require that foods meet strict definitions if their packaging includes the terms "low-fat" or "high in fibre" (see below). Health claims such as "good source of dietary fibre" or "low in saturated fat" on packages are signals that those products can wisely be included in your diet. Overall, the food label is an important tool to help you choose a diet that conforms to the Food Guide.

continued

1. Serving size: Determine how many servings there are in the food package and compare it to how much you actually eat. You may need to adjust the rest of the nutrient values based on your typical serving size.

2. Calories and calories from fat: Note whether a serving is high in calories and fat. The sample food shown here is low in fat, with only 30 of its 235 calories from fat.

3. Daily Values: Based on a 2000-calorie diet, Daily Value percentages tell you whether the nutrients in a serving of food contribute a lot or a little to your total daily diet.

> 5% or less is low
> 20% or more is high

4. Limit these nutrients: Look for foods low in fat, saturated fat, trans fat, cholesterol, and sodium.

5. Get enough of these nutrients: Look for foods high in dietary fibre, vitamin A, vitamin C, calcium, and iron.

Nutrition Facts

Serving Size 1 cup (265g)
Servings per Container 2

Amount per Serving

Calories 235   Calories from Fat 30

	% Daily Value*
Total Fat 3g	5%
Saturated Fat 1g	5%
Trans Fat 0.5g	
Cholesterol 30mg	10%
Sodium 775mg	32%
Total Carbohydrate 34g	11%
Dietary Fiber 9g	36%
Sugars 5g	
Protein 18g	

Vitamin A 25%	•	Vitamin C 0%	
Calcium 12%	•	Iron 20%	

*Percent Daily Values are based on a 2,000 calorie diet. Your daily values may be higher or lower depending on your calorie needs:

	Calories	2,000	2,500
Total Fat	Less than	65g	80g
Sat Fat	Less than	20g	25g
Cholesterol	Less than	300mg	300mg
Sodium	Less than	2,400mg	2,400mg
Total Carbohydrate		300g	375g
Dietary Fiber		25g	30g

Calories per gram:
Fat 9 • Carbohydrate 4 • Protein 4

Footnote: This section shows recommended daily intake for two levels of calorie consumption and values for dietary calculations. It's the same on all labels.

Selected Nutrient Claims and What They Mean

The Canadian Food Inspection Agency has set out guidelines based on which the Nutrition Labels are permitted to include health claims. Listed below are some of the more common health claims you may see on foods. For a full listing of the regulations, please see http://www.inspection.gc.ca.

Source of energy. Food provides at least 100 calories per serving.

Reduced or fewer. At least 25% less of a nutrient than a similar product; can be applied to fat ("reduced fat"), saturated fat, cholesterol, sodium, and calories.

Low calorie. 40 calories or less per serving.

Fat-free/nonfat. Less than 0.5 grams of fat per serving.

Low-fat. 3 grams or less of fat per serving.

Saturated fatty acids-free. Less than 0.2 grams of saturated fat and 0.2 grams of trans fatty acids per serving.

Low in saturated fatty acids. 2 grams or less of saturated fatty acids and trans fatty acids combined per serving.

Cholesterol-free. Less than 2 milligrams of cholesterol and 2 grams or less of saturated fat per serving.

Low cholesterol. 20 milligrams or less of cholesterol and 2 grams or less of saturated fat per serving.

Sugar. Keep in mind that sugar does not always appear as "sugar." Typically words on the ingredients list ending in "ose" imply that those sources are in fact, sugar sources.

Source of fibre. 2 grams or more fibre per serving.

High in fibre. 4 grams or more fibre per serving.

Low sodium. 140 milligrams or less of sodium per serving.

Low in protein. Contains no more than 1 gram of protein per 100 grams of the food.

Source of protein. Food has a protein rating of 20 or more. Foods such as proteins can be assigned a biological value (BV), or in this case protein rating, identifying an approximate percentage of the nutrient that the body is able to use.

High in protein. Food has a protein rating of 40 or more.

Lean. Meat or poultry that has not been ground, marine or fresh water animals or a product of any of these; and contains 10% or less fat.

Extra-lean. Meat or poultry that has not been ground, marine or fresh water animals or a product of any of these; and contains 7.5% or less fat.

Because most meat, poultry, fish, fruits, and vegetables are not processed, they were not covered by the 2003 law. You can obtain information on the nutrient content of these items from the Internet, basic nutrition books, registered dietitians, nutrient analysis computer software, and the companies that produce or distribute these foods. Also, supermarkets often have large posters or pamphlets listing the nutrient contents of these foods. Lab 7.3 gives you the opportunity to compare foods using the information provided on their labels.

Reading Dietary Supplement Labels

Dietary supplements include vitamins, minerals, amino acids, herbs, enzymes, and other compounds. Although dietary supplements are often thought of as safe and natural, they contain powerful bioactive chemicals that have the potential for harm. About one-quarter of all pharmaceutical drugs are derived from botanical sources, and even essential vitamins and minerals can have toxic effects if consumed in excess.

A 2010 Ipsos-Reid survey shows that 73% of Canadians regularly take natural health products (NHPs) like vitamins and minerals, herbal products, and homeopathic medicines. In Canada, these supplements are regulated by the Natural Health Products Regulations. Before they are approved by Health Canada and put on the market, all supplements undergo assessment to determine if they are safe, effective, and of a high quality. Products are then given a product licence and can be sold in Canada.

Food Additives

Today, some 3000 substances are intentionally added to foods to maintain or improve nutritional quality, to maintain freshness, to help in processing or preparation, or to alter taste or appearance. The most widely used additives in food are sugar, salt, and corn syrup; these three, plus citric acid, baking soda, vegetable colours, mustard, and pepper, account for 98% by weight of all food additives used in North America.

Food additives pose no significant health hazard to most people because the levels used are well below any that could produce toxic effects. Two additives of potential concern for some people are sulfites, which are used to keep vegetables from turning brown, and monosodium glutamate (MSG), used as a flavour enhancer. To protect yourself, eat a variety of foods in moderation. If you have any sensitivity to an additive, check food labels when you shop and ask questions when you eat out.

Wellness Tip

To get produce as clean as possible, rub it with a soft brush while holding it under running water.

Foodborne Illness

Many people worry about additives or pesticide residues in their food. However, a greater threat comes from microorganisms that cause foodborne illnesses. Raw or undercooked animal products, such as chicken, hamburger, and oysters, pose the greatest risk for contamination. Health Canada and the Centers for Disease Control in the United States estimate that 2.2 million Canadians and 48 million Americans become sick each year as a result of foodborne illness. Symptoms include diarrhea, vomiting, fever, and weakness. Although the effects of foodborne illness are usually not serious, some groups, such as children, pregnant women, and older people, are at risk for severe complications, including rheumatic diseases, kidney failure, seizures, blood poisoning, and death.

Causes of Foodborne Illnesses

Most cases of foodborne illness are caused by pathogens, disease-causing microorganisms that contaminate food, usually from improper handling. The threats are numerous and varied; among them are the sometimes deadly *Escherichia coli (E. coli)* O157:H7 in meat and water; *Salmonella* in eggs, on vegetables, and on poultry; *Vibrio* in shellfish; *Cyclospora* and *hepatitis A* virus on fruit; *Cryptosporidium* in drinking water; *Campylobacter jejuni* in meat and poultry; and *Listeria monocytogenes* in lunch meats, sausages, and hot dogs.

You can't tell by taste, smell, or sight whether a food is contaminated. Although most pathogens are usually destroyed during cooking, it is important to recognize that your handling of foods before cooking can be critical. In addition, while foodborne illness outbreaks associated with food-processing plants make headlines, most cases of illness trace back to poor food handling in the home or in food-service establishments. The Canadian Partnership for Consumer Food Safety Education is taking steps to bring down levels of contamination by educating Canadians about the importance of food safety in the home. See the box Safe Food Handling for more information.

Take CHARGE

SAFE FOOD HANDLING

Shopping

- Don't buy food in containers that leak, bulge, or are severely dented. Refrigerated foods should be cold, and frozen foods should be solid.
- Check the food label for an expiration date and for safe-handling instructions.
- Place meat, poultry, and seafood in plastic bags, and separate foods in your grocery cart.
- Select cold and frozen food last to ensure they stay refrigerated until just before checkout.

Storing Food

- Store raw meat, poultry, fish, and shellfish in containers in the refrigerator so that the juices don't drip onto other foods. Keep these items away from other foods, surfaces, utensils, or serving dishes to prevent cross-contamination.

- Store eggs in the coldest part of the refrigerator, not in the door, and use them within three to five weeks.
- Keep hot foods hot (60°C or above) and cold foods cold (4.5°C or below); harmful bacteria can grow rapidly between these two temperatures.
- Refrigerate foods within two hours of purchase or preparation, and within one hour if the air temperature is above 32°C. Refrigerate foods at or below 5°C and freeze at or below –18°C. Use refrigerated leftovers within three to four days.

Preparing Food

- Thoroughly wash your hands with warm soapy water for 20 seconds before and after handling food, especially raw meat, fish, poultry, or eggs.
- Make sure counters, cutting boards, dishes, and other equipment are thoroughly cleaned before and after use using hot, soapy water. Wash dishcloths and kitchen towels frequently.
- Use separate cutting boards for meat, poultry, and seafood and for foods that will be eaten raw, such as fruits and vegetables. Replace cutting boards once they become worn or develop hard-to-clean grooves.
- Thoroughly rinse and scrub fruits and vegetables with a brush, if possible, or peel off the skin.
- Don't eat raw animal products, including raw eggs in home-made hollandaise sauce, eggnog, or cookie dough. Use only pasteurized milk and juice, and look for pasteurized eggs.
- Thaw frozen food in the refrigerator, in cold water, or in the microwave, not on the kitchen counter. Cook foods immediately after thawing.

Cooking

- Cook foods thoroughly, especially beef, poultry, fish, pork, and eggs; cooking kills most microorganisms. Use a food thermometer to ensure that foods are cooked to a safe temperature. Hamburgers should be cooked to 71°C. Turn or stir microwaved food to make sure it is heated evenly throughout.
- Cook stuffing separately from poultry; or wash poultry thoroughly, stuff immediately before cooking, and transfer the stuffing to a clean bowl immediately after cooking. The temperature of cooked stuffing should reach 75°C.
- Cook eggs until they're firm and fully cook foods containing eggs.
- To protect against *Listeria,* reheat ready-to-eat foods like hot dogs and cold cuts until steaming hot.
- Because of possible contamination with *E. coli* O157:H7 and *Salmonella,* avoid raw sprouts.

Treating Foodborne Illness

If you think you may be having a bout of foodborne illness, drink plenty of clear fluids to prevent dehydration and rest to speed recovery. To prevent further contamination, wash your hands often and always before handling food until you recover. A fever higher than 39°C, blood in the stool, or dehydration deserves a physician's evaluation, especially if the symptoms persist for more than two or three days. In cases of suspected botulism—characterized by symptoms such as double vision, paralysis, dizziness, and vomiting—consult a physician immediately.

Irradiated Foods—A Technique of Biotechnology

Food irradiation is the treatment of foods with gamma rays, X-rays, or high-voltage electrons to kill potentially harmful pathogens, including bacteria, parasites, insects, and fungi that cause foodborne illness. It also reduces spoilage and extends shelf life. Even though irradiation has been generally endorsed by agencies such as the World Health Organization and the Centers for Disease Control and Prevention, few irradiated foods are currently on the market due to consumer resistance and skepticism. Studies indicate that when consumers are given information about the process of irradiation and the benefits of irradiated foods, most want to purchase them.

> **food irradiation** The treatment of foods with gamma rays, X rays, or high-voltage electrons to kill potentially harmful pathogens and increase shelf life.

All primary irradiated foods (meat, vegetables, and so on) are labelled with the flowerlike radura symbol and a brief information label; spices and foods that are merely ingredients do not have to be so labelled. Proper handling of irradiated foods is still critical for preventing foodborne illness.

Organic Foods—Stricter Standards for a Booming Industry

Some people who are concerned about pesticides and other environmental contaminants choose to buy foods that are **organic**. Since 2009, the Canadian Organics Products Regulations (OPR), of the Canadian Food Inspection Agency, have been responsible for certifying foods as organic according to strict production, processing, handling, and labelling criteria. Food certified as organic carries the Biologique Canada Organic logo below.

> **organic** A designation applied to foods grown and produced according to strict guidelines limiting the use of pesticides, nonorganic ingredients, hormones, antibiotics, genetic engineering, irradiation, and other practices.

 Organic foods are not necessarily free of chemicals; they may be contaminated with pesticides used on neighbouring lands or on foods transported in the same train or truck. Nevertheless, they tend to have lower levels of pesticide residues than conventionally grown crops. Some experts recommend that consumers who want to buy organic fruits and vegetables spend their money on those that carry lower pesticide residues than their conventional counterparts (the "dirty dozen"): apples, bell peppers, celery, cherries, imported grapes, nectarines, peaches, pears, potatoes, red raspberries, spinach, and strawberries. Experts also recommend buying organic beef, poultry, eggs, dairy products, and baby food. Fruits and vegetables that carry little pesticide residue whether grown conventionally or organically include asparagus, avocadoes, bananas, broccoli, cauliflower, corn, kiwi, mangoes, onions, papaya, pineapples, and peas. All foods are subject to strict pesticide limits; the debate about the health effects of small amounts of residue is ongoing.

Whether organic foods are better for your health cannot be said for certain, but organic farming is better for the environment. It helps maintain biodiversity of crops and replenish the Earth's resources. It is less likely to degrade soil, contaminate water, or expose farm workers to toxic chemicals. As multinational food companies get into the organic food business, consumers who want to support environmentally friendly farming methods should look for foods that are not only organic, but also locally grown.

Guidelines for Fish Consumption

A specific area of concern has been possible mercury contamination in fish. Overall, fish and shellfish are healthy sources of protein, omega-3 fats, and other nutrients, and experts continue to encourage consumption of both wild-caught and farmed fish. Prudent choices can minimize the risk of any possible negative health effects. High mercury concentrations are most likely to be found in predator fish—large fish that eat smaller fish. Mercury can cause brain damage to fetuses and young children. According to Health Canada guidelines, women who are or who may become pregnant and nursing mothers should follow these guidelines to minimize their exposure to mercury:

- Limit your consumption of tuna (fresh and frozen), shark, swordfish, marlin, orange roughy, and escolar to no more than 150 grams per month.

- Eat 150 grams a week of a variety of fish and shellfish that are lower in mercury, such as shrimp, canned light tuna, salmon, pollock, and catfish. Limit consumption of albacore tuna to no more than 300 grams per week.

LO5 7.4 A Personal Plan: Applying Nutritional Principles

There probably is an ideal diet for you based on your particular nutrition and health status, but there is no single type of diet that provides optimal health for everyone. Many cultural dietary patterns can meet people's nutritional requirements (see the box Ethnic Foods). Every individual needs to customize a food plan based on age, gender, weight, activity level, medical risk factors, and personal tastes.

DIVERSITY Matters

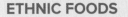

ETHNIC FOODS

Every diet has its advantages and disadvantages and, within each cuisine, some foods are better choices. As the table below shows, the dietary guidelines described in this chapter can be applied to any ethnic cuisine.

	Choose More Often	Choose Less Often
Chinese	Dishes that are steamed, poached (jum), boiled (chu), roasted (kow), barbecued (shu), or lightly stir-fried Hoisin sauce, oyster sauce, wine sauce, plum sauce, velvet sauce, or hot mustard Fresh fish and seafood, skinless chicken, tofu Mixed vegetables, Chinese greens steamed rice, steamed spring rolls, soft noodles	Fried wontons or egg rolls Crab rangoon Crispy (Peking) duck or chicken Sweet-and-sour dishes made with breaded and deep-fried meat, poultry, or fish Fried rice Fried or crispy noodles
French	Dishes prepared au vapeur (steamed), en brochette (skewered and broiled), or grillé (grilled) Fresh fish, shrimp, scallops, or mussels or skinless chicken, without sauces Clear soups	Dishes prepared à la crème (in cream sauce), au gratin or gratinée (baked with cream and cheese), or en croûte (in pastry crust) Drawn butter, hollandaise sauce, and remoulade (mayonnaise-based sauce)

continued

Greek	Dishes that are stewed, broiled, or grilled, including shish kabobs (souvlaki) Dolmas (grape leaves) stuffed with rice Tzatziki (yogourt, cucumbers, and garlic) Tabouli (bulgur-based salad) Pita bread, especially whole wheat	Moussaka, saganaki (fried cheese) Vegetable pies such as spanakopita and tyropita Baba ghanoush (eggplant and olive oil) Deep-fried falafel (chickpea patties) Gyros stuffed with ground meat Baklava
Indian	Dishes prepared masala (curry), tandoori (roasted in a clay oven), or tikke (pan roasted), and kabobs Raita (yogourt and cucumber salad) and other yogourt-based dishes and sauces Dal (lentils), pullao or pilau (basmati rice) Chapati (baked bread)	Ghee (clarified butter) Korma (meat in cream sauce) Samosas, pakoras (fried dishes) Molee and other coconut milk-based dishes Poori, bhatura, or paratha (fried breads)
Italian	Pasta primavera or pasta, polenta, risotto, or gnocchi with marinara, red or white wine, white or red clam, or light mushroom sauce Dishes that are grilled or prepared cacciatore (tomato-based sauce), marsala (broth and wine sauce), or piccata (lemon sauce) Cioppino (seafood stew) Vegetable soup, minestrone or fagioli (beans)	Antipasto (cheese, smoked meats) Dishes that are prepared alfredo, frito (fried), crema (creamed), alla panna (with cream), or carbonara Veal scaloppini Chicken, veal, or eggplant parmigiana Italian sausage, salami, and prosciutto Buttered garlic bread Cannoli
Japanese	Dishes prepared nabemono (boiled), shabu-shabu (in boiling broth), mushimono (steamed), nimono (simmered), yaki (broiled), or yakimono (grilled) Sushi or domburi (mixed rice dish) Steamed rice or soba (buckwheat), udon (wheat), or rice noodles	Tempura (battered and fried) Agemono (deep fried) Katsu (fried pork cutlet) Sukiyaki Fried tofu
Mexican	Soft corn or wheat tortillas Burritos, fajitas, enchiladas, soft tacos, and tamales filled with beans, vegetables, or lean meats Refried beans, nonfat or low-fat, rice and beans Ceviche (fish marinated in lime juice) Gazpacho, menudo, or black bean soup Fruit or flan for dessert	Crispy, fried tortillas Dishes that are fried, such as chile rellenos, chimichangas, flautas, and tostadas Nachos and cheese, chili con queso, and other dishes made with cheese or cheese sauce Refried beans made with lard Fried ice cream
Thai	Dishes that are barbecued, sautéed, broiled, boiled, steamed, braised, or marinated Sàté (skewered and grilled meats) Fish sauce, basil sauce, chili or hot sauces Bean thread noodles, Thai salad	Coconut milk soup Peanut sauce or dishes topped with nuts Mee-krob (crispy noodles) Red, green, and yellow curries, which typically contain coconut milk

SOURCES: National Heart, Lung, and Blood Institute. 2006. Guidelines on Overweight and Obesity: Electronic Textbook (http://www.nhlbi.nih.gov/guidelines/obesity/e_txtbk/appndx/6a3b.htm, retrieved December 10, 2011); and Duyff, R.L. 2006. The American Dietetic Association's Complete Food and Nutrition Guide, 2nd ed. Hoboken, NJ: Wiley.

Assessing and Changing Your Diet

The first step in planning a healthy diet is to examine what you currently eat. Labs 7.1 and 7.2 are designed to help you analyze your current diet and compare it with optimal dietary goals. This analysis can be completed using a nutritional analysis software program or one of several websites.

To put your plan into action, use the behavioural self-management techniques and tips described in Chapter 1. If you identify several changes you want to make, focus on one at a time. You might start, for example, by substituting nonfat or low-fat milk for whole milk. When you become used to that, try substituting whole-wheat bread for white bread. The information on eating behaviour in Lab 7.1 will help you identify and change unhealthy patterns of eating.

Staying Committed to a Healthy Diet

Beyond knowledge and information, you also need support in difficult situations. Refer back to the Cycle of Behaviour Change presented in Chapter 1 to help you construct a plan that will be easier to maintain. Use the following tips to help keep yourself on track:

- Choose and prepare your own food at home to help you keep to your plan.

- Consider using a meal plan such as the 100-Mile diet, which is based on the efforts of two residents of northern British Columbia who, for one year, restricted their diets to only foods grown within 100 miles (160 kilometres) of their residence. In addition to assisting the local community and helping the environment, the 100-Mile diet is also thought to be safer and more nutritious.

- Keep in mind that advance planning is the key. Map out meals and shopping appropriately, cook in advance when possible, and prepare enough food for leftovers later in the week. A tight budget does not necessarily make it more difficult to eat healthy meals. It makes good health sense and good budget sense to use only small amounts of meat and to have a few meatless meals each week.

- Remain focused on your goals when eating out in restaurants, when keeping to food plan goals can become somewhat more difficult. Portion sizes in restaurants tend to be larger than serving sizes of the Food Guide, but you can eat only part of your meal and take the rest home for a meal later in the week. Don't hesitate to ask questions when you're eating in a restaurant. Most restaurant personnel are glad to explain how menu selections are prepared and to make small adjustments, such as serving salad dressings and sauces on the side so they can be avoided or used sparingly. To limit your fat intake, order meat or fish broiled or grilled rather than fried or sautéed, choose rice or a plain baked potato over french fries, and select a clear soup rather than a creamy one. Desserts that are irresistible can, at least, be shared.

Strategies like these can be helpful, but small changes cannot change a fundamentally high-fat, high-calorie meal into a moderate, healthful one. Often, the best advice is to bypass a large steak with potatoes au gratin for a flavourful but low-fat entrée. Many of the selections offered in ethnic restaurants are healthy choices (refer to the Ethnic Foods box for suggestions).

Tips for Today and the Future

Opportunities to improve your diet present themselves every day, and small changes add up.

RIGHT NOW YOU CAN

- Substitute a healthy snack—an apple, a banana, or plain popcorn—for a bag of chips or cookies.

- Drink a glass of water and put a bottle of water in your backpack for tomorrow.

continued

- Plan to make healthy selections when you eat out, such as a baked potato instead of french fries or salmon instead of steak.

IN THE FUTURE, YOU CAN

- Visit the Canada's Food Guide site at http://www.hc-sc.gc.ca/fn-an/food-guide-aliment/index-eng.php and use the online tools to create a personalized nutrition plan and begin tracking your eating habits.

- Learn to cook healthier meals. There are hundreds of free websites and low-cost cookbooks that provide recipes for healthy dishes.

Common Questions ANSWERED

Q **Canada's Food Guide seems to recommend such a large number of servings. How can I possibly follow its recommendations without gaining weight?**

A First of all, consider how many servings from each food group are appropriate for you. The suggested number of servings is given as a range: three to eight servings of grain products, four to ten of fruits and vegetables, and so on. The smaller number of servings is for people who consume about 1800 calories a day, such as many sedentary women. The larger number is for those who consume about 3200 calories a day, such as active men. If the smaller number of servings is appropriate for you, concentrate on choosing nutrient-dense foods—those that are rich in nutrients but relatively low in calories, such as most grains, fruits, and vegetables.

Second, compare the serving sizes of the foods you eat with those used in the Food Guide. Some of the Food Guide's serving sizes are smaller than what you might typically eat. For example, many people eat a cup or more of pasta or rice in a meal, which would correspond to two or more servings from the grain products group. You'll probably find that your current diet already includes the minimum number of servings from most of the food groups. If not, you may find that you are eating too many servings from one group and not enough from another. Make small changes in your eating habits and food choices to bring your diet into line with the recommendations in the Guide, paying particular attention to your consumption of fat and added sugars. The Food Guide is designed to help you balance your food choices to ensure good health. (Strategies for successful weight management are described in detail in Chapter 8.)

Q **What exactly are genetically modified foods? Are they safe? How can I recognize them on the shelf, and how can I know when I'm eating them?**

A Genetic engineering involves altering the characteristics of a plant, animal, or microorganism by adding, rearranging, or replacing genes in its DNA; the result is a genetically modified (GM) organism. New DNA may come from related species or organisms or from entirely different types of organisms. Many GM crops are already grown in Canada: About 60% of all processed food in Canada contain some genetic modifications. Products made with GM organisms include juice, carbonated drinks, nuts, tuna, frozen pizza, spaghetti sauce, canola oil, chips, salad dressing, and soup.

The potential benefits of GM foods cited by supporters include improved yields overall and in difficult growing conditions, increased disease resistance, improved nutritional content, lower prices, and less use of pesticides. Critics of biotechnology argue that unexpected effects may occur: Gene manipulation could elevate levels of naturally occurring toxins or allergens, permanently change the gene pool and reduce biodiversity, and produce pesticide-resistant insects through the transfer of genes. In 2000, a form of GM corn approved for use only in animal feed was found to have commingled with other varieties of corn and to have been used in human foods; this mistake sparked fears of allergic reactions and led to recalls. Opposition to GM foods is particularly strong in Europe. In many developing nations that face food shortages, responses to GM crops have tended to be more positive.

There is currently no Canadian legislation governing the labelling of GM foods in Canada, meaning that Canadians will have virtually no knowledge of their consumption of GM foods. The one exception to this rule is when a food's composition has changed significantly and in such a way that a known allergen is introduced. For example, soybeans that contain a gene from a peanut would have to be labelled because peanuts are a common allergen. The only foods guaranteed not to contain GM ingredients are those certified as organic.

Q How can I tell if I'm allergic to a food?

A A true food allergy is a reaction of the body's immune system to a food or food ingredient, usually a protein. This immune reaction can occur within minutes of ingesting the food, resulting in symptoms such as hives, diarrhea, difficulty breathing, or swelling of the lips or tongue. The most severe response is a systemic reaction called anaphylaxis, which involves a potentially life-threatening drop in blood pressure. Food allergies affect only about 2% of the adult population and about 4–6% of infants. Just a few foods account for most of the food allergies in Canada: cow's milk, eggs, peanuts, tree nuts (e.g., walnuts, cashews, and so on), soy, wheat, fish, and shellfish.

Many people who believe they have food allergies may actually suffer from a food intolerance, a much more common source of adverse food reaction that typically involves problems with metabolism rather than with the immune system. The body may not be able to adequately digest a food or the body may react to a particular food compound. Food intolerances have been attributed to lactose (milk sugar), gluten (a protein in some grains), tartrazine (yellow food colouring), sulfite (a food additive), MSG, and the sweetener aspartame. Although symptoms of a food intolerance may be similar to those of a food allergy, they are typically more localized and not life-threatening. Many people with a food intolerance can safely and comfortably consume small amounts of the food that affects them.

If you suspect you have a food allergy or intolerance, a good first step is to keep a food diary. Note everything you eat or drink, any symptoms you develop, and how long after eating the symptoms appear. Then make an appointment with your physician to go over your diary and determine if any additional tests are needed. People at risk for severe allergic reactions must diligently avoid trigger foods and carry medications to treat anaphylaxis.

SUMMARY

- The six classes of nutrients are carbohydrates, proteins, fats, vitamins, minerals, and water.

- The nutrients essential to humans are released into the body through digestion. Nutrients in foods provide energy, measured in kilocalories (commonly called calories); build and maintain body tissues; and regulate body functions.

- Protein, an important component of body tissue, is composed of amino acids; nine are essential to a diet. Foods from animal sources provide complete proteins, while plants provide incomplete proteins.

- Fats, a major source of energy, also insulate the body and cushion the organs; just 3 to 4 teaspoons of vegetable oil per day supplies the essential fats. For most people, dietary fat intake should be 20–35% of total calories, and unsaturated fats should be favoured over saturated and trans fats.

- Carbohydrates provide energy to the brain, nervous system, and blood and to muscles during high-intensity exercise. Naturally occurring simple carbohydrates and unrefined complex carbohydrates should be favoured over added sugars and refined carbohydrates.

continued

- Fibre includes plant substances that are impossible for the human body to digest. It helps reduce cholesterol levels and promotes the passage of wastes through the intestines.

- The 13 essential vitamins are organic substances that promote specific chemical and cell processes and act as antioxidants. The 17 known essential minerals are inorganic substances that regulate body functions, aid in growth and tissue maintenance, and help in the release of energy from food. Deficiencies in vitamins and minerals can cause severe symptoms over time, but excess doses are also dangerous.

- Water aids in digestion and food absorption, allows chemical reactions to take place, serves as a lubricant or cushion, helps regulate body temperature, flushes toxins, and eliminates wastes.

- Foods contain other substances, such as phytochemicals, that may not be essential nutrients but that may protect against chronic diseases.

- The Dietary Reference Intakes and Canada's Food Guide for Healthy Eating provide standards and recommendations for getting all essential nutrients from a varied, balanced diet and for eating in ways that protect against chronic disease.

- A vegetarian diet requires special planning but can meet all nutritional needs.

- Different population groups, such as university/college students and athletes, face special dietary challenges and should plan their diets to meet their particular needs.

- Consumers can get help applying nutritional principles by reading the standardized labels that appear on all packaged foods and on dietary supplements.

- Although nutritional basics are well established, no single diet provides wellness for everyone. Individuals should focus on their particular needs and adapt general dietary principles to meet them.

FOR FURTHER EXPLORATION

Organizations and Websites

Canadian Food Inspection Agency. Delivers information related to food, animal health, and plant protection. Includes allergy alerts and food releases important to Canadians.

http://www.inspection.gc.ca

Dietitians of Canada. Provides a variety of educational materials and self-awareness activities on nutrition.

http://dietitians.ca

FDA Center for Food Safety and Applied Nutrition. Offers information about topics such as food labelling.

https://www.fda.gov/AboutFDA/CentersOffices/OfficeofFoods/CFSAN/default.htm

Gateways to Government Nutrition Information. Provides access to government resources relating to food safety, including consumer advice and information on specific pathogens.

http://www.nutrition.gov

http://www.foodsafety.gov

Harvard School of Public Health: Nutrition Source. Offers advice on interpreting news on nutrition and suggestions for building a healthy diet.

http://www.hsph.harvard.edu/nutritionsource

Health Canada—Food and Nutrition. Details all relevant areas of food and nutrition including labelling, genetically modified foods, and Canada's Food Guide to Healthy Eating.

http://www.hc-sc.gc.ca/fn-an/nutrition/index_e.html

Heart and Stroke Foundation of Canada. Provides information about heart and stroke and healthy living in Canada.

http://heartandstroke.ca

MedlinePlus: Nutrition. Includes links to information from government agencies and major medical associations on a wide variety of nutrition topics.

http://www.nlm.nih.gov/medlineplus/nutrition.html

Osteoporosis Society of Canada. Provides resources and support networks for those suffering from osteoporosis.

http://www.osteoporosis.ca/

USDA Food and Nutrition Information Center. Contains a variety of materials relating to the Dietary Guidelines, food labels, Food Guide Pyramid, and many other topics.

http://www.nal.usda.gov/fnic

Vegetarian Resource Group. Includes information and links for vegetarians and people interested in learning more about vegetarian diets.

http://www.vrg.org

See also the resources listed in Chapter 8, Chapter 10, and Chapter 11.

Nutrition Resources

TABLE 1

Dietary Reference Intakes (DRIs): Recommended Levels for Individual Intake

Life Stage	Group	Biotin (µg/day)	Choline (mg/day)a	Folate (µg/day)b	Niacin (mg/day)c	Pantothenic Acid (mg/day)	Riboflavin (mg/day)	Thiamin (mg/day)	Vitamin A (µg/day)d	Vitamin B-6 (mg/day)	Vitamin B-12 (µg/day)	Vitamin C (mg/day)e	Vitamin D (µg/day)f	Vitamin E (mg/day)g
Infants	0–6 months	5	125	65	2	1.7	0.3	0.2	400	0.1	0.4	40	5	4
	7–12 months	6	150	80	4	1.8	0.4	0.3	500	0.3	0.5	50	5	5
Children	1–3 years	8	200	150	6	2	0.5	0.5	300	0.5	0.9	15	5	6
	4–8 years	12	250	200	8	3	0.6	0.6	400	0.6	1.2	25	5	7
Males	9–13 years	20	375	300	12	4	0.9	0.9	600	1.0	1.8	45	5	11
	14–18 years	25	550	400	16	5	1.3	1.2	900	1.3	2.4	75	5	15
	19–30 years	30	550	400	16	5	1.3	1.2	900	1.3	2.4	90	5	15
	31–50 years	30	550	400	16	5	1.3	1.2	900	1.3	2.4	90	5	15
	51–70 years	30	550	400	16	5	1.3	1.2	900	1.7	2.4h	90	10	15
	>70 years	30	550	400	16	5	1.3	1.2	900	1.7	2.4h	90	15	15
Females	9–13 years	20	375	300	12	4	0.9	0.9	600	1.0	1.8	45	5	11
	14–18 years	25	400	400i	14	5	1.0	1.0	700	1.2	2.4	65	5	15
	19–30 years	30	425	400i	14	5	1.1	1.1	700	1.3	2.4	75	5	15
	31–50 years	30	425	400i	14	5	1.1	1.1	700	1.3	2.4	75	5	15
	51–70 years	30	425	400i	14	5	1.1	1.1	700	1.5	2.4h	75	10	15
	>70 years	30	425	400	14	5	1.1	1.1	700	1.5	2.4h	75	15	15
Pregnancy	≤18 years	30	450	600i	18	6	1.4	1.4	750	1.9	2.6	80	5	15
	19–30 years	30	450	600i	18	6	1.4	1.4	770	1.9	2.6	85	5	15
	31–50 years	30	450	600i	18	6	1.4	1.4	770	1.9	2.6	85	5	15
Lactation	≤18 years	35	550	500	17	7	1.6	1.4	1200	2.0	2.8	115	5	19
	19–30 years	35	550	500	17	7	1.6	1.4	1300	2.0	2.8	120	5	19
	31–50 years	35	550	500	17	7	1.6	1.4	1300	2.0	2.8	120	5	19
Tolerable Upper Intake Levels for Adults (19–70)			3500	1000k	35k				3000	100		2000	50	1000k

Note: The table includes values for the type of DRI standard—Adequate Intake (AI) or Recommended Dietary Allowance (RDA)—that has been established for that particular nutrient and life stage; RDAs are shown in **bold type**. The final row of the table shows the Tolerable Upper Intake Levels (ULs) for adults; refer to the full DRI report for information on other ages and life stages. A UL is the maximum level of daily nutrient intake that is likely to pose no risk of adverse effects. There is insufficient data to set ULs for all nutrients, but this does not mean that there is no potential for adverse effects; source of intake should be from food only to prevent high levels of intake of nutrients without established ULs. In healthy individuals, there is no established benefit from nutrient intakes above the RDA or AI.

a Although AIs have been set for choline, there are few data to assess whether a dietary supply of choline is needed at all stages of the life cycle, and it may be that the choline requirement can be met by endogenous synthesis at some of these stages.

b As dietary folate equivalents (DFE): 1 DFE = 1 µg food folate = 0.6 µg folate from fortified food or as a supplement consumed with food = 0.5 µg of a supplement taken on an empty stomach.

c As niacin equivalents (NE): 1 mg niacin = 60 mg tryptophan.

TABLE 1

Dietary Reference Intakes (DRIs): Recommended Levels for Individual Intake (continued)

Life Stage	Group	Vitamin K (µg/day)	Calcium (mg/day)	Chromium (µg/day)	Copper (µg/day)	Fluoride (mg/day)	Iodine (mg/day)	Iron (mg/day)	Magnesium (mg/day)	Manganese (mg/day)	Molybdenum (µg/day)	Phosphorus (mg/day)	Selenium (µg/day)	Zinc (mg/day)
Infants	0–6 months	2.0	210	0.2	200	0.01	110	0.27	30	0.003	2	100	15	2
	7–12 months	2.5	270	5.5	220	0.5	130	11	75	0.6	3	275	20	3
Children	1–3 years	30	500	11	340	0.7	90	7	80	1.2	17	460	20	3
	4–8 years	55	800	15	440	1	90	10	130	1.5	22	500	30	5
Males	9–13 years	60	1300	25	700	2	120	8	240	1.9	34	1250	40	8
	14–18 years	75	1300	35	890	3	150	11	410	2.2	43	1250	55	11
	19–30 years	120	1000	35	900	4	150	8	400	2.3	45	700	55	11
	31–50 years	120	1000	35	900	4	150	8	420	2.3	45	700	55	11
	51–70 years	120	1200	30	900	4	150	8	420	2.3	45	700	55	11
	>70 years	120	1200	30	900	4	150	8	420	2.3	45	700	55	11
Females	9–13 years	60	1300	21	700	2	120	8	240	1.6	34	1250	40	8
	14–18 years	75	1300	24	890	3	150	15	360	1.6	43	1250	55	9
	19–30 years	90	1000	25	900	3	150	18	310	1.8	45	700	55	8
	31–50 years	90	1000	25	900	3	150	18	320	1.8	45	700	55	8
	51–70 years	90	1200	20	900	3	150	8	320	1.8	45	700	55	8
	>70 years	90	1200	20	900	3	150	8	320	1.8	45	700	55	8
Pregnancy	≤18 years	75	1300	29	1000	3	220	27	400	2.0	50	1250	60	13
	19–30 years	90	1000	30	1000	3	220	27	350	2.0	50	700	60	11
	31–50 years	90	1000	30	1000	3	220	27	360	2.0	50	700	60	11
Lactation	≤18 years	75	1300	44	1300	3	290	10	360	2.6	50	1250	70	14
	19–30 years	90	1000	45	1300	3	290	9	310	2.6	50	700	70	12
	31–50 years	90	1000	45	1300	3	290	9	320	2.6	50	700	70	12
Tolerable Upper Intake Levels for Adults (19–70)			2500		10 000	10	1100	45	350*	11	2000	4000	400	40

[d] As retinol activity equivalents (RAEs). 1 RAE = 1 µg retinol, 12 µg β-carotene, or 24 µg α-carotene or β-cryptoxanthin. Preformed vitamin A (retinol) is abundant in animal-derived foods; provitamin A carotenoids are abundant in some dark yellow, orange, red, and deep-green fruits and vegetables. For preformed vitamin A and for provitamin A carotenoids in supplements, 1RE = 1 RAE; for provitamin A carotenoids in foods, divide the REs by 2 to obtain RAEs. The UL applies only to preformed vitamin A.

[e] Individuals who smoke require an additional 35 mg/day of vitamin C over that needed by nonsmokers; nonsmokers regularly exposed to tobacco smoke should ensure they meet the RDA for vitamin C.

[f] As cholecalciferol: 1 µg cholecalciferol = 40 IU vitamin D. DRI values are based on the absence of adequate exposure to sunlight.

[g] As α-tocopherol. Includes naturally occurring RRR-α-tocopherol and the 2R-stereoisomeric forms from supplements; does not include the 2S-stereoisomeric forms from supplements.

[h] Because 10–30% of older people may malabsorb food-bound B12, those over age 50 should meet their RDA mainly with supplements or foods fortified with B12.

[i] In view of evidence linking folate intake with neural tube defects in the fetus, it is recommended that all women capable of becoming pregnant consume 400 µg from supplements or fortified foods in addition to consuming folate from a varied diet.

[j] It is assumed that women will continue consuming 400 µg from supplements or fortified food until their pregnancy is confirmed and they enter prenatal care, which ordinarily occurs after the end of the periconceptional period—the critical time for formation of the neural tube.

[k] The UL applies only to intake from supplements, fortified foods, and/or pharmacological agents and not to intake from foods.

[l] Because the absorption of iron from plant foods is low compared to that from animal foods, the RDA for strict vegetarians is approximately 1.8 times higher than the values established for omnivores (14 mg/day for adult male vegetarians; 33 mg/day for premenopausal female vegetarians). Oral contraceptives (OCs) reduce menstrual blood losses, so women taking them need less daily iron; the RDA for premenopausal women taking OCs is 10.9 mg/day. For more on iron requirements for other special situations, refer to *Dietary Reference Intakes for Vitamin A, Vitamin K, Arsenic, Boron, Chromium, Copper, Iodine, Iron, Manganese, Molybdenum, Nickel, Silicon, Vanadium, and Zinc* (visit http://www.nap.edu for the complete report).

[m] Zinc absorption is lower for those consuming vegetarian diets so the zinc requirement for vegetarians is approximately twofold greater than for those consuming a nonvegetarian diet.

TABLE 1

Dietary Reference Intakes (DRIs): Recommended Levels for Individual Intake (continued)

Life Stage	Group	Potassium (g/day)	Sodium (g/day)	Chloride (g/day)	Carbohydrate RDA/AI (g/day)	Carbohydrate AMDR[n] (%)	Total Fibre RDA/AI (g/day)	Total Fat AMDR[o] (%)	Linoleic Acid RDA/AI (g/day)	Linoleic Acid AMDR[o] (%)	Alpha-linolenic Acid RDA/AI (g/day)	Alpha-linolenic Acid AMDR[o] (%)	Protein[n] RDA/AI (g/day)	Protein AMDR[o] (%)	Water[p] (L/day)
Infants	0–6 months	0.4	0.12	0.18	60	ND[q]	ND	r	4.4	ND[q]	0.5	ND[q]	9.1	ND[q]	0.7
	7–12 months	0.7	0.37	0.57	95	ND[q]	ND	r	4.6	ND[q]	0.5	ND[q]	13.5	ND[q]	0.8
Children	1–3 years	3.0	1.0	1.5	130	45–65	19	30–40	7	5–10	0.7	0.6–1.2	13	5–20	1.3
	4–8 years	3.8	1.2	1.9	130	45–65	25	25–35	10	5–10	0.9	0.6–1.2	19	10–30	1.7
Males	9–13 years	4.5	1.5	2.3	130	45–65	31	25–35	12	5–10	1.2	0.6–1.2	34	10–30	2.4
	14–18 years	4.7	1.5	2.3	130	45–65	38	25–35	16	5–10	1.6	0.6–1.2	52	10–30	3.3
	19–30 years	4.7	1.5	2.3	130	45–65	38	20–35	17	5–10	1.6	0.6–1.2	56	10–35	3.7
	31–50 years	4.7	1.5	2.3	130	45–65	38	20–35	17	5–10	1.6	0.6–1.2	56	10–35	3.7
	51–70 years	4.7	1.3	2.0	130	45–65	30	20–35	14	5–10	1.6	0.6–1.2	56	10–35	3.7
	>70 years	4.7	1.2	1.8	130	45–65	30	20–35	14	5–10	1.6	0.6–1.2	56	10–35	3.7
Females	9–13 years	4.5	1.5	2.3	130	45–65	26	25–35	10	5–10	1.0	0.6–1.2	34	10–30	2.1
	14–18 years	4.7	1.5	2.3	130	45–65	26	25–35	11	5–10	1.1	0.6–1.2	46	10–30	2.3
	19–30 years	4.7	1.5	2.3	130	45–65	25	20–35	12	5–10	1.1	0.6–1.2	46	10–35	2.7
	31–50 years	4.7	1.5	2.3	130	45–65	25	20–35	12	5–10	1.1	0.6–1.2	46	10–35	2.7
	51–70 years	4.7	1.3	2.0	130	45–65	21	20–35	11	5–10	1.1	0.6–1.2	46	10–35	2.7
	>70 years	4.7	1.2	1.8	130	45–65	21	20–35	11	5–10	1.1	0.6–1.2	46	10–35	2.7
Pregnancy	≤18 years	4.7	1.5	2.3	175	45–65	28	20–35	13	5–10	1.4	0.6–1.2	71	10–35	3.0
	19–30 years	4.7	1.5	2.3	175	45–65	28	20–35	13	5–10	1.4	0.6–1.2	71	10–35	3.0
	31–50 years	4.7	1.5	2.3	175	45–65	28	20–35	13	5–10	1.4	0.6–1.2	71	10–35	3.0
Lactation	≤18 years	5.1	1.5	2.3	210	45–65	29	20–35	13	5–10	1.3	0.6–1.2	71	10–35	3.8
	19–30 years	5.1	1.5	2.3	210	45–65	29	20–35	13	5–10	1.3	0.6–1.2	71	10–35	3.8
	31–50 years	5.1	1.5	2.3	210	45–65	29	20–35	13	5–10	1.3	0.6–1.2	71	10–35	3.8
Tolerable Upper Intake Level for Adults (19–70)			2.3	3.6											

[n] Daily protein recommendations are based on body weight for reference body weights. To calculate for a specific body weight, use the following values: 1.5 g/kg for infants, 1.1 g/kg for 1–3 years, 0.95 g/kg for 4–13 years, 0.85 g/kg for 14–18 years, 0.8 g/kg for adults, and 1.1 g/kg for pregnant (using pre-pregnancy weight) and lactating women.

[o] Acceptable Macronutrient Distribution Range (AMDR), expressed as a percent of total daily calories, is the range of intake for a particular energy source that is associated with reduced risk of chronic disease while providing intakes of essential nutrients. If an individual consumes in excess of the AMDR, there is a potential for increasing the risk of chronic diseases and/or insufficient intakes of essential nutrients.

[p] Total water intake from fluids and food.

[q] Not determinable due to lack of data of adverse effects in this age group and concern with regard to lack of ability to handle excess amounts. Source of intake should be from food only to prevent high levels of intake.

[r] For infants, adequate Intake of total fat is 31 grams/day (0–6 months) and 30 grams per day (7–12 months) from breast milk and, for infants 7–12 months, complementary food and beverages.

* Reprinted with permission from *Dietary Reference Intakes Applications in Dietary Planning.* Copyright © 2004 by the National Academy of Sciences. Reprinted with permission from the National Academies Press, Washington, DC.

SOURCE: Food and Nutrition Board, Institute of Medicine, National Academies. 2004. Dietary Reference Intakes Tables. Washington, D.C.: National Academics Press. The complete Dietary Reference Intake reports are available from the National Academy Press (http://www.nap.edu).

Laboratory Activities

Name _____ Section _____ Date _____

Lab 7.1 Your Daily Diet versus the Food Guide

![McGraw Hill Education] connect

Keep a record of everything you eat for three consecutive days. Record all foods and beverages you consume, breaking each food item into its component parts (e.g.,, a turkey sandwich would be listed as two slices of bread, 100 grams of turkey, 1 tsp of mayonnaise, and so on) and list them separately in the column labelled "Food." Complete the first two columns of the chart during the course of the day; fill in the remaining information at the end of the day using Figure 7.3 and the *Canada's Food Guide* section of this chapter.

(Note: This lab can also be completed using nutritional analysis software or websites.)

DAY 1

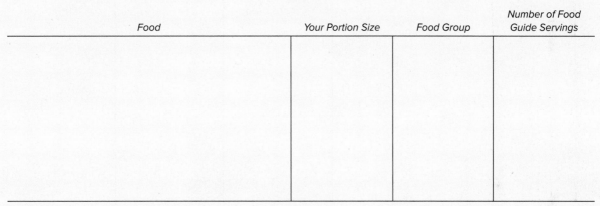

Food	Your Portion Size	Food Group	Number of Food Guide Servings

Daily Total

Food Group	Number of Servings
Milk, yogourt, cheese	
Meat, poultry, fish, dry beans, eggs, nuts	
Fruits	
Vegetables	
Breads, cereals, rice, pasta	
Water	
Other foods, e.g., soft drinks, unhealthy snacks	

* Your portion sizes may be smaller or larger than the serving sizes given in the Food Guide. List the actual number of Food Guide servings contained in the foods you eat.

DAY 2

Food	Your Portion Size	Food Group	Number of Food Guide Servings*

Daily Total

Food Group	Number of Servings
Milk, yogourt, cheese	
Meat, poultry, fish, dry beans, eggs, nuts	
Fruits	
Vegetables	
Breads, cereals, rice, pasta	
Water	
Other foods, e.g., soft drinks, unhealthy snacks	

* Your portion sizes may be smaller or larger than the serving sizes given in the Food Guide. List the actual number of Food Guide servings contained in the foods you eat.

DAY 3

Food	Your Portion Size	Food Group	Number of Food Guide Servings*

Daily Total

Food Group	Number of Servings
Milk, yogourt, cheese	
Meat, poultry, fish, dry beans, eggs, nuts	
Fruits	
Vegetables	
Breads, cereals, rice, pasta	
Water	
Other foods, e.g., soft drinks, unhealthy snacks	

* Your portion sizes may be smaller or larger than the serving sizes given in the Food Guide. List the actual number of Food Guide servings contained in the foods you eat.

Next, average your serving totals for the three days and enter them in the chart below. Fill in the recommended serving totals that apply to you from Figure 7.3.

Food Group	Recommended Number of Daily Servings	Actual (Average) Number of Daily Servings
Milk, yogourt, cheese		
Meat, poultry, fish, dry beans, eggs, nuts		
Fruits		
Vegetables		
Breads, cereals, rice, pasta		
Water		
Other foods, e.g., soft drinks, unhealthy snacks		

Using Your Results

How did you score? How close is your diet to that recommended by the Food Guide? Are you at all surprised by the actual number of servings you're consuming from each food group?

_____

_____

_____

What should you do next? If the results of the assessment indicate that you could boost your level of wellness by improving your diet, set realistic goals for change. Do you need to increase or decrease your consumption of any food groups? Be sure to use the information on portion sizes in this chapter. List any areas of concern below, along with a goal for change and strategies for achieving the goal you've set. If you see that you are falling short in one food group, such as fruits or vegetables, you might try increasing those servings by consuming an apple, a bunch of grapes, or some baby carrots. Think carefully about the reasons behind your food choices. For example, if you eat doughnuts for breakfast every morning because you feel rushed, make a list of ways to save time to allow for a healthier breakfast.

Problem:

_____

_____

Goal:

_____

Strategies for change:

_____

_____

Problem:

_____

_____

Goal:

_____

Strategies for change:

_____

_____

Problem:

_____

_____

Goal:

_____

Strategies for change:

_____

_____

Enter the results of this lab in the Preprogram Assessment column in Appendix B. If you've set goals and identified strategies for change, begin putting your plan into action. After several weeks of your program, complete this lab again and enter the results in the Postprogram Assessment column of Appendix B. How do the results compare?

_____

_____

_____

Name _____ Section _____ Date _____

Lab 7.2 Dietary Analysis

connect

You can complete this activity using either a nutrition analysis software program or the charts printed below. Information about the nutrient content of foods is also available online; see the For Further Exploration section for recommended websites. (This lab asks you to analyze one day's diet. For a more complete and accurate assessment of your diet, analyze the results from several different days, including a weekday and a weekend day.)

DATE _____   **DAY: M Tu W Th F Sa Su**

Food	Amount	Calories	Protein (g)	Carbohydrate (g)	Dietary fibre (g)	Fat, total (g)	Saturated fat (g)	Cholesterol (mg)	Sodium (mg)	Vitamin A (mg)	Vitamin C (mg)	Calcium (mg)	Iron (mg)
Recommended totals[a]			10–30%	45–65%	25–38 g	20–35%	≤10%	≤300 mg	≤2300 mg	RE	mg	mg	mg
Actual totals[b]		cal	g / %	g / %	g	g / %	g / %	mg	mg	RE	mg	mg	mg

[a] Fill in the appropriate DRI values for vitamin A, vitamin C, calcium, and iron from Table 1 in the Nutrition Resources section.

[b] Total the values in each column. To calculate the percentage of total calories from protein, carbohydrates, fat, and saturated fat, use the formulas from the Setting Intake Goals for Protein, Fat, and Carbohydrates box. Protein and carbohydrate provide 4 calories per gram; fat provides 9 calories per gram. For example, if you consume a total of 270 grams of carbohydrate and 2000 calories, your percentage of total calories from carbohydrate would be (270 g × 4 cal/g) ÷ 2000 cal = 54%. Do not include data for alcoholic beverages in your calculations. Percentages may not total 100% due to rounding.

Using Your Results

How did you score? How close is your diet to that recommended by the Dietary Reference Intakes, and other guidelines? Are you surprised by any of the results of this assessment?

_____

_____

_____

What should you do next? Enter the results of this lab in the Preprogram Assessment column in Appendix B. If your daily diet meets all the recommended intakes, congratulations—and keep up the good work. If the results of the assessment pinpoint areas of concern, then work with your food record on the previous page to determine what changes you could make to meet all the guidelines. Make changes, additions, and deletions until it conforms to all or most of the guidelines. Or, if you prefer, start from scratch to create a day's diet that meets the guidelines. Use the chart below to experiment and record your final, healthy sample diet for one day. Then put what you learned from this exercise into practice in your daily life. After several weeks of your program, complete this lab again and enter the results in the Postprogram Assessment column of Appendix B. How do the results compare?

_____

_____

_____

DATE _____   **DAY: M Tu W Th F Sa Su**

Food	Amount	Calories	Protein (g)	Carbohydrate (g)	Dietary fibre (g)	Fat, total (g)	Saturated fat (g)	Cholesterol (mg)	Sodium (mg)	Vitamin A (mg)	Vitamin C (mg)	Calcium (mg)	Iron (mg)
Recommended totals[a]			10–30%	45–65%	25–38 g	20–35%	≤10%	≤300 mg	≤2300 mg	RE	mg	mg	mg
Actual totals[b]		cal	g / %	g / %	g	g / %	g / %	mg	mg	RE	mg	mg	mg

Name _____   Section _____   Date _____

Lab 7.3 Informed Food Choices
Mc Graw Hill Education connect·

Part I Using Nutrition Labels

Choose three food items to evaluate. You might want to select three similar items, such as regular, low-fat, and nonfat salad dressing, or three very different items. Record the information from their nutrition labels in the table below.

Food Items			
Serving size			
Calories	cal	cal	cal
Total fat—grams	g	g	g
% Daily Value	%	%	%
Saturated fat—grams	g	g	g
% Daily Value	%	%	%
Trans fat—grams	g	g	g
Cholesterol—milligrams	mg	mg	mg
Sodium—milligrams	mg	mg	mg
% Daily Value	%	%	%
Carbohydrates (total)—grams	g	g	g
% Daily Value	%	%	%
Fibre—grams	g	g	g
% Daily Value	%	%	%
Sugars—grams	g	g	g
Protein—grams	g	g	g
Vitamin A—% Daily Value	%	%	%
Vitamin C—% Daily Value	%	%	%
Calcium—% Daily Value	%	%	%
Iron—% Daily Value	%	%	%

How do the items you chose compare? You can do a quick nutrient check by totalling the Daily Value percentages for nutrients you should limit (total fat, sodium) and the nutrients you should favour (fibre, vitamin A, vitamin C, calcium, iron) for each food. Which food has the largest percent Daily Value sum for nutrients to limit? For nutrients to favour?

_____
_____
_____

Food Items			
Calories	cal	cal	cal
% Daily Value total for nutrients to limit (total fat, sodium)	%	%	%
% Daily Value total for nutrients to favour (fibre, vitamin A, vitamin C, calcium, iron)	%	%	%

Part II Evaluating Fast Food

Use the information from the links in Appendix A, Nutritional Content of Popular Items from Fast-Food Restaurants, to complete the chart below for the last fast-food meal you ate. Add up your totals for the meal. Compare the values for fat, protein, carbohydrate, cholesterol, and sodium content for each food item and for the meal as a whole with the levels suggested by Health Canada and the Food and Nutrition Board. Calculate the percentage of total calories derived from fat, saturated fat, protein, and carbohydrates using the formulas given.

If you haven't recently been to one of the restaurants included in the appendix, fill in the chart for any sample meal you might eat from one of the restaurants listed.

Food Items

	AMDR							Total[b]
Serving size (g)		g	g	g	g	g	g	g
Calories		cal	cal	cal	cal	cal	cal	cal
Total fat—grams		g	g	g	g	g	g	g
% calories[a]	20–35%	%	%	%	%	%	%	%
Saturated fat—grams		g	g	g	g	g	g	g
% calories[a]	≤10%	%	%	%	%	%	%	%
Protein—grams		g	g	g	g	g	g	g
% calories[a]	10–30%	%	%	%	%	%	%	%
Carbohydrate—grams		g	g	g	g	g	g	g
% calories[a]	45–65%	%	%	%	%	%	%	%
Cholesterol[c]	100 mg	mg	mg	mg	mg	mg	mg	mg
Sodium[c]	800 mg	mg	mg	mg	mg	mg	mg	mg

[a] To calculate the percentage of total calories from each food energy source (fat, carbohydrate, protein), use the following formula:

$$\frac{\text{(number of grams of energy source)} \times \text{(number of calories per gram of energy source)}}{\text{(total calories in serving of food item)}}$$

(Note: Fat and saturated fat provide 9 calories per gram; protein and carbohydrate provide 4 calories per gram.) For example, the percentage of total calories from protein in a 150-calorie dish containing 10 grams of protein is

$$\frac{\text{(10 grams of protein)} \times \text{(4 calories per gram)}}{\text{(150 calories)}} = \frac{40}{510} = 0.27, \text{ or } 27\% \text{ of total calories from protein}$$

[b] For the Total column, add up the total grams of fat, carbohydrate, and protein contained in your sample meal and calculate the percentages based on the total calories in the meal. (Percentages may not total 100% due to rounding.) For cholesterol and sodium values, add up the total number of milligrams.

[c] Recommended daily limits of cholesterol and sodium are divided by 3 here to give an approximate recommended limit for a single meal.

Using Your Results

Consider your nutritional intake from fast food and compare it to your intake of a meal that was not fast food. What differences did you notice in the proportion of nutrients that came from each nutrient group?

_____

_____

_____

What changes do you need to make to your fast food intake to enhance your nutritional intake?

_____

_____

_____

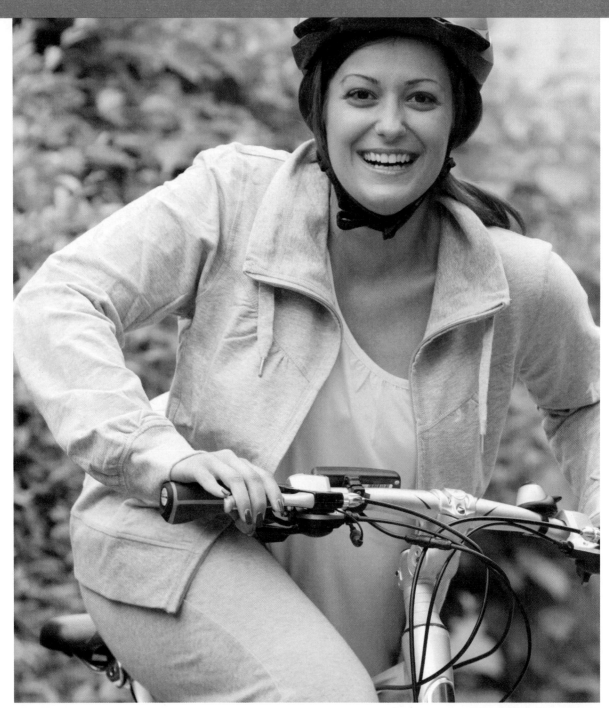

© altrendo images / Getty Images RF

CHAPTER 8

Weight Management

LEARNING OBJECTIVES

After reading this chapter, you should be able to

LO1 Explain the health risks associated with overweight and obesity

LO2 Explain the factors that may contribute to a weight problem, including genetic, physiological, lifestyle, and psychosocial factors

LO3 Describe lifestyle factors that contribute to weight gain and loss, including the role of diet, exercise, and emotional factors

LO4 Design a personal plan for successfully managing body weight

LO5 Identify and describe the symptoms of eating disorders and the health risks associated with them

TEST YOUR KNOWLEDGE

1. **About what percentage of Canadian adults are at an increased health risk due to excess weight?**
   a. 26%
   b. 36%
   c. 53%

2. **Approximately what percentage of those with eating disorders are women?**
   a. 50%
   b. 70%
   c. 90%

3. **The consumption of low-calorie sweeteners has helped Canadians control their weight.**

   True or false?

ANSWERS

1. **C.** About 53% of Canadian adults are overweight or obese, thus dramatically increasing their risk for health complications as a result of excess weight.

2. **C.** 90%. Health Canada reports that over 152 000 Canadian women suffer from either anorexia nervosa or bulimia, with many developing the disorder between the ages of 14 and 25.

3. **FALSE.** Since the introduction of low-calorie sweeteners, both total calorie intake and total sugar intake have increased, as has the proportion of Canadians who are overweight.

Achieving and maintaining a healthy body weight is a serious public health challenge in Canada and a source of distress for many people. The 2012 Canadian Community Health Survey reported that 34% of Canadians are considered overweight and about 2% are underweight. In addition, trends for the past 25 years suggest a 9% increase in the number of Canadian adults reported to be obese.[1] Canadian figures now mimic those of the United States in overall numbers of overweight adults. In terms of obese adults, there are fewer Canadian men (19%) and women (18%) who are obese compared to American men (34.6%) and women (35.9%).[2]

And while millions struggle to lose weight, some fall into dangerous eating patterns such as binge eating or self-starvation. Being overweight or obese is linked to serious health problems, such as heart disease and type 2 diabetes, and it is linked to rising health-care costs. It is not total weight but body composition—the proportion of fat to fat-free mass—that is critical for health (see Chapter 6). Most people who are overweight are also overfat (having more than a healthy amount of body fat), and the health risks they face are due to being overfat.

Although this chapter uses the common terms *weight management* and *weight loss*, the goal for wellness is to adopt healthy behaviours and achieve an appropriate body composition, not to conform to rigid standards of total body weight. A reasonable goal for body composition—body weight in relation to body shape—must take into account heredity, sex, weight history, social circumstances, metabolic rate, and psychological well-being. Adopting a wellness lifestyle that includes regular exercise and a healthy dietary pattern can help you achieve and maintain a healthy body weight and shape.

Managing body weight is not a mysterious process. The "secret" is balancing calories consumed with calories expended in daily activities—in other words, eating a moderate diet and using up that energy in regular physical activity and body processes.

As more and more people are becoming unhappy with their bodies (body image) and obsessed with their weight, a large number of people also seem to contradict what they believe and practise about their body image. Even as the Canadian National Obesity Survey reminded Canadians that those who are overweight and obese are twice as likely as healthy-weight Canadians to suffer from conditions such as high blood pressure and type 2 diabetes, 70% of respondents said they are satisfied with their weight. It is also slightly perplexing that overweight Canadians are as likely as healthy-weight Canadians to believe that being overweight might lead to a greater risk of suffering from these health conditions.[3] Dissatisfaction with body weight and shape may also be associated with dangerous eating patterns such as binge eating or self-starvation and with eating disorders.

This chapter explores the factors that contribute to the development of overweight and obesity, as well as eating disorders. It also takes a closer look at weight management through lifestyle and suggests specific strategies for reaching and maintaining a healthy weight.

LO1 8.1 Health Implications of Overweight and Obesity

As rates of overweight and obesity have risen in Canada, so has the prevalence associated health conditions—including a more than 33% rise in the rate of type 2 diabetes in just the past decade. It's estimated that inactivity and overweight account for more than 21 000 premature deaths annually in Canada,[4] and at least $4.6 billion per year is spent treating obesity-related health problems.[5] Overweight and obesity are two of the most serious and widespread challenges to wellness.

Defining Overweight and Obesity

As described in Chapter 6, overweight is usually defined as total body weight above the recommended range for good health, as determined by large-scale population surveys. Obesity is defined as a more serious degree of overweight that carries multiple health risks. Both terms are used to identify weight ranges that are associated with increased risk of certain diseases and health problems. When looking at body composition, the most important consideration is the proportion of the body's total weight that is fat—the percent body fat. For example, two men may both be 170 centimetres tall and weigh 170 pounds, but they may differ in percent body fat—one might have 12% body fat, and the other 22% body fat. In this case, only the second man would be considered overfat. Assessment methods based on body weight are less accurate than those based on body fat, but they are commonly used because body weight is easier to measure than body fat.

Body mass index (BMI) is a measure of body weight that is useful for estimating a person's weight status and for classifying the health risks of body weight if more sophisticated methods aren't available. BMI is often used in surveys and studies, and it is the basis for the population statistics presented in this chapter. BMI is a fairly accurate measure of the health risks of body weight for most average people; it is less accurate for muscular athletes, people under 5 feet tall, older adults with little muscle mass, and certain other groups. BMI is calculated by dividing your body weight (in kilograms) by the square of your height (in meters); an alternative equation based on pounds and inches is the following:

$$BMI = (weight \div [height \times height]) \times 703$$

(Space for calculations and a complete BMI chart appear in Labs 6.1 and 6.2.)

Waist measurement helps provide an assessment of body fat distribution; visceral fat, fat stored around the internal organs, is more harmful to health than subcutaneous fat, fat stored under the skin. For classifying your health risks, use the combination of BMI and waist measurement in Table 8.1, or complete one of the more sophisticated body composition assessment methods presented in Chapter 6.

TABLE 8.1

Body Mass Index, Waist Circumference, and Disease Risk.

Disease Risk* Relative to Normal Weight and Waist Circumference				
	BMI (kg/m²)	Obesity Class	Men: Waist 40 in (102 cm) or less Women: Waist 35 in (88 cm) or less	Men: Waist >40 in (102 cm) Women: Waist >35 in (88 cm)
Underweight	<18.5		–	–
Normal	18.5–24.9		–	–
Overweight	25.0–29.9		Increased	High
Obesity	30.0–34.9	I	High	Very High
	35.0–39.9	II	Very High	Very High
Extreme Obesity	40.0+	III	Extremely High	Extremely High

*Disease risk for type 2 diabetes, hypertension, and CVD.
Note: Increased waist circumference also can be a marker for increased risk, even in persons of normal weight.
SOURCE: National Heart, Lung, and Blood Institute. 1998. *Clinical Guidelines on the Identification, Evaluation, and Treatment of Overweight and Obesity in Adults: The Evidence Report. Bethesda,* Md.: National Institutes of Health.

Overweight, Obesity, and Specific Health Risks

Many studies have confirmed that obesity and—to a lesser extent—overweight shorten lives. Obesity is one of six major controllable risk factors for heart disease, and it also increases the risk for other forms of cardiovascular disease (CVD), hypertension, certain forms of cancer, gallbladder disease, respiratory problems, joint diseases, skin problems, impaired immune function, and sleep disorders. Obesity is strongly linked to the development of insulin resistance and type 2 diabetes; nearly 90% of people with type 2 diabetes are overweight when diagnosed.

Gaining weight over the years has also been found to be dangerous. A recent study found that women who gained more than 10 kilograms since they were 18 years old had a sevenfold increase in the risk of heart disease. Gaining weight, especially as a young adult, is also strongly linked to risk for type 2 diabetes.

Is obesity itself a disease? The 2015 decision by the Canadian Medical Association to declare obesity a chronic medical disease has benefits as well as disadvantages. Health care providers must now exert greater focus on the problem, which may help more people lose more weight. On the other hand, as we have discussed, the measurement of obesity must be carried out with a low degree of error to ensure that the diagnosis is correct.

Can Someone Be Overfat and Fit?

The general answer is yes. Recent research at the Cooper Institute in the United States indicates that those who are fit (based on cardiovascular testing) have a lower mortality risk than those who are unfit, even if they are overweight or obese. While it is important to focus some attention on increasing obesity rates, many suggest that we then neglect the benefits of exercise and fitness. As a rule, lower body fat levels are preferred, but it is possible to have higher, and in some cases overfat or obese levels of fat, and still be considered fit.

Benefits of Weight Loss

Even modest weight loss can have a significant positive impact on health. Modest weight loss improves blood levels of good cholesterol (HDL), triglycerides, and glucose, as well as blood pressure. A weight loss of just 5–10% in obese individuals can reduce the risk of weight-related health conditions and increase life expectancy.

LO2 8.2 Factors Contributing to Excess Body Fat

Several factors determine body weight and composition. These factors can be grouped into genetic, physiological, lifestyle, and psychosocial factors.

Genetic Factors

Estimates of the genetic contribution to obesity vary widely, from about 25–40% of an individual's body fat. More than 600 genes have been linked to obesity, but their actions are still under study. Genes can influence body size and shape, body fat distribution, and metabolic rate. Genetic factors may also affect the ease with which weight is gained as a result of overeating and where on the body extra weight is added.

If both parents are overweight, their children have an 80% risk of being obese; children with one obese parent face a 40% risk of becoming obese.[6] In studies that compared adoptees and their biological parents, the weights of the adoptees were found to be more like those of the biological parents than the adoptive parents, again indicating a strong genetic link.

Hereditary influences, however, must be balanced against the contribution of environmental factors. Not all children of obese parents become obese, and normal-weight parents can have overweight children. Environmental factors like diet and exercise are probably responsible for such differences. Thus, the tendency to develop obesity may be inherited, but the expression of this tendency is affected by environmental influences.

Physiological Factors

Metabolism is a key physiological factor in the regulation of body fat and body weight, and hormones also play a role. A few other physiological factors have been proposed as causes for weight gain, such as carbohydrate craving due to low levels of the neurotransmitter serotonin, but research on this and other theories has so far been inconclusive.

Metabolism and Energy Balance

Metabolism is the sum of all the vital processes by which food energy and nutrients are made available to and used by the body. The largest component of metabolism, **resting metabolic rate (RMR)**, is the energy required to maintain vital body functions, including respiration, heart rate, body temperature, and blood pressure, while the body is at rest. As shown in Figure 8.1, RMR accounts for 65–70% of daily energy expenditure. The energy required to digest food accounts for an additional ±10% of daily energy expenditure. The remaining 20–30% is expended during physical activity.

resting metabolic rate (RMR)   The energy required (in calories) to maintain vital body functions, including respiration, heart rate, body temperature, and blood pressure, while the body is at rest.

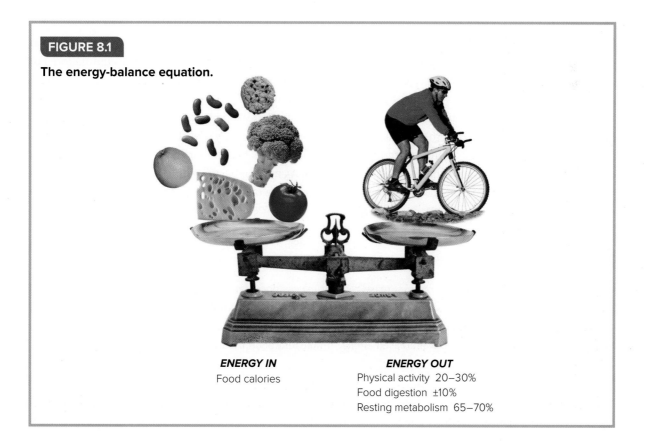

FIGURE 8.1

The energy-balance equation.

ENERGY IN
Food calories

ENERGY OUT
Physical activity 20–30%
Food digestion ±10%
Resting metabolism 65–70%

Both heredity and behaviour affect metabolic rate. Men, who have a higher proportion of muscle mass than women, have a higher RMR since muscle tissue is more metabolically active than fat. In addition, some individuals inherit a higher or lower RMR than others. A higher RMR means that a person burns more calories while at rest and can therefore take in more calories without gaining weight.

Weight loss or gain also affects metabolic rate. When a person loses weight, both RMR and the energy required to perform physical tasks decrease; the reverse occurs when weight is gained. One of the reasons exercise is so important during a weight-loss program is that exercise, especially resistance training, helps maintain muscle mass and metabolic rate.

Exercise has a positive effect on metabolism. When people exercise, they slightly increase their RMR, the number of calories their bodies burn at rest. In fact, a 2011 study of college-age men showed that following 45 minutes of vigorous exercise, the participants' resting metabolic rate remained elevated for 14 hours—during which the men burned an additional 200 calories while at rest or performing normal, everyday activities. People who regularly exercise increase their muscle mass, which is associated with a higher metabolic rate. The exercise itself also burns calories, raising total energy expenditure; the higher the energy expenditure, the more the person can eat without gaining weight.

The energy-balance equation is the key to weight management. If you burn the same amount of energy as you take in (a *neutral* [isocaloric] energy balance), your weight remains constant. If you consume more calories than you expend (a *positive* energy balance), your weight increases. If you burn more calories than you consume (a *negative* energy balance), your weight decreases.

To create a negative energy balance and lose weight and body fat, you can increase the amount of energy you burn by increasing your level of physical activity and/or decrease the amount of energy you take in by consuming fewer calories.

Hormones

Hormones clearly play a role in the accumulation of body fat, especially for females. Hormonal changes at puberty, during pregnancy, and at menopause contribute to the amount and location of fat accumulation. For example, during puberty, hormones cause the development of secondary sex characteristics, including larger breasts, wider hips, and a fat layer under the skin. This addition of body fat at puberty is normal and healthy.

One hormone thought to be linked to obesity is *leptin.* Secreted by the body's fat cells, leptin is carried to the brain, where it appears to let the brain know how big or small the body's fat stores are. With this information, the brain can regulate appetite and metabolic rate accordingly. Researchers hope to use these hormones to develop treatments for obesity based on appetite control. As most of us will admit, however, hunger is often not the primary reason we overeat. Cases of obesity based solely or primarily on hormone abnormalities do exist, but they are rare.

LO3 Lifestyle Factors

Genetic and physiological factors may increase risk for excess body fat, but they are not sufficient to explain the increasingly high rate of obesity seen in Canada. The gene pool has not changed dramatically in the past 40 years, but the rate of obesity among Canadians has nearly tripled. Clearly, other factors are at work—particularly lifestyle factors such as increased energy intake and decreased physical activity.

Eating

North Americans generally have access to an abundance of highly palatable and calorie-dense foods, and many have eating habits that contribute to weight gain. Most overweight adults will admit to eating more than they should of high-fat, high-sugar, high-calorie foods. People eat out more frequently now than in the past, and we rely more heavily on fast food and packaged convenience foods. Restaurant and convenience food portion sizes tend to be very large, and the foods themselves are more likely to be high in fat, sugar, and calories and low in nutrients. The Neilsen Company reported that 24% of Canadians eat at a restaurant once or twice a week, 9% eat out three to six times a week, and 2% report they eat out every day. Interestingly, Canadians report the largest percentage of consumers in the world who choose breakfast as the meal they usually eat out. Studies of adults have also found that the more people eat out, the more calories they consume, especially when they choose a fast-food restaurant.[7]

Research has also consistently found that people underestimate portion sizes (i.e., believing they are smaller than they actually are) by as much as 25%. When participants in one study were asked to report their food intake over the previous 24 hours, the majority underestimated their intake by about 600 calories.

According to the Dietitians of Canada, the average calorie intake by Canadians has increased by over 400 calories per day since 1991. Coupled with a decline in the levels of physical activity, the net result has been a substantial increase in the number of Canadians who are overweight. Even small increases in energy intake make a difference. For example, 150 additional calories per day, the number of calories in one can of pop or beer, can translate into a 7-kilogram weight gain in one year (7700 calories corresponds to 1 kilogram of body fat).

Compared to 1991, Canadians today consume significantly more carbohydrates (about 50 more grams per day), a lot more fat, and about the same amount of protein. The additional carbohydrate calories do not come from the fruits, vegetables, and whole grains recommended by health experts, but rather from salty snacks, soft drinks, pizza, and sweet desserts. Other factors contributing to increased calorie intake include increased portion sizes and consumption of more high-calorie meals away from home.

Physical Activity

Activity levels among Canadians are declining, beginning in childhood and continuing throughout life. Many schools have cut back on physical education classes and even recess. Most adults drive to work, sit all day, and then relax in front of the TV (or continue working) at night. Internet use has fast become the "new" TV, while other modern conveniences such as remote controls, elevators, and power mowers have also reduced daily physical activity. This increase in sedentary lifestyles can also lead to an increased risk for obesity. In fact, the Canadian Community Health Survey (CCHS) reported that 27% of sedentary men were obese, compared with only 20% of active men.[8]

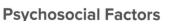

Wellness Tip

Looking for an easy way to cut calories? Cut down on soft drinks or beer. A 355 mL can of regular pop or beer contains about 150 calories. Reduce your consumption by just one can a day, and you can lose about 7 kilograms in a year!

Psychosocial Factors

Many people have learned to use food as a means of coping with stress and negative emotions. Eating can provide a powerful distraction from difficult feelings such as loneliness, anger, boredom, anxiety, shame, sadness, or inadequacy. It can also be used to combat low moods, low energy levels, and low self-esteem. When eating becomes the primary means of regulating emotions, **binge eating** or other unhealthy eating patterns can develop.

binge eating   A pattern of eating in which normal food consumption is interrupted by episodes of high consumption.

Obesity is strongly associated with socioeconomic status. The CCHS found that more women tend to be obese at lower income levels, while more men are obese at higher income levels.[9] These differences may reflect the greater sensitivity and concern for a slim physical appearance among upper-income women, as well as greater access to information about nutrition and to low-fat and low-calorie foods. It may also reflect the greater acceptance of obesity among certain ethnic groups, in addition to different cultural values related to food choices.

In some families and cultures, food is used as a symbol of love and caring. It is an integral part of social gatherings and celebrations. In such cases, it may be difficult to change established eating patterns because they are linked to cultural and family values.

Strengthening Mental Wellness

Is anyone in your family overweight? If so, can you identify factors that may contribute to this weight problem, such as heredity, eating patterns, or psychosocial factors? Has the person tried to address the problem? How is the issue handled in your family? How do family members help the situation or make it worse?

LO4 8.3 Adopting a Healthy Lifestyle for Successful Weight Management

When all the research has been assessed, it is clear that most weight problems are lifestyle problems. Even though more and more young people are developing weight problems, most arrive at early adulthood with the advantage of having a normal body weight—neither too fat nor too thin. In fact, many young adults get away with very poor eating and exercise habits and don't develop a weight problem. But as the rapid growth of adolescence slows and family and career obligations increase, maintaining a healthy weight becomes a greater challenge. Slow weight gain is a major cause of overweight and obesity, so weight management is important for everyone, not just for people who are currently overweight. A good time to develop a lifestyle for successful weight management is during early adulthood, when healthy behaviour patterns have a better chance of taking hold.

Permanent weight loss is not something you start and stop. You need to adopt healthy behaviours that you can maintain throughout your life, including eating habits, physical activity and exercise, an ability to think positively and manage your emotions effectively, and the coping strategies you use to deal with the stresses and challenges in your life.

Diet and Eating Habits

In contrast to dieting, which involves some form of food restriction, the term *diet* refers to your daily food choices. Everyone has a diet, but not everyone is dieting. It is important to develop a diet that you enjoy and that enables you to maintain a healthy body composition.

Use Canada's Food Guide as the basis for planning a healthy diet (see Chapter 7) and choose the healthiest options within each food group. For weight management, you may need to pay special attention to total calories, portion sizes, energy density, fat and carbohydrate intake, and eating habits.

Total Calories

Canada's Food Guide suggests we choose foods from the food groups that will permit us to consume between 1600 calories (for many smaller, sedentary women and some older adults) and 2800 calories (for teenage boys, many active men, and some very active women) a day. However, the precise number of calories needed to maintain weight will vary from individual to individual based on heredity, fitness status, level of physical activity, and other factors. Focus more on individual energy balance than on a general recommendation for daily calorie intake. To calculate your approximate daily caloric needs, complete the calculations in Lab 8.1.

The best approach for weight loss is combining an increase in physical activity with moderate calorie restriction (see the box Is Any Diet Best for Weight Loss? on the next page). Don't go on a crash diet. You need to eat and drink enough to meet your need for essential nutrients. To maintain weight loss you will probably have to maintain some degree of the calorie restriction you used to lose the weight, so it is important that you adopt a level of food intake that you can live with over the long term. For most people, maintaining weight loss is more difficult than losing the weight in the first place. To identify weight-loss goals and ways to meet them, complete Lab 8.2.

Portion Sizes

Overconsumption of total calories is closely tied to portion sizes. Many Canadians are unaware that the portion sizes of packaged foods and of foods served at restaurants have increased in size, and most of us significantly underestimate the amount of food we eat. In fact, one study found that the larger the meal, the greater the underestimation of calories.[10] Limiting portion sizes to those recommended in the Food Guide is critical for weight management. For many people, concentrating on portion sizes is easier than counting calories. (See Chapter 7 for more information and hints on choosing appropriate portion sizes.)

Energy (Calorie) Density

Experts recommend that you pay attention to *energy density*—the number of calories per gram or ounce of weight in a food. Studies suggest that it isn't consumption of a certain amount of fat or calories in food that reduces hunger and leads to feelings of fullness and satisfaction, but rather it is consumption of a certain weight of food. Foods that are low in energy density have more volume and bulk—that is, they are relatively heavy but have few calories (Table 8.2). For example, for the same 100 calories, you could eat 20 baby

TABLE 8.2

Examples of Foods Low in Energy Density

Food	Amount	Calories
Carrot, raw	1 medium	25
Popcorn, air popped	2 cups	62
Apple	1 medium	72
Vegetable soup	1 cup	72
Plain instant oatmeal	½ cup	80
Fresh blueberries	1 cup	80
Corn on the cob (plain)	1 ear	80
Cantaloupe	½ melon	95
Light (fat-free) yogourt with fruit	170 mL	100
Unsweetened apple sauce	1 cup	100
Pear	1 medium	100
Corn flakes	1 cup	101
Sweet potato, baked	1 medium	120

Critical CONSUMER

IS ANY DIET BEST FOR WEIGHT LOSS?

Many popular weight-loss plans promote specific food choices and macronutrient combinations. Research findings have been mixed, but two points are clear: Total calorie intake matters, and the best diet is probably the one you can stick with.

Low-Carbohydrate Diets

Some low-carb diets advocate fewer than 10% of total calories from carbohydrates, compared to the 45–65% recommended by Health Canada. Some suggest a daily carbohydrate intake below the 130 grams needed to provide essential carbohydrates in the diet. Low-carb diets that advocate switching to complex carbohydrates are better for you than the more extreme versions, which may eliminate cereals or grains.

Low-Fat Diets

Many experts advocate diets that are relatively low in fat, high in carbohydrates, and moderate in protein. If you try a low-fat, high-carb diet, you still need to pay attention to the quality of the carbohydrates you consume, focusing on whole grains and your total calorie intake. A low-fat diet is not a licence to consume excess calories, even in low-fat foods.

High-Protein Diets

High-protein diets advocate high protein intake, moderate fat, and low carbohydrate intake. These diets can be low in fibre, whole grains, vegetables, and fruits, so they may lack some essential nutrients. Diets high in protein and saturated fat have been linked to an increased risk of heart disease, high blood pressure, and cancer. One study found that following a diet with a normal protein-to-carbohydrate ratio (1 gram of protein to 2 grams of carbohydrate) promoted more improvements in body fat, waist circumference, and waist-to-hip ratio than following either a low-protein diet (1 gram of protein to 4 grams of carbohydrate) or a high-protein diet (1 gram of protein to 1 gram of carbohydrate). A normal protein-to-carbohydrate ratio is probably superior in reducing long-term chronic disease risk.

How Do Popular Diets Measure Up?

A study comparing weight loss among adults assigned to one of four reduced-calorie diets differing in percentages of protein, carbohydrate, and fat found that weight loss at two years was similar for all four diets (about 4 kilograms). Weight loss was strongly associated with attendance at group sessions. Other studies have also found little difference in weight loss among popular reduced-calorie diets; most resulted in modest weight loss and reduced heart disease risk factors. The more closely people adhered to each diet, the more weight they lost.

Energy Balance Counts: Healthy Living Unit—Public Health Agency of Canada

Future research may determine that certain macronutrient patterns are somewhat more helpful for disease reduction in people with particular risk profiles. In terms of weight loss, however, such differences among diets are likely overshadowed by the importance of total calorie intake and physical activity. Important lessons about energy balance can be drawn from the Public Health Agency of Canada's Healthy Living Unit (https://www.canada.ca/en/public-health/services/health-promotion/healthy-living/healthy-living-unit.html). Here you can learn about ways to manage your energy balance through the development of proper eating habits and the incorporation of physical activity into your daily routine.

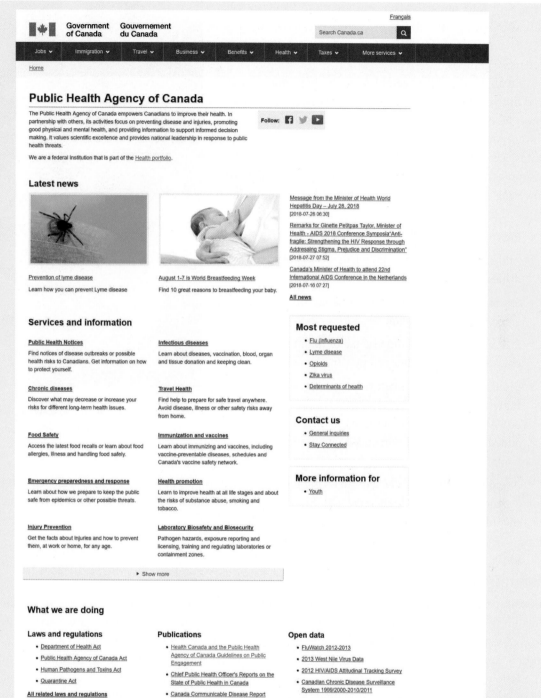

SOURCES: Naude, C. E., et al. 2014. Low carbohydrate versus isoenergetic balanced diets for reducing weight and cardiovascular risk: A systemic review and meta-analysis. *PLoS One* 9(7): e100652; Papadaki, A., et al. 2013. Impact of weight loss and maintenance with ad libitum diets varying in protein and glycemic index content on metabolic syndrome. *Nutrition* 30(4): 410–417; Campbell, D. D., and K. A. Meckling. January 2012. Effect of the protein:carbohydrate ratio in hypoenergetic diets on metabolic syndrome risk factors in exercising overweight and obese women. *British Journal of Nutrition* 16: 1–14; Sacks, F. M., et al. 2009. Comparison of weight loss diets with different compositions of fat, protein, and carbohydrates. *The New England Journal of Medicine* 360: 859–873.

carrots or four pretzel twists; you are more likely to feel full after eating the serving of carrots because it weighs 10 times that of the serving of pretzels (about 300 grams versus 30 grams).

Fresh fruits and vegetables, with their high water and fibre content, are low in energy density, as are whole-grain foods. Fresh fruits contain fewer calories and more fibre than fruit juices or drinks. Meat, ice cream, potato chips, croissants, crackers, and cakes and cookies are examples of foods high in energy density. Strategies for lowering the energy density of your diet include the following:

* Eat fruit with breakfast and for dessert.
* Add extra vegetables to sandwiches, casseroles, stir-fry dishes, pizza, pasta dishes, and fajitas.
* Start meals with a bowl of broth-based soup; include a green salad or fruit salad.
* Snack on fresh fruits and vegetables rather than crackers, chips, or other energy-dense snack foods.
* Limit serving sizes of energy-dense foods such as butter, mayonnaise, cheese, chocolate, fatty meats, croissants, and snack foods that are fried or high in added sugars (including reduced-fat products), or that contain trans fat.

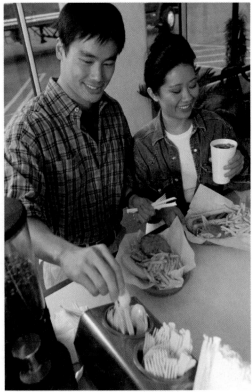

© Photodisc / Alamy

When fast food is the only available option, it can be difficult to make healthy lifestyle changes.

* Avoid processed foods, which can be high in fat and sodium. Even processed foods labelled "fat-free" or "reduced fat" may be high in calories. Such products may contain sugar and fat substitutes, which often include as many calories as the nutrients they replace.

Eating Habits

Equally important to weight management is eating small, frequent meals—four or five meals per day including breakfast and snacks—on a regular schedule. Skipping meals leads to excessive hunger; feelings of deprivation, and increased vulnerability to binge eating or snacking. Establish a regular pattern of eating, and set some rules governing food choices. Rules governing breakfast, for example, might include the following: Choose a sugar-free, high-fibre cereal with nonfat milk and fruit most of the time; have a hard-boiled egg no more than three times a week; and save pancakes or waffles for special occasions. For effective weight management, it is better to consume the majority of calories during the day rather than in the evening.

Decreeing some foods off-limits generally sets up a rule to be broken. The better principle is "everything in moderation." No foods need to be entirely off-limits, though some should be eaten judiciously. (See the box Supplementing your Intake for information on using supplements.)

In FOCUS

SUPPLEMENTING YOUR INTAKE

Eating healthy and maintaining a healthy lifestyle can be a challenging prospect given our busy lives. In an effort to help, Canadians often turn to supplements to get enough essential nutrients, to maintain or improve their health, or to aid in their body's ability to train.

Nutritional Supplements

Statistics Canada reports that almost 50% of Canadians use at least one nutritional supplement. Vitamin D, multivitamins, and Omega-3 fatty acids are the most common nutritional supplements used by Canadians in an effort to ensure they are maintaining a healthy lifestyle.

Vitamin D is an important supplement in bone density and is more commonly used by Canadians as they age. Older Canadians (70 years of age and older) are the largest consumers of Vitamin D.

Multivitamins contain three or more vitamins and may include minerals. They are the most commonly used nutritional supplement by Canadians. Omega-3 fatty acids contribute to visual and neural development and because they cannot be produced by the body, we must consume them as supplements.

Be sure to check the section Should You Take Supplements in Chapter 7 before starting a nutritional supplement regime.

WORKOUT SUPPLEMENTS

Many Canadians also consider the use of Natural Health Products to increase muscle mass, speed recovery from training, overcome fatigue, or to aid weight control. These substances are controlled by Canada's Department of Justice's Natural Health Products Regulations (http://laws-lois.justice.gc.ca/eng/regulations/SOR-2003-196/). Before using workout supplements, be sure to check the list of products that have received a license for use in Canada.

8.4 Physical Activity and Exercise

Making significant cuts in food intake in order to lose weight is a difficult strategy to maintain; increasing your physical activity is a much better strategy. Physical activity and exercise burn calories and keep the metabolism geared to using food for energy instead of storing it as fat. Regular physical activity also protects against weight gain and is essential for maintaining weight loss.

Physical Activity

All physical activity will help you manage your weight. The first step in becoming more active is to incorporate more physical activity into your daily life. If you are currently sedentary, follow the recommendations of Health Canada by accumulating short bouts of moderate-intensity physical activity—walking, gardening, doing housework, and so on—or 75 minutes of vigorous-intensity physical activity—e.g., jogging, aerobics—or a combination of the two for a total of 150 minutes or more every week. Even a small increase in activity level can help maintain your current weight or help you lose a moderate amount of weight (see Table 8.3 on the next page). In fact, research suggests that fidgeting—stretching, squirming, standing

TABLE 8.3

Calorie Costs of Selected Physical Activities*

To determine how many calories you burn when you engage in a particular activity, multiply the calorie multiplier given below by your body weight (in pounds) and then by the number of minutes you exercise.

Activity	Cal/lb/min	×	Body Weight	×	Min	=	Total Calories
Cycling (21 km/h)	.071		_____		_____		_____
Dancing (popular)	.049		_____		_____		_____
Digging	.062		_____		_____		_____
Driving a car	.020		_____		_____		_____
Housework	.029		_____		_____		_____
Painting a house	.034		_____		_____		_____
Shovelling snow	.052		_____		_____		_____
Sitting quietly	.009		_____		_____		_____
Sleeping and resting	.008		_____		_____		_____
Standing quietly	.012		_____		_____		_____
Typing or writing	.013		_____		_____		_____
Walking briskly (7 km/h)	.048		_____		_____		_____

*See Chapter 9 for the energy costs of fitness activities.

SOURCE: Adapted from Kusinitz, I. and M. Fine. 1995. *Your Guide to Getting Fit,* 3d ed. Mountain View, Calif.: Mayfield.

up, and so on—may help prevent weight gain in some people. Short bouts of activity (no less than 10 minutes each) spread throughout the day can produce many of the same health benefits as continuous physical activity.

If you are overweight and want to lose weight, or if you are trying to maintain a lower weight following weight loss, a greater amount of physical activity can help. Researchers have found that people who lose weight and don't regain it typically burn about 2800 calories per week in physical activity—the equivalent of about one hour of brisk walking per day.

Fitness Tip

When you watch TV, turn commercial breaks into exercise breaks. When commercials come on, get off the couch and move: Do jumping jacks, push-ups, curl-ups, run in place, or just walk around. During a two-hour program, you can accumulate about 30 minutes of physical activity!

Exercise

After you become more active every day, begin a formal exercise program that includes cardiorespiratory endurance exercise, resistance training, and stretching exercises. (See the box What Is the Best Way to Exercise for Weight Loss?.) Moderate-intensity endurance exercise, if performed frequently for a relatively long duration, can burn a significant number of calories. Endurance training also increases the rate at which your body uses calories after your exercise session is over—burning an additional 5 to 180 extra calories, depending on the intensity of exercise. Resistance training builds muscle mass, and more muscle translates into a higher metabolic rate. Resistance training can also help you maintain your muscle mass during a period of weight loss, helping you avoid the significant drop in RMR associated with weight loss.

The Evidence *for* EXERCISE

WHAT IS THE BEST WAY TO EXERCISE FOR WEIGHT LOSS?

If weight loss is your primary goal, the guidelines for planning a fitness program can vary depending on your weight, body composition, and current level of fitness. For example, there is some dispute among fitness experts about the best target heart rate (THR) zone to use when exercising for weight loss. Some experts recommend exercising at a moderate THR (55–69% of maximum heart rate) because the body burns fat at a slightly more efficient rate at this level of exertion. Others recommend exercising vigorously (70–90% of maximum heart rate) because exercise at this intensity burns more calories overall. According to some estimates, for example, a 30-minute workout at 80–85% of maximum heart rate burns about 30% more calories overall than a 30-minute workout at 60–65% maximum heart rate—but the lower-intensity workout burns roughly 20% more fat calories than the higher-intensity workout.

Regardless, if you are obese or your fitness level is very low, start with a lower-intensity workout (55% of maximum heart rate) and stick with it until your cardiorespiratory fitness level improves enough to support short bouts of higher-intensity exercise. This way, you will burn more fat, reduce the risk of injury and strain on your heart, and improve your chances of staying with your program. Even if your primary goal is to lose weight, you are also improving your cardiorespiratory fitness. Any amount of exercise, even at low to moderate intensity, will help you achieve both goals. But patience is required, especially if you need to lose a great deal of weight.

For weight loss to occur, exercise at lower intensities has to be offset by longer and/or more frequent exercise sessions. About 60 to 90 minutes of daily exercise is recommended for anyone who needs to lose weight or maintain weight loss. If you cannot fit such a large block of activity into your daily schedule, break your workouts into short segments—as little as 10 to 15 minutes each. This approach is probably best for someone who has been sedentary because it allows the body to become accustomed to exercise at a gradual pace while preventing injury and avoiding strain on the heart.

Many research studies have shown that walking is an ideal form of exercise for losing weight and avoiding weight gain. A landmark 15-year study by the University of North Carolina at Charlotte showed that, over time, people who did not walk gained 8 kilograms more than people who walked just 30 minutes per day. Those who regularly walked farther were better able to lose or maintain weight. Other studies have found that people who walked 30 minutes five times per week lost an average of 2.25 kilograms in 6

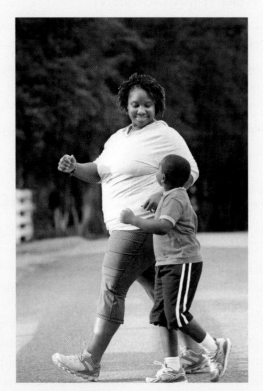

© Ariel Skelley / Getty Images

continued

to 12 months, without dieting, watching what they ate, or exercising intensely. You can lose even more weight if you eat sensibly and walk farther and faster.

A 75-kilogram (165-pound) adult who walks at a speed of 5 kilometres per hour for 60 minutes a day, five days a week, can lose about one-quarter kilogram of body weight per week. Regular walking is the simplest and most effective health habit for controlling body weight and promoting health. Even if you're sedentary, a few months of walking can increase your fitness level to the point where more vigorous types of exercise—and even greater health benefits—are possible.

SOURCES: Gordon-Larsen, P., et al. 2009. Fifteen-year longitudinal trends in walking patterns and their impact on weight change. *American Journal of Clinical Nutrition* 89(1): 19–26; Levine, J.A., et al. 2008. The role of free-living daily walking in human weight gain and obesity. *Diabetes* 57(3): 548–554; Nelson, M.E., and S.C. Folta. 2009. Further evidence for the benefits of walking. *American Journal of Clinical Nutrition* 89(1): 15–16; Physical Activity Guidelines Advisory Committee. 2008. *Physical Activity Guidelines Advisory Committee Report, 2008.* Washington, DC: U.S. Department of Health and Human Services.

Regular physical activity, maintained throughout life, makes weight management easier. The sooner you establish good habits, the better. The key to success is making exercise an integral part of a lifestyle you can enjoy now and will enjoy in the future.

CAREER OPTIONS FOR...

WEIGHT MANAGEMENT

Community: weight loss consultant, lifestyle coach, provincial sport or active living organization, physical activity journalist

Recreation and Leisure: commercial recreation (e.g., hotel, cruise ship, or workplace recreation), youth program manager (e.g., YMCA/YWCA, Boys and Girls Clubs), provincial and federal government (e.g., tourism promotion or national/territorial park employee)

SOURCE: Physical and Health Education Canada (http://www.phecanada.ca).

8.5 Thoughts and Emotions

The way you think about yourself and your world influences, and is influenced by, how you feel and how you act. In fact, research on people who have a weight problem indicates that low self-esteem and the negative emotions that accompany it are significant problems. People with low self-esteem mentally compare the actual self to an internally held picture of the "ideal self," an image based on perfectionist goals and beliefs about how they and others should be. The more these two pictures differ, the larger the impact on self-esteem and the more likely the presence of negative emotions.

Besides the internal picture we carry of ourselves, all of us carry on an internal dialogue about events happening to us and around us. This *self-talk* can be either deprecating or positively motivating, depending on our beliefs and attitudes. Having realistic beliefs and goals and engaging in positive self-talk and problem solving support a healthy lifestyle. (Chapter 12 and Activity 11 in the Behaviour Change Workbook include strategies for developing realistic self-talk.)

Coping Strategies

Appropriate coping strategies help you deal with the stresses of life; they are also an important lifestyle factor in weight management. Many people use eating as a way to cope, while others may use drugs, alcohol, smoking, or gambling. Those who overeat might use food to alleviate loneliness or fatigue, as an antidote to boredom, or as a distraction from problems. Some people even overeat to punish themselves for real or imagined transgressions.

Those who recognize that they are misusing food in such ways can analyze their eating habits with fresh eyes. They can consciously attempt to find new coping strategies and begin to use food appropriately—to fuel life's activities, to foster growth, and to bring pleasure, but *not* to manage stress. For a summary of the components of weight management through healthy lifestyle choices, see the box Lifestyle Strategies for Successful Weight Management.

Take CHARGE

LIFESTYLE STRATEGIES FOR SUCCESSFUL WEIGHT MANAGEMENT

Food Choices

- Focus on making good choices from each food group.
- Choose foods with a *low energy (calorie) density* and a *high nutrient density*
- Check labels for serving sizes, calories, and nutrients. (See Chapter 8 for more on food labelling.)
- Watch for hidden calories. Reduced-fat foods often have as many calories as their full-fat versions.
- Drink fewer calories in the form of soft drinks, fruit drinks, sports drinks, alcohol, and speciality coffees and teas. Water and nonfat or low-fat milk are good beverage choices.

Planning and Serving

- Keep a log of what you eat, as described earlier in the text.
- Eat four to five meals/snacks daily, *including breakfast,* to distribute calories throughout your day.
- Fix more meals yourself and eat out less often.
- Keep low-calorie snacks on hand to combat the "munchies." Fresh fruits and vegetables are good choices.
- When shopping, make a list and stick to it. Don't shop when you're hungry. Avoid aisles that contain problem foods.
- Consume the majority of your daily calories during the day, not in the evening.
- Pay attention to portion sizes. Use measuring cups and spoons and a food scale to become familiar with portion sizes.
- Serve meals on small plates and in small bowls to help you eat smaller portions without feeling deprived. (Research has shown that using a larger plate makes food portions appear smaller, so people serve themselves more food and overeat.)
- Eat only in specifically designated spots. Remove food from other areas of your home.
- When you eat, just eat. Don't do anything else.
- Avoid late-night eating, a behaviour specifically associated with weight gain among college and university students.
- Eat slowly. It takes time for your brain to get the message that your stomach is full. Take small bites and chew food thoroughly. Pay attention to every bite, and enjoy your food.

Special Occasions

- When you eat out, choose a restaurant where you can make healthy food choices.
- Ask the server not to put bread and butter on the table before the meal, and request that sauces and salad dressings be served on the side.

continued

- If portion sizes are large, take half your food home for a meal later in the week. Don't choose supersized meals.
- If you're eating at a friends home, eat a little and leave the rest. Don't eat to be polite.

Physical Activity and Stress Management

- Increase your level of daily physical activity as slowly as necessary based on your current fitness level.
- Begin an exercise program that includes cardiorespiratory endurance exercise, strength training, and stretching.
- Develop techniques for handling stress. (See Chapter 12 for more on stress management.)
- Develop strategies for coping with nonhunger cues to eat, such as boredom, sleepiness, or anxiety. Try calling a friend, taking a shower, or reading a magazine.
- Tell family members and friends that you're changing your eating and exercise habits. Ask them to be supportive.

8.6 Approaches to Overcoming a Weight Problem

Each year, Canadians spend more than $6 billion on various weight-loss surgeries, pills, special diets, and meal replacement products. If you are overweight, you may already be creating a plan to lose weight and keep it off. You have many options.

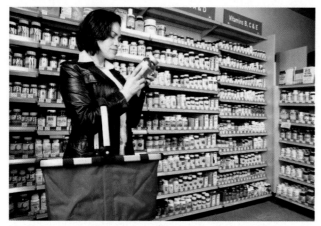

(c) VStock LLC / Tanya Constantine / Getty Images

There are many plans and supplements promoted for weight loss, but few have any research supporting their effectiveness for long-term weight management.

Doing It Yourself

If you need to lose weight, focus on adopting the healthy lifestyle described throughout this book. The "right" weight for you will naturally evolve, and you won't have to diet. Combine modest cuts in energy intake with exercise, and avoid very-low-calorie diets. (In general, a low-calorie diet should provide 1200 to 1500 calories per day, whereas an average adult calorie diet provides 1800 to 3000 calories.) By achieving a negative energy balance of 250 to 1000 calories per day, you'll produce the recommended weight loss of about 0.25 to 1 kilogram per week.

Most low-calorie diets cause a rapid loss of body water at first. When this phase passes, weight loss declines. As a result, people are often misled into believing that their efforts are not working. They give up, not realizing that smaller losses later in the diet are actually better than the initial big losses, because later loss is mostly fat loss, whereas initial loss is primarily fluid. For someone who is overweight, reasonable weight loss is 8–10% of body weight over six months.

For many people, maintaining weight loss is a bigger challenge than losing weight. Most weight lost during a period of dieting is regained. When planning a weight management program, include strategies that you can maintain over the long-term, both for food choices and for physical activity. Weight-management is a lifelong project. A registered dietitian or nutritionist can recommend an appropriate plan for you when you want to lose weight on your own. For more tips on losing weight on your own, we will discuss creating an individual weight-management plan later in the chapter.

Diet Books

Many people who try to lose weight by themselves fall prey to one or more of the dozens of diet books on the market. Although some books contain useful advice and motivational tips, most make empty promises. Accept books that advocate a balanced approach to diet plus exercise and sound nutritional advice, but reject any book that does the following:

- Advocates an unbalanced way of eating, such as high-carbohydrate-only diets or low-carbohydrate high-protein diets, or promotes a single food, such as cabbage or grapefruit.

- Claims to be based on a "scientific breakthrough" or to have the "secret" to success.

- Uses gimmicks, such as matching eating to blood type, hyping insulin resistance as the single cause of obesity or combining foods in special ways to achieve weight loss.

- Promises quick weight loss or limits the selection of foods.

Many diets cause weight loss if maintained; the real difficulty is finding a safe and healthy pattern of food choices and physical activity that results in long-term maintenance of a healthy body weight and reduced risk of chronic disease (see the box High-Tech Weight Management).

Wellness *in the* DIGITAL AGE

HIGH-TECH WEIGHT MANAGEMENT

Technology is making inroads into the area of weight management at an ever-quickening pace. Once the domain of clinical weight-loss programs, digital tools are now available for consumers who want to lose weight or keep it off.

At the clinical level, new research shows that overweight patients who are equipped with high-tech monitoring devices (which monitor their energy intake and output) lose at least as much weight as patients who participate only in in-person weight-management counselling sessions. When person-to-person counselling is added to the use of digital monitors, patients lose even more weight and manage to keep it off longer.

A wide and ever-growing range of portable devices and weight-loss applications is also available to consumers. There are dozens of Smartphone apps that can help you keep a nutrition journal and calculate your daily intake of calories and nutrients. Such apps often pair with other programs that can help track your physical activity level and calculate the number of calories you burn throughout the day. Some of these apps can upload your daily data to a website that lets you track energy intake and output over the course of time. Many such programs can also help you set goals, provide dietary or exercise advice, or let you join communities of users who are also trying to manage their weight.

Internet-based weight-loss programs have proliferated over the last decade. Most such websites offer a cross between self-help and group support through chat rooms, bulletin boards, and e-newsletters. Many sites offer online self-assessment for diet and physical activity habits as well as a meal plan;

continued

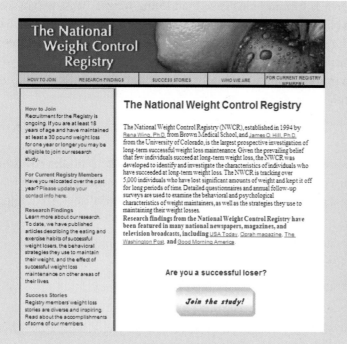

some provide access to a staff professional for individualized help. Many are free, but some charge a weekly or monthly fee.

An example of a particularly successful online weight-management program is the US National Weight Control Registry. This site is part of an ongoing study of people who have lost significant amounts of weight and kept it off. Most follow moderate-calorie diets that are relatively low in fat and fried foods, and users monitor their body weight and their food intake frequently. Participants engage in an average of 60 minutes of moderate physical activity daily.

SOURCE: The National Weight Control Registry. (http://www.nwcr.ws). Screen reprinted by permission.

Dietary Supplements and Diet Aids

The number of dietary supplements and other weight-loss aids on the market has also increased in recent years. Promoted in advertisements, magazines, direct mail campaigns, infomercials, and websites, these products typically promise a quick and easy path to weight loss. Most of these products are marketed as dietary supplements and so are subject to fewer regulations than over-the-counter (OTC) medications. According to the US Federal Trade Commission, more than half of the advertisements for weight-loss products make representations that are likely to be false. Although the Competition Bureau of Canada does not report full data like this, consumers are urged to critically evaluate any product that sounds too good to be true.

The bottom line on nonprescription diet aids is *caveat emptor* (let the buyer beware). There is no quick and easy way to lose weight. The most effective approach is to develop healthy diet and exercise habits and to make them a permanent part of your lifestyle. The following sections describe some commonly marketed OTC products for weight loss.

Formula Drinks and Food Bars

Canned diet drinks, powders used to make shakes, and diet food bars and snacks are meal replacements. They are designed to help you lose weight by substituting for some or all of your daily food intake. Meal replacements are convenient, however most people find it difficult to use these products for long periods. Although they sometimes result in rapid short-term weight loss, the weight is typically regained because users don't learn to change their eating and lifestyle behaviours.

Herbal Supplements

As described in Chapter 7, herbs are marketed as dietary supplements, so there is little information about their effectiveness, proper dosage, drug interactions, and side effects. In addition, labels may not accurately reflect the ingredients and dosages present, and safe manufacturing practices are not guaranteed. For example, the substitution of a toxic herb for another compound during the manufacture of a Chinese herbal weight-loss preparation caused more than 100 cases of kidney damage and cancer among users in Europe.

There are currently no guidelines for the sale of herbal supplements for weight loss in Canada. If you are considering using an herbal supplement, check its ingredients carefully and be sure to consult with your doctor before starting your supplement regime.

Other Supplements

Fibre is another common ingredient in OTC diet aids, promoted for appetite control. However, dietary fibre acts as a bulking agent in the large intestine, not the stomach, so it doesn't have a pronounced effect on appetite. In addition, many diet aids contain less than 3 grams of fibre, which does not contribute much toward the recommended daily intake of 25 to 38 grams.

Other popular dietary supplements include conjugated linoleic acid, carnitine, chromium, pyruvate, calcium, B vitamins, chitosan, and a number of products labelled "fat absorbers," "fat blockers," or "starch blockers." Research has not found these products to be effective, and many have potentially adverse side effects.

Weight-Loss Programs

Weight-loss programs come in a variety of types, including noncommercial support organizations, commercial programs, websites, and medically supervised clinical programs.

Noncommercial Weight-Loss Programs

Noncommercial programs such as TOPS (Take Off Pounds Sensibly) and Overeaters Anonymous (OA) mainly provide group support. They do not advocate any particular diet, but they do recommend seeking professional advice for creating an individualized diet and exercise plan. Like Alcoholics Anonymous, OA is a 12-step program with a spiritual orientation that promotes "abstinence" from compulsive overeating. These types of programs are generally free. Your physician or a registered dietitian can also provide information and support for weight loss.

Strengthening Mental Wellness

An interesting phenomenon regarding weight-loss interventions among university/college students has recently been observed: Groups of students who shared certain characteristics did better at losing and managing weight than groups of dissimilar students. The study grouped students according to common psychosocial factors (such as emotional eating), which contribute to weight gain. These clusters of similar students were able to lose more weight and keep more weight off than were groups of students who did not share common dietary or psychosocial characteristics. The findings of this study may help shape group-oriented weight-loss programs in the future, whether such programs are commercial, noncommercial, or clinical. Speak to your university/college or community support network (counsellors, health clinicians, nurses) to learn more about weight-loss interventions.

Commercial Weight-Loss Programs

Commercial programs typically provide group support, nutrition education, physical activity recommendations, and behaviour modification advice. Some also make available packaged foods to assist in following dietary advice. Many Canadian commercial programs voluntarily belong to the Partnership for Healthy Weight Management established by the US Federal Trade Commission in 1999. By doing so, they agree to provide clients with information on staff training and education, the risks associated with overweight and obesity, the risks associated with each program or product, the costs of the program, and the expected outcomes of the program, including rates of success.

A responsible and safe weight-loss program should have the following features:

- The recommended diet should be safe and balanced, include all the food groups, and meet the Recommended Nutrient Intake (RNIs) for all nutrients. Physical activity and exercise should be strongly encouraged.

- The program should promote slow, steady weight loss averaging 0.25 to 1 kilogram per week. (There may be rapid weight loss initially due to fluid loss.)

- If a participant plans to lose more than 10 kilograms, has any health problems, or is taking medication on a regular basis, physician evaluation and monitoring should be recommended. The staff of the program should include qualified counsellors and health professionals.

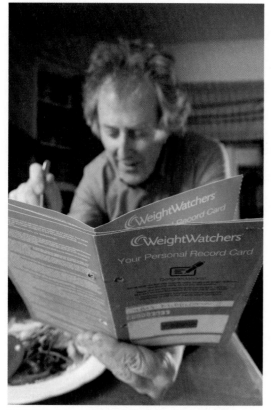

© Jeff Gilbert / Alamy Stock Photo

A variety of commercial weight-loss programs are available. These programs yield mixed results, but most provide nutritional counselling and support for people who are serious about losing weight.

- The program should include plans for weight maintenance after the weight-loss phase is over.

- The program should provide information on all fees and costs, including those of supplements and prepackaged foods, as well as data on risks and expected outcomes of participating in the program.

You should also consider whether a program fits your lifestyle and whether you are truly ready to make a commitment to it. A strong commitment and a plan for maintenance are especially important because only 10–15% of program participants maintain their weight loss; the rest gain back all or more than they had lost. One study of participants found that regular exercise was the best predictor of maintaining weight loss, and frequent television viewing was the best predictor of weight gain.

Clinical Weight-Loss Programs

Medically supervised clinical programs are usually located in a hospital or other medical setting. Designed to help those who are severely obese, these programs typically involve a closely monitored very-low-calorie diet. The cost of a clinical program is usually high, but insurance often covers part of the fee.

Prescription Drugs

For a medicine to cause weight loss, it must reduce energy consumption, increase energy expenditure, and/

or interfere with energy absorption. The medications most often prescribed for weight loss are appetite suppressants that reduce feelings of hunger or increase feelings of fullness. Appetite suppressants usually work by increasing levels of catecholamine or serotonin, two brain chemicals that affect mood and appetite.

Only two weight-loss drugs are legal for long-term use in Canada: orlistat (Xenical) and liraglutide (Saxenda). While both work to help people reduce obesity by different methods, they also both have potential side effects, including sleeplessness, nervousness, and euphoria; increases in blood pressure and heart rate; headaches; constipation or diarrhea; and dry mouth. Be sure to confirm a drug's legality and safety with Health Canada's website before using weight-loss drugs.

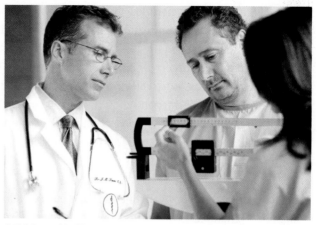

© Rick Gomez / Corbis

Severely obese people may get the most benefit from a clinical weight-loss program, where diet and activity are monitored closely by health professionals.

Prescription drugs for weight-loss work best in conjunction with behaviour modification. Appetite suppressants produce modest weight loss—about 2 to 10 kilograms above the loss expected with nondrug obesity treatments. Individuals respond differently, however, and some experience more weight loss than others. Weight loss tends to level off or reverse after four to six months on a medication, and many people regain the weight they've lost if they stop taking the drugs.

Prescription weight-loss drugs are not for people who just want to lose a few kilograms. The latest federal guidelines advise people to try lifestyle modification for at least six months before trying drug therapy. Prescription drugs are recommended—in conjunction with lifestyle changes—only in certain cases: for people who have been unable to lose weight with nondrug options and who have a BMI over 30 (or over 27 if two or more additional risk factors such as diabetes and high blood pressure are present).

Surgery

It is estimated that about 3% of adult Canadians have a BMI greater than 40, which qualifies them as severely, or morbidly obese.[11] The number of severely obese people has nearly tripled in the last two decades. Morbid obesity is a serious medical condition that is often complicated by other health problems, such as diabetes, sleep disorders, heart disease, and arthritis. Surgical intervention—known as *bariatric surgery*—may be necessary as a treatment of last resort. Bariatric surgery may be recommended for patients with a BMI greater than 40, or greater than 35 with obesity-related illnesses.

Due to the increasing prevalence of severe obesity, surgical treatment of obesity is growing worldwide. Obesity-related health conditions, as well as risk of premature death, generally improve after surgical weight loss. Surgery, however, carries risks. Patients with poor cardiorespiratory fitness prior to surgery experience more postoperative complications—including stroke, kidney failure, and even death—than patients with higher fitness levels.

Bariatric surgery reduces the size of the stomach. One method partitions the stomach with staples or a band, and another modifies the way the stomach drains (gastric bypass). In either type of surgical intervention, the goal is to promote weight loss by reducing the amount of food the patient can eat. Potential complications from surgery include nutritional deficiencies, fat intolerance, nausea, vomiting, and reflux. As many as 10–20% of patients may require follow-up surgery to address complications.

Weight loss from surgery generally ranges between 40% and 70% of total body weight over the course of a year. The key to success is to have adequate follow-up and to stay motivated so that life behaviours and eating patterns are changed permanently.

The surgical technique of liposuction involves the removal of small amounts of fat from specific locations. Liposuction is not a method for treating obesity.

Psychological Help

When concern about body weight and shape have developed into an eating disorder, professional help is recommended. Therapists who help people with these disorders should have experience working with weight management, body image issues, eating disorders, addictions, and abuse issues.

8.7 Body Image

Defined as the collective picture of the body as seen through the mind's eye, **body image** consists of perceptions, images, thoughts, attitudes, and emotions. A negative body image is characterized by dissatisfaction with the body in general or some part of the body in particular.

> **body image**   The mental representation a person holds about their body at any given moment in time, consisting of perceptions, images, thoughts, attitudes, and emotions about the body.

Developing a positive body image is an important aspect of psychological wellness and successful weight management. Dissatisfaction with body size and shape comes from external, cultural forces as well as internal, psychological perceptions that are specific to life stages. For example, a cultural ideal of female body shape in Western society has become progressively thinner, whereas actual female body size continues to increase. How we individually perceive these norms and act on them, for example by not eating enough or avoiding appearing in a bathing suit, represents our psychological response.

> **Fitness Tip**
>
> It may not be possible to be "too fit," but it is possible to exercise too much. This is a common problem among people who are obsessed with their weight or body image.
> Track your exercise habits for a week; if they seem excessive and you can't seem to cut back, talk to a professional counsellor or your doctor to find out if you have a body image problem.

LO5 Severe Body Image Problems

Poor body image can cause significant psychological distress. A person can become preoccupied by a perceived defect in appearance, thereby damaging self-esteem and interfering with relationships. Adolescents and adults who have a negative body image are more likely to diet restrictively, eat compulsively, or develop some other form of disordered eating.

When dissatisfaction becomes extreme, the condition is called body dysmorphic disorder (BDD). BDD usually begins before age 18 but can begin in adulthood. Sufferers are overly concerned with physical appearance, often focusing on slight flaws that are not obvious to others. Individuals with BDD may spend hours every day thinking about their defect and looking at themselves in mirrors; they may also desire and seek repeated cosmetic surgeries. BDD is related to obsessive-compulsive disorder and can lead to depression, social phobia, and suicide if left untreated. Medication and psychotherapy can help people with BDD.

In some cases, body image may bear little resemblance to fact. People suffering from the eating disorder anorexia nervosa typically have a severely distorted body image, believing themselves to be fat even when they have become emaciated (see the next section for more on anorexia). Distorted body image is also a hallmark of *muscle dysmorphia*, a disorder experienced by some body builders in which they see themselves as small and out of shape despite being very muscular. People with muscle dysmorphia may let obsessive bodybuilding interfere with their work and relationships. They may also use steroids and other potentially dangerous muscle-building drugs.

To assess your own body image, complete the body image self-test in Lab 8.3.

Acceptance and Change

There are limits to the changes that can be made to body weight and body shape, both of which are influenced by heredity. Knowing when the limits to healthy change have been reached—and learning to accept those limits—is crucial for overall wellness. Women in particular tend to measure self-worth in terms of their appearance; when they don't measure up to an unrealistic cultural ideal, they may see themselves as defective, and their self-esteem falls. The result can be negative body image, disordered eating, or even a full-blown eating disorder (see the box Gender, Ethnicity, and Body Image).

Weight management needs to take place in a positive and realistic atmosphere. For an obese person, losing as few as 4 kilograms can reduce blood pressure and improve mood. The hazards of excessive dieting and overconcern about body weight need to be countered by a change in attitude. A reasonable weight must take into account a person's weight history, social circumstances, metabolic profile, and psychological well-being.

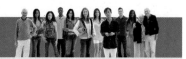

DIVERSITY Matters

GENDER, ETHNICITY, AND BODY IMAGE

Body Image and Gender

Women are much more likely than men to be dissatisfied with their bodies, often wanting to be thinner than they are. Body weight perception has been found to begin in girls as young as seven years old. Approximately 50% of girls and undergraduate women report being dissatisfied with their bodies. Girls and women are much more likely than boys and men to diet and develop eating disorders, and to be obese.

The image of the "perfect" woman presented in the media is often unrealistic and even unhealthy. In a review of BMI data for Miss America pageant winners since 1922, researchers noted a significant decline in BMI over time, with an increasing number of recent winners having BMIs in the "underweight" category. The average fashion model is 10 to 18 centimetres taller and 8 kilograms lighter than the average North American woman.

Our culture may be promoting an unattainable masculine ideal as well. Researchers have found that males who form their ideals from media-generated images show a preference for thinness and muscularity. Researchers studying male action figures noted that they have become increasingly muscular. A recent Batman action figure, if projected onto a man of average height, would result in someone with a 75-centimetre waist, 142-centimetre chest, and 67-centimetre biceps. Such media messages can be demoralizing, and although not as common, boys and men also suffer from body image problems.

continued

Body Image and Ethnicity

Although some groups espouse thinness as an ideal body type, others do not. In many traditional African societies, for example, full-figured women's bodies are seen as symbols of health, prosperity, and fertility. African-Canadian teenage girls have a much more positive body image than European-Canadian girls; in one survey, two-thirds of them defined beauty as "the right attitude," whereas European-Canadian girls were more preoccupied with weight and body shape. In another study about pressure to look like idealized images, Latina women reported the greatest pressure (over white or black women) to be physically attractive.

Nevertheless, recent evidence indicates that African-Canadian women are as likely to engage in disordered eating behaviour, especially binge eating and vomiting, as their First Nations, Métis, Inuit, and white counterparts. This finding underscores the complex nature of eating disorders and body image.

Avoiding Body Image Problems

To minimize your risk of developing a body image problem, keep the following strategies in mind:

- Focus on healthy habits and good physical health.
- Put concerns about physical appearance in perspective. Your worth as a human being does not depend on how you look.
- Practise body acceptance. You can influence your body size and type through lifestyle to some degree, but the basic fact is that some people are genetically designed to be bigger or heavier than others.
- Find things to appreciate in yourself besides an idealized body image. People who can learn to value other aspects of themselves are more accepting of the physical changes that occur naturally with age.
- View eating as a morally neutral activity—eating dessert isn't "bad" and doesn't make you a bad person.
- See the beauty and fitness industries for what they are. Realize that one of their goals is to prompt dissatisfaction with yourself so you will buy their products.

8.8 Eating Disorders

Problems with body weight and weight control are not limited to excessive body fat. A growing number of people, especially adolescent girls and young women, experience **eating disorders**, characterized by severe disturbances in eating patterns and eating-related behaviour. Based on population data, it is estimated that nearly one million Canadians meet the criteria for suffering from an eating disorder (2–3% of the population). Many more people have abnormal eating habits and attitudes about food that, although not meeting the criteria for a full-blown eating disorder, do disrupt their lives. To assess your eating habits, complete Lab 8.3.

eating disorder   A serious disturbance in eating patterns or eating-related behaviour, characterized by a negative body image and concerns about body weight or body fat.

Although many different explanations for the development of eating disorders have been proposed, they share one central feature: a dissatisfaction with body image and body weight. Such dissatisfaction is created by distorted thinking, including perfectionistic beliefs, unreasonable demands for self-control, and excessive self-criticism. Dissatisfaction with body weight leads to dysfunctional attitudes about eating, such as fear of fat, preoccupation with food, and problematic eating behaviours. Eating disorders are classified as mental disorders.

Anorexia Nervosa

People with **anorexia nervosa** have an intense fear of gaining weight or becoming fat. Although they may express a great interest in food, they do not eat enough food to maintain a reasonable body weight. They may engage in compulsive behaviours or rituals that help them keep from eating. Anorexia affects over 38 000 Canadians, 90% of them female. Although it can occur later, anorexia typically develops between the ages of 14 and 25 years.[12] People with anorexia are typically introverted, emotionally reserved, and socially insecure. Their entire sense of self-esteem may be tied up in their evaluation of their body shape and weight.

anorexia nervosa An eating disorder characterized by a refusal to maintain body weight at a minimally healthy level and an intense fear of gaining weight or becoming fat; self-starvation.

Anorexia nervosa has been linked to a variety of medical complications, including disorders of the cardiovascular, gastrointestinal, and endocrine systems. Because of extreme weight loss, females with anorexia often stop menstruating. When body fat is virtually gone and muscles are severely wasted, the body turns to its own organs in a desperate search for protein. Death can occur from heart failure caused by electrolyte imbalances. About one in ten women with anorexia dies of starvation, cardiac arrest, or other medical complications—one of the highest death rates for any psychiatric disorder. Depression is also a serious risk, and about half the fatalities relating to anorexia are suicides.[13]

Bulimia Nervosa

A person with **bulimia nervosa** engages in recurrent episodes of binge eating followed by **purging**. Bulimia is often difficult to recognize because sufferers conceal their eating habits and usually maintain a normal weight, although they may experience weight fluctuations of 4 to 7 kilograms. Although bulimia usually begins in adolescence or young adulthood, it has recently begun to emerge at increasingly younger (11–12 years) and older (40–60 years) ages. Research suggests that about 5% of university/college-age women have bulimia.

bulimia nervosa An eating disorder characterized by recurrent episodes of binge eating and then purging to prevent weight gain.
purging The use of vomiting, laxatives, excessive exercise, restrictive dieting, enemas, diuretics, or diet pills to compensate for food that has been eaten and that the person fears will produce weight gain.

A bulimic person may rapidly consume thousands of calories during a binge. This is followed by an attempt to get rid of the food by purging, usually by vomiting or using laxatives or diuretics. During a binge, bulimics feel as though they have lost control and cannot stop or limit how much they eat. Some binge and purge only occasionally; others do so many times every day. Binges may be triggered by a major life change or other stressful event. Binge eating and purging may become a way of dealing with difficult feelings such as anger and disappointment.

The binge-purge cycle of bulimia places a tremendous strain on the body and can have serious health effects, including tooth decay, esophageal damage and chronic hoarseness, menstrual irregularities, depression, liver and kidney damage, and cardiac arrhythmia. About 114 000 Canadian women suffer from bulimia.[14]

Binge-Eating Disorder

Binge-eating disorder is characterized by uncontrollable eating without any compensatory purging behaviours. Common eating patterns are eating more rapidly than normal, eating until uncomfortably full, eating when not hungry, and preferring to eat alone. Uncontrolled eating is usually followed by weight gain and feelings of guilt, shame, and depression. Many people with binge-eating disorder mistakenly see rigid dieting as the only solution to their problem, but this usually causes feelings of deprivation and a return to overeating.

> **binge-eating disorder** An eating disorder characterized by binge eating and a lack of control over eating behaviour in general.

Compulsive overeaters rarely eat because of hunger. Instead, they use food to cope with stress, conflict, and other difficult emotions or to provide solace or entertainment. Binge eaters are almost always obese, so they face all the health risks associated with obesity. In addition, binge eaters may have higher-than-average rates of depression and anxiety. Although Canadian statistics have not been collected, binge-eating disorder is the most prevalent eating disorder among Americans, with 2–5% of all US adults suffering from the disorder.[15]

Borderline Disordered Eating

People with *borderline disordered eating* have some symptoms of eating disorders—for example, excessive dieting or occasional bingeing or purging—but do not meet the full diagnostic criteria for anorexia, bulimia, or binge-eating disorder. Meaningful statistics about borderline disordered eating are hard to come by, in part because it is difficult to define exactly when eating habits cross the line between normal and disordered. However, many experts feel that the majority of Canadians, particularly women, have at least some unhealthy attitudes and behaviours in relation to food and self-image. Concerns about weight and dieting are so common that they are considered culturally normal for many North Americans.

Ideally, our relationship to food should be a happy one. The biological urge to satisfy hunger is one of our most basic drives, and eating is associated with many pleasurable sensations. For some of us, food triggers pleasant memories of good times, family, holidays, and fun. But for too many people, food is a source of anguish rather than pleasure. Eating results in feelings of guilt and self-loathing rather than satisfaction, causing tremendous disruption in the lives of affected individuals.

How do you know if you have disordered eating habits? When thoughts about weight and food dominate your life, you have a problem. If you're convinced that your worth as a person hinges on how you look and how much you weigh, it's time to get help. Self-induced vomiting or laxative use after meals, even if only once in a while, is reason for concern. Do you feel compelled to overexercise to compensate for what you've eaten? Do you routinely restrict your food intake and sometimes eat nothing in an effort to feel more in control? These are all danger signs and could mean that you are developing a serious problem. Lab 8.3 can help you determine whether you are at risk for an eating disorder.

Treating Eating Disorders

The treatment of eating disorders must address both problematic eating behaviours and the misuse of food to manage stress and emotions. Treatment for anorexia nervosa first involves averting a medical crisis by restoring adequate body weight; then the psychological aspects of the disorder can be addressed. The treatment of bulimia nervosa or binge-eating disorder involves first stabilizing the eating patterns, then identifying and changing the patterns of thinking that lead to disordered eating. Treatment usually involves a combination of psychotherapy, medication, and medical management. Friends and family members often want to know what they can do to help someone with an eating disorder. For suggestions, see the box If Someone You Know Has an Eating Disorder....

People with milder patterns of disordered eating may benefit from getting a nutrition checkup with a registered dietitian. A professional can help determine appropriate body weight and calorie intake, and offer advice on how to budget calories into a balanced, healthy diet.

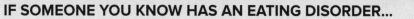

Take CHARGE

IF SOMEONE YOU KNOW HAS AN EATING DISORDER...

Secrecy and denial are two hallmarks of eating disorders, so it can be hard to know if someone has anorexia or bulimia. Signs that a friend may have anorexia include sudden weight loss, excessive dieting or exercise, guilt or preoccupation with food and eating, frequent weighing, fear of becoming fat despite being thin, and wearing baggy or layered clothes to conceal weight loss. Signs that someone may have bulimia include excessive eating without weight gain; secretiveness about food (stealing, hiding, or hoarding food); self-induced vomiting (bathroom visits during or after a meal); swollen glands or puffy face; erosion of tooth enamel; and use of laxatives, diuretics, or diet pills to control weight.

If you decide to approach a friend with your concerns, here are some tips to follow:

- Find out about treatment resources in your community. (See For Further Exploration for suggestions.) You may want to consult a professional at your school clinic or counselling centre about the best way to approach the situation.
- Arrange to speak with your friend in a private place, and allow enough time to talk.
- Express your concerns, with specific observations of your friend's behaviour. Expect them to deny or minimize the problem and possibly to become angry with you. Stay calm and nonjudgmental, and continue to express your concern.
- Avoid giving simplistic advice about eating habits. Listen if your friend wants to talk, and offer your support and understanding. Give your friend the information you found about where they can get help, and offer to go along.
- If the situation is an emergency—if your friend has fainted, for example, or attempted suicide—call 911 for help immediately.
- If you are upset about the situation, consider talking to someone yourself. The professionals at the clinic or counselling centre are there to help you. Remember, you are not to blame for another person's eating disorder.

Tips for Today and the Future

Many weight management approaches work, but the simplest formula is moderate food intake coupled with regular exercise.

RIGHT NOW YOU CAN

- Assess your weight-management needs. Do you need to gain weight, lose weight, or stay at your current weight?
- List five things you can do to add more lifestyle activity (not exercise) to your daily routine.
- Identify the foods you regularly eat that may be sabotaging your ability to manage your weight.

IN THE FUTURE YOU CAN

- Make an honest assessment of your current body image. Is it accurate and fair, or is it unduly negative and unhealthy? If your body image presents a problem, consider getting professional advice on how to view yourself realistically.
- Keep track of your energy needs to determine whether your energy-balance equation is correct. Use this information as part of your long-term weight-management efforts.

Common Questions ANSWERED

Q How can I safely gain weight?

A Just as for losing weight, a program for weight gain should be gradual and should include both exercise and dietary changes. The foundation of a successful and healthy program for weight gain is a combination of strength training and a high-carbohydrate, high-calorie diet. Strength training is critical because it will help you add weight as muscle rather than fat.

Energy balance is also important in a program for gaining weight. You need to consume more calories than your body needs in order to gain weight, but you need to choose those extra calories wisely. Fatty, high-calorie foods may seem like an obvious choice, but consuming additional calories as fat can jeopardize your health and your weight-management program. A diet high in fat carries health risks, including increased risk of cardiovascular disease and certain types of cancer. A better strategy is to consume additional calories as complex carbohydrates from whole grains, fruits, and vegetables.

A diet for weight gain should contain about 60–65% of total daily calories from carbohydrates. You probably do not need to be concerned with protein; although protein requirements increase when you exercise, the protein consumption of most Canadians is already well above the Recommended Nutrient Intake (RNI).

In order to gain primarily muscle weight instead of fat, a gradual program of weight gain is your best bet. Try these strategies for consuming extra calories:

- Don't skip any meals.
- Add two or three snacks to your daily eating routine.
- Try a sports drink or supplement that has at least 60% of calories from carbohydrates, as well as significant amounts of protein, vitamins, and minerals. (But don't use supplements to replace meals, because they don't contain all food components.)

Q How can I achieve a "perfect" body?

A The current cultural ideal of an ultrathin, ultrafit body is impossible for most people to achieve. A reasonable goal for body weight and body shape must take into account your heredity, weight history, social circumstances, metabolic rate, and psychological well-being. Don't set goals based on movie stars or fashion models. Modern photographic techniques can make people look much different on film or in magazines than they do in person. Many of these people are also genetically endowed with body shapes that are impossible for us to emulate. The best approach is to work with what you've got. Adopting a wellness lifestyle that includes regular exercise and a healthy diet will naturally result in the best possible body shape for you. Obsessively trying to achieve unreasonable goals can lead to problems such as eating disorders, overtraining, and injuries.

SUMMARY

- Excess body weight increases the risk of numerous diseases, particularly cardiovascular disease, cancer, and diabetes.

- Although genetic factors help determine a person's weight, the influence of heredity can be overcome.

- Physiological factors involved in the regulation of body weight and body fat include metabolic rate and hormones.

- Energy-balance components that an individual can control are calories taken in and calories expended in physical activity.

- Nutritional guidelines for weight management and wellness include controlling consumption of total calories, unhealthy fats, carbohydrates, and protein; monitoring portion sizes and calorie density; increasing consumption of whole grains, fruits, and vegetables; and developing an eating schedule based on rules.

- Activity guidelines for weight control emphasize engaging in moderate-intensity physical activity for 150 minutes or more per week; regular, prolonged endurance exercise and weight training can burn a significant number of calories while maintaining muscle mass.

- The sense of well-being that results from a well-balanced diet can reinforce commitment to weight control; improve self-esteem; and lead to realistic, as opposed to negative, self-talk. Successful weight management results in not using food as a way to cope with stress.

- In cases of extreme obesity, weight loss requires medical supervision; in less extreme cases, people can set up individual programs, perhaps getting guidance from reliable books, or they can get help by joining a formal weight-loss program.

- Dissatisfaction with body image and body weight can lead to physical problems and serious eating disorders, including anorexia nervosa, bulimia nervosa, and binge-eating disorder.

FOR FURTHER EXPLORATION

Organizations and Websites

Canadian Mental Health Association: Eating Disorders. Includes information on a number of eating disorders and answers commonly asked questions about dealing with eating disorders.

http://www.cmha.ca/mental-health/understanding-mental-illness/eating-disorders/

Canadian Obesity Network. Consists of news, events, and resources related to obesity in Canada.

http://www.obesitynetwork.ca/

Health Canada—Food and Nutrition. Answers questions dealing with food consumption, active lifestyles, and other relevant areas.

http://www.hc-sc.gc.ca/fn-an/index_e.html

MedlinePlus: Obesity and Weight Loss. Offers news and links to reliable information from government agencies and key professional associations.

http://www.nlm.nih.gov/medlineplus/obesity.html

http://www.nlm.nih.gov/medlineplus/weightcontrol.html

Public Health Agency of Canada. Includes timely, trusted, and credible information on healthy living.

http://www.phac-aspc.gc.ca/index-eng.php

World Health Organizaation. Provides information on WHO's global strategy on diet and physical activity.

http://www.who.int/dietphysicalactivity/en

There are also many resources for people concerned about body image and eating disorders, such as:

MedlinePlus: Eating Disorders

http://www.nlm.nih.gov/medlineplus/eatingdisorders.html

National Eating Disorder Information Centre

http://www.nedic.ca/

See also the listings in Chapter 1, Chapter 6, and Chapter 7.

Laboratory Activities

Name _____ **Section** _____ **Date** _____

Lab 8.1 Calculating Daily Energy Needs

connect

Part I Estimating Current Energy Intake from a Food Record

If your weight is stable, your current daily energy intake is the number of calories you need to consume to maintain your weight at your current activity level. For women, average calorie requirements are 1600 to 2400 calories per day; for men, 2000 to 3000. The low end of the range is for sedentary individuals, while the high end is for active individuals. In addition, caloric needs tend to decrease with age.

If you completed Lab 7.2, you should have a record of your current energy intake; if you didn't complete the lab, keep a careful and complete record of everything you eat for one day, and then total the calories in all the foods and beverages you consumed. Record your total energy intake below.

Current energy intake (from food record): _____ Calories per day

Part II Estimating Daily Energy Requirements Using Food and Nutrition Board Formulas

Many people underestimate the size of their food portions, so energy goals based on estimates of current calorie intake from food records can be inaccurate. You can also estimate your daily energy needs using a formula. To use the appropriate formula for your sex, plug the following values into the equation below:

- age (in years)
- weight (in pounds)
- height (in inches)
- physical activity coefficient (PA) from the table below

To help estimate your physical activity level, consider the following guidelines: Someone who typically engages in 30 minutes of moderate-intensity activity, equivalent to walking 3.2 kilometres in 30 minutes, in addition to the activities in maintaining a sedentary lifestyle is considered "low active"; someone who typically engages in the equivalent of 90 minutes of moderate-intensity activity is rated as "active." You might find it helpful to refer back to Lab 2.2 to estimate your physical activity level.

	Physical Activity Coefficient (PA)	
Physical Activity Level	Men	Women
Sedentary	1.00	1.00
Low active	1.12	1.14
Active	1.27	1.27
Very active	1.54	1.45

Estimated Daily Energy Requirement for Weight Maintenance in Men

$$864 - (9.72 \times age) + (PA \times [(6.39 \times weight) + (12.78 \times height)])$$

1. $9.72 \times$ _____ Age (years) = _____

2. $864 -$ _____ Result from step 1 = _____ [result may be a negative number]

3. 6.39 × _____ Weight (pounds) = _____

4. 12.78 × _____ Height (inches) = _____

5. _____ result from step 3 + _____ result from step 4 = _____

6. _____ PA (from table) × _____ result from step 5 = _____

7. _____ result from step 2 + _____ result from step 6 = _____
calories per day

Estimated Daily Energy Requirement for Weight Maintenance in Women

$$387 - (7.31 \times \text{age}) + (PA \times [(4.91 \times \text{weight}) + (16.78 \times \text{height})])$$

1. 7.31 × _____ Age (years) = _____

2. 387 − _____ Result from step 1 = _____ [result may be a negative number]

3. 4.91 × _____ Weight (pounds) = _____

4. 16.78 × _____ Height (inches) = _____

5. _____ result from step 3 + _____ result from step 4 = _____

6. _____ PA (from table) × _____ result from step 5 = _____

7. _____ result from step 2 + _____ result from step 6 = _____
calories per day

Daily energy needs for weight maintenance (from formula): _____ calories/day

Part III Determining an Individual Daily Energy Goal for Weight Maintenance

If you calculated values for daily energy needs based on both methods, examine the two values. Some difference is likely—people tend to underestimate their food intake and overestimate their level of physical activity—but if the two values are very far off, check your food record and your physical activity estimate for accuracy and make any necessary adjustments. For an individualized estimate of daily calorie needs, average the two values:

Daily energy needs = (food record result _____ calories/day + formula result _____ calories/day)
÷ 2 = _____ calories/day

Using Your Results

How did you score? Are you surprised by the value you calculated for your approximate daily energy needs? If so, is the value higher or lower than you expected?

_____

_____

_____

What should you do next? Enter the results of this lab in the Preprogram Assessment column in Appendix B. If you wish to change your energy balance to lose weight, complete Lab 8.2 to set goals and develop specific strategies for change. (If your goal is weight gain, see the Common Questions Answered section of this chapter for basic guidelines.)

One of the best ways to tip your energy balance toward weight loss is to increase your daily physical activity. If you include increases in activity as part of your program, then you can use the results of this lab to chart changes in your daily energy expenditure (and needs). Look for ways to increase the amount of time you spend in physical activity, thus increasing your physical activity coefficient. After several weeks of your program, complete this lab again, and enter the results in the Postprogram Assessment column of Appendix B. How do the results compare? Did your program for boosting physical activity show up as an increase in your daily energy expenditure and need?

SOURCE: Estimating Daily Energy Requirements Using Food and Nutrition Board Formulas Part II: Reprinted with permission from *Dietary Reference Intakes for Energy, Carbohydrate, Fiber, Fat, Fatty Acids, Cholesterol, Protein, and Amino Acids (Macronutrients)*. Reprinted with permission from the National Academies Press, Copyright 2005, National Academy of Sciences.

Name _____ Section _____ Date _____

Lab 8.2 Identifying Weight-Loss Goals and Ways to Meet Them

connect

Negative Calorie Balance

Complete the following calculations to determine your weekly and daily negative calorie balance goals and the number of weeks to achieve your target weight.

Current weight _____ kg − target weight (from Lab 6.2) _____ kg = total weight to lose _____ kg

Total weight to lose _____ kg ÷ weight to lose each week _____ kg = time to achieve target weight _____ weeks

Weight to lose each week _____ kg × 7700 cal/kg = weekly negative calorie balance _____ cal/week

Weekly negative calorie balance _____ cal/week ÷ 7 days/week = daily negative calorie balance _____ cal/day

To keep your weight-loss program on schedule, you must achieve the daily negative calorie balance by either decreasing your calorie consumption (eating less) or increasing your calorie expenditure (being more active). Combining the two strategies may be most successful.

Changes in Activity Level

Adding a few minutes of exercise every day is a good way of expending calories. Use the calorie costs for different activities listed in either the table below or Table 8.2 to plan ways for raising your calorie expenditure level.

Activity	Cal/lb/min	×	Body weight	×	min	=	Total calories
Aerobic dance	.046		_____		_____		_____
Basketball (half ct.)	.045		_____		_____		_____
Bicycling (casual)	.049		_____		_____		_____
Bicycling (13 mph)	.071		_____		_____		_____
Elliptical exercise	.049		_____		_____		_____
Football (touch)	.049		_____		_____		_____
Hiking	.051		_____		_____		_____
Housework	.029		_____		_____		_____
Jogging	.060		_____		_____		_____
Rope skipping	.071		_____		_____		_____
Rowing	.032		_____		_____		_____
Skating	.049		_____		_____		_____
Soccer	.052		_____		_____		_____
Swimming	.032		_____		_____		_____
Walking (normal pace)	.029		_____		_____		_____
Walking (briskly)	.048		_____		_____		_____

continued

Activity	Duration	**Calories Used**
_____	_____	_____
_____	_____	_____
_____	_____	_____
	Total calories expended:	_____

Changes in Diet

Look closely at your diet from one day, as recorded in Lab 7.2. Identify ways to cut calorie consumption by eliminating certain items or substituting lower-calorie choices. Be realistic in your cuts and substitutions; you need to develop a plan you can live with.

Food Item	Substitute Food Item	Calorie Savings
_____	_____	_____
_____	_____	_____
_____	_____	_____
	Total calories expended:	_____

Total calories expended _____ + Total calories cut _____ = Total negative calorie balance _____

Have you met your required negative energy balance? If not, revise your dietary and activity changes to meet your goal.

Common Problem Eating Behaviours

For each of the groups of statements that appear below, check those that are true for you. If you check several statements for a given pattern or problem, it will probably be a significant factor in your weight-management program. One possible strategy for dealing with each type of problem is given. For those eating problems you identify as important, add your own ideas to the strategies listed.

1. _____ I often skip meals.

   _____ I often eat a number of snacks in place of a meal.

   _____ I don't have a regular schedule of meal and snack times.

   _____ I make up for missed meals and snacks by eating more at the next meal.

   Problem: Irregular eating habits

   Possible solutions:

- Write out a plan for each day's meals in advance. Carry it with you and stick to it.

- _____

- _____

2. _____ I eat more than one sweet dessert or snack each day.

   _____ I usually snack on foods high in calories and fat (chips, cookies, ice cream).

   _____ I drink regular (not sugar-free) soft drinks.

   _____ I choose types of meat that are high in fat.

   _____ I consume more than one alcoholic beverage a day.

Problem: Poor food choices

Possible solutions:

• Keep a supply of raw fruits or vegetables handy for snacks.

• _____

• _____

3. _____ I always eat everything on my plate.

_____ I often go back for seconds and thirds.

_____ I take larger helpings than most people.

_____ I eat up leftovers instead of putting them away.

Problem: Portion sizes too large

Possible solutions:

• Measure all portions with a scale or measuring cup.

• _____

• _____

Name _____   Section _____   Date _____

Lab 8.3 Checking for Body Image Problems and Eating Disorders

connect

Assessing Your Body Image

	Never	Sometimes	Often	Always
1. I dislike seeing myself in mirrors.	0	1	2	3
2. When I shop for clothing, I am more aware of my weight problem, and consequently I find shopping for clothes somewhat unpleasant.	0	1	2	3
3. I'm ashamed to be seen in public.	0	1	2	3
4. I prefer to avoid engaging in sports or public exercise because of my appearance.	0	1	2	3
5. I feel somewhat embarrassed about my body in the presence of someone of the other sex.	0	1	2	3
6. I think my body is ugly.	0	1	2	3
7. I feel that other people must think my body is unattractive.	0	1	2	3
8. I feel that my family or friends may be embarrassed to be seen with me.	0	1	2	3
9. I find myself comparing myself with other people to see if they are heavier than I am.	0	1	2	3
10. I find it difficult to enjoy activities because I am self-conscious about my physical appearance.	0	1	2	3
11. Feeling guilty about my weight problem preoccupies most of my thinking.	0	1	2	3
12. My thoughts about my body and physical appearance are negative and self-critical.	0	1	2	3

Now add up the number of points you have circled in each column: _____   _____ + _____ + _____ + _____

Score Interpretation

The lowest possible score is 0, and this indicates a positive body image. The highest possible score is 36, and this indicates an unhealthy body image. A score higher than 14 suggests a need to develop a healthier body image.

SOURCE: Nash, J.D. 1997. *The New Maximize Your Body Potential.* Palo Alto, CA: Bull Publishing. Reprinted with permission of the publisher.

Eating Attitudes Test to Evaluate Eating Disorder Risk

To help determine whether you might have an eating disorder that needs professional attention, answer the questions as accurately, honestly, and completely as possible; there are no right or wrong answers.

Part I. Eating Attitudes Test (EAT-26)

Circle a response for each of the following statements.

	Always	Usually	Often	Sometimes	Rarely	Never
1. Am terrified about being overweight.	3	2	1	0	0	0
2. Avoid eating when I am hungry.	3	2	1	0	0	0
3. Find myself preoccupied with food.	3	2	1	0	0	0
4. Have gone on eating binges where I feel that I may not be able to stop.	3	2	1	0	0	0
5. Cut my food into small pieces.	3	2	1	0	0	0

		Always	Usually	Often	Sometimes	Rarely	Never
6.	Aware of the calorie content of foods that I eat.	3	2	1	0	0	0
7.	Particularly avoid food with a high carbohydrate content (i.e. bread, rice, potatoes, etc.).	3	2	1	0	0	0
8.	Feel that others would prefer if I ate more.	3	2	1	0	0	0
9.	Vomit after I have eaten.	3	2	1	0	0	0
10.	Feel extremely guilty after eating.	3	2	1	0	0	0
11.	Am preoccupied with a desire to be thinner.	3	2	1	0	0	0
12.	Think about burning up calories when I exercise.	3	2	1	0	0	0
13.	Other people think that I am too thin.	3	2	1	0	0	0
14.	Am preoccupied with the thought of having fat on my body.	3	2	1	0	0	0
15.	Take longer than others to eat my meals.	3	2	1	0	0	0
16.	Avoid foods with sugar in them.	3	2	1	0	0	0
17.	Eat diet foods.	3	2	1	0	0	0
18.	Feel that food controls my life.	3	2	1	0	0	0
19.	Display self-control around food.	3	2	1	0	0	0
20.	Feel that others pressure me to eat.	3	2	1	0	0	0
21.	Give too much time and thought to food.	3	2	1	0	0	0
22.	Feel uncomfortable after eating sweets.	3	2	1	0	0	0
23.	Engage in dieting behaviour.	3	2	1	0	0	0
24.	Like my stomach to be empty.	3	2	1	0	0	0
25.	Have the impulse to vomit after meals.	3	2	1	0	0	0
26.	Enjoy trying new rich foods.	0	0	0	1	2	3

Total the points for your responses to determine your EAT-26 score: _____

Part II. Behavioural Questions

Answer the following questions according to your behaviour in the past 6 months. Circle the most appropriate response.

In the past 6 months have you:	Never	Once a month or less	2-3 times a month	Once a week	2-6 times a week	Once a day or more
1. Gone on eating binges where you feel that you may not be able to stop?*			✓	✓	✓	✓
2. Made yourself sick (vomited) to control your weight or shape?		✓	✓	✓	✓	✓
3. Used laxatives, diet pills or diuretics (water pills) to control your weight or shape?		✓	✓	✓	✓	✓
4. Exercised more than 60 minutes a day to lose or to control your weight?						✓
5. Lost 20 pounds or more in the past 6 months	YES ✓			NO		

Interpreting Your Results

If you meet one or more of the following criteria, evaluation by a qualified professional is recommended:

- a score of 20 or higher on EAT-2
- a score in any of the checked boxes in the Behavioural Questions section
- a body mass index (BMI) that classifies you as underweight or very underweight using norms for sex and age (see the following table)

This screening is not designed to make a diagnosis of an eating disorder or take the place of a professional consultation. A high score on the EAT-26 assessment does not mean that you have an eating disorder, but it does indicate that you should seek the advice of a qualified mental health professional who has experience with treating eating disorders. If you have a low score on the EAT-26, you still could have problems with eating behaviour or body image; if you are suffering from feelings that are causing you concern or interfering with your daily functioning, seek help.

Body Mass Index (BMI) Cutoffs for Classification of Underweight

Age (years)	Females					Males			
	18	19	20	20+		18	19	20	20+
Very underweight	≤ 17.5	≤ 17.5	≤ 17.5	≤ 18.5		≤ 18.0	≤ 18.5	≤ 19.0	≤ 19.5
Underweight	17.6–18.0	17.6–18.0	17.6–18.5	18.6–19.0		18.1–18.5	18.6–19.0	19.1–19.5	19.6–20.0

SOURCE: © Copyright: EAT-26: (Garner et al. 1982. *Psychological Medicine, 12,* 871–878); adapted by D. Garner with permission.

Using Your Results

How did you score? Are you surprised by your scores? Do the results of either assessment indicate that you may have a problem with body image or disordered eating?

_____

_____

_____

What should you do next? If your results are borderline, consider trying some of the self-help strategies suggested in the chapter. If body image or disordered eating is a significant problem for you, get professional advice; a physician, therapist, and/or registered dietitian can help. Make an appointment today.

CHAPTER 9

Putting Together a Complete Fitness Program

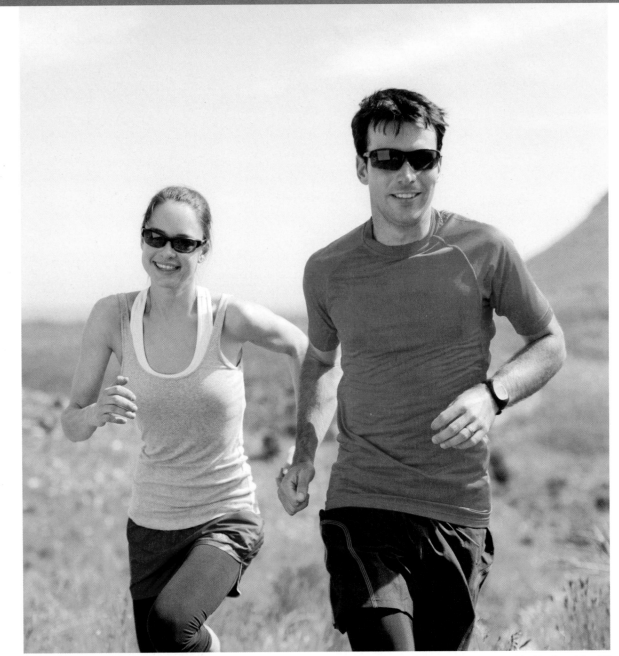

© Paul Bradbury / Getty RF

LEARNING OBJECTIVES

After reading this chapter, you should be able to

LO1 List the steps for putting together a successful personal fitness program

LO2 Describe strategies that can help you maintain a fitness program over the long term

LO3 Tailor a fitness program to accommodate different life stages

TEST YOUR KNOWLEDGE

1. **Swimming is a total fitness activity that develops all the components of health-related fitness.**

   True or false?

2. **Older adults should avoid exercise to protect themselves against falls and injuries.**

   True or false?

3. **Which of the following physical activities is considered a vigorous-intensity exercise?**
   a. uphill hiking
   b. singles tennis
   c. jumping rope

ANSWERS

1. **FALSE.** Swimming is excellent for developing cardiorespiratory endurance and muscular endurance, but because it is not a weight-bearing activity, it tends to reduce bone density. Swimmers are advised to include weight training in their exercise program to maintain bone mass.

2. **FALSE.** Older adults receive the same health benefits from exercise as younger adults, including improvements in strength, body composition, cardiorespiratory health, flexibility, balance, stability, and cognitive functioning. A far greater danger is posed by inactivity.

3. **ALL THREE.** According to the Canadian Society for Exercise Physiology, adults can perform any of these activities for 75 minutes per week to obtain health and wellness benefits.

Understanding the benefits of physical fitness, as explained in Chapters 1 to 8, is the first step toward creating a well-rounded exercise program. The next challenge is to choose activities and combine them into a program that develops all the components of fitness and helps you stay motivated. This chapter presents a step-by-step plan for creating and maintaining a well-rounded fitness program. At the end of this chapter, you'll find sample programs based on popular activities. These programs provide a structure that can be helpful if you're beginning an exercise program for the first time.

LO1 9.1 Developing a Personal Fitness Plan

If you're ready to create a complete fitness program based on the activities you enjoy most, begin by preparing the program plan and agreement in Lab 9.1. By carefully developing your plan and signing an agreement, you'll increase your chances of success. The step-by-step procedure outlined here will guide you through the steps in Lab 9.1 to create an exercise program that's right for you. (See Figure 9.1 for a sample personal fitness program plan and agreement.)

For additional help in setting up your program, choose one of the sample programs at the end of this chapter. Sample programs are provided for walking/jogging, cycling, swimming, and rowing. They include detailed instructions for starting a program and developing and maintaining fitness.

1. Set Goals

Ask yourself, "What do I want from my fitness program?" Develop different types of goals—general and specific, long term and short term. General or long-term goals might include things like lowering your risk for chronic disease, improving posture, having more energy, and improving the fit of your clothes.

It's a good idea to also develop some specific, short-term goals based on measurable factors. Specific goals might include the following:

- raise your cardiorespiratory capacity ($\dot{V}O_{2\,max}$) by 10%
- reduce the time it takes you to jog 5 kilometres from 22 minutes to 19 minutes
- increase the number of push-ups you can do from 15 to 25
- lower your BMI from 26 to 24.5

Having specific goals will allow you to track your progress and enjoy the measurable changes brought about by your fitness program. Finally, break your specific goals into several smaller steps (mini-goals), such as those shown in Figure 9.1. For example, instead of dwelling on losing 20 or 30 pounds, try losing 2 pounds. Remember, yard by yard is hard; inch by inch is a cinch. (For detailed discussions of goals and goal setting in a behaviour change or fitness program, refer back to Chapter 1 and Chapter 2.)

Physical fitness assessment tests—as described in Chapters 3 to 6—are essential to determining your goals. They help you decide which types of exercise you should emphasize, and they help you understand the relative difficulty of attaining specific goals. If you have health problems, such as high blood pressure, heart disease, obesity, or serious joint or muscle disabilities, see your physician before taking assessment tests. Measure your progress by taking these tests about every three months.

FIGURE 9.1

A sample personal fitness program plan and agreement.

A. I [Tracie Kaufman] am contracting with myself to follow a physical
   (name)
   fitness program to work toward the following goals:

Specific or short-term goals

1. Improving cardiorespiratory fitness by raising my $\dot{V}O_{2max}$ from 34 to 37 ml/kg/min
2. Improving upper body muscular strength and endurance rating from fair to good
3. Improving body composition (from 28% to 25% body fat)
4. Improving my tennis game (hitting 20 playable shots in a row against the ball machine)

General or long-term goals

1. Developing a more positive attitude about myself
2. Improving the fit of my clothes
3. Building and maintaining bone mass to reduce my risk of osteoporosis
4. Increasing my life expectancy and reducing my risk for diabetes and heart disease

B. **My program plan is as follows:**

Activities	Components (Check X)					Time	Frequency (Check X)							Intensity*
	CRE	MS	ME	F	BC		M	Tu	W	Th	F	S	S	
Swimming	X	X	X	X	X	35min	X		X		X			140–170 bpm
Tennis	X	X	X	X	X	90min						X		RPE } 13–16
Weight training		X	X	X	X	30min		X		X		X		see Lab 4.3
Stretching				X		25min	X		X		X	X		—

*List your target heart rate range or an RPE value if appropriate.

C. My program will begin on [Sept.] [*] [21] My program includes the following schedule
   of mini-goals. For each step in my program, I will give myself the reward listed.

Completing 2 full weeks of program (mini-goal 1)	Oct.	5	movie with friends (reward)
$\dot{V}O_{2max}$ of 35 ml/kg/min (mini-goal 2)	Nov.	2	new app or game (reward)
Completing 10 full weeks of program (mini-goal 3)	Nov.	30	new sweater (reward)
Percent body fat of 27% (mini-goal 4)	Dec.	22	weekend away (reward)
$\dot{V}O_{2max}$ of 36 ml/kg/min (mini-goal 5)	Jan.	18	new app or game (reward)

D. My program will include the addition of physical activity to my daily routine (such
   as climbing stairs or walking to class):

1. Walking to and from campus job
2. Taking the stairs to dorm room instead of elevator
3. Bicycling to the library instead of driving
4. Taking a drop-in fitness class at the campus recreation center

E. My program will include the following strategies for reducing sedentary time:

1. Setting "move" reminders on phone and laptop
2. Moving during television commercial breaks or between programs
3. Standing or walking during phone calls

F. I will use the following tools to monitor my program and my progress toward
   my goals:

I'll use a chart that lists the number of laps and minutes I swim and the
charts for strength and flexibility from Labs 4.3 & 5.2.

I sign this contract as an indication of my personal commitment to reach my goal.

Tracie Kaufman
(your signature)   [Sep.] [10]

I have recruited a helper who will witness my contract and

swim with me three days per week

(list any way your helper will participate in your program)

Russell Walker
(witness's signature)   [Sep.] [10]

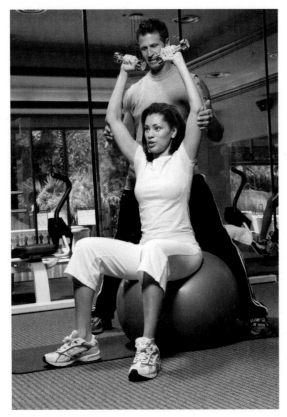

© Chris Clinton / Getty Images

An overall fitness program includes exercises to develop all the components of physical fitness.

2. Select Activities

If you have already chosen activities and used the FITT principle to create separate program plans for different fitness components in Chapters 3 to 5, you can put those plans together into a single program. It's usually best to include exercises to develop each of the health-related components of fitness. The components (with abbreviations used in Figure 9.1, section B) are as follows:

- Cardiorespiratory endurance (CRE) is developed by activities that involve continuous rhythmic movements of large-muscle groups like those in the legs (see Chapter 3).

- Muscular strength and endurance (MS and ME) are developed by training against resistance (see Chapter 4).

- Flexibility (F) is developed by stretching the major muscle groups (see Chapter 5).

- Healthy body composition (BC) can be developed by combining a sensible diet and a program of regular exercise, including cardiorespiratory endurance exercise to burn calories and resistance training to build muscle mass (see Chapter 6).

Fitness Tip

Although some research indicates that pre-workout stretching can reduce muscle power and interfere with motor control, there are benefits to stretching after running. You can increase flexibility by doing stretching exercises as part of your cool-down.

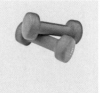

The Conference Board of Canada reported that Canadians participate in a vast number of sports but tend to concentrate their energy expenditures on a few—ice hockey, golf, baseball, skiing, and soccer are the top five sports.[1]

Table 9.1 shows the intensity levels of several popular activities that promote health. Check the ratings of the activities you're considering to make sure the program you put together will help you achieve your goals. The Public Health Agency of Canada also provides age-specific recommendations on its website at http://www.phac-aspc.gc.ca/hp-ps/hl-mvs/pa-ap/index-eng.php.

TABLE 9.1

Examples of Different Aerobic Activities and Their Intensities

Moderate-Intensity Activities	Vigorous-Intensity Activities
• Walking briskly (5 km/h per hour [3 m/h], but not race-walking)	• Race-walking, jogging, or running
• Water aerobics	• Swimming laps
• Bicycling slower than 16 km/h [10 m/h]	• Bicycling 16 km/h [10 m/h] or faster
• Doubles tennis	• Singles tennis
• Ballroom dancing	• Aerobic dancing
• General gardening	• Heavy gardening (continuous digging or hoeing)
• Basketball	• Jumping rope
• Elliptical trainer	• Hiking uphill or with a heavy backpack

SOURCE: Physical Activity Guidelines Advisory Committee. 2008. *Physical Activity Guidelines Advisory Committee Report, 2008.* Washington, DC: U.S. Department of Health and Human Services.

Ask Yourself

QUESTIONS FOR CRITICAL THINKING AND REFLECTION

Consider the list of physical activities and sports in Table 9.1. Given your current fitness and skill level, which ones could you reasonably incorporate into your exercise program?

If you select activities that support your commitment rather than activities that turn exercise into a chore, your program will provide plenty of incentive for continuing. Consider the following factors in making your choices:

- **Fun and interest.** Your fitness program is much more likely to be successful if you choose activities that you currently engage in and enjoy doing. Often you can modify your current activities to fit your fitness program. If you want to add a new activity to your program, try it for a while before committing to it. Table 9.2 (on the next page) shows a few popular recreational activities you may enjoy.

- **Current skill and fitness level.** Although many activities are appropriate for beginners, some sports and activities require a moderate level of skill to obtain fitness benefits. For example, if you are a beginning tennis player, you will probably not be able to sustain rallies long enough to develop cardiorespiratory endurance. A better choice might be a walking program while you improve your tennis game. To build skill for a particular activity, consider taking a class or getting some instruction from a coach or fellow participant.

- **Time and convenience.** You are more likely to maintain a long-term exercise program if you can easily fit exercise into your daily routine. As you consider activities, think about whether a special location or facility is required. Can you participate in the activity close to your home, school, or job? Are the necessary facilities available at convenient times (see Lab 9.2)? Can you participate in the activity year-round, or will you need to find an alternative during the summer or winter? Would a home treadmill make you more likely to exercise regularly?

TABLE 9.2 VITAL STATISTICS

Popular Recreational Activities of Canadians

Activity	Reported by % of Sample
Walking for exercise	71%
Gardening, yard work	49%
Home exercise	33%
Swimming	22%
Bicycling	20%
Social dancing	18%

SOURCE: "Popularity of Physical Recreation Activities of Adults, Age 20+ ." Statistics Canada, Canadian Community Health Survey, 2005. Table 13100086; Formerly CANSIM Table 105-0400. Contains information licensed under the Open Government Licence – Canada.

- **Cost.** Some sports and activities require equipment, fees, or some type of membership investment. If you are on a tight budget, limit your choices to activities that are inexpensive or free. Investigate the facilities on your campus, which you may be able to use at little or no cost. Many activities require no equipment beyond an appropriate pair of shoes. Chapter 4 provides examples of exercises you can do at home without equipment.

- **Special health needs.** If you have a particular health problem, choose activities that will conform to your needs and enhance your ability to cope. Ask your physician about how best to tailor an exercise program to your particular needs and goals.

3. Set a Target Frequency, Intensity, and Time (Duration) for Each Activity

The next step is to apply the FITT principle and set a starting frequency, intensity, and time (duration) for each type of activity you've chosen (see the sample in Figure 9.1 and the summary in Figure 9.2).

FIGURE 9.2

A summary of the FITT principle for the health-related components of fitness.

	Cardiorespiratory endurance training	Strength training	Flexibility training
Frequency	3–5 days per week	2–3 nonconsecutive days per week	2–3 days per week (minimum); 5–7 days per week (ideal)
Intensity	55/65–90% of maximum heart rate	Sufficient resistance to fatigue muscles	Stretch to the point of tension
Time	20–60 minutes in sessions lasting 10 minutes or more	8–12 repetitions of each exercise, 1 or more sets	2–4 repetitions of each exercise, held for 15–30 seconds
Type	Continuous rhythmic activities using large muscle groups	Resistance exercises for all major muscle groups	Stretching exercises for all major joints

Cardiorespiratory Endurance Exercise

As noted in earlier chapters, the Public Health Agency of Canada has concluded that most health benefits occur with at least 150 minutes per week of moderate-intensity physical activity (such as brisk walking) or 75 minutes per week of vigorous-intensity activity (such as jogging). Additional benefits occur with more exercise. An appropriate frequency for cardiorespiratory endurance exercise is three to five times per week. For intensity, note your target heart rate zone or RPE value (see Chapter 3). Your target total workout time (duration) should be about 20 to 60 minutes, depending on the intensity of the activity. You can exercise in a single session or in multiple sessions of 10 or more minutes. New research on high-intensity interval training suggests that you can exercise for shorter durations if you train at maximal intensities.

Fitness Tip

Want to lift weights without going to a gym? Try using resistance bands. Research shows that resistance bands are just as effective as weight machines or free weights for increasing muscular strength, especially for young women.

Muscular Strength and Endurance Training

Experts recommend doing strength training for at least two nonconsecutive days per week. As described in Chapter 4, a general fitness strength training program includes one or more sets of 8 to 12 repetitions of 8 to 10 exercises that work all major muscle groups. For intensity, choose a weight that is heavy enough to fatigue your muscles but not so heavy that you cannot complete the full number of repetitions with proper form. Exercises that use body weight for resistance also build strength and muscle endurance. A note of caution: Years of weight training can lead to stiffer blood vessels. Some studies show that doing aerobics after weight training helps to prevent blood vessel stiffening.

Flexibility Training

You should perform stretches at least two to three days per week when your muscles are warm (five to seven days per week is ideal). The stretches should work all major muscle groups. For each exercise, stretch to the point of slight tension or mild discomfort and hold the stretch for 15 to 30 seconds; do two to four repetitions of each exercise.

4. Set Up a System of Mini-Goals and Rewards

To keep your program on track, set up a system of goals and rewards. Break your specific goals into several steps, and set a target date for each step. For example, if one of the goals of an 18-year-old male student's program is to improve upper-body strength and endurance, he could use the push-up test in Lab 4.2 to set intermediate goals. If he can currently perform 15 push-ups (for a rating of "very poor"), he might set intermediate goals of 17, 20, 25, and 30 push-ups (for a final rating of "fair"). By allowing several weeks between mini-goals and specifying rewards, he'll be able to track his progress and reward himself as he moves toward his final goal. Reaching a series of small goals is more satisfying than working toward a single, more challenging goal that may take months to achieve. For more on choosing appropriate rewards, refer to Chapter 1 and Activity 4 in the Behaviour Change Workbook.

5. Include Lifestyle Physical Activity in Your Program

Daily physical activity is a simple but important way to improve your overall wellness. As part of your fitness program plan, specify ways to be more active during your daily routine, such as by taking the stairs up to class rather than taking an elevator. In addition, develop specific strategies to reduce the amount of time you spend being sedentary (see the box The Importance of Reducing Sedentary Time). You may find it helpful to first use your health journal to track your activities for several days. Review the records in your journal, identify routine opportunities to be more active, and add these to your program plan in Lab 9.1.

The Evidence *for* EXERCISE

THE IMPORTANCE OF REDUCING SEDENTARY TIME

Does a 45-minute workout make up for the effects of 8 hours of sitting time? The answer to this question appears to be no. A complete exercise program focused on the health-related components of fitness provides many benefits. But researchers have found that too much sedentary time—sitting too much—is detrimental to health, regardless of whether an individual meets the physical activity goals set by the Public Health Agency of Canada. A 2015 review found that sedentary time was associated with the following, independent of participation in physical activity:

- deaths from all causes
- cardiovascular disease
- cancer (breast, colon, colorectal, endometrial, and certain types of ovarian cancers)
- type 2 diabetes

The risk of negative outcomes from sedentary time was lower among people with higher levels of physical activity, but they were not eliminated.

How does sedentary time impact health? Although not completely understood, sedentary time is associated with markers of poor metabolic functioning, including unhealthy levels of blood glucose, insulin, and blood fats, as well as a large waist circumference. A study that looked at the impact of increased sedentary time in moderately active individuals found that sitting for more than 30 or 60 minutes at a time resulted in significantly elevated glucose and insulin levels. Sedentary time also affects blood fats and markers for inflammation. All these factors have the potential to contribute to the development of type 2 diabetes, metabolic syndrome, heart disease, and cancer.

What does this mean for an individual? Studies have found that the average American adult spends more than half their waking day in sedentary activities, such as using a computer or watching television. Luckily, evidence so far suggests that frequent breaks from sedentary time—2 minutes every 20 or 30 minutes, for example—protect against some of the impacts of sedentary time. So, it is important to take frequent breaks when you are engaged in sedentary activities, whether at work or school or during leisure time. To help stick with your plan, include your strategies as part of your overall fitness program plan.

SOURCES: Biswas, A., et al. 2015. Sedentary time and its association with risk for disease incidence, mortality, and hospitalization in adults: A systematic review and meta-analysis. *Annals of Internal Medicine* 162: 123–132; Lyden, K., et al. 2015. Discrete features of sedentary behaviors impact cardiometabolic risk factors. *Medicine and Science in Sports and Exercise* 47(5): 1079–1086; President's Council on Fitness, Sports & Nutrition. 2012. Too much sitting: Health risks of sedentary behavior and opportunities for change. *Research Digest Series* 13, Number 3.

6. Develop Tools for Monitoring Your Progress

A record that tracks your daily progress will help remind you of your ongoing commitment to your program and give you a sense of accomplishment. Figure 9.3 shows you how to create a general program log and record the activity type, frequency, and time (duration). Or if you wish, complete specific activity logs like those in Lab 3.2, Lab 4.3, and Lab 5.2 in addition to, or instead of, a general log. Post your log in a place where you'll see it often as a reminder and as an incentive for improvement. If you have specific, measurable goals, you can also graph your weekly or monthly progress toward your goal (Figure 9.4). To monitor the overall progress of your fitness program, you may choose to reassess your fitness every three months or so during the improvement phase of your program. Because the results of different fitness tests vary, be sure to compare results for the same assessments over time.

FIGURE 9.3

A sample program log.

Name   Tracie Kaufman

Enter time, distance, or another factor (such as heart rate or perceived exertion) to track your progress.

Activity/Date	M	Tu	W	Th	F	Sa	Su	Weekly Total	M	Tu	W	Th	F	Sa	Su	Weekly Total
1 Swimming	730 m		660 m		730 m			2125 m	730 m		730 m		775 m			2240 m
2 Tennis					90 min			90 min						95 min		95 min
3 Weight Training		X		X		X				X		X			X	
4 Stretching	X		X		X	X			X			X	X	X	X	

FIGURE 9.4

A sample program progress chart.

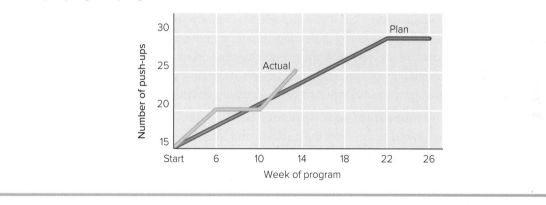

---

7. Make a Commitment

Your final step in planning your program is to make a commitment by signing a contract. Find a witness for your contract—preferably one who will be actively involved in your program. Keep your contract in a visible spot to remind you of your commitment.

LO2 9.2 Putting Your Plan into Action

After you've developed a detailed plan and signed your agreement, you are ready to begin your fitness program. Refer to the specific training suggestions provided in Chapters 2 to 5 for advice on beginning and maintaining your program. Many people find it easier to plan a program than to put their plan into action and stick with it over time. For that reason, adherence to healthy lifestyle programs has become an important area of study for psychologists and health researchers. The guidelines below and in the next section reflect research into strategies that help people succeed in sticking with an exercise program.

- **Start slowly and increase fitness gradually**. Overzealous exercising can result in discouraging discomforts and injuries. Your program is meant to last a lifetime. The important first step is to break your established pattern of inactivity. Be patient and realistic. Once your body has adjusted to your starting level of exercise, slowly increase the amount of overload. Small increases are the key—achieving a large number of small improvements will eventually result in substantial gains in fitness. It's usually best to increase duration and frequency before increasing intensity.

- **Find an exercise buddy**. The social side of exercise is an important factor for many regular exercisers. Working out with a friend will make exercise more enjoyable and increase your chances of sticking with your program. Find an exercise partner who shares your goals and general fitness level. On days when a partner isn't available, a Smartphone or MP3 player can be your workout buddy; see the box Digital Motivation for more information.

- **Ask for support from others**. Consistent exercise requires the support of important people in your life, such as parents, spouse, partner, and friends. Talk with them about your program, and let them know the importance of exercise and wellness in your life. Exercise needs to be a critical component of your day—just like sleeping and eating. Good communication will help others become more supportive of and enthusiastic about the time you spend on your wellness program.

- **Vary your activities**. You can make your program more fun over the long term if you participate in a variety of different activities that you enjoy. You can also add interest by using strategies such as varying the routes you take when walking, finding a new tennis or racquetball partner, or switching to a new volleyball or basketball court. Varying your activities, a strategy known as *cross-training*, has other benefits. It can help you develop balanced, total body fitness. For example, by alternating running with swimming, you build both upper- and lower-body strength. Cross-training can reduce the risk of injury and overtraining because the same muscles, bones, and joints are not continuously subjected to the stresses of the same activity. You can cross-train by either choosing different activities on different days or by alternating activities within a single workout.

- **Cycle the duration and intensity of your workouts**. Olympic athletes use a training technique called *periodization of training*, meaning they vary the duration and intensity of their workouts. Sometimes they exercise very intensely; at other times they train lightly or rest. You can use the same technique to improve fitness more quickly and make your training program more varied and enjoyable. For example, if your program consists of walking, weight training, and stretching, pick one day a week for each activity to train a little harder or longer than you normally do. If you usually walk 3 kilometres at 10 minutes per kilometre, increase the pace to 9 minutes per kilometre once a week. If you lift weights twice a week, train more intensely during one of the workouts by using more resistance or performing multiple sets.

- **Adapt to changing environments and schedules**. Most people are creatures of habit and have trouble adjusting to change. Don't use bad weather or a new job as an excuse to give up your exercise program. If you walk in the summer, put on a warm coat and walk in the winter. If you can't go out because of darkness, join a gym and walk on a treadmill. Review the results of Lab 2.2 on overcoming barriers to activity to develop additional strategies.

- **Expect fluctuations and lapses**. On some days your progress will be excellent, but on others you'll barely be able to drag yourself through your scheduled activities. Don't let off-days or lapses discourage you or make you feel guilty. Instead, feel a renewed commitment for your fitness program (see the box Getting Your Fitness Program Back on Track on page 410).

- **Choose other healthy lifestyle behaviours**. Exercise provides huge benefits for your health, but other behaviours are also important. Choose a nutritious diet, and avoid harmful habits like smoking and overconsumption of alcohol. Be sure to stay hydrated with water or other healthy beverages (see the box Choosing Healthy Beverages on the next page). Don't skimp on sleep, which has a mutually beneficial relationship with exercise. Physical activity improves sleep, and adequate sleep can improve physical performance.

Wellness *in the* DIGITAL AGE

DIGITAL MOTIVATION

If you ever have trouble getting inspired to work out, motivation may be as close as your Smartphone.

Since the iPhone's advent, dozens of interactive motivational applications (apps) have been developed for use on smart cellphones. Coaching and motivational recordings are available for use on MP3 players as well. These apps and recordings can substitute for an exercise partner when your workout buddy isn't around and can inspire you to keep your program on track. Some Smartphone apps can monitor your workouts, track your progress, and even provide on-the-spot coaching to help you keep going.

The following are just a few examples of low-cost or free Smartphone apps that can help you keep exercising.

- **Nike Training Club.** This training app designs programs according to your goals and experience. Goals include "get lean"—high-intensity cardio exercise to promote weight loss; "get toned"—light weight training and interval training; "get strong"—weight training to build strength and muscle mass; and "get focused"—15-minute workouts that target specific areas of the body. The app shows specific exercises, paces, and repetitions for the person exercising. It also has tools for motivating you to exercise, such as workout music and a clock that keeps track of the workout time. It is a digital personal trainer at an affordable price.
- **The "Fu" series.** Featuring titles like "CrunchFu" and "PushupFu," each app in this series focuses on one type of exercise and motivates you to excel at it. Using the motion sensors built into your Smartphone, these apps can count your reps and monitor your speed as you exercise. A built-in coach offers suggestions and can challenge you to improve your performance.
- **Cyclemeter.** Use this highly motivational app for cycling, running, and walking. It brings detailed statistics to your workouts by keeping track of peak and average speed, caloric expenditure, rest times, elevation changes, and environmental conditions. You can store the results on the cloud or email them to yourself, friends, or social media. You can also integrate the app with a heart rate monitor. The GPS function gives you a map or satellite view of your route.
- **Endomondo.** This app uses GPS to keep track of routes used during running, walking, cycling, skating, or cross-country skiing. It also helps people share their workouts with social media, which promotes social accountability as a way to stick with the program.
- **NexTrack.** Track exercise and weight loss with this app and win "mPoints" for completing workouts. Many apps award mPoints for using their products, and you can cash them in for gift cards to companies such as Amazon. Several studies have found that rewards such as money or gift cards are effective for helping people with their fitness or weight loss goals.

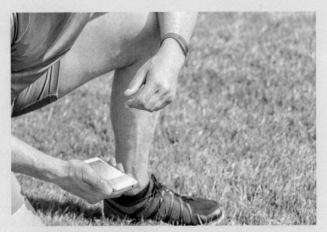

© mezzotint_alamy / Alamy Stock Photo

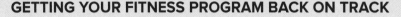

Take CHARGE

GETTING YOUR FITNESS PROGRAM BACK ON TRACK

Lapses are a normal part of any behaviour change program. The important point is to move on and avoid becoming discouraged. Try again, and keep trying. Know that continued effort will lead to success. Here are some tips to help you keep going:

- Don't judge yourself harshly, especially in comparison with others. Some people make faster gains in fitness than others. Focus on the improvements you've already obtained from your program and how good you feel after exercise—both physically and mentally.
- Visualize what it will be like to reach your goals. Keep these pictures in your mind as an incentive to stick with your program.
- Use your exercise journal to identify thoughts and behaviours that are causing noncompliance. Devise strategies to combat these problematic patterns. If needed, make additional changes in your environment or obtain more social support. For example, call a friend to walk with you, or keep exercise clothes in your car or backpack.
- Make changes in your plan and reward system to help renew your enthusiasm and commitment to your program. Try changing fitness activities or your exercise schedule. Build in more opportunities to reward yourself.
- Plan ahead for difficult situations. Think about what circumstances might make it tough to keep up your fitness routine. Develop strategies to increase your chances of sticking with your program. For example, figure out ways to continue your program during vacation, travel, bad weather, and so on.
- If you're in a bad mood or just don't feel like exercising, remind yourself that physical activity is probably the one thing you can do that will make you feel better. Even if you can only do half your scheduled workout, you'll boost your energy, improve your mood, and help keep your program on track.

Strengthening Mental Wellness

How do you typically deal with setbacks? For example, if you have trouble getting motivated to study for exams, what strategies do you use to get back on track? Could those strategies work for keeping your fitness program moving forward? If so, how?

In FOCUS

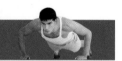

CHOOSING HEALTHY BEVERAGES

As discussed in other chapters, it's important to stay hydrated at all times, but especially when you are exercising. Too little water intake can leave you feeling fatigued, reduce your body's performance, and leave you vulnerable to heat-related sicknesses in hot weather. But *what* you drink is as significant as how much you drink, both when you are exercising and when you are going about your normal routine.

The Great Water Controversy

Wherever you see people exercising, you will see bottled water in abundance. For several years, a debate has been raging about the quality and safety of commercially bottled water. Recently, evidence has emerged showing that most bottled waters are no better for you than regular tap water, and some bottled waters may actually be bad for you. To make matters worse, bottled water costs up to 1900 times more than tap water.

In a 2011 analysis of 173 bottled water products, the Environmental Working Group found 38 different contaminants in ten popular brands of bottled water. Contaminants included heavy metals such as arsenic, pharmaceutical residues and other pollutants commonly found in urban wastewater, and a variety of industrial chemicals. Bottled-water companies are notoriously secretive about their products. Overall, 18% of bottled waters fail to list the location of their source, and 32% disclose nothing about the treatment or purity of the water.

Many commercially bottled water products are, in fact, tap water drawn from municipal water systems. Such revelations have caused some bottlers to put statements on their products' labels, identifying them as having been drawn from a standard water supply. These products, priced many times higher than water from a residential tap, provide no benefit over standard tap water.

An even bigger issue is that plastic water bottles have become a huge environmental problem, with billions of bottles now filling landfills and floating in the world's oceans. Some types of plastic take years to biodegrade, and many kinds of plastic bottles will never decompose at all. Newer types of plastic bottles can decompose significantly faster than older bottles, but fast-degrading plastics have not yet come into widespread use in the bottled-water industry.

Experts say that when you're exercising, the cheapest and safest way to stay hydrated is to drink filtered tap water. If you need to carry water with you, buy a reusable container (preferably made of stainless steel) that can be cleaned after each use. If you drink from plastic bottles, be sure they are recyclable and dispose of them by recycling.

Other Choices

Instead of water, many people choose to drink carbonated beverages, juice, tea, or flavoured water. While these kinds of beverages have their place, it's important not to drink them too often or in large amounts, especially if they are high in sugar or caffeine. Sugary drinks add empty calories to your diet, and caffeine is a psychoactive drug with a variety of side effects.

Regular (nondiet) carbonated beverages are now one of the leading sources of calories in the Canadian diet. Most people don't count the calories from beverages as part of their daily caloric intake, leading them to underestimate their total intake. For this reason and others, many experts believe that soft drink consumption is a major factor in the increasing levels of obesity, metabolic syndrome, diabetes, and other chronic diseases among North Americans.

If you're concerned that the liquid portion of your diet is not as healthy as it should be, choose water, fat-free milk, or unsweetened herbal tea more often. Avoid regular carbonated beverages, sweetened bottled ice tea, flavoured water, and fruit beverages made with little fruit juice. To make water more appealing, try adding slices of citrus fruit with sparkling water. With some imagination, you can make sure you stay hydrated without consuming excess calories, spending money unnecessarily, or hurting the environment.

SOURCE: Adapted from Leiba, N., et al. 2011. The Environmental Working Group's 2011 Bottled Water Scorecard (https://static.ewg.org/reports/2010/bottledwater2010/pdf/2011-bottledwater-scorecard-report.pdf, retrieved April 5, 2011).

LO3 9.3 Exercise Guidelines for Life Stages

A fitness program may need to be adjusted to accommodate the requirements of different life stages.

Children and Adolescents

Only 7% of Canadian children and youth between the ages of 5 and 17 years are physically active enough to meet Canada's Physical Activity Guidelines of at least 60 minutes of moderate to vigorous physical activity per day.[2] Lack of physical activity has led to alarming increases in overweight and obesity in children and adolescents. If you have children or are in a position to influence children, keep these guidelines in mind:

- Provide opportunities for children and adolescents to exercise every day. Minimize sedentary activities, such as watching television or computer use. Children and adolescents should aim for 60 minutes of moderate activity every day.

- During family outings, choose dynamic activities. For example, go for a walk, or park away from a mall and then walk to the stores.

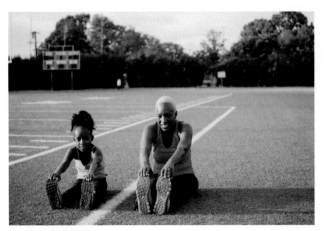

© Shestock / Blend Images LLC

People of all ages benefit from exercise. Simply by playing actively with their children, parents can set a positive example that will lead to a lifetime of physical activity.

- For children younger than 12 years, emphasize skill development and fitness rather than excellence in competitive sports. For adolescents, combine participation and training in lifetime sports with traditional, competitive sports.

- Make sure children are developmentally capable of participating in an activity. For example, catching skills are difficult for young children because their nervous system is not developed enough to fully master the skill. Gradually increase the complexity of the skill once the child has mastered the simpler skill.

- Make sure children get plenty of water when exercising in the heat. Make sure they are dressed properly when doing sports in the cold.

Pregnancy

Exercise is important during pregnancy, but women should be cautious because some types of exercise can pose increased risk to the mother and the unborn child. Pregnant women should consider these guidelines when exercising:

- See your physician about possible modifications needed for your particular pregnancy.

- Continue mild-to-moderate exercise routines at least three times a week (for most women, this means maintaining an exercise heart rate of 100 to 160 beats per minute). Avoid exercising vigorously or to exhaustion, especially in the third trimester. Monitor exercise intensity by assessing how you feel rather than by monitoring your heart rate; RPE levels of 11 to 13 are appropriate.

- Favour non- or low-weight-bearing exercises such as swimming or cycling over weight-bearing exercises, which can carry increased risk of injury.

- Avoid exercise in a supine position—lying on your back—after the first trimester. This position restricts blood flow to the uterus. Also avoid prolonged periods of motionless standing.

- Avoid exercise that could cause loss of balance, especially in the third trimester, and exercise that might injure the abdomen, stress the joints, or carry a risk of falling (such as contact sports, vigorous racquet sports, skiing, and in-line skating).

- Avoid activities involving extremes in barometric pressure, such as scuba diving and mountain climbing.

- Especially during the first trimester, drink plenty of fluids and exercise in well-ventilated areas to avoid heat stress.

- Do three to five sets of 10 Kegel exercises daily. These exercises involve tightening the muscles of the pelvic floor for 5 to 15 seconds. Kegel exercises are thought to help prevent incontinence (involuntary loss of urine) and speed recovery after giving birth.

- After giving birth, resume pre-pregnancy exercise routines gradually, based on how you feel.

Older Adults

Older people readily adapt to endurance exercise and strength training. Exercise principles are the same as for younger people, but the following specific guidelines apply:

- The Public Health Agency and CSEP recommend that older adults (those over 65 years of age) take part in at least 2.5 hours of moderate- to vigorous-intensity aerobic activity each week.

- For strength training, it is recommended that older adults add bone and muscle strengthening activities involving the major muscle groups at least twice each week.

- Older adults should perform flexibility exercises at least two days per week for at least 10 minutes. Exercises that improve balance should also be performed two days per week.

- Drink plenty of water and avoid exercising in excessively hot or cold environments. Wear clothes that speed heat loss in warm environments and that prevent heat loss in cold environments.

- Warm up slowly and carefully. Increase intensity and duration of exercise gradually.

- Cool down slowly, continuing very light exercise until the heart rate is below 100 beats per minute.

- If you have physical disabilities or limitations and cannot meet the recommendation of at least 150 minutes per week of moderate-intensity exercise, do as much exercise as you can.

Tips for Today and the Future

A complete fitness program includes activities to build and maintain cardiorespiratory endurance, muscular strength and endurance, and flexibility.

RIGHT NOW YOU CAN

- Get a journal to track your daily physical activity and exercise routine.
- Put away your remote control devices—every bit of physical activity can benefit your health.
- Set a firm time for your next workout with your training partner.
- Plan to go to bed 15 minutes earlier than usual.

IN THE FUTURE YOU CAN

- Create a schedule that incorporates your workouts into your daily routine. Each week, update the schedule for the upcoming week.

- Learn more about the importance of sleep to good health. If you consistently have trouble sleeping, consult with your physician about seeing a sleep specialist or undergoing a sleep evaluation.

Common Questions ANSWERED

Q Should I exercise every day?

A Some daily exercise is beneficial, and health experts recommend that you engage in at least 30 minutes of moderate physical activity at least five days per week. However, if you train intensely every day without giving yourself a rest, you will likely injure yourself or overtrain. When strength training, for example, rest at least 48 hours between workouts before exercising the same muscle group. For cardiorespiratory endurance exercise, rest or exercise lightly the day after an intense or long-duration workout. Balancing the proper amount of rest and exercise will help you feel better and improve your fitness faster.

Q I'm just starting an exercise program. How much activity should I do at first?

A Be conservative. Walking is a good way to begin almost any fitness program. At first, walk for about 10 minutes, and then increase the distance and pace. After several weeks, progress to something more vigorous. Let your body be your guide. If the intensity and duration of a workout seem easy, increase them a little the next time. The key is to be progressive; don't try to achieve physical fitness in one or two workouts. Build your fitness gradually.

SUMMARY

- Steps for putting together a complete fitness program include: (1) setting realistic goals; (2) selecting activities to develop all the health-related components of fitness; (3) setting a target frequency, intensity, and time (duration) for each activity; (4) setting up a system of mini-goals and rewards; (5) making lifestyle physical activity a part of the daily routine; (6) developing tools for monitoring progress; and (7) making a commitment.

- In selecting activities, consider fun and interest, your current skill and fitness levels, time and convenience, cost, and any special health concerns.

- Keys to beginning and maintaining a successful program include starting slowly, increasing intensity and duration gradually, finding a buddy, varying the activities and intensity of the program, and expecting fluctuations and lapses.

- Regular exercise is appropriate and highly beneficial for people in all stages of life, although program modifications may be necessary for safety.

FOR FURTHER EXPLORATION

Organizations and Websites

Canadian Orthopaedic Association. Provides information about injury care and treatment as well as resources for professionals.

http://coa-aco.org/

Healthy Active Kids Canada. Includes resources and information on active children and promotes increased physical activity participation in Canadian children.

http://activehealthykids.ca/

ParticipAction Canada. Promotes ways to include physical activity in any lifestyle.

http://www.participaction.com/en-us/Get-Moving/Easy-Ways-To-Start.aspx

The Society of Obstetricians and Gynaecologists of Canada. Provides guidelines for promoting healthy pregnancy and postpartum recovery, including exercise during pregnancy.

https://sogc.org/

The following sections present sample programs based on different types of cardiorespiratory activities—walking/jogging/running and calisthenics circuit training. Each sample program includes regular cardiorespiratory endurance exercise, resistance training, and stretching. Read the descriptions of the programs you're considering, and decide which will work best for you based on your present routine, the potential for enjoyment, and adaptability to your lifestyle. If you choose one of these programs, complete the personal fitness program plan in Lab 9.1, just as if you had created a program from scratch.

No program will produce enormous changes in your fitness level in the first few weeks. Follow the specifics of the program for three to four weeks. Then if the exercise program doesn't seem suitable, make adjustments to adapt it to your particular needs. But retain the basic elements of the program that make it effective for developing fitness.

GENERAL GUIDELINES

The following guidelines can help make the activity programs more effective for you:

- **Frequency and time**. Exercise for 20 to 60 minutes at least three times a week to experience training effects.

- **Intensity**. To work effectively for cardiorespiratory endurance training or to improve body composition, you must raise your heart rate into its target zone. Monitor your pulse or use rates of perceived exertion (RPE) to monitor your intensity. If you've been sedentary, begin very slowly. Give your muscles a chance to adjust to their increased workload. It's probably best to keep your heart rate below target until your body has had time to adjust to new demands. At first you may not need to work very hard to keep your heart rate in its target zone, but as your cardiorespiratory endurance improves, you will probably need to increase intensity.

- **Interval training**. Some of the sample programs provided involve continuous activity. Others rely on interval training, which calls for alternating a relief interval with exercise (walking after jogging, for example, or coasting after biking uphill). Interval training is an effective way of progressive overload and improves fitness rapidly (see Chapter 3).

- **Resistance training and stretching guidelines**. For the resistance training and stretching parts of the program, remember the general guidelines for safe and effective exercise. See the summary of FITT principle guidelines in Figure 9.2.

- **Warm-up and cool-down**. Begin each exercise session with a 10-minute warm-up. Begin your activity at a slow pace and work up gradually to your target heart rate. Always slow down gradually at the end of your exercise session to bring your system back to its normal state. It's a good idea to do stretching exercises to increase your flexibility after cardiorespiratory exercise or strength training because your muscles will be warm and ready to stretch. More information regarding warm-up and cool-down are included in Chapter 2. Follow the guidelines presented in Chapter 3 for exercising in hot or cold weather. Drink enough liquids to stay adequately hydrated, particularly in hot weather.

- **Record keeping**. After each exercise session, record your daily distance or time on a progress chart.

WALKING/JOGGING/RUNNING SAMPLE PROGRAM

Walking is the perfect exercise. It increases longevity, builds fitness, expends calories, prevents weight gain, and protects against heart disease, stroke, and back pain. You don't need to join a gym, and you can walk almost anywhere. People who walk 30 minutes five times per week will lose an average of 2.5 kilograms in 6 to 12 months—without dieting, watching what they eat, or exercising intensely.

Jogging takes walking to the next level. Jogging only 75 minutes per week will increase fitness, promote weight control, and provide health benefits that will prevent disease and increase longevity. Your ultimate goal for promoting wellness is to walk at a moderate intensity for 150 to 300 minutes per week or jog at 70% effort or more for 75 to 150 minutes per week.

It isn't always easy to distinguish among walking, jogging, and running. For clarity and consistency, we'll consider walking to be any on-foot exercise of less than 8 kilometres per hour, jogging to be any pace between 8 and 12 kilometres per hour, and running to be any pace faster than that. The faster your pace or the longer you exercise, the more calories you burn (see Table 1). The greater the number of calories burned, the higher the potential training effects of these activities. Table 2 (on the next page) provides a sample walking/jogging fitness program.

Equipment and Technique

These activities require no special skills, expensive equipment, or unusual facilities. Comfortable clothing, well-fitted walking or running shoes (see Chapter 3), and a stopwatch or ordinary watch with a second hand are all you need.

When you advance to jogging, use proper technique as outlined below:

- Run with your back straight and your head up. Look straight ahead, not at your feet. Shift your pelvis forward and tuck your buttocks in.

- Hold your arms slightly away from your body. Your elbows should be bent so your forearms are parallel to the ground. You may cup your hands, but do not clench your fists. Allow your arms to swing loosely and rhythmically with each stride.

- Let your heel hit the ground first in each stride. Then roll forward onto the ball of your foot and push off for the next stride. If you find this difficult, you can try a more flat-footed style, but don't land on

TABLE 1

Estimated Calories Expended by a 75 kilogram (165-pound) Adult at Different Intensities of Walking and Running for 150 and 300 minutes per week (min/wk)

	Speed (Kilometres per Hour)	Speed (Minutes per Kilometre)	Calories Expended Exercising 150 Min/Wk	Calories Expended Exercising 300 Min/Wk
	Rest	—	190	380
Walking	6.5	9.0	565	1130
	7.8	7.6	620	1240
	10.4	5.8	940	1880
	11.2	5.4	1125	2250
Jogging/Running	13.0	4.6	1500	3000
	15.6	3.8	1875	3750
	18.2	3.3	2155	4310
	20.8	2.6	2530	5060
	26.0	2.3	3000	6000

NOTE: Heavier people will expend slightly more calories, while lighter people will expend slightly fewer.

SOURCE: Adapted from Physical Activity Guidelines Advisory Committee. 2008. *Physical Activity Guidelines Advisory Committee Report, 2008*. Washington, DC: U.S. Department of Health and Human Services.

TABLE 2

Sample Walking/Jogging Fitness Program

Day	Activities
Monday	• **Walking/Jogging:** Walk briskly for 30 minutes or jog for 25 minutes.
	• **Stretching:** Stretch major muscle groups for 10 minutes after exercise. Do each exercise 2 times; hold stretch for 15–30 seconds.
Tuesday	• **Resistance workout:** Using body weight for resistance, perform the following exercises: • Push-ups: 2 sets, 20 reps per set • Pull-ups: 2 sets, 5 reps per set • Unloaded squats: 2 sets, 10 reps per set • Curl-ups: 2 sets, 20 reps per set • Side bridges: 3 sets, 10-second hold (left and right sides) • Spine extensions: 3 sets, 10-second hold (left and right sides)
Wednesday	• Repeat Monday activities.
Thursday	• Repeat Tuesday activities.
Friday	• Repeat Monday activities.
Saturday	• **Rest**
Sunday	• **Rest**

the balls of your feet. More of a forefoot landing is recommended in barefoot running or with minimal footwear.

• Keep your steps short by allowing your foot to strike the ground in line with your knee. Keep your knees bent at all times.

• Breathe deeply through your mouth. Try to use your abdominal muscles rather than just your chest muscles to take deep breaths.

• Stay relaxed.

Find a safe, convenient place to walk or jog. Exercise on a trail, path, or sidewalk to stay clear of bicycles and cars. Make sure your clothes are brightly coloured so others can see you easily.

Developing Cardiorespiratory Endurance

The four variations of the basic walking/jogging/running sample program that follow are designed to help you regulate the intensity, duration, and frequency of your program. Use the following guidelines to choose the variation that is right for you:

• **Variation 1: Walking (Starting).** Choose this program if you have medical restrictions, are recovering from illness or surgery, tire easily after short walks, are obese, or have a sedentary lifestyle, and if you want to prepare for the advanced walking program to improve cardiorespiratory endurance, body composition, and muscular endurance.

• **Variation 2: Advanced Walking.** Choose this program if you already can walk comfortably for 30 minutes and if you want to develop and maintain cardiorespiratory fitness, a lean body, and muscular endurance.

• **Variation 3: Preparing for a Jogging Program.** Choose this program if you already can walk comfortably for 30 minutes and if you want to prepare for the jogging/running program to improve cardiorespiratory endurance, body composition, and muscular endurance.

- **Variation 4: Jogging/Running.** Choose this program if you already can jog comfortably without muscular discomfort, if you already can jog for 15 minutes without stopping or 30 minutes with brief walking intervals within your target heart rate range, and if you want to develop and maintain a high level of cardiorespiratory fitness, a lean body, and muscular endurance.

Variation 1: Walking (Starting)

FIT—frequency, intensity, and time.   Walk for 15 minutes at a pace that keeps your heart rate below your target zone. Gradually increase to 30-minute sessions. You will probably travel a distance of 2 to 4 kilometres. At the beginning, walk every other day. You can gradually increase to daily walking if you want to burn more calories (which is helpful if you want to change body composition).

Calorie cost.   Work up to using 90 to 135 calories in each session (see Table 1). To increase calorie costs to the target level, walk for a longer time or for a longer distance rather than sharply increasing speed.

Beginning a walking/jogging program.   Start slowly if you have not been exercising, are overweight, or are recovering from an illness or surgery. At first, walk for 15 minutes at a slow pace, below your target heart rate zone. Gradually increase to 30-minute sessions. You will probably cover 1.5 to 3 kilometres. At the beginning, walk every other day.

You can gradually increase to walking each day of the week if you want to expend more calories (which is helpful if you want to change body composition). Depending upon your weight, you will expend ("burn") 90 to 135 calories during each 30-minute walking session. To increase the calories that you expend, walk for a longer time or for a longer distance instead of sharply increasing speed.

Start at the level of effort that is most comfortable for you. Maintain a normal, easy pace and stop to rest as often as you need to. Never prolong a walk past the point of comfort. When walking with a friend (a good motivator), let a comfortable conversation be your guide to pace. If you find that you cannot carry on a conversation without getting out of breath, then you are walking too quickly.

Once your muscles have become adjusted to the exercise program, increase the duration of your sessions by no more than 10% each week. Keep your heart rate just below your target zone. Don't be discouraged by a lack of immediate progress, and don't try to speed things up by overdoing it. Remember that pace and heart rate can vary with the terrain, the weather, and other factors.

Variation 2: Advanced Walking

Advanced walking involves walking more quickly for longer times. You should feel an increased perception of effort, but the exercise intensity should not be too stressful. Vary your pace to allow for intervals of slow, medium, and fast walking. Keep your heart rate toward the lower end of your target zone with brief periods in the upper levels. At first, walk for 30 minutes and increase your walking time gradually until eventually you reach 60 minutes at a brisk pace and can walk 3 to 6.5 kilometres. Try to walk at least five days per week. Vary your program by changing the pace and distance or by walking routes with different terrains and views. You can expect to burn 200 to 350 calories or more during each advanced walking session.

Variation 3: Preparing for a Jogging Program

Increase the intensity of exercise by gradually introducing jogging into your walking program. During a 3-kilometre walk, for example, periodically jog for 100 metres and then resume walking. Increase the number and distance of your jogging segments until you can jog continuously for the entire distance. More physically fit people may be capable of jogging without walking first. However, people unaccustomed to jogging should initially combine walking with short bouts of jogging.

A good strategy is to exercise on a 400-metre track at a local high school or university. Begin by jogging the straight-aways and walking the turns for 800 metres (two laps). Progress to walking 200 metres (half a lap) and jogging 200 metres; jogging 400 metres and walking 200 metres; jogging 800 metres and walking 800 metres; and jogging 1200 metres and walking 400 metres. Continue until you can run 3 kilometres without stopping.

Variation 4: Jogging/Running

During the transition to jogging, adjust the ratio of walking to jogging to keep within your target heart rate zone as much as possible. Most people who sustain a continuous jog/run program will find that they can stay within their target heart rate zone with a speed of 9 to 12 kilometres per hour (5 to 7 minutes per kilometre). Exercise at least every other day. Increasing frequency by doing other activities on alternate days will place less stress on the weight-bearing parts of your lower body than will a daily program of jogging/running.

Developing Muscular Strength and Endurance and Flexibility

Walking, jogging, and running provide muscular endurance workouts for your lower body; they also develop muscular strength of the lower body to a lesser degree. If you'd like to increase your running speed and performance, you might want to focus your program on lower-body exercises. (Don't neglect upper-body strength; it is important for overall wellness.) For flexibility, pay special attention to the hamstrings and quadriceps, which are not worked through their complete range of motion during walking or jogging.

Staying with Your Walking/Jogging Program

Health experts have found that simple motivators such as using a pedometer, walking a dog, parking farther from the office or grocery store, or training for a fun run helps people stay with their programs. Use a pedometer or GPS exercise device to track your progress and help motivate you to increase distance and speed. Accurate pedometers for walking, such as those made by Omron, Yamax, and New Lifestyles, cost $20 to $40 and are accurate to about 5%. Sophisticated GPS-based devices made by Polar and Garmin keep track of your exercise speed and distance via satellite, monitor heart rate, and store data that can be downloaded wirelessly to your computer. Several of these units can be plugged into programs such as Google Earth, which can give you a satellite view of your walking or jogging route.

A pedometer can also help you increase the number of steps you walk each day. Most sedentary people take only 2000 to 3000 steps per day. Adding 1000 steps per day and increasing gradually until you reach 10 000 steps can increase fitness and help you manage your weight. Once you reach 10 000 steps, continue to increase the effectiveness of those steps by reducing the time it takes to complete them!

BICYCLING SAMPLE PROGRAM

Bicycling can also lead to large gains in physical fitness. For many people, cycling is a pleasant and economical alternative to driving and a convenient way to build fitness.

Equipment and Technique

Cycling has its own special array of equipment, including helmets, lights, safety gear, and biking shoes. The bike is the most expensive item, ranging from about $100 to $1000 or more. Avoid making a large investment until you're sure you'll use your bike regularly. While investigating what the marketplace has to offer, rent or borrow a bike. Consider your intended use of the bike. Most cyclists who are interested primarily in fitness are best served by a sturdy 10-speed rather than a mountain bike or sport bike. Stationary cycles are good for rainy days and areas that have harsh winters.

Clothing for bike riding shouldn't be restrictive or binding; nor should it be so loose that it catches the wind and slows you down. Shirts that wick moisture away from your skin and padded biking shorts make a ride more comfortable. Wear glasses or goggles to protect your eyes from dirt, small objects, and irritation from wind. Wear a pair of well-padded gloves if your hands tend to become numb while riding or if you begin to develop blisters or calluses.

To avoid saddle soreness and injury, choose a soft or padded saddle, and adjust it to a height that allows your legs to almost reach full extension while pedaling. To prevent backache and neck strain, warm up thoroughly and periodically shift the position of your hands on the handlebars and your body in the saddle. Keep your arms relaxed and don't lock your elbows. To protect your knees from strain, pedal with your feet pointed straight ahead or very slightly inward, and don't pedal in high gear for long periods.

Bike riding requires a number of precise skills that become automatic through practice. If you've never ridden before, consider taking a course. In fact, many courses are not just for beginners; they'll help you develop skills in braking, shifting, and handling emergencies, as well as teach you ways of caring for and repairing your bike. For safe cycling, follow these rules:

- Always wear a helmet.

- Keep on the correct side of the road. Bicycling against traffic is usually illegal and always dangerous.

- Obey all the same traffic signs and signals that apply to autos.

- On public roads, ride in single file, except in low-traffic areas (if the law permits). Ride in a straight line; don't swerve or weave in traffic.

- Be alert; anticipate the movements of other traffic and pedestrians. Listen for approaching traffic that is out of your line of vision.

- Slow down at street crossings. Check both ways before crossing.

- Use hand signals—the same as for automobile drivers—if you intend to stop or turn. Use audible signals to warn those in your path.

- Maintain full control. Avoid anything that interferes with your vision. Don't jeopardize your ability to steer by carrying anything (including people) on the handlebars.

- Keep your bicycle in good shape. Brakes, gears, saddle, wheels, and tires should always be in good condition.

- See and be seen. Use a headlight at night and equip your bike with rear reflectors. Use side reflectors on pedals, front and rear. Wear light-coloured clothing or use reflective tape at night; wear bright colours or use fluorescent tape by day.

- Be courteous to other road users. Anticipate the worst and practise preventive cycling.

- Use a rear-view mirror.

Developing Cardiorespiratory Endurance

Cycling is an excellent way to develop and maintain cardiorespiratory endurance and a healthy body composition.

FIT—frequency, intensity, and time.   If you've been inactive for a long time, begin your cycling program at a heart rate that is 10–20% below your target zone. Beginning cyclists should pedal at about 80 to 100 revolutions per minute; adjust the gear so you can pedal at that rate easily. You can equip your bicycle with a cycling computer that displays different types of useful information, such as speed, distance travelled, heart rate, altitude, and revolutions per minute.

Once you feel at home on your bike, try cycling 1 kilometre at a comfortable speed, and then stop and check your heart rate. Increase your speed gradually until you can cycle at 20 to 25 kilometres per hour (2.5 to 3 minutes per kilometre), a speed fast enough to bring most new cyclists' heart rate into their target zone. Allow your pulse rate to be your guide: More highly fit individuals may need to ride faster to achieve their target heart rate. Cycling three days a week for at least 20 minutes will improve your fitness.

Beginning a bicycling program.   It may require several outings to get the muscles and joints of your legs and hips adjusted to this new activity. Begin each outing with a 10-minute warm-up. When your muscles are warm, stretch your hamstrings and your back and neck muscles. Until you become a skilled cyclist, select routes with the fewest hazards and avoid heavy automobile traffic.

As you progress.   Interval training is also effective with bicycling. Simply increase your speed for periods of 4 to 8 minutes or for specific distances, such as 2 to 3 kilometres. Then coast for 2 to 3 minutes. Alternate the speed intervals and slow intervals for a total of 20 to 60 minutes, depending on your level of fitness. Biking over hilly terrain is also a form of interval training.

Developing Muscular Strength and Endurance and Flexibility

Bicycling develops a high level of endurance and a moderate level of strength in the muscles of the lower body. If one of your goals is to increase your cycling speed and performance, be sure to include exercises for the quadriceps, hamstrings, and buttocks muscles in your strength training program. For flexibility, pay special attention to the hamstrings and quadriceps, which are not worked through their complete range of motion during bike riding, and to the muscles in your lower back, shoulders, and neck.

SWIMMING SAMPLE PROGRAM

Swimming works every major muscle group in the body. It increases upper-and lower-body strength, promotes cardiovascular fitness, and is excellent for rehabilitating athletic injuries and preventing day-to-day aches and pains. It promotes weight control; builds powerful lungs, heart, and blood vessels; and promotes metabolic health. People weigh only 2 to 2.5 kilograms in the water, so swimming places less stress on the knees, hips, and back than jogging, hiking, volleyball, or basketball.

Swimming is one of the most popular recreational and competitive sports in the world. Over a million Canadians swim regularly and swimming ranked third (behind golf and hockey) in a StatsCan study of most-practised sports. You don't need a backyard pool to swim. Almost every town and city in Canada has a public pool. Pools are standard in many health clubs, YMCAs/YWCAs, and schools. Ocean and lake swimming may be options in the summer. High-tech wet suits make it possible to swim outdoors even in the middle of winter in many parts of the country.

Training Methods

Improved fitness from swimming depends on the quantity, quality, and frequency of training. Most swimmers use interval training to increase swimming fitness, speed, and endurance. Interval training calls for repeated fast swims at fixed distances followed by rest. Continuous distance or endurance training builds stamina and mental toughness. Interval and distance training each play important and different roles in improving fitness for swimming. Interval training improves overall swimming speed and the ability to swim fast at the beginning of a swim. Endurance training helps to maintain a faster average pace during a swim without becoming overly fatigued. Endurance training becomes more important when you want to compete in long open-water swims or triathlons.

In swimming workouts, however, quality is better than quantity. Thirty years ago, elite swimmers from East Germany sometimes swam as much as 20 000 metres in a single workout (more than 12 miles). Recent studies found that competitive athletes who swam 4000 to 6000 metres per workout produced results similar to those who swam much farther. Likewise, recreational swimmers can improve fitness, strength, and power by swimming 1000 to 2000 metres (about 1100 to 2200 yards) per workout. Swim fast to get maximum benefits, but maintain good technique to maximize efficiency and minimize the risk of injury.

Interval training.   Interval training increases sprinting speed so you can accelerate faster at the beginning of a swim. It also helps the body cope with metabolic waste products so you can maintain your speed during the workout. To increase speed, swim intervals between 25 and 200 metres (or yards) at 80–90% effort. An example of a beginning program might be to swim four sets of 50 metres using the sidestroke at 70% of maximum effort, with a 1-minute rest between sets. A more advanced program would be to swim 10 sets of 100 metres using the freestyle stroke at 85–95% maximum effort with 30 seconds of rest between sets.

Endurance training.   Include longer swims—1000 metres or more at a time—to build general stamina for swimming. Endurance training will improve aerobic capacity and help your cells use fuels and clear metabolic wastes. This will allow you to swim faster and longer. Longer swims promote metabolic health and build physical fitness.

Cross-training.   Cross-training combines more than one type of endurance exercise, such as swimming and jogging, in your program. It also includes exercises that build strength, power, and skill. It is a good training method for people who prefer swimming but don't have daily access to a swimming pool or open water. Including multiple exercises, such as swimming and running, stair stepping, cycling, weight training exercises, and callisthenics, adds variety to the program. It also prepares you for a greater variety of physical challenges. See Chapter 3 for a discussion of cross-training and a description of typical workouts.

Technique: The Basic Swimming Strokes for General Conditioning

The best strokes for conditioning are the freestyle and side-stroke. Competitive athletes also swim the breaststroke, butterfly, and backstroke (but not the sidestroke). Learning efficient swimming strokes helps increase enjoyment and results in better workouts. Take a class from the Red Cross, a local recreation department, or a private coach if you are not a strong swimmer or need help with the basic strokes.

Freestyle.   While freestyle technically includes any unregulated stroke (such as the sidestroke), it generally refers to the front (Australian) crawl or overhand stroke. Freestyle is the fastest stroke and is best for general conditioning. Swim this stroke in a prone (face-down) position with arms stretched out in front and legs extended to the back. Move through the water by pulling first with the right arm and then with the left, while performing a kicking motion generated from the hips. During the stroke, rotate the thumb and palm 45 degrees toward the bottom of the pool. Pull in a semicircle downward toward the centre of the body with the elbow higher than the hand. When the hand reaches the beginning of the rib cage, push the palm backward underneath the body as far as possible. Don't begin to stroke with the other hand until the first stroke is completed. Maximize the distance with each stroke by pulling fully and maintaining good posture.

The crawl uses a flutter kick, which involves moving the legs alternately with the force generated from the hips and a slight bend of the knees. Maintain a neutral spine during the stroke. A strong kick is important to minimize body roll during the stroke. For this reason, some of your training should include kicking without using the arms.

Breathing is almost always a problem for novice swimmers. Don't hold your breath! You will fatigue rapidly if you have poor air exchange during swimming. Breathe by turning the head to the side of a recovering stroke. Do not lift the head out of the water. Exhale continuously through the nose and mouth between breaths. Beginners should breathe on the same side following each stroke cycle (left and right arm strokes).

Sidestroke.   Even novices can get a good workout with minimal skill using the sidestroke. This is a good choice for beginners because you keep your head out of water and can swim great distances without fatigue. Lie in the water on your right side and stretch your right arm and hand in front of you in the direction you want to swim and place your left hand across your chest. Draw your right arm toward you, pulling at the water until your hand reaches your waist. At the same time, make a scissors kick with your legs. Repeat the stroke as your forward speed slows. Swim half the distance on your right side and the rest on your left side.

Beginning Swim Program

Take swimming lessons from a certified teacher or coach if you are a nonswimmer or have not used swimming as your primary form of exercise. A swim teacher can help you develop good technique, make more rapid progress, and avoid injuries.

To assess your starting fitness, take the 12-minute swim test described in Lab 3.1. Use the swim test table to help you measure progress in your program. Take the test every one or two months to help establish short-term goals.

Start your program by swimming one length (one-half lap) at a time, using either freestyle or sidestroke. If you can't swim the length of a standard pool (25 metres or yards), begin by swimming the width. As soon as you can, swim one length of the pool, rest for 30 seconds, and then repeat. Build up your capacity until you can swim 20 lengths with a short rest interval between each length. If you start your program with the sidestroke, try to switch to the freestyle stroke as quickly as you can.

Increase the distance of each swim to a full lap (50 metres or yards) with 30 to 60 seconds of rest between laps. Build up until you can swim 20 sets of 50-metre swims with 30 seconds of rest between sets. Gradually increase the distance of each set to 100-metre swims. You are ready for the next level when you can swim 10 sets of 100 metres with 30 seconds of rest between sets.

Swimming Program for Higher Levels of Fitness

This program includes a warm-up, specific conditioning drills for strokes and kicking, and a cool-down. It involves interval training three days a week and distance training two days per week.

Warm up before each workout by swimming 2 to 4 laps at an easy pace. It is also a good idea to warm up your legs and hips by holding on to the side of the pool and gently moving your legs using a flutter-kick motion. At the end of the workout, cool down by swimming 100 to 200 metres at a slow pace.

On Monday, Wednesday, and Friday, do interval training. Your goal is to swim intervals totalling 2000 metres per workout (20 sets of 100 metres each) at a fast pace with 30 seconds of rest between each set, or interval (i.e., swim 100 metres, rest, swim 100 metres, rest, etc.). Every fifth interval, swim 25 metres using your legs alone, with your arms extended in front of you. Have someone watch you during the legs-only swims to make sure you are kicking mainly from the hips and maintaining a neutral spine. Add variety to your interval training workouts by using gloves, swim paddles, or fins.

If you are unable to do the interval workout at first, modify it by increasing rest intervals, decreasing speed, or decreasing the number of sets as you gradually increase the volume and intensity.

On Tuesday and Thursday, do distance training. Swim 1000 to 2000 metres continuously at a comfortable pace. Although distance days will help develop endurance, they are used mainly to help you recover from intense interval training days.

Rest on Saturday and Sunday. Rest is very important to help your muscles and metabolism recover and build fitness. Rest will also prevent overtraining and overuse injuries. Include two rest days per week. Rest days can be consecutive (such as Saturday and Sunday) or interspersed during the normal workout schedule.

Integrating Swimming into a Total Fitness Program

Develop fitness and maintain interest in continuing your exercise program by varying the structure of your workouts. Incorporate kick boards, pull-buoys, hand paddles, and fins into some of your training sessions. Cross-training is a good option for developing well-rounded fitness. Swimming results in moderate gains in strength and large gains in endurance.

Because swimming is not a weight-bearing activity and is not done in an upright position, it elicits a lower heart rate per minute. Therefore, swimmers need to adjust their target heart rate zone. To calculate your target heart rate for swimming, use this formula:

Maximum swimming heart rate (MSHR) $= 205 - $ age
Target heart rate zone $= 65-90\%$ of MSHR

For example, a 19-year-old swimmer would calculate their target heart rate zone for swimming as follows:

MSHR: $205 - 19 = 186$ bpm
65% intensity: $0.65 \times 186 = 121$ bpm
90% intensity: $0.90 \times 186 = 167$ bpm

Swimming does not preserve bone density as you age, so swimmers are advised to include weight training in their exercise program. Perform at least one set of 10 repetitions for 8 to 10 exercises that use the major muscle groups in the body. To improve swimming performance, include exercises that work key muscles. For example, if you primarily swim the freestyle stroke, include exercises to increase strength in your shoulders, arms, upper back, and hips. Training the muscles you use during swimming can also help prevent injuries. In your flexibility training, pay special attention to the muscles you use during swimming, particularly the shoulders, hips, and back. Table 3 shows a basic sample swimming program that incorporates all these types of exercises.

TABLE 3

Sample Swimming Program

Day	Activities
Monday	• **Warm-up:** Swim 100–200 metres (2–4 laps of a standard pool) at an easy pace. • **Intervals:** Swim 10–20 sets of 100-metre swims at 90% effort, with 30 seconds of rest between sets. After every 5 sets, swim 25 metres using your legs alone. • **Cool-down:** Swim 100–200 metres at a slow pace. • **Weight training:** Do at least 1 set of 10 repetitions of 8–10 exercises that work the body's major muscle groups. • **Flexibility:** Do standard stretching exercises for the shoulders, chest, back, hips, and thighs.
Tuesday	• **Distance:** Swim 1000–2000 metrers continuously at a comfortable pace.
Wednesday	• Repeat Monday activities.
Thursday	• Repeat Tuesday activities.
Friday	• Repeat Monday activities.
Saturday	• **Rest**
Sunday	• **Rest**

Rowing is a whole-body exercise that overloads the cardiorespiratory system and strengthens the major muscles of the body. The beauty and serenity of rowing on flat water in the morning is indescribable, but few people have access to a lake and rowing shell. Fortunately, sophisticated rowing machines simulate the rowing motion and make it possible to do this exercise at the fitness centre or at a health club.

Modern rowing machines are very much like the real thing, providing resistance with hydraulic pistons, magnets, air, or water. The best machines are solid and comfortable, provide a steady stroke, and allow you to maintain a neutral spine so you don't injure your back. Many rowing machines come with LCD displays that show heart rate, stroke rate, power output, and estimated caloric expenditure. They are also preprogrammed with workouts for interval training, cardiovascular conditioning, and moderate-intensity physical activity. Good rowing mechanics are essential because, if done incorrectly, rowing can cause severe overuse injuries that can damage the back, hips, knees, elbows, and shoulders.

Technique: Basic Rowing Movement

Most of the power for rowing comes from the thigh and hip muscles and finishes with a pulling motion with the upper body. Maintain a neutral spine (that is, with normal curves) during the movement. Hinge at the hips and not at the back during the rowing motion.

The rowing movement includes the following phases:

- **The catch.** Slide the seat forward on the track with arms straight as far as you can while keeping the spine neutral.

- **The drive.** Push with the legs and keep your arms straight.

- **The finish**. Lean back slightly (still maintaining a neutral spine) and pull the handle to your abdomen.

- **The recovery**. Extend your arms forward, hinging forward at the hips with a neutral spine, and slide forward again on the seat for another "catch."

Training Methods

Your rowing program should include both continuous training and interval training. Continuous training calls for rowing for a specific amount of time—typically 20 to 90 minutes without stopping. Most people enjoy rowing at about 70% of maximum heart rate.

Interval training involves a series of exercise bouts followed by rest. The method manipulates distance, intensity, repetitions, and rest. An example of an interval workout would be to row for eight sets of 4-minute exercise bouts at 85% effort with 2 minutes of rest between intervals, or sets. During interval training, changing one factor affects the others. For example, if you increase the intensity of exercise, you will need more rest between intervals and won't be able to do as many repetitions. High-intensity exercise builds fitness best but also increases the risk of injury and loss of motivation. Make intervals challenging but not so difficult that you get injured or discouraged.

Beginning Rowing Program

During the first few workouts, start conservatively by rowing for 10 minutes at a rate of about 20 strokes per minute with a moderate resistance. Exercise at about 60% effort. Do this workout three times during the first week. The movement is deceptively easy and invigorating. You are, however, using all the major muscle groups in the body and are probably not ready for a more intense exercise program.

After the first workout, do a series of 5-minute intervals during the first few weeks of training. For example, row for 5 minutes, rest 3 minutes, row 5 minutes, then rest 3 minutes. Build up until you can do four to six repetitions of 5-minute exercise intervals, resting only 1 minute between sets. Gradually, increase the time for each interval to 15 minutes and vary the rowing cadence from 20 to 25 strokes per minute. Your first short-term goal is to complete 30 minutes of continuous rowing without stopping.

Rowing Program for Higher Levels of Fitness

Vary your training methods after you can row continuously for 30 minutes, gain some fitness, and are used to the technique. Alternate between interval training and distance training. Doing both will help you develop fitness rapidly and improve rowing efficiency. A good strategy is to row continuously at about 70% effort for 30 to 60 minutes three days per week and practise interval training at 80–90% effort for two days per week. Do resistance and flexibility training two to three days per week. A basic but complete rowing machine program that includes continuous and interval training as well as resistance and flexibility exercises is shown in Table 4.

TABLE 4

Sample Rowing Machine Fitness Program

Day	Activities
Monday	• **Warm-up:** Row at low intensity for 2 minutes. • **Continuous rowing:** Row for 30 minutes at 70% effort (20–22 strokes per minute). • **Weight training (1–2 sets of 10 repetitions):** Squats, leg curls,bench press, lat pulls, raises, biceps curls, triceps extensions, curl-ups, side bridge (10 seconds per side), spine extensions (10 seconds per side). • **Stretching:** Do static stretching exercises for the shoulders, chest, back, hips, and thighs. Hold each stretch for 10–30 seconds.
Tuesday	• Warm-up: Row at low intensity for 2 minutes. • Continuous rowing: Row at 60–70% of maximum effort for 5 minutes. Rest for 3 minutes. • Interval rowing: Row 6 sets, for 5 minutes per set, at 25 strokes per minute (90% effort). Rest for 3 minutes between intervals.
Wednesday	• **Warm-up:** Row at low intensity for 2 minutes. • **Continuous rowing:** Row for 45 minutes at 70% effort (20–22 strokes per minute). • **Stretching:** Repeat Monday stretches.
Thursday	• **Warm-up:** Row at low intensity for 2 minutes. • **Continuous rowing:** Row for 30 minutes at 70% effort (20–22 strokes per minute). • **Weight training (1–2 sets of 10 repetitions):** Repeat Monday weight training exercises.
Friday	• **Warm-up:** Row at low intensity for 2 minutes. • **Continuous rowing:** Row for 30 minutes at 70% effort (20–22 strokes per minute). • **Stretching:** Repeat Monday stretches.
Saturday	• **Rest**
Sunday	• **Rest**

Laboratory Activities

Name _____ Section _____ Date _____

Lab 9.1 A Personal Fitness Program Plan and Agreement

Mc Graw Hill Education connect

A. I, _____, am making an agreement with myself to follow a
(name)

physical fitness program to work toward the following goals.

Specific or short-term goals (include current status for each):

1. _____

2. _____

3. _____

4. _____

General or long-term goals:

1. _____

2. _____

3. _____

4. _____

B. My program plan is as follows:

Activities	Components (Check √)					Frequency (Check √)							Intensity*	Time (duration)
	CRE	MS	ME	F	BC	M	Tu	W	Th	F	Sa	Su		

***Conduct** activities for achieving CRE goals in your target range for heart rate or RPE.

CRE = cardiorespiratory endurance; MS = muscular strength; ME = muscular endurance; F = flexibility; BC = body composition

C. My program will begin on _____. My program includes the following schedule of
(date)

mini-goals. For each step in my program, I will give myself the reward listed.

_____	_____	_____
(mini-goal 1)	(date)	(reward)
_____	_____	_____
(mini-goal 2)	(date)	(reward)
_____	_____	_____
(mini-goal 3)	(date)	(reward)
_____	_____	_____
(mini-goal 4)	(date)	(reward)
_____	_____	_____
(mini-goal 5)	(date)	(reward)

D. My program will include the addition of physical activity to my daily routine (such as climbing stairs or walking to class):

1. _____

2. _____

3. _____

4. _____

5. _____

E. I will use the following tools to monitor my program and my progress toward my goals:

_____

(list any charts, graphs, or journals you plan to use)

_____

_____

I sign this agreement as an indication of my personal commitment to reach my goal.

_____   _____

(your signature)   (date)

I have recruited a helper who will witness my agreement and _____

_____

_____

_____   _____

(witness's signature)   (date)

Name _____   Section _____   Date _____

Lab 9.2 Getting to Know Your Fitness Facility

connect

To help create a successful training program, take time out to learn more about the fitness facility you plan to use.

Basic Information

Name and location of facility: _____

Hours of operation: _____

Times available for general use:_____

Times most convenient for your schedule:_____

Can you obtain an initial session or consultation with a trainer to help you create a program?

yes _____ no _____

If so, what does the initial planning session involve? _____

_____

Are any of the staff certified? Do any have special training? If yes, list/describe: _____

_____

What types of equipment are available for the development of cardiorespiratory endurance? Briefly list/
describe: _____

_____

_____

Are any group activities or classes available? If so, briefly describe: _____

_____

_____

What types of weight training equipment are available for use? _____

_____

Yes	No	
_____	_____	Is there a fee for using the facility? If so, how much? $ _____
_____	_____	Is a student ID required for access to the facility?
_____	_____	Do you need to sign up in advance to use the facility or any of the equipment?
_____	_____	Is there typically a line or wait to use the equipment during the times you use the facility?
_____	_____	Is there a separate area with mats for stretching and/or cool-down?
_____	_____	Do you need to bring your own towel?
_____	_____	Are lockers available? If so, do you need to bring your own lock? yes _____ no _____
_____	_____	Are showers available? If so, do you need to bring your own soap and shampoo?
		yes _____ no _____
_____	_____	Is drinking water available? (If not, be sure to bring your own bottle of water.)

Describe any other amenities, such as vending machines or saunas, that are available at the facility.

_____

_____

Information about Equipment

Fill in the specific equipment and exercise(s) that you can use to develop cardiorespiratory endurance and each of the major muscle groups. For cardiorespiratory endurance, list the type(s) of equipment and a sample starting workout: frequency, intensity, time, and other pertinent information (such as a setting for resistance or speed). For muscular strength and endurance, list the equipment, exercises, and indicate the order in which you'll complete them during a workout session. Remember, you don't have to use equipment—you can use body weight or elastic bands as resistance.

Cardiorespiratory Endurance Equipment

Equipment	Sample Starting Workout

Muscular Strength and Endurance Equipment

Order	Muscle Groups	Equipment	Exercise(s)
	Neck		
	Chest		
	Shoulders		
	Upper back		
	Front of arms		
	Back of arms		
	Buttocks		
	Abdomen		
	Lower back		
	Front of thighs		
	Back of thighs		
	Calves		
	Other:		
	Other:		

CHAPTER 10

Cardiovascular Health

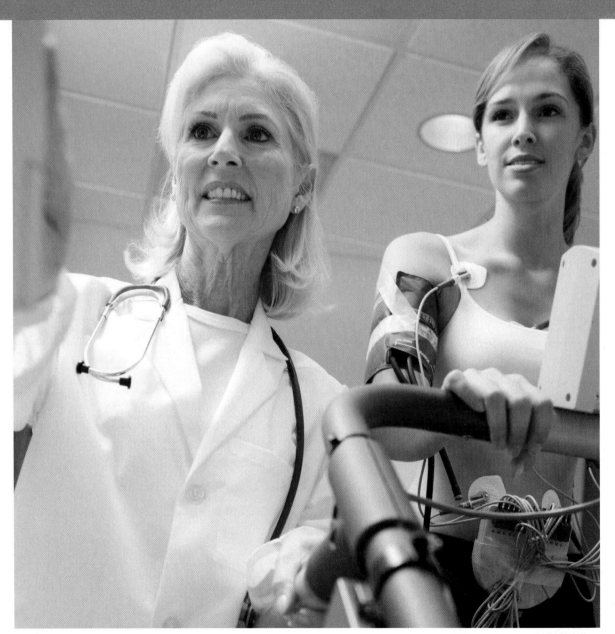

© MBI / Alamy

LEARNING OBJECTIVES

After reading this chapter, you should be able to

LO1 Discuss the major forms of cardiovascular disease and how they develop

LO2 Describe the controllable and uncontrollable risk factors associated with cardiovascular disease

LO3 List the steps you can take now to lower your personal risk of developing cardiovascular disease

TEST YOUR KNOWLEDGE

1. **Women are about as likely to die of cardiovascular disease as they are to die of breast cancer.**
   True or false?

2. **On average, how much earlier does heart disease develop in people who don't exercise regularly than in people who do?**
   a. 6 months
   b. 2 years
   c. 6 years

3. **Which of the following foods would be a good choice for promoting heart health?**
   a. whole grains
   b. salmon
   c. bananas

ANSWERS

1. **FALSE.** Cardiovascular disease kills far more. Among Canadian women, more than one in three deaths are due to cardiovascular disease, and heart disease and stroke will kill seven times as many Canadian women as breast cancer. In addition, more women than men die each year from cardiovascular disease.

2. **C.** Both endurance exercise and strength training significantly reduce the risk for cardiovascular disease.

3. **ALL THREE.** Whole grains (e.g., whole wheat, oatmeal, rye, barley, and brown rice), foods with omega-3 fatty acids (e.g., salmon), and foods high in potassium and low in sodium (e.g., bananas) all improve cardiovascular health.

Cardiovascular disease (CVD) is the second leading cause of death in Canada (see Table 1.1); one-third of all Canadians alive today will die from CVD. The Heart Research Institute estimates that 90% of Canadians have at least one risk factor for heart disease or stroke. Heart disease is the leading cause of death for both men and women, and Aboriginal-Canadians are 1.5 to 2 times more likely to develop heart disease than the general population. Among the life-threatening manifestations of CVD, strokes ranks third on the list of the leading causes of death among Canadians. High blood pressure, which is both a form of CVD and a risk factor for other types of disease, affects nearly 1 in 4 adults, while another 1 in 5 Canadian adults have blood pressure numbers that are higher than normal but not yet in the high blood pressure range.

> **cardiovascular disease (CVD)** A collective term for various diseases of the heart and blood vessels.

CVD is largely due to our way of life. Too many Canadians are overweight and sedentary, smoke cigarettes, manage stress ineffectively, have uncontrolled high blood pressure or high cholesterol levels, and don't know the signs of CVD. Not all risk factors for CVD are controllable—some people have an inherited tendency toward high cholesterol levels, for example—but many are within the control of the individual.

This chapter explains the major forms of CVD, including hypertension, atherosclerosis, and stroke. It also considers the factors that put people at risk for CVD. Most important, it explains the steps individuals can take to protect their hearts and promote cardiovascular health throughout their lives.

🔲 LO1 10.1 Major Forms of Cardiovascular Disease

Cardiovascular diseases kill over 47 000 people a year in Canada alone. The financial burden of CVD, including the costs of medical treatments and lost productivity, exceeds $20 billion annually. Although the main forms of CVD are interrelated and have elements in common, we treat them separately here for the sake of clarity. Hypertension, which is both a major risk factor and a form of CVD, is discussed later in the chapter.

Atherosclerosis

Atherosclerosis is a form of arteriosclerosis, or thickening and hardening of the arteries. In atherosclerosis, arteries become narrowed by deposits of fat, cholesterol, and other substances. The process begins when the cells lining the arteries (endothelial cells) become damaged, often through a combination of factors such as smoking, high blood pressure, high insulin or glucose levels, and deposits of oxidized LDL particles. The body's response to this damage results in inflammation and changes in the artery lining. Deposits, called **plaques**, accumulate on artery walls; the arteries lose their elasticity and their ability to expand and contract, restricting blood flow. Once narrowed by a plaque, an artery is vulnerable to blockage by blood clots (Figure 10.1). The risk of life-threatening clots and heart attacks increases if the fibrous cap covering a plaque ruptures.

> **atherosclerosis** A form of CVD in which the inner layers of artery walls are made thick and irregular by plaque deposits; arteries become narrowed, and blood supply is reduced.
> **plaque** A deposit of fatty (and other) substances on the inner wall of the arteries.

If the heart, brain, and/or other organs are deprived of blood, and the oxygen it carries, the effects of atherosclerosis can be deadly. Coronary arteries, which supply the heart with blood, are particularly susceptible to plaque buildup, a condition called **coronary heart disease (CHD)**, or *coronary artery disease*. The blockage of a coronary artery causes a heart attack. If a cerebral artery (leading to the brain) is blocked, the result

> **coronary heart disease (CHD)** Heart disease caused by atherosclerosis in the arteries that supply blood to the heart muscle; also called coronary artery disease.

FIGURE 10.1

Stages of plaque development.

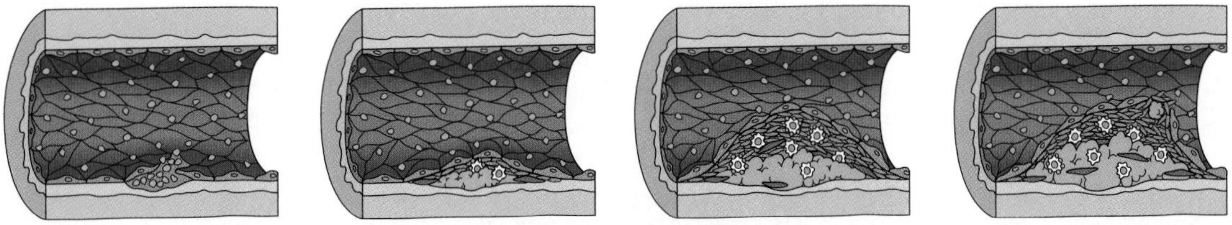

Plaque buildup begins when endothelial cells lining the arteries are damaged by smoking, high blood pressure, oxidized LDL, and other causes; excess cholesterol particles collect beneath these cells.

In response to the damage, platelets and other types of cells collect at the site; a fibrous cap forms, isolating the plaque within the artery wall. An early-stage plaque is called a fatty streak.

Chemicals released by cells in and around the plaque cause further inflammation and buildup; an advanced plaque contains LDL, white blood cells, connective tissue, smooth muscle cells, platelets, and other compounds.

The narrowed artery is vulnerable to blockage by clots. The risk of blockage and heart attack rises if the fibrous cap cracks (probably due to destructive enzymes released by white blood cells within the plaque).

---

is a stroke. The main risk factors for atherosclerosis are cigarette smoking, physical inactivity, high levels of blood cholesterol, high blood pressure, and diabetes.

Heart Disease and Heart Attacks

The Heart and Stroke Foundation estimates that 70 000 heart attacks occur in Canada each year and that almost 16 000 Canadians die as a result.[1] Although a **heart attack**, or myocardial infarction (MI), may come without warning, it is usually the end result of a long-term disease process. The heart requires a steady supply of oxygen-rich blood to function properly (see Figure 10.2 on the next page). If one of the coronary arteries that supplies blood to the heart becomes blocked, a heart attack results. A heart attack caused by a clot is called a *coronary thrombosis*. During a heart attack, part of the heart muscle (myocardium) may die from lack of oxygen.

> **heart attack**   Damage to, or death of, heart muscle, resulting from a failure of the coronary arteries to deliver enough blood to the heart; also known as *myocardial infarction* (MI).

Chest pain called **angina pectoris** is a signal that the heart isn't getting enough oxygen to supply its needs. Although not actually a heart attack, angina—felt as an extreme tightness in the chest and heavy pressure behind the breastbone or in the shoulder, neck, arm, hand, or back—is a warning that the heart is overloaded.

> **angina pectoris**   A condition in which the heart muscle does not receive enough blood, causing severe pain in the chest and often in the arm and shoulder.

If the electrical impulses that control heartbeat are disrupted, the heart may beat too quickly, too slowly, or in an irregular fashion, a condition known as **arrhythmia**. The symptoms of arrhythmia range from imperceptible to severe and even fatal. **Sudden cardiac death**, also called *cardiac arrest*, is most often caused by an arrhythmia called *ventricular fibrillation*, a kind of "quivering" of the ventricle that makes it ineffective in pumping blood. If ventricular fibrillation continues for more than a few minutes, it is generally fatal. Cardiac

> **arrhythmia**   A change in the normal pattern of the heartbeat.
> **sudden cardiac death**   A nontraumatic, unexpected death from sudden cardiac arrest, most often due to arrhythmia; in most instances, victims have underlying heart disease.

FIGURE 10.2

Blood supply to the heart. Blood is supplied to the heart from the right and left coronary arteries, which branch off the aorta. If a coronary artery becomes blocked by plaque buildup or a blood clot, a heart attack occurs; part of the heart muscle may die due to lack of oxygen.

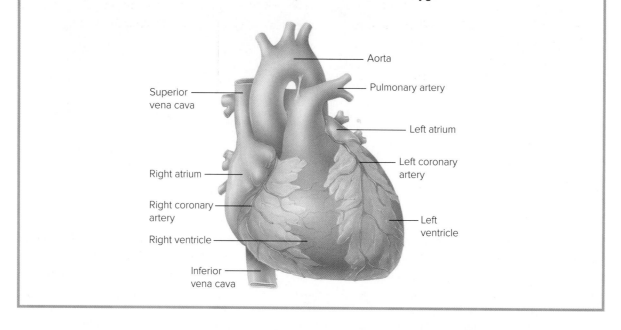

defibrillation, in which an electrical shock is delivered to the heart, can jolt the heart into a more efficient rhythm. This shock can be administered with an automated external defibrillator (AED), a first-aid device that is available in many public places in case someone experiences a heart attack.

Heart attack symptoms may include pain or pressure in the chest; pain in the arm, neck, or jaw; difficulty breathing; excessive sweating; nausea and vomiting; and loss of consciousness. But not all heart attacks involve sharp chest pain. Women, in particular, are more likely to have different symptoms, including shortness of breath, weakness, unusual fatigue, cold sweat, and dizziness.

If symptoms of heart trouble do occur, it is critical to contact the emergency medical service or go immediately to the nearest hospital or clinic (see the box Warning Signs of Heart Attack, Stroke, and Cardiac Arrest). Many experts also suggest that the heart attack victim chew and swallow one adult aspirin tablet (325 mg); aspirin has an immediate anti-clotting effect. If someone having a heart attack gets to the emergency room quickly enough, a clot-dissolving agent can be injected to dissolve a clot in the coronary artery, reducing the amount of damage to the heart muscle.

Physicians have a variety of diagnostic tools and treatments for heart disease. Patients may undergo a stress or exercise test, where they run on a treadmill or pedal a stationary cycle while being monitored with an electrocardiogram (ECG or EKG). Certain characteristic changes in the heart's electrical activity while it is under stress can reveal particular heart problems, such as restricted blood flow to the heart muscle. Tools that allow the physician to visualize a patient's heart and arteries include magnetic resonance imaging (MRI), electron beam computed tomography (EBCT), echocardiograms, and others.

If tests indicate a problem or if a person has already had a heart attack, several treatments are possible. Along with a low-fat diet, regular exercise, and smoking cessation, many patients are also advised to take a low-dose aspirin tablet (81 mg) daily. Aspirin has an anti-clotting effect, discouraging platelets in the blood from sticking to arterial plaques and forming clots; it also reduces inflammation. Low-dose aspirin therapy appears to help prevent first heart attacks in men, second heart attacks in men and women, and strokes in women over age 65. In addition to aspirin, prescription drugs can also help reduce the strain on the heart.

Several surgical treatments are available to treat certain forms of heart disease. *Balloon angioplasty* involves threading a catheter with an inflatable balloon tip through a coronary artery until it reaches the area of blockage. The balloon is then inflated, flattening the plaque and widening the arterial opening. Many surgeons permanently implant coronary stents—flexible stainless steel tubes—to prop the artery open and prevent reclogging after angioplasty. In *coronary bypass surgery*, healthy blood vessels from the person are grafted to coronary arteries to bypass the blockages.

Wellness Tip

Automated external defibrillators (AEDs) have very simple instructions printed on them; public AEDs are so easy to use that no training is required. If you are assisting a heart attack victim and an AED is nearby, use it.

Stroke

A **stroke**, also called a *cerebrovascular accident (CVA)*, occurs when the blood supply to the brain is cut off. If brain cells are deprived of blood for more than a few minutes, they die. Once brain cells begin dying, about 2 million cells are lost every minute that blood flow is not restored. Nerve cells control sensation and most body movements; depending on the area of the brain affected, a stroke may cause paralysis, walking disability, speech impairment, memory loss, and changes in behaviour. Prompt treatment of stroke can greatly decrease the risk of permanent disability. Of the over 62 000 Canadians who have strokes each year, 24% will die and those that survive will have double the risk of suffering from dementia.[2]

stroke   An impeded blood supply to some part of the brain resulting in the destruction of brain cells; also called cerebrovascular accident (CVA).

There are two major types of strokes: ischemic and hemorrhagic. An *ischemic stroke* is caused by a blockage in a blood vessel. They are the more common type and account for 87% of all strokes.There are two types of ischemic strokes:

- A *thrombotic stroke* is caused by a blood clot that forms in a cerebral or carotid artery that has been narrowed or damaged by atherosclerosis.
- An *embolic stroke* is caused by an embolus, a wandering blood clot that is carried in the bloodstream and may become wedged in a cerebral artery.

A *hemorrhagic stroke* occurs when a blood vessel in the brain bursts, spilling blood into the surrounding tissue. Cells normally nourished by the vessel are deprived of blood and cannot function. In addition, accumulated blood from the burst vessel may put pressure on surrounding brain tissue, causing damage and even death. There are two types of hemorrhagic strokes:

- In an *intracerebral hemorrhage*, a blood vessel ruptures within the brain.
- In a *subarachnoid hemorrhage*, a blood vessel on the brain's surface ruptures and bleeds into the space between the brain and the skull.

Hemorrhages can be caused by head injuries or the bursting of a malformed blood vessel, or *aneurysm*, which is a blood-filled pocket that bulges out from a weak spot in the artery wall. Aneurysms in the brain may remain stable and never break. But when they do, the result is a hemorrhagic stroke. Aneurysms may be caused or worsened by hypertension.

Effective treatment requires the prompt recognition of symptoms and correct diagnosis of the type of stroke that has occurred. Treatment may involve the use of clot-dissolving and antihypertensive drugs. Even if brain tissue has been damaged or destroyed, nerve cells in the brain can make new pathways, and some functions can be taken over by other parts of the brain.

Many people have strokes without knowing it, however, so they do not realize they may need treatment or evaluation for the risk of a full-blown stroke in the future. These silent strokes do not cause any noticeable symptoms while they are occurring. Although they may be mild, silent strokes leave their victims at a higher risk for subsequent and more serious strokes later in life. They also contribute to loss of mental and cognitive skills. (See the box Warning Signs of Heart Attack, Stroke, and Cardiac Arrest for more information.)

Take CHARGE

WARNING SIGNS OF HEART ATTACK, STROKE, AND CARDIAC ARREST

Heart Attack Warning Signs

The most common warning symptoms of a heart attack for both men and women are the following:

- **Chest discomfort** in the centre or left side of the chest that usually lasts for more than a few minutes or goes away and comes back. It can feel like pressure, squeezing, fullness, or pain. It also can feel like heartburn or indigestion. It can be mild or severe.
- **Upper body discomfort** in one or both arms, the back, shoulders, neck, jaw, or upper part of the stomach (above the navel).
- **Shortness of breath** may be the only symptom or it may occur before or along with chest pain or discomfort. It can occur when you are resting or doing mild physical activity.

But remember these additional facts:

- Heart attacks can start slowly and cause only mild pain or discomfort. Symptoms can be mild or more intense and sudden. Symptoms also may come and go over several hours.
- People who have high blood sugar (diabetes) may have no symptoms or very mild ones. Heart attacks without symptoms or with very mild symptoms are called silent heart attacks.
- The most common symptom, in both men and women, is chest pain or discomfort.
- Women are somewhat more likely to have shortness of breath, nausea and vomiting, unusual tiredness (sometimes for days), and pain in the back, shoulders, and jaw.
- Other possible symptoms include breaking out in a cold sweat, light-headedness or sudden dizziness, or a change in the pattern of usual symptoms.

The signs and symptoms of a heart attack can develop suddenly or slowly—within hours, days, or weeks of a heart attack. If you think you or someone you know might be having heart attack symptoms or a heart attack, don't ignore it or feel embarrassed to call for help. **Call 9-1-1 right away.** Here's why:

- Acting fast can save your life. Every minute matters. Never delay calling 9-1-1 to do anything you think might help.
- An ambulance is the best and safest way to get to the hospital. Emergency medical services (EMS) personnel start lifesaving treatments right away. People who arrive by ambulance often receive faster treatment at the hospital.
- The 9-1-1 operator or EMS technician can give you advice. You might be told to crush or chew an aspirin if you're not allergic, unless there is a medical reason for you not to take one.

Stroke Warning Signs

The symptoms of stroke are distinctive because they happen quickly. They include the following:

- sudden numbness or weakness of the face, arm, or leg (especially on one side of the body)
- sudden confusion, trouble speaking or understanding speech
- sudden trouble seeing in one or both eyes

- sudden trouble walking, dizziness, loss of balance or coordination
- sudden severe headache with no known cause

If you experience any of these symptoms, **call 9-1-1 immediately**. Health Canada has approved the clot-busting drug called tPA to be used within three hours from the time symptoms begin. However, emerging science is now showing that tPA could be effective up to four-and-a-half hours afterwards. As a result, the Canadian Stroke Strategy has issued Canadian Best Practices Recommendations for Stroke Care, which have included this new treatment time. Still, it will be up to the attending emergency doctors to determine when tPA may be administered or if it is appropriate to the situation.

A transient ischemic attack (TIA) has the same signs and symptoms as a stroke. However, TIA symptoms usually last less than 1 to 2 hours (although they may last up to 24 hours). A TIA may occur only once in a person's lifetime or more often and can be a warning sign for future strokes. At first, it may not be possible to tell whether someone is having a TIA or stroke. All stroke-like symptoms require medical care.

Sudden Cardiac Arrest Signs

In sudden cardiac arrest (SCA), the heart suddenly and unexpectedly stops beating. As a result, blood stops flowing to the brain and other vital organs. The patient suddenly becomes unresponsive and stops breathing, and if they are not treated within minutes, death occurs. Some people may have a racing heartbeat or feel dizzy or light-headed just before they faint. Within an hour before SCA, some people have chest pain, shortness of breath, nausea, or vomiting. Usually, however, the first sign of SCA is loss of consciousness (fainting). At the same time, no heartbeat (or pulse) can be felt.

If you are with someone who suddenly experiences these symptoms, **call 9-1-1 and begin CPR immediately**. (Visit your local Heart and Stroke Foundation, or http://www.heartandstroke.ca, to find out how to sign up to become certified in CPR). If an automated external defibrillator (AED) is available and someone trained to use it is nearby, involve them.

SOURCES: Heart and Stroke Foundation, 2018. Signs of heart attack, cardiac arrest, sudden arrhythmia death syndrome (SADS). http://www.heartandstroke.ca/heart/emergency-signs; National Heart, Lung, and Blood Institute. 2013. What are the symptoms of a heart attack? http://www.nhlbi.nih.gov/health/health-topics/topics/heartattack/signs; National Institute of Neurological disorders and Stroke. 2013. Know stroke. Know the signs. Act in time. http://www.ninds.nih.gov/disorders/stroke/knowstroke.htm; National Heart, Lung, and Blood Institute. 2011. What is sudden cardiac arrest? http://www.nhlbi.nih.gov/health/health-topics/topics/scda

Congestive Heart Failure

The heart's pumping mechanism can be damaged by a number of conditions, including high blood pressure, heart attack, atherosclerosis, viral infections, rheumatic fever, and birth defects. When the heart cannot maintain its regular pumping rate and force, fluids begin to back up. When extra fluid seeps through capillary walls, edema (swelling) results, usually in the legs and ankles, but sometimes in other parts of the body as well. Fluid can collect in the lungs and interfere with breathing, particularly when a person is lying down. This condition is called *pulmonary edema*, and the entire process is known as **congestive heart failure**. Treatment includes reducing the workload on the heart, modifying salt intake, and using drugs that help the body eliminate excess fluid.

congestive heart failure   A condition resulting from the heart's inability to pump out all the blood that returns to it. Blood backs up in the veins leading to the heart, causing an accumulation of fluid in various parts of the body.

LO2 10.2 Risk Factors for Cardiovascular Disease

Researchers have identified a variety of factors associated with an increased risk of developing CVD. They are grouped into two categories: major risk factors linked to controllable aspects of lifestyle (or health conditions that can be altered), and major risk factors that are beyond an individual's control. (You can evaluate your personal CVD risk factors in Part I of Lab 10.1.)

Major Risk Factors That Can Be Altered

The Canadian Heart Health Initiative and the Heart and Stroke Foundation of Canada have identified two kinds of controllable risk factors: lifestyle-related and health conditions. The six lifestyle-related risk factors for CVD that can be changed are tobacco use, unhealthy diet, physical inactivity, unhealthy weight, drug and alcohol abuse, and stress. It is estimated that almost 80% of premature heart disease and strokes could be prevented by engaging in healthy lifestyle behaviours.

The four health conditions that can be changed are high blood pressure, high cholesterol, diabetes, and atrial fibrillation. Most Canadians, including young adults, have at least one of these ten controllable risk factors for CVD. For example, among adult Canadians, close to 35% have high cholesterol levels,[3] 25% have high blood pressure,[4] 19% smoke,[5] and more than 32% are overweight.[6]

Tobacco Use

Your risk of developing CVD increases with the length and intensity of your exposure to cigarette smoke. Smokers are two to four times more likely to develop CVD than non-smokers. In addition, Canadians who smoke have a 70% greater chance of dying from CVD than non-smokers. Women who smoke double their risk for cervical cancer, triple their risk of dying from CVD, and are five times more likely to die from a stroke than women who do not smoke.[7]

Smoking harms the cardiovascular system in several ways:

- It damages the linings of arteries.
- It reduces the level of *high-density lipoproteins (HDL)*, or "good" cholesterol.
- It raises the levels of triglycerides and *low-density lipoproteins (LDL)*, or "bad" cholesterol.
- Nicotine increases blood pressure and heart rate.
- The carbon monoxide in cigarette smoke displaces oxygen in the blood, reducing the amount of oxygen available to the body.
- It causes **platelets** to stick together in the blood stream, leading to clotting.
- It speeds the development of fatty deposits in the arteries.

platelets Cell fragments in the blood that are necessary for the formation of blood clots.

You don't have to smoke to be affected. The risk of developing heart disease increases up to 30% among people exposed to environmental tobacco smoke (ETS)—also known as *secondhand smoke*. Researchers estimate that about 800 nonsmokers die from heart disease each year as a result of exposure to ETS.

Unhealthy Diet

Two areas of concern in terms of diet increase the risk for CVD for Canadians: not understanding the basics of healthy eating, and not recognizing the impact of processed foods. Healthy eating involves ensuring the intake of 7 to 10 servings of fruit and vegetable per day, increasing fibre intake through the consumption of whole grains, and providing enough protein for both brain and heart health. Processed foods are often dangerous as they not only contain little nutritional value, but at the same time, they provide added salt and sugar that are often not needed. (Chapter 7 provides plenty of advice for meal planning to reduce the risk for CVD.)

Physical Inactivity

Almost 60% of Canadians are so sedentary that they are at high risk for developing CVD. Exercise is thought to be the closest thing we have to a "magic bullet" against heart disease. It lowers CVD risk by helping decrease blood pressure, increase HDL levels, maintain desirable weight, improve the condition of the blood vessels, and prevent or control diabetes. In fact, introducing exercise to your daily routine dramatically reduces your risk for stroke.[8] One study found that women who accumulated at least three hours of brisk walking each week cut their risk of heart attack and stroke by more than half. (See Chapter 3 for more information on the physical and psychological effects of exercise.)

Unhealthy Weight

The risk of death from CVD is two to three times higher in obese people (BMI > 30) than it is in lean people (BMI 18.5–24.9). For every five-unit increment of BMI, a person's risk of death from coronary heart disease increases by 30%. Excess weight increases the strain on the heart by contributing to high blood pressure and high cholesterol. It can also lead to diabetes, another CVD risk factor (explored later in this section). As discussed in Chapter 6, distribution of body fat is significant: Fat that collects in the abdomen is more dangerous than fat that collects around the hips. Obesity in general, and abdominal obesity in particular, is significantly associated with narrowing of the coronary arteries, even in young adults in their 20s. A sensible diet and regular exercise are the best ways to achieve and maintain a healthy body weight.

Fitness Tip

Weight training should be part of any fitness program, but it can raise your blood pressure, at least temporarily. Be sure to balance weight training with aerobic exercise, which can lower blood pressure over the long term.

Drug and Alcohol Abuse

Stimulant drugs, particularly cocaine and methamphetamines, along with associated stimulants such as designer drugs like ecstasy (MDMA), can also cause serious cardiac problems, including heart attack, stroke, and sudden cardiac death. In addition, injection drug use can cause heart infections that can significantly increase your risk for stroke.

Excessive use of any type of alcohol will increase your risk for heart disease and stroke. Limit your alcohol consumption to moderate amounts and follow suggestions outlined in Chapter 14 to avoid excessive use.

Stress

As noted in Chapter 12, people who suffer from prolonged or high levels of stress often experience an increased risk for high blood pressure and CVD. Look for ways to manage your stress to reduce those possible effects.

Strengthening Mental Wellness

Being diagnosed with heart disease can sometimes be an additional stressor. The Heart and Stroke Foundation provides resources to help those dealing with the emotions and feelings that come with this diagnosis. See their website at http://www.heartandstroke.ca/services-and-resources/social-and-peer-support for helpful resources.

High Blood Pressure

In addition to being a form of CVD in itself, high blood pressure, or **hypertension**, is a risk factor for many forms of cardiovascular disease, including heart attacks and strokes.

hypertension Sustained abnormally high blood pressure.

Blood pressure, the force exerted by the blood on blood vessel walls, is created by the pumping action of the heart. High blood pressure occurs when too much force is exerted against the walls of the arteries. Short periods of high blood pressure—such as in response to excitement or exertion—are normal, but chronic high blood pressure is a health risk.

Blood pressure is expressed as two numbers—for example, 120 over 80—and is measured in millimetres of mercury (mm Hg). The first number is systolic blood pressure; the second is diastolic blood pressure. A normal blood pressure reading for a healthy young adult is in the range of 115 to 120 systolic over 75 to 80 diastolic. CVD risk increases when blood pressure rises above this level. Canadian Hypertension Guidelines define high blood pressure in adults as equal to or greater than 140 over 90. Health care professionals measure blood pressure with a stethoscope and an instrument called a *sphygmomanometer*. Professional measurement is needed for a diagnosis of hypertension, but you can track your own blood pressure at a drugstore or at home with an inexpensive monitor.

Wellness Tip

Always relax a few minutes before checking your blood pressure; doing so will help your blood pressure settle to its normal level. You may get a false reading if you take your blood pressure when you're agitated or moving around.

High blood pressure results from either an increased output of blood by the heart or from increased resistance to blood flow in the arteries. The latter condition can be caused by the constriction of smooth muscle surrounding the arteries or by atherosclerosis, a disease process that causes arteries to become clogged and narrowed. High blood pressure also scars and hardens arteries, making them less elastic and further increasing blood pressure. When a person has high blood pressure, the heart must work harder than normal to force blood through the narrowed and stiffened arteries, straining both the heart and the arteries. Eventually the strained heart weakens and tends to enlarge, which weakens it even more.

High blood pressure is often called a "silent killer" because it usually has no symptoms. A person may have hypertension for years without realizing it. But during that time, it damages vital organs and increases the risk of heart attack, congestive heart failure, stroke, kidney failure, and blindness. In fact, the Heart and Stroke Foundation of Canada reports that high blood pressure is the most important controllable risk factor for stroke.

Recent research has shed new light on the importance of lowering blood pressure to improve cardiovascular health. The risk of death from heart attack or stroke begins to rise when blood pressure is above 115 over 75, well below the traditional 140 over 90 cutoff for hypertension. People with blood pressures in the prehypertension range (defined as systolic pressure of 120 to 139 and diastolic pressure of 80 to 89), are at increased risk of heart attack and stroke as well as at significant risk of developing full-blown hypertension.

Hypertension is common, occurring in about one in four adults. Its incidence rises dramatically with age; however, it can also occur among children and young adults. There are currently no statistics identifying the number of Canadians suffering from prehypertension. In most cases hypertension cannot be cured, but it can be controlled. The key to avoiding the complications is to have your blood pressure tested at least once every two years—more often if you have other CVD risk factors.

Lifestyle changes are recommended for anyone with prehypertension and hypertension, including the following:

- weight reduction

- regular physical activity

- a healthy diet—the DASH diet (https://www.nhlbi.nih.gov/health-topics/dash-eating-plan) is recommended specifically for people with high blood pressure; it emphasizes fruits, vegetables, and whole grains, foods that are rich in potassium and fibre, both of which may reduce blood pressure; sodium restriction is also helpful

- moderate consumption of alcohol

Many people are "salt-sensitive," meaning their blood pressure will decrease significantly when salt intake is restricted. Most experts feel that restricting sodium intake is a good strategy for all people, whether or not they have hypertension. Health Canada guidelines state that adequate intake of sodium is 1500 milligrams per day (about two-thirds of a teaspoon of salt); the upper intake limit is set at 2300 milligrams per day (about 1 teaspoon of salt). Statistics Canada data suggest that Canadians consume, on average, nearly 3100 milligrams of salt a day, though that figure is actually low because it does not include the salt people add to their food.[9]

Recent research has shown that lowering your blood pressure through healthy lifestyle changes improves cardiovascular health even if your current blood pressure is already below 140 over 90. For people whose blood pressure isn't adequately controlled with lifestyle changes, medication is prescribed.

Wellness Tip

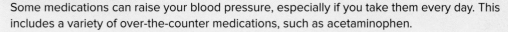

Some medications can raise your blood pressure, especially if you take them every day. This includes a variety of over-the-counter medications, such as acetaminophen.

Unhealthy Cholesterol Levels

Cholesterol is a fatty, waxlike substance that circulates through the bloodstream and is an important component of cell membranes, sex hormones, vitamin D, the fluid that coats the lungs, and the protective sheaths around nerves. Adequate cholesterol is essential for the proper functioning of the body. Excess cholesterol, however, can clog arteries and increase the risk of CVD (see Figure 10.3 on the next page). Your liver manufactures cholesterol; you also get cholesterol from foods.

Good versus Bad Cholesterol Cholesterol is carried in the blood by protein-lipid packages called **lipoproteins**, which range in size from 10 to 1000 nanometers (nm). **Low-density lipoproteins (LDLs)** (26 nm) shuttle cholesterol from the liver to the organs and tissues that require it. LDL is known as "bad" cholesterol because if there is more than the body can use, the excess is deposited in the blood vessels. LDL that accumulates and becomes trapped in artery walls may be oxidized by free radicals, speeding inflammation and damage to artery walls and increasing the likelihood that an artery will become blocked, causing a heart attack or stroke.

lipoproteins   Protein-and-lipid substances in the blood that carry fats and cholesterol; classified according to size, density, and chemical composition.

low-density lipoprotein (LDL)   A lipoprotein containing a moderate amount of protein and a large amount of cholesterol; "bad" cholesterol.

High-density lipoproteins (HDLs), or "good" cholesterol, are the smallest of the lipoproteins (6–12.5 nm). They shuttle unused cholesterol back to the liver for recycling. By removing cholesterol from blood vessels, HDLs help protect against atherosclerosis.

high-density lipoprotein (HDL)   A lipoprotein containing relatively little cholesterol that helps transport cholesterol out of the arteries; "good" cholesterol.

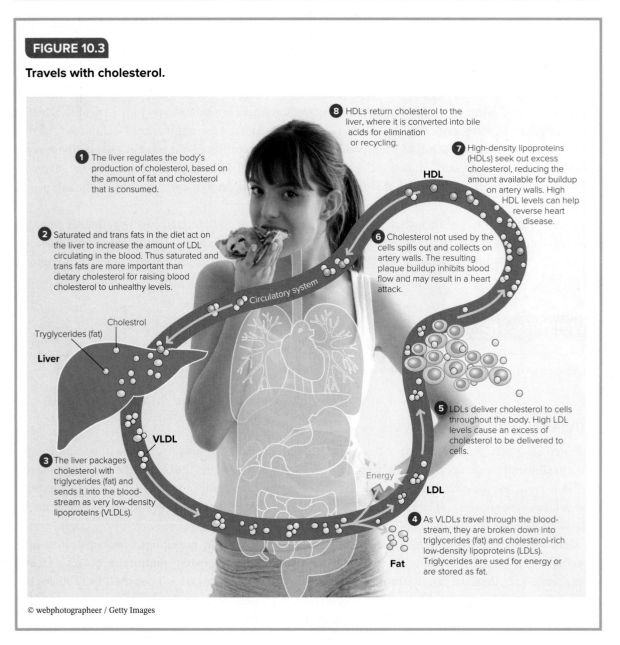

FIGURE 10.3

Travels with cholesterol.

1 The liver regulates the body's production of cholesterol, based on the amount of fat and cholesterol that is consumed.

2 Saturated and trans fats in the diet act on the liver to increase the amount of LDL circulating in the blood. Thus saturated and trans fats are more important than dietary cholesterol for raising blood cholesterol to unhealthy levels.

3 The liver packages cholesterol with triglycerides (fat) and sends it into the blood-stream as very low-density lipoproteins (VLDLs).

4 As VLDLs travel through the blood-stream, they are broken down into triglycerides (fat) and cholesterol-rich low-density lipoproteins (LDLs). Triglycerides are used for energy or are stored as fat.

5 LDLs deliver cholesterol to cells throughout the body. High LDL levels cause an excess of cholesterol to be delivered to cells.

6 Cholesterol not used by the cells spills out and collects on artery walls. The resulting plaque buildup inhibits blood flow and may result in a heart attack.

7 High-density lipoproteins (HDLs) seek out excess cholesterol, reducing the amount available for buildup on artery walls. High HDL levels can help reverse heart disease.

8 HDLs return cholesterol to the liver, where it is converted into bile acids for elimination or recycling.

Circulatory system

Cholestrol

Tryglycerides (fat)

Liver

VLDL

HDL

LDL

Energy

Fat

© webphotographeer / Getty Images

Recommended Blood Cholesterol Levels The risk for CVD increases with increasing blood cholesterol levels, especially LDL. The Heart and Stroke Foundation of Canada does not advocate cholesterol testing for all Canadians. Rather, those with a strong family history of elevated cholesterol or premature heart disease and those who have other coronary heart disease risk factors should consider having their cholesterol levels tested on a regular basis. Visit your doctor to assess your need for a cholesterol test. The recommended test is a lipoprotein profile that measures total cholesterol, LDL cholesterol, HDL cholesterol, and triglycerides (another blood fat).

General cholesterol and triglyceride guidelines are given in Table 10.1. In general, high LDL, total cholesterol and triglyceride levels, and low HDL levels are associated with a high risk for CVD; lowering LDL, total cholesterol, and triglycerides can lower risk. Raising HDL is also important because a high HDL level seems to offer protection from CVD even in cases where total cholesterol is high, especially for women.

TABLE 10.1

Cholesterol Guidelines

Total Cholesterol	
Ideal:	less than 5.2 mmol/L
Borderline High:	5.2–6.2 mmol/L
High:	6.2 mmol/L or more
HDL Cholesterol (Good Cholesterol)	
Desired:	more than 1.5 mmol/L
LDL Cholesterol (Bad Cholesterol)	
Ideal:	less than 3.3 mmol/L
Borderline High:	3.4–4.1 mmol/L
High:	4.1–4.9 mmol/L
Triglycerides	
Ideal:	less than 1.7 mmol/L
Borderline High:	1.7–2.2 mmol/L
High:	2.3–5.6 mmol/L

SOURCE: Cholesterol Guidelines, Mayo Clinic. www.mayoclinic.com, Used with permission.

As shown in Table 10.1, LDL levels below 3.3 mmol/L and total cholesterol levels below 5.2 mmol/L are desirable. It is estimated that close to 45% of Canadians have total cholesterol levels of 5.2 mmol/L or higher.[10] The CVD risk associated with elevated cholesterol levels also depends on other factors. For example, an above optimal level of LDL would be of more concern for an individual who also smoked and had high blood pressure than for an individual without these additional CVD risk factors.

Improving Cholesterol Levels Your primary goal should be to reduce LDL to healthy levels. Important dietary changes for reducing LDL levels include choosing unsaturated fats instead of saturated and trans fats and increasing fibre intake. Decreasing saturated and trans fats is particularly important because they promote the production and excretion of cholesterol by the liver. Exercising regularly and eating more fruits, vegetables, and whole grains also help. Many experts believe that cholesterol-lowering foods may be most effective when eaten in combination rather than separately. You can raise your HDL levels by exercising regularly, losing weight if you are overweight, quitting smoking, and altering the amount and type of fat you consume.

Diabetes

As described in Chapter 6, diabetes is a disorder in which the metabolism of glucose is disrupted, causing a buildup of glucose in the bloodstream. People with diabetes are at increased risk for CVD, partly because elevated blood glucose levels can damage the lining of arteries, making them more vulnerable to atherosclerosis; diabetics also often have other risk factors, including hypertension, obesity, unhealthy cholesterol and triglyceride levels, and platelet and blood coagulation abnormalities. Even people whose diabetes is under control face an increased risk of CVD. Therefore, careful control of other risk factors is critical for people with diabetes. People with pre-diabetes also face a significantly increased risk of CVD.

Major Risk Factors That Can't Be Changed

A number of major risk factors for CVD cannot be changed, such as heredity, aging, being male, ethnicity, and inflammation.

Heredity

Multiple genes contribute to the development of CVD and its risk factors. Having an unfavourable set of genes increases your risk, but risk is modifiable by lifestyle factors such as whether you smoke, exercise, or eat a healthy diet. People who inherit a tendency for CVD are not destined to develop it, but they may have to work harder than other people to prevent it.

Aging

The risk of heart attack increases dramatically after age 65. Over 90% of Canadians over the age of 65 have at least one major risk factor for CVD, and the highest percentage of Canadians with two or more risk factors falls in this age demographic.[11] For people over 55, the incidence of stroke increases by close to 30% in each successive decade. However, many people in their 30s and 40s, especially men, have heart attacks.

Being Male

Although CVD is the leading killer of both men and women in Canada, men show a greater prevalence (than women) of risk factors for CVD such as hypertension and obesity.[12] Estrogen production, highest during the childbearing years, may offer premenopausal women some protection against CVD (see the box Sex and CVD). By age 75, the gender gap nearly disappears.

DIVERSITY Matters

SEX AND CVD

CVD is the leading cause of death for all North Americans, but significant differences exist between men and women in the incidence, diagnosis, and treatment of this deadly disease.

CVD in Women

CVD has been thought of as a "man's disease," but it actually kills about the same number of women as it does men. Polls indicate that women vastly underestimate their risk of dying of a heart attack and overestimate their risk of dying of breast cancer. In reality, nearly one in three women dies of CVD, while one in 34 dies of breast cancer. Although CVD typically does not develop in women younger than age 50, recent research suggests that the number of CVD deaths in women aged 35 to 45 may be increasing.

The hormone estrogen, produced naturally by a woman's ovaries until menopause, improves blood lipid concentrations and reduces other CVD risk factors. For several decades, many physicians encouraged menopausal women to take hormone replacement therapy (HRT) to relieve menopause symptoms and presumably to reduce their risk of CVD. However, some studies have found that HRT actually *increases* a woman's risk for heart disease and other health problems, including breast cancer. Some newer studies have found that the increased risk of CVD in women who start HRT may be age dependent; women in the early stages of menopause or ages 50 to 59 did not appear to have excess risk. This suggests that outcomes may depend on several factors, including the timing of hormone use. For

continued

this reason, the use of HRT for the prevention of chronic diseases such as CVD may not be recommended for some women.

When women have heart attacks, they are more likely than men to die within a year. One reason is that since they develop heart disease at older ages, they are more likely to have other health problems that complicate treatment. Women also have smaller hearts and arteries than men, possibly making diagnosis and treatment more difficult.

Women presenting with CVD are just as likely as men to report chest pain, but they are also likely to report non-chest-pain symptoms, which may obscure their diagnosis. These symptoms include fatigue, weakness, shortness of breath, nausea, vomiting, and pain in the abdomen, neck, jaw, and back. Women are also more likely to have pain at rest, during sleep, or with mental stress. A woman who experiences these symptoms should be persistent in seeking accurate diagnosis and appropriate treatment.

Careful diagnosis of cardiac symptoms is also key in avoiding unnecessary invasive procedures in cases of stress cardiomyopathy ("broken heart syndrome"), which occurs much more commonly in women than in men. In this condition, hormones and neurotransmitters associated with a severe stress response stun the heart, producing heart-attack-like symptoms and decreased pumping function of the heart, but no damage to the heart muscle. Typically, the condition reverses quickly.

Women should be aware of their CVD risk factors and consult with a physician to assess their risk and determine the best way to prevent CVD.

SOURCES: Heart and Stroke Foundation, 2018. *Signs of heart attack, cardiac arrest, sudden arrhythmia death syndrome (SADS).* http://www.heartandstroke.ca/heart/emergency-signs; National Heart, Lung, and Blood Institute. 2013. What are the symptoms of a heart attack? http://www.nhlbi.nih.gov/health/health-topics/topics/heartattack/signs; National Institute of Neurological disorders and Stroke. 2013. Know Stroke. Know the Signs. Act in Time. http://www.ninds.nih.gov/disorders/stroke/knowstroke.htm; National Heart, Lung, and Blood Institute. 2011. What is Sudden Cardiac Arrest? http://www.nhlbi.nih.gov/health/health-topics/topics/scda.

Ethnicity

Death rates from heart disease vary among ethnic groups in Canada. The 1999 First Nations and Inuit Regional Health Survey found the self-reported rate of CVD in this group to be approximately three times higher than that in the Canadian population as a whole.[13] Canadians of both European and South Asian origin have also been shown to have relatively high rates of CVD. Overall trends among the groups indicate that mortality rates from CVD are converging in the three groups––suggesting that lifestyle and environmental factors may be playing a role.[14] In fact, the Heart and Stroke Foundation of Canada reports that as immigrant groups begin to adopt more and more unhealthy lifestyle habits, their risk for CVD increases.[15] The rate at which immigrants are adopting those unhealthy habits is nearing, and in some cases has surpassed, those born in Canada (see Figure 10.4 on the next page).

Inflammation

Inflammation plays a key role in the development of CVD. When an artery is injured by hypertension, smoking, cholesterol, or other factors, the body's response is to produce inflammation. A substance called C-reactive protein (CRP) is released into the bloodstream during the inflammatory response, and high levels of CRP indicate a substantially elevated risk for heart attack and stroke. CRP may also be harmful to the coronary arteries themselves. Gum disease involves another type of inflammation that may moderately influence the progress of coronary heart disease.

Lifestyle changes and certain drugs can reduce CRP levels. Statin drugs, widely prescribed to lower cholesterol, also decrease inflammation; this may be one reason that statin drugs seem to lower CVD risk even in people with normal blood lipid levels.

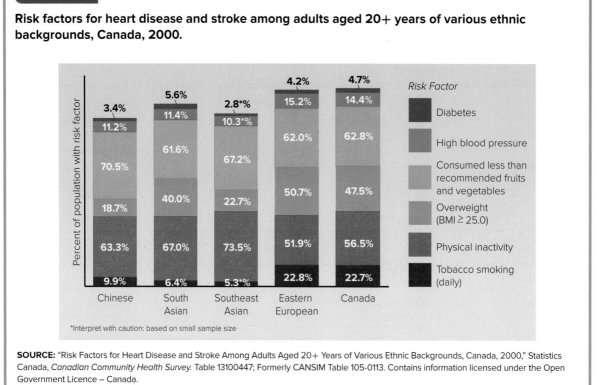

FIGURE 10.4

Risk factors for heart disease and stroke among adults aged 20+ years of various ethnic backgrounds, Canada, 2000.

*Interpret with caution: based on small sample size

SOURCE: "Risk Factors for Heart Disease and Stroke Among Adults Aged 20+ Years of Various Ethnic Backgrounds, Canada, 2000," Statistics Canada, *Canadian Community Health Survey.* Table 13100447; Formerly CANSIM Table 105-0113. Contains information licensed under the Open Government Licence – Canada.

Possible Risk Factors Currently Being Studied

In recent years, a number of other possible risk factors for cardiovascular disease have been identified. Elevated blood levels of homocysteine, an amino acid that may damage the lining of blood vessels, are associated with an increased risk of CVD. Men generally have higher homocysteine levels than women, as do individuals with diets low in folic acid, vitamin B12, and vitamin B6. Most people can lower homocysteine levels easily by adopting a healthy diet rich in fruits, vegetables, and grains. Severe vitamin D deficiency has also been associated with heart dysfunction, independent of homocysteine levels.

Several infectious agents, including *Chlamydia pneumoniae, cytomegalovirus,* and *Helicobacter pylori,* have also been identified as possible risk factors for CVD. *Chlamydia pneumoniae,* a common cause of flu-like respiratory infections, has been found in sections of clogged, damaged arteries but not in sections of healthy arteries. This effect may be secondary to the inflammation that many infectious agents produce in the body.

Gum disease has long been suspected to be linked to CVD. Gingivitis, the beginning stages of gum disease, occurs when bacteria accumulate on the teeth, causing gums to become inflamed and to bleed easily; thus both gum disease and CVD are inflammatory processes. The exact linkages are still unknown, but studies suggest a potential relationship between oral disease and CVD, so it makes sense to practise good oral hygiene. For recommendations on good dental self-care, visit the Canadian Dental Association Oral Health—Good For Life website at http://www.cda-adc.ca/en/oral_health/cfyt/good_for_life/.

QUESTIONS FOR CRITICAL THINKING AND REFLECTION

What risk factors do you have for cardiovascular disease? Which ones are factors you have control over, and which are factors you can't change? If you have risk factors you cannot change (such as a family history of CVD), were you aware that you can make lifestyle adjustments to reduce your risk? Do you think you will make them? Why or why not?

LO3 10.3 Protecting Yourself against Cardiovascular Disease

You can take several important steps right now to lower your risk of developing CVD in the future (Figure 10.5). Reducing CVD risk factors when you are young can pay off with many extra years of life and health.

FIGURE 10.5

Strategies for reducing your risk of cardiovascular disease.

Do More

- Eat a diet rich in fruits, vegetables, whole grains, and low-fat or fat-free dairy products. Eat five to nine servings of fruits and vegetables each day.
- Eat several servings of high-fibre foods each day.
- Eat two or more servings of fish per week; try a few servings of nuts and soy foods each week.
- Choose unsaturated fats rather than saturated and trans fats.
- Be physically active; do both aerobic exercise and strength training on a regular basis.
- Achieve and maintain a healthy weight.
- Develop effective strategies for handling stress and anger. Nurture old friendships and family ties, and make new friends; pay attention to your spiritual side.
- Obtain recommended screening tests and follow your physician's recommendations.

Do Less

- Don't use tobacco in any form: cigarettes, spit tobacco, cigars and pipes, bidis and clove cigarettes.
- Limit consumption of fats, especially trans fats and saturated fats.
- Limit consumption of salt to no more than 2300 mg of sodium per day (1500 mg if you have or are at high risk for hypertension).
- Avoid exposure to environmental tobacco smoke.
- Avoid excessive alcohol consumption— no more than one drink per day for women and two drinks per day for men.
- Limit consumption of cholesterol, added sugars, and refined carbohydrates.
- Avoid excess stress, anger, and hostility.

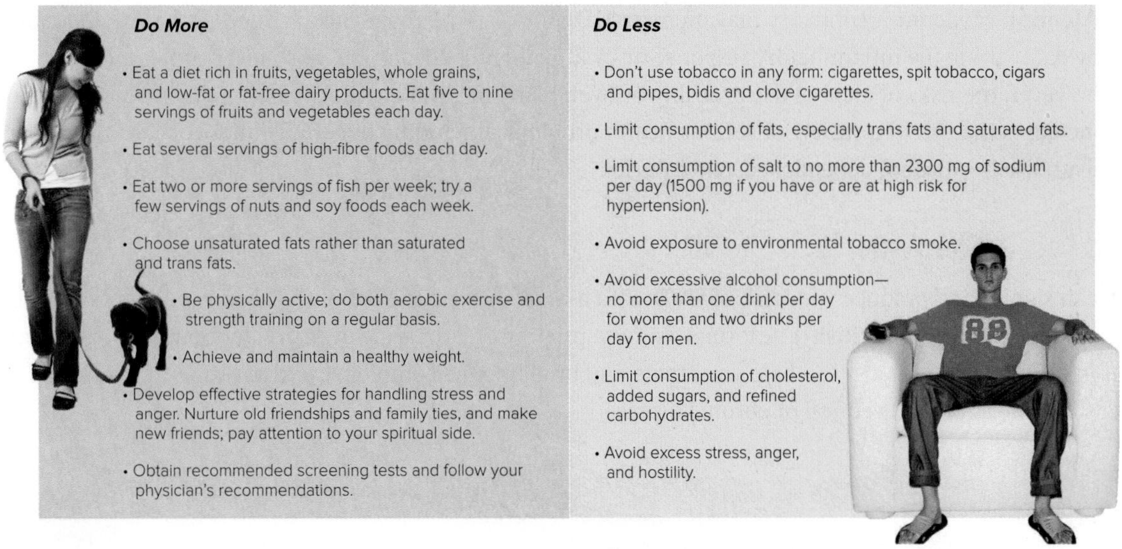

(left), © Jessica Peterson / Rubberball Production / Getty Images; (right), © Stockbyte / PunchStock

Eat a Heart-Healthy Diet

For most Canadians, changing to a heart-healthy diet involves cutting total fat intake, substituting unsaturated fats for saturated and trans fats, and increasing intake of whole grains and fibre. Several aspects of nutrition apply directly to heart health.

- **Fats.** Health Canada recommends that all Canadians adopt a diet in which total fat consumption is no more than 30% of total daily calories, with no more than one-third of those fat calories (10% of total daily calories) coming from saturated fat. For people with heart disease or high LDL levels, a total fat intake of 25–35% of total daily calories and a saturated fat intake of less than 7% of total calories is recommended. Trans fats should be avoided. The majority of fats in your diet should be unsaturated, from sources such as vegetable oils, fish, and nuts.

- **Fibre.** Studies have shown that a high-fibre diet is associated with a 40–50% reduction in the risk of heart attack and stroke. To get the recommended 25 to 38 grams of dietary fibre a day, eat whole grains, fruits, and vegetables. Good sources of fibre include oatmeal, some breakfast cereals, barley, legumes, and most fruits and vegetables.

Wellness Tip

Oatmeal can actually lower your level of LDL cholesterol. Oatmeal contains soluble fibre, which prevents LDL particles from entering the bloodstream.

- **Sodium and potassium.** Reducing sodium intake to recommended levels, while also increasing potassium intake, can help reduce blood pressure for many people. The recommended limit for sodium intake is 2300 milligrams per day; for population groups at special risk, including those with hypertension, middle-aged and older adults, and some ethnic groups, the recommended limit is 1500 milligrams per day. Recommended potassium intake is 4700 milligrams per day for those over 14 years of age.

- **Alcohol.** Moderate alcohol use may increase HDL cholesterol; it may also reduce stroke risk, possibly by dampening the inflammatory response or by affecting blood clotting. For most people under age 45, however, the risks of alcohol use probably outweigh any health benefit. Excessive alcohol consumption increases the risk of a variety of serious health problems, including hypertension, stroke, some cancers, liver disease, alcohol dependence, and injuries.

Exercise Regularly

You can significantly reduce your risk of CVD with a moderate amount of physical activity (see the box How Does Exercise Affect CVD Risk?). A formal exercise program can provide even greater benefits. The information in Chapters 2 to 5 and 9 can help you create and implement a complete exercise program that meets your needs for fitness and prevention of chronic disease.

The Evidence *for* EXERCISE

HOW DOES EXERCISE AFFECT CVD RISK?

Regular exercise directly and indirectly benefits your cardiovascular health and can actually help you avoid having a heart attack or stroke. The evidence comes from dozens of large-scale, population-based studies conducted over the past several decades. There is so much evidence about the cardiovascular health benefits of exercise, in fact, that physicians regard physical activity as a magic bullet against heart disease.

Physical activity has an inverse relationship with cardiovascular health, meaning that the more exercise you get, the less likely you are to develop or die from CVD. Compared to sedentary individuals, people who engage in regular, moderate physical activity lower their risk of CVD by 20% or more.

People who get regular, vigorous exercise reduce their risk of CVD by 30% or more. This positive benefit applies regardless of sex, age, race, or ethnicity.

Most studies focus on various aerobic endurance exercises, such as walking, running on a treadmill, or biking. As noted in Chapter 1, the type of exercise performed is less important than the amount of energy expended during the activity: The greater the energy expenditure, the greater the health benefits.

Exercise affects heart health via many mechanisms, all of which are being studied. For example, exercise helps people lose weight and improve body composition. Weight loss can improve heart health by reducing the amount of stress on the heart. Changing body composition to a more positive ratio of fat to fat-free mass boosts resting metabolic rate. Exercise directly strengthens the heart muscle itself, and it improves the balance of fats in the blood by boosting HDL and reducing LDL and triglyceride levels.

Exercise can also prevent metabolic syndrome and reverse many of its negative effects on the body. For example, exercise improves the health and function of the endothelial cells—the inner lining of the arteries. These cells secrete nitric oxide, which regulates blood flow, improves nerve function, strengthens the immune system, enhances reproductive health, and suppresses inflammation. Exercise training also improves the function of cell sodium-potassium pumps, which regulate fluid and electrolyte balance and cellular communication throughout the body.

One of the clearest positive effects of exercise is on hypertension. Many studies, involving thousands of people, have shown that physical activity reduces both systolic and diastolic blood pressure. These studies showed that people who engaged in regular aerobic exercise lowered their resting blood pressure by 2–4%, on average. Lowered blood pressure itself reduces the risk of other kinds of cardiovascular disease.

Fewer studies have been conducted on exercise and risk of stroke. Even with limited evidence, however, there appears to be a similar inverse relationship between physical activity and stroke. According to a handful of studies, the most physically active people reduced their risk of both ischemic and hemorrhagic strokes by up to 30%. Although this benefit appears to apply equally to men and women, there is not sufficient evidence that it applies equally across races or ethnicities.

Of course, exercise isn't possible for everyone and may actually be dangerous for some people. Anyone who has CVD or serious risk factors for heart disease should work with their physician to determine whether or how to exercise.

Effective Means of Keeping Physically Active

Keep these guidelines in mind as you strive to reduce CVD risk factors:

- **Set goals.** Not physiological goals (e.g., to improve LDL cholesterol levels), but to target a behaviour (such as exercising for 30 minutes per day).

- **Monitor yourself.** Self-monitoring increases your awareness of physical cues and behaviours and helps you identify the barriers to changing a behaviour.

- **Schedule follow-up exercise sessions.** Multiple sessions are more effective than single sessions.

- **Get feedback from your health care provider.** Feedback can encourage healthy choices by giving you an external measuring stick you can use to monitor your progress.

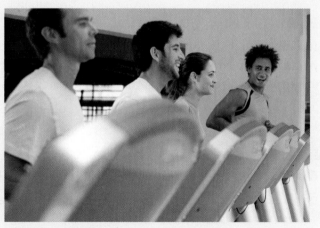

© Juice Images/Alamy RF

continued

- **Keep a positive outlook on your progress.** A feeling of accomplishment is very important in motivating you to initiate new behaviours and continue your efforts once begun.

SOURCES: Eckel, R.H., et al. 2014. 2013 AHA/ACC Guideline on lifestyle management to reduce cardiovascular risk: A report of the American College of Cardiology/American Heart Association Task Force on practice guidelines. *Journal of the American College of Cardiology* 63(25_PA); Lackland, D. T., and J. H. Voeks. 2014. Metabolic syndrome and hypertension: Regular exercise as part of lifestyle management. *Current Hypertension Reports* 16(11): 492; Artinian N.T., et al. 2010. Interventions to promote physical activity and dietary lifestyle changes for cardiovascular risk factor reduction in adults: A scientific statement from the American heart association. *Circulation.* 10:406–441; Cornelissen, V. A., and R. H. Fagard. 2005. Effect of resistance training on resting blood pressure: A meta-analysis of randomized controlled trials. *Journal of Hypertension* 23(2): 251–259; Physical Activity Guidelines Advisory Committee. 2008. *Physical Activity Guidelines Advisory Committee Report, 2008.* Washington, D.C.: U.S. Department of Health and Human Services.

Avoid Tobacco

The number-one risk factor for CVD that you can control is smoking. If you smoke, quit. If you don't smoke, don't start. If you live or work with people who smoke, encourage them to quit—for their sake and yours. If you find yourself breathing in smoke, take steps to prevent or stop this exposure.

Know and Manage Your Blood Pressure

Currently, nearly 43% of the 5 million Canadians with hypertension are not even aware that they may have blood pressure problems.[14] If you have no CVD risk factors, have your blood pressure measured at least once every two years; yearly tests are recommended if you have other risk factors. If your blood pressure is high, follow your physician's advice on lowering it.

Know and Manage Your Cholesterol Levels

Everyone age 20 and over should have their cholesterol checked at least once every five years. Your goal for LDL depends in part on how many of the following major risk factors you have: cigarette smoking, high blood pressure, low HDL cholesterol (less than 0.9 mmol/L), a family history of heart disease, and age above 45 years for men and 55 years for women. After you know your baseline numbers, you and your physician can develop a treatment and lifestyle plan.

Develop Ways to Handle Stress and Anger

To reduce the psychological and social risk factors for CVD, develop effective strategies for handling the stress in your life. Shore up your social support network, and, if anger and hostility are problems for you, try some of the techniques described in Chapter 12 for managing stress and anger.

Ask Yourself
QUESTIONS FOR CRITICAL THINKING AND REFLECTION

Do you know what your blood pressure and cholesterol levels are, on average? If not, is there a reason you don't know? Is there something preventing you from getting this information about yourself? How can you motivate yourself to have these easy but important health checks?

Tips for Today and the Future

Because cardiovascular disease is a long-term process that can begin when you're young, it's important to develop heart-healthy habits early in life.

RIGHT NOW YOU CAN

- Make an appointment to have your blood pressure and cholesterol levels checked.

- List the key stressors in your life, and decide what to do about the ones that bother you most.

- Plan to replace one high-fat item in your diet with one that is high in fibre. For example, replace a doughnut with a bowl of whole-grain cereal or a cup of yogourt with fruit.

IN THE FUTURE YOU CAN

- Track your eating habits for one week, then compare them to the Dietary Reference Intakes (DRIs). Make adjustments to bring your diet closer to the DRIs.

- Sign up for a class in CPR. A CPR certification equips you with valuable life-saving skills you can use to help someone who is choking, having a heart attack, or experiencing cardiac arrest. Many CPR classes also include training in the use of an AED.

Common Questions ANSWERED

Q I know what foods to avoid to prevent CVD, but are there any foods I should eat to protect myself from CVD?

A The most important dietary change for CVD prevention is a negative one: cutting back on foods high in saturated and trans fat. However, certain foods can be helpful. The positive effects of unsaturated fats, soluble fibre, and alcohol on heart health were discussed earlier in the chapter. Other potentially beneficial foods include those rich in the following:

- **Omega-3 fatty acids**. Found in fish, shellfish, and some nuts and seeds, omega-3 fatty acids reduce clotting and inflammation and may lower the risk of fatal arrhythmia.
- **Folic acid, vitamin B6, and vitamin B12**. These vitamins may affect CVD risk by lowering homocysteine levels; see Table 7.4 for a list of food sources.
- **Plant stanols and sterols**. Plant stanols and sterols, found in some types of trans-free margarines and other products, reduce the absorption of cholesterol in the body and help lower LDL levels.
- **Soy protein**. Replacing some animal protein with soy protein can lower LDL cholesterol. Soy-based foods include tofu, tempeh, and soy-based beverages.
- **Calcium**. Diets rich in calcium may help prevent hypertension and possibly stroke by reducing insulin resistance and platelet aggregation. Low-fat or nonfat dairy products are rich in calcium; refer to Chapter 7 for other sources.

Q The advice I hear from the media about protecting myself from CVD seems to be changing all the time. What am I supposed to believe?

A Health-related research is now described in popular newspapers and magazines rather than just medical journals, meaning that more and more people have access to the information. Researchers do not deliberately set out to mislead or confuse people. However, news reports may oversimplify the results of research studies, leaving out some of the qualifications and questions the researchers present with their findings. In addition, news reports may not differentiate between a preliminary finding and a result that has been verified by a large number of long-term studies. And researchers themselves must strike a balance between reporting promising preliminary findings to the public,

continued

thereby allowing people to act on them, and waiting 10 to 20 years until long-term studies confirm (or disprove) a particular theory. Although you cannot become an expert on all subjects, there are some general strategies you can use to assess the health advice that appears in the media; see the box Evaluating Sources of Health Information in Chapter 1.

Q What's a heart murmur, and is it dangerous?

A A heart murmur is an extra or altered heart sound heard during a routine medical exam. The source is often a problem with one of the heart valves that separate the chambers of the heart. Congenital defects and certain infections can cause abnormalities in the valves. The most common heart valve disorder is mitral valve prolapse (MVP), which occurs in about 4% of the population. MVP is characterized by a "billowing" of the mitral valve, which separates the left ventricle and left atrium, during ventricular contraction; in some cases, blood leaks from the ventricle into the atrium. Most people with MVP have no symptoms; they are able to exercise and live as long as people without MVP.

MVP can be confirmed with echocardiography. Treatment is usually unnecessary, although surgery may be needed in the rare cases where leakage through the faulty valve is severe. Experts disagree over whether patients with MVP should take antibiotics prior to dental procedures. This precautionary step is sometimes used to prevent bacteria, which may be dislodged into the bloodstream during some types of dental and surgical procedures, from infecting the defective valve. Most often, only those patients with significant blood leakage are advised to take antibiotics.

Although MVP usually requires no treatment, more severe heart valve disorders can impair blood flow through the heart. Treatment depends on the location and severity of the problem. More serious defects may be treated with surgery to repair or replace a valve.

Q How does stress contribute to cardiovascular disease?

A With stress, the brain tells the adrenal glands to secrete cortisol and other hormones and neurotransmitters, which in turn activate the sympathetic nervous system—causing the fight-or-flight response. This response increases heart rate and blood pressure so that more blood is distributed to the heart and other muscles in anticipation of physical activity. Blood glucose concentrations and cholesterol also increase to provide a source of energy, and the platelets become activated so that they will be more likely to clot in case of injury. Such a response can be adaptive if you're being chased by a hungry lion but may be more detrimental than useful if you're sitting at a desk taking an exam or feeling frustrated by a task given to you by your boss.

If you are healthy, you can tolerate the cardiovascular responses that take place during stress, but if you already have CVD, stress can lead to adverse outcomes such as abnormal heart rhythms, heart attacks, and sudden cardiac death. It has long been known that an increase in heart rhythm problems and deaths is associated with acute mental stress. For example, the rate of potentially life-threatening arrhythmias in patients who already had underlying heart disease doubled during the month after the September 11 terrorist attacks in 2001; this increase was not limited to people in close proximity to Manhattan.

Because avoiding all stress is impossible, having healthy mechanisms to cope with it is your best defence. Instead of adopting unhealthy habits such as smoking, drinking, or overeating to deal with stress, try healthier coping techniques such as exercising, getting enough sleep, and talking to family and friends.

SUMMARY

- The major controllable risk factors for CVD that are related to lifestyle are tobacco use, unhealthy diet, physical inactivity, unhealthy weight, excessive drug and alcohol abuse, and stress. The four major controllable risk factors associated with health conditions are high blood pressure, high cholesterol levels, diabetes, and atrial fibrillation.

- Major risk factors for CVD that can't be changed are heredity, aging, being male, and ethnicity.

- Hypertension weakens the heart and scars and hardens arteries, causing resistance to blood flow. It is defined as blood pressure equal to or higher than 140 over 90.

- Atherosclerosis is a progressive hardening and narrowing of arteries that can lead to restricted blood flow and even complete blockage.

- Heart attacks, strokes, and congestive heart failure are the results of a long-term disease process; hypertension and atherosclerosis are usually involved.

- Reducing heart disease risk involves eating a heart-healthy diet, exercising regularly, avoiding tobacco, managing blood pressure and cholesterol levels, and handling stress and anger.

FOR FURTHER EXPLORATION

Organizations and Websites

Canadian Cardiovascular Society. Includes research-based information on cardiovascular issues.

   http://www.ccs.ca

Dieticians of Canada. Provides nutrition information for professionals and consumers.

   http://www.dieticians.ca

The Heart: The Engine of Life. Contains information on the structure and function of the heart, how to monitor your heart's health, and how to maintain a healthy heart as part of an online museum exhibit.

   https://www.fi.edu/heart-engine-of-life

Heart and Stroke Foundation of Canada. Provides information on the prevention and control of heart disease and stroke. Includes risk assessments and articles for reducing the risks associated with heart disease and stroke.

   http://www.heartandstroke.ca

Government of Canada. Offers information about healthy living, food and nutrition, and health services.

   https://www.canada.ca/en.html

MedlinePlus: Heart and Circulation Topics. Provides links to reliable sources of information on cardiovascular health.

   http://www.nlm.nih.gov/medlineplus/bloodheartandcirculation.html

   See also the listings for Chapter 8 and Chapter 13.

Laboratory Activities

Name _____ **Section** _____ **Date** _____

Lab 10.1 Cardiovascular Health

![Mc Graw Hill Education] connect

Part I CVD Risk Assessment

Your chances of suffering a heart attack or stroke before age 55 depend on a variety of factors, many of which are within your control. To help identify your risk factors, circle the response for each risk category that best describes you.

1. Sex and Age

  0 Female age 55 or younger; male age 45 or younger
  2 Female over age 55; male over age 45

2. Heredity/Family History

  0 Neither parent suffered a heart attack or stroke before age 60
  3 One parent suffered a heart attack or stroke before age 60
  7 Both parents suffered a heart attack or stroke before age 60

3. Smoking

  0 Never smoked
  3 Quit more than 2 years ago and lifetime smoking is less than 5 pack-years*
  6 Quit less than 2 years ago and/or lifetime smoking is greater than 5 pack-years*
  8 Smoke less than ½ pack per day
  13 Smoke more than ½ pack per day
  15 Smoke more than 1 pack per day

4. Environmental Tobacco Smoke (ETS)

  0 Do not live or work with smokers
  2 Exposed to ETS at work
  3 Live with smoker
  4 Both live and work with smokers

5. Blood Pressure

(If available, use the average of the last three readings.)

0 120/80 or below	1 121/81–130/85
3 Don't know blood pressure	5 131/86–150/90
9 151/91–170/100	13 Above 170/100

6. Total Cholesterol

0 Lower than 5.2	1 5.3–5.4
2 Don't know	3 5.5–5.7
4 5.8–5.9	5 6.0–6.1
6 Over 6.2	

7. HDL Cholesterol

    0 Over 0.9 mmol/L   1 0.7–0.8

    2 Don't know   12 Lower than 0.9

8. Exercise

    0 Exercise three times a week   1 Exercise once or twice a week

    2 Occasional exercise less than once a week   7 Rarely exercise

9. Diabetes

    0 No personal or family history   2 One parent with diabetes

    6 Two parents with diabetes   9 Type 2 diabetes

   13 Type 1 diabetes

10. Body Mass Index (kg/m^2)

    0 <23.0   1 23.0–24.9

    2 25.0–28.9   3 29.0–34.9

    5 35.0–39.9   7 $\leq$40.0

11. Stress

    0 Relaxed most of the time   1 Occasionally stressed and angry

    2 Frequently stressed and angry   3 Usually stressed and angry

* Pack-years can be calculated by multiplying the number of packs you smoked per day by the number of years you smoked. For example, if you smoked a pack and a half a day for 5 years, you would have smoked the equivalent of $1.5 \times 5 = 7.5$ pack-years.

Scoring

Total your risk factor points. Refer to the list below to get an approximate rating of your risk of suffering an early heart attack or stroke. Whether your risk is low or extremely high, you should be aware of the factors that contribute to that risk and seek health care advice in reducing its effect on your health.

Score	Estimated Risk
Less than 20	Low risk
20–29	Moderate risk
30–45	High risk
Over 45	Extremely high risk

Part II Hostility Assessment

Are you too hostile? To help answer that question, Duke University researcher Redford Williams, M.D., has devised a short self-test. It is not a scientific evaluation, but it does offer a rough measure of hostility. Are the following statements true or false for you?

1. I often get annoyed at checkout cashiers or the people in front of me when I'm waiting in line.

2. I usually keep an eye on the people I work or live with to make sure they do what they should.

3. I often wonder how homeless people can have so little respect for themselves.

4. I believe that most people will take advantage of you if you let them.

5. The habits of friends or family members often annoy me.

6. When I'm stuck in traffic, I often start breathing faster and my heart pounds.

7. When I'm annoyed with people, I really want to let them know it.

8. If someone does me wrong, I want to get even.

9. I'd like to have the last word in any argument.

10. At least once a week, I have the urge to yell at or even hit someone.

According to Williams, five or more "true" statements suggest that you're excessively hostile and should consider taking steps to mellow out.

Using Your Results

How did you score? What is your CVD risk assessment score? Are you at all surprised by your score?

_____
_____
_____

Are you satisfied with your CVD risk rating? If not, set a specific goal:

_____
_____
_____

What is your hostility assessment score? Are you at all surprised by the result?

_____
_____
_____

Are you satisfied with your hostility rating? If not, set a specific goal:

_____
_____
_____

What should you do next? Enter the results of this lab in the Preprogram Assessment column in Appendix B. If you've set a goal for the overall CVD risk assessment score, identify a risk area that you can change, such as smoking, exercise, or stress. Then list three steps or strategies for changing the risk area you've chosen.

Risk area:_____

_____
_____
_____

Strategies for change:

_____
_____
_____

If you've set a goal for the hostility assessment score, review the anger management strategies in Chapter 12 and select several that you will try to use to manage your own angry responses. Strategies for anger management:

_____
_____
_____

Next, begin to put your strategies into action. After several weeks of a program to reduce CVD risk or hostility, do this lab again and enter the results in the Postprogram Assessment column of Appendix B. How do the results compare?

_____

_____

_____

SOURCE: Hostility quiz from *Life Skills* by Virginia Williams and Redford Williams. New York: Times Books. Reprinted by permission of the authors.

Cancer

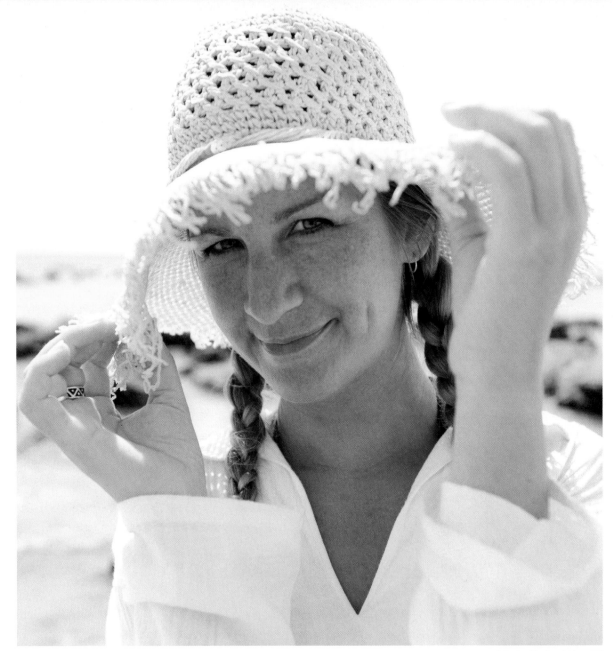

LEARNING OBJECTIVES

After reading this chapter, you should be able to

LO1   Explain what cancer is and how it spreads

LO2   Discuss some of the causes of cancer and how they can be avoided or minimized

LO3   List and describe common cancers, including their risk factors, signs and symptoms, treatments, and approaches to prevention

LO4   Describe how cancer can be detected, diagnosed, and treated

LO5   List specific actions you can take to lower your risk of cancer

TEST YOUR KNOWLEDGE

1. **Eating which of these foods may help prevent cancer?**
   a. chili peppers
   b. broccoli
   c. oranges

2. **Using a sunscreen with an SPF rating of 15 means that you**
   a. can stay in the sun for 15 minutes without getting burned.
   b. can stay in the sun 15 times longer without getting burned than if you didn't use it.
   c. are protected against the full range of ultraviolet (UV) radiation.

3. **The use of condoms during sexual intercourse can prevent cancer in women.**

   True or false?

ANSWERS

1. **ALL THREE.** These and many other fruits and vegetables are rich in phytochemicals, naturally occurring substances that may have anticancer effects.

2. **B.** Choose a sunscreen that has an SPF rating of 15 or higher and that protects against both UVA and UVB rays. Apply it generously; most people use less than half the recommended amount.

3. **TRUE.** The primary cause of cervical cancer is infection with the human papillomavirus (HPV), a sexually transmitted pathogen. The use of condoms can prevent HPV infection.

It is estimated that cancer caused more than 80 800 deaths in Canada in 2017,[1] and it is currently the most common cause of death. Evidence indicates that more than 60% of all cancers in Canada could be prevented by simple changes in lifestyle.[2] In Canada, tobacco use is responsible for about one-third of all cancer deaths. Diet and exercise, including their relationship with obesity, account for a similar proportion of deaths in those with prostate cancer.[3]

📍LO1 11.1 What Is Cancer?

Cancer is the abnormal, uncontrolled growth of cells, which can ultimately cause death if left untreated.

> **cancer**   Abnormal, uncontrolled multiplication of cells.

Tumours

Most cancers take the form of tumours, although not all tumours are cancerous. A **tumour** (or neoplasm) is a mass of tissue that serves no physiological purpose. It can be benign, like a wart, or malignant, like most lung cancers.

> **tumour**   A mass of tissue that serves no physiological purpose; also called a *neoplasm.*

Benign (noncancerous) **tumours** are made up of cells similar to the surrounding normal cells and are enclosed in a membrane that prevents them from penetrating neighbouring tissues. They are dangerous only if their physical presence interferes with body functions. A benign brain tumour, for example, can cause death if it blocks the blood supply to the brain.

> **benign tumour**   A tumour that is not cancerous.

The term **malignant tumour** is synonymous with cancer. A malignant tumour can invade surrounding structures, including blood vessels, the **lymphatic system**, and nerves. It can also spread to distant sites via the blood and lymphatic circulation, producing invasive tumours in almost any part of the body. A few cancers, like leukemia (cancer of the blood), do not produce a mass but still have the fundamental property of rapid, uncontrolled cell proliferation.

> **malignant tumour**   A tumour that is cancerous and capable of spreading.
> **lymphatic system**   A system of vessels that returns proteins, lipids, and other substances from fluid in the tissues to the circulatory system.

Every case of cancer begins as a change in a cell that allows it to grow and divide when it should not. A malignant cell divides without regard for normal control mechanisms and gradually produces a mass of abnormal cells, or a tumour. It takes about a billion cells to make a mass the size of a pea, so a single tumour cell must go through many divisions, often taking years, before the tumour grows to a noticeable size. Eventually, a tumour produces a sign or symptom that is detected. In an accessible location (such as a testicle), a tumour may be felt as a lump. In less accessible locations (such as the lungs), a tumour may be noticed only after considerable growth has taken place and may then be detected only by an indirect symptom, such as a persistent cough or unexplained bleeding or pain.

Metastasis

Metastasis, the spreading of cancer cells, occurs because cancer cells do not stick to each other as strongly as normal cells do and therefore may not remain at the site of the *primary tumour*, the original location. They break away and can pass through the lining of lymph or blood vessels to invade nearby tissue. They can also drift to distant parts of the body, where they establish new colonies of cancer cells. This travelling and seeding process is called *metastasizing*, and the new tumours are called *secondary tumours*, or *metastases*.

> **metastasis**   The spread of cancer cells from one part of the body to another.

This ability of cancer cells to metastasize makes early cancer detection critical. To control the cancer, every cancerous cell must be removed. Once cancer cells enter either the lymphatic system or the bloodstream, it is extremely difficult to stop their spread to other organs.

LO2 11.2 The Causes of Cancer

Although scientists do not know everything about what causes cancer, they have identified genetic, environmental, and lifestyle factors that may influence a person's risk for cancer Lab 11.1 gives you the opportunity to consider two areas of cancer prevention over which you have individual control: diet and sun exposure. There are usually several steps in the transformation of a normal cell into a cancer cell, and different factors may work together in the development of cancer.

The Role of DNA

Heredity and genetics are important factors in a person's risk of cancer. Certain genes may predispose some people to cancer, and specific gene mutations have been associated with cancer.

DNA Basics

The nucleus of each cell in your body contains 23 pairs of **chromosomes**, which are made up of tightly packed coils of **DNA** (deoxyribonucleic acid). Each chromosome contains thousands of **genes**; you have about 25 000 genes in all. Each of your genes controls the production of a particular protein. By making different proteins at different times, genes can act as switches to alter the ways a cell works. Some genes are responsible for controlling the rate of cell division, and these genes often play a critical role in the development of cancer.

> **chromosomes**   The threadlike bodies in a cell nucleus that contain molecules of DNA; most human cells contain 23 pairs of chromosomes.
> **DNA**   Deoxyribonucleic acid, a chemical substance that carries genetic information.
> **gene**   A section of a chromosome that contains the instructions for making a particular protein; the basic unit of heredity.

DNA Mutations and Cancer

A *mutation* is any change in the makeup of a gene. Some mutations are inherited; others are caused by environmental agents known as *mutagens*. Mutagens include radiation, certain viruses, and chemical substances in the air we breathe. When a mutagen also causes cancer, it is called a **carcinogen**. Some mutations are the result of copying errors that occur when DNA replicates itself as part of cell division.

> **carcinogen**   Any substance that causes cancer.

A mutated gene no longer contains the proper code for producing its protein. It usually takes several mutational changes before a normal cell takes on the properties of a cancer cell. Genes in which mutations are associated with the conversion of a normal cell into a cancer cell are known as **oncogenes**. In their undamaged form, many oncogenes play a role in controlling or restricting cell growth; they are called *tumour suppressor genes*. Mutational damage to suppressor genes releases the brake on growth and leads to rapid and uncontrolled cell division—a precondition for the development of cancer.

> **oncogene**   A gene involved in the transformation of a normal cell into a cancer cell.

An example of an inherited mutated oncogene is BRCA1 (breast cancer gene 1). Women who inherit a damaged copy of this suppressor gene face a significantly increased risk of breast and ovarian cancer. In most cases, however, mutational damage occurs after birth. For example, only about 5–10% of breast cancer cases can be traced to inherited copies of a damaged BRCA1 gene. In addition, lifestyle factors are important even for those who have inherited a damaged suppressor gene. Testing and identification of hereditary cancer risks can be helpful for some people, especially if it leads to increased attention to controllable risk factors and better medical screening.

Cancer Promoters

Substances known as cancer promoters make up another important piece of the cancer puzzle. They don't directly produce DNA mutations, but they accelerate the growth of cells, which means less time for a cell to repair DNA damage caused by other factors. Estrogen, which stimulates cellular growth in the female reproductive organs, is an example of a cancer promoter.

Tobacco Use

Smoking is responsible for up to 85% of lung cancers and for about 30% of all cancer deaths. In addition to lung and bronchial cancer, tobacco use is linked to cancer of the larynx, mouth, pharynx, esophagus, stomach, pancreas, kidneys, bladder, and cervix. The Canadian Cancer Society estimates that the average smoker will die about 10 years earlier than someone who has never smoked.

Dietary Factors

Diet is one of the most important factors in cancer prevention, but it is also one of the most complex and controversial. Your food choices can affect your cancer risk by exposing you to potentially dangerous compounds, while also depriving you of potentially protective ones. The following dietary factors may affect cancer risk.

Dietary Fat and Meat

Diets high in fat and meat may contribute to certain cancers, including colon, stomach, and prostate. Certain types of fats may be riskier than others. Omega-6 poly-unsaturated fats are associated with a higher risk of certain cancers; omega-3 fats are not. (See Chapter 7 for more information on types of fatty acids.)

Alcohol

Alcohol is associated with an increased incidence of several cancers. For example, an average alcohol intake of three drinks a day is associated with a doubling in the risk of breast cancer. Alcohol and tobacco interact as risk factors for oral cancer. Heavy users of both alcohol and tobacco have a risk for oral cancer many times greater than that of people who don't drink or use tobacco.

Foods Cooked at High Temperatures

Scientists have found high levels of the chemical acrylamide (a probable human carcinogen) in starch-based foods that have been fried or baked at high temperatures, especially french fries and certain types of snack chips and crackers. Acrylamide is also found in high concentrations in tobacco. When muscle meats (e.g., beef, pork, fish, and poultry) are cooked at high temperatures, such as when grilled over an open flame or pan fried, different types of cancer-causing chemicals can form.

Fibre

Various potential cancer-fighting actions have been proposed for fibre, but none has been firmly established. Further study is needed to clarify the relationship between fibre intake and cancer risk, but experts still recommend a high-fibre diet for its overall positive effect on health.

Fruits and Vegetables

Canada's Food Guide encourages individuals to eat a plant-based diet containing numerous servings of vegetables and fruits every day, and to choose whole grains over processed grains. A massive number of epidemiological studies provide evidence that high consumption of fruits and vegetables reduces the risk of many cancers. Exactly which constituents of fruits and vegetables are responsible for reducing cancer risk is not clear, but researchers have identified many mechanisms by which food components may act against cancer. Some may prevent carcinogens from forming in the first place or block them from reaching or acting on target cells, while others boost enzymes that detoxify carcinogens and render them harmless. Some essential nutrients act as anticarcinogens. For example, vitamin C, vitamin E, selenium, and the **carotenoids** (vitamin A precursors) may help block cancer by acting as antioxidants.

> **carotenoids**   Any group of yellow-to-red plant pigments that can be converted to vitamin A by the liver; many act as antioxidants or have other anti-cancer effects. Carotenoids include beta-carotene, lutein, lycopene, and zeaxanthin.

Many other anticancer agents in the diet fall under the broader heading of **phytochemicals**, substances in plants that help protect against chronic diseases (see Table 11.1). One of the first to be identified was sulforaphane, a potent anticarcinogen found in broccoli.

> **phytochemicals**   Naturally occurring substances found in plant foods that may help prevent chronic diseases such as cancer and heart disease; *phyto* means plant.

TABLE 11.1

Foods with Phytochemicals

Food	Phytochemical	Potential Anticancer Effects
Chili peppers (*Note:* Hotter peppers contain more capsaicin.)	Capsaicin	Neutralizes effect of nitrosamines; may block carcinogens in cigarette smoke from acting on cells
Oranges, lemons, limes, onions, apples, berries, eggplant	Flavonoids	Act as antioxidants; block access of carcinogens to cells; suppress malignant changes in cells; prevent cancer cells from multiplying
Citrus fruits, cherries	Monoterpenes	Help detoxify carcinogens; inhibit spread of cancer cells
Cruciferous vegetables (broccoli, cabbage, bok choy, cauliflower, kale, Brussels sprouts, collards)	Isothiocyanates	Boost production of cancer-fighting enzymes; suppress tumour growth; block effects of estrogen on cell growth
Garlic, onions, leeks, shallots, chives	Allyl sulfides	Increase levels of enzymes that break down potential carcinogens; boost activity of cancer-fighting immune cells
Grapes, red wine, peanuts	Resveratrol	Acts as an antioxidant; suppresses tumour growth
Green, oolong, and black teas (*Note:* Drinking burning hot tea may *increase* cancer risk.)	Polyphenols	Increase antioxidant activity; prevent cancer cells from multiplying; help speed excretion of carcinogens from body
Orange, deep yellow, red, pink, and dark green vegetables; some fruits	Carotenoids	Act as antioxidants; reduce levels of cancer-promoting enzymes; inhibit spread of cancer cells
Soy foods, whole grains, flax seeds, nuts	Phytoestrogens	Block effects of estrogen on cell growth; lower blood levels of estrogen
Whole grains, legumes	Phytic acid	Binds iron, which may prevent it from creating cell-damaging free radicals

Obesity and Inactivity

It is important to maintain a healthy weight throughout life by balancing caloric intake with physical activity and achieving and maintaining a healthy weight if currently overweight or obese. Several common types of cancer (colon, breast,[4] endometrium, kidney, prostate) are associated with being overweight or obese,[5] and gaining weight over time (Figure 11.1). Physical activity reduces the risk of cancer of the breast, colon, and uterus, as well as advanced prostate cancer. The Canadian Cancer Society guidelines encourage everyone to adopt a physically active lifestyle (see the box How Does Exercise Affect Cancer Risk?).

FIGURE 11.1

Adult weight gain and risk of cancer. Gaining weight over time is a risk factor for several types of cancer, including cancers of the breast and colon. Preventing weight gain during adulthood is a key lifestyle cancer prevention strategy.

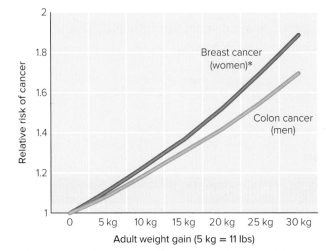

*Postmenopausal women not taking hormone replacement therapy.

SOURCE: Keum, N., et al. 2015. Adult weight gain and adiposity-related cancers: A dose-response meta-analysis of prospective observational studies. *Journal of the National Cancer Institute 107*(2): djv088.

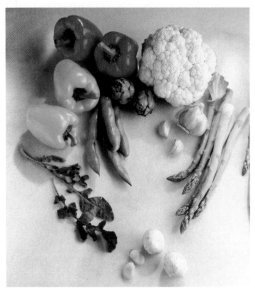

Ed Carey / Cole Group / Getty Images

Your food choices significantly affect your risk of cancer. Red bell peppers, chili peppers, and garlic are just a few of the foods containing cancer-fighting phytochemicals.

The Evidence *for* EXERCISE

HOW DOES EXERCISE AFFECT CANCER RISK?

According to statistics from the International Agency for Research on Cancer (IARC), as many as 25% of cancers are due to overweight, obesity, and physical inactivity. Increasing levels of physical activity can potentially ward off several types of cancer.

The links between exercise and cancer prevention are not entirely clear. However, experts have associated increased physical activity with a reduced risk of several specific types of cancer. Studies show, for example, that people who do moderate aerobic exercise for three to four hours per week reduce their risk of colon cancer by 30%. Women who do the same amount of exercise can reduce their risk of breast cancer by as much as 40%, with some studies suggesting that women who meet certain criteria can reduce their breast cancer risk by up to 80%. Evidence also shows that, when compared with sedentary people, active people can reduce their risk of lung cancer (20%), endometrial cancer (30%), and ovarian cancer (20%). Researchers are continually trying to establish similar connections between exercise and other types of cancer.

As is the case with cardiovascular disease, physical activity appears to have an inverse relationship with the types of cancer just listed. That is, the more you exercise, the lower your risk of developing these kinds of cancer. Energy balance also seems to be a factor, at least in relation to a few types of cancer, meaning that people who burn at least as many calories as they take in may further reduce their risk of some cancers. This positive effect may be due to the fact that reducing body fat (through exercise and a healthy diet) lowers the chemical and hormonal activities of adipose (fat) tissue—activities that may encourage some cancers to develop.

In addition to reducing the biological influences of adipose tissue, physical activity is known to reduce the inflammatory response and to boost immune function. Chronic inflammation, which can have many causes, leaves body tissues more vulnerable to infection. The immune system is the body's first line of defence against cancer, so supporting immune function through exercise may help prevent some cancers.

Emerging data also indicate that physical activity can help improve health outcomes in people who have cancer or are cancer survivors. For example, physical activity appears to restore cardiorespiratory fitness at least to some degree in patients whose heart muscles have been weakened by cancer treatments. This positive outcome was found in 13 separate studies, many of which found significant improvements in heart function among cancer survivors who performed moderate-intensity exercise for 20 to 40 minutes three times per week. The benefits were similar across several forms of aerobic exercise, including walking, yoga, and tai chi. A handful of studies have also found that exercise improves muscular strength and endurance and flexibility in patients whose muscles and joints have been weakened by cancer treatments.

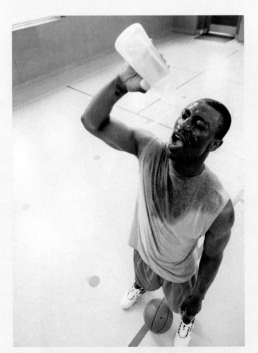

© Andersen Ross / Blend Images LLC / GettyRF

SOURCES: Mishra, S.I., et al. 2012. Exercise interventions on health-related quality of life for people with cancer during active treatment. *Clinical Otolaryngology* 37(5): 390–392.; Irwin, M.L., and S.T. Mayne. 2008. Impact of nutrition and exercise on cancer survival. *Cancer Journal* 14(6): 435–441; Morris, G.S., et al. 2009. Pulmonary rehabilitation improves functional status in oncology patients. *Archives of Physical Medicine and Rehabilitation* 90(5): 837–841; Physical Activity Guidelines Advisory Committee. 2008. *Physical Activity Guidelines Advisory Committee Report, 2008.* Washington, DC: U.S. Department of Health and Human Services.

Carcinogens in the Environment

Some carcinogens occur naturally in the environment, like the sun's UV rays. Others are manufactured or synthetic substances that show up occasionally in the general environment, but occur more often in the work environments of specific industries.

Ingested Chemicals

The food industry uses preservatives and other additives to prevent food from becoming spoiled or stale. Some of these compounds are antioxidants that may actually decrease any cancer-causing properties the food might have. Other compounds, like the nitrates and nitrites found in processed meats, are potentially more dangerous. Although nitrates and nitrites are not themselves carcinogenic, they can combine with dietary substances in the stomach and be converted to nitrosamines, which are highly potent carcinogens. Foods cured with nitrites, as well as those cured by salt or smoke, have been linked to esophageal and stomach cancer, and they should be eaten only in modest amounts.

Wellness Tip

Grilling meats at high temperatures can produce cancer-causing compounds. If you regularly eat grilled foods, cut away and avoid eating any charred parts. Reduce the formation of these cancer-causing chemicals by marinating before grilling, turning meat frequently, and reducing grilling time by pre-cooking meat in the microwave before finishing on the grill.

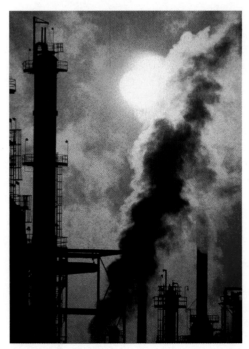

Tom Mareschal / Getty Images

Environmental pollution can raise the risk of heart and lung diseases, but it appears to account for only 2% of cancer deaths.

Environmental and Industrial Pollution

The best available data indicate that less than 2% of cancer deaths are caused by general environmental pollution, such as substances in our air and water. Exposure to carcinogenic materials in the workplace is a more serious problem. Occupational exposure to specific carcinogens may account for up to 5% of cancer deaths. With increasing industry and government regulations, industrial sources of cancer risk should continue to diminish.

Radiation

All sources of radiation are potentially carcinogenic, including medical X-rays, radioactive substances (radioisotopes), and UV radiation from the sun. Most physicians and dentists are quite aware of the risk of radiation, and successful efforts have been made to reduce the amount of radiation needed for mammography, dental X-rays, and other necessary medical X-rays. Sunlight is also a potential carcinogen, and care should be taken to avoid excessive exposure.

Microbes

About 15% of the world's cancers are caused by microbes, including viruses, bacteria, and parasites, although the percentage is much lower in developed countries like Canada. Certain types of HPV are known to cause oropharyngeal cancer, cervical cancer, and other cancers, and the *Helicobacter pylori* bacterium has been definitively linked to stomach cancer.

The Epstein-Barr virus, best known for causing mononucleosis, is also suspected of contributing to Hodgkin's disease, cancer of the nasopharynx, and some stomach cancers. Human herpes virus 8 has been linked to Kaposi's sarcoma and certain types of lymphoma. Hepatitis virus B and C together cause as many as 80% of the world's liver cancers.

Ask Yourself

QUESTIONS FOR CRITICAL THINKING AND REFLECTION

Has anyone you know had cancer? If so, what type of cancer was it? What were its symptoms? Based on the information presented so far in this chapter, did the person have any of the known risk factors for the disease?

LO3 11.3 Common Cancers

The Canadian Cancer Society estimates that more than 206 200 Canadians were diagnosed with cancer in 2017; of those, 80 800 will die from the disease.[6] While 90% of new cases are diagnosed in those aged 50 and over, at current Canadian rates, 49% of men and 45% of women will develop cancer at some point in their lives.

Cancer is an intriguing disease in that it has many origins and it affects numerous parts of the body. In addition, treatment for the different kinds of cancer can vary. Figure 11.2 (on the next page) describes those areas of the body that cancer can strike and the rate of death from those cancer sites.

A discussion of all types of cancer is beyond the scope of this book. This section looks at the most common cancers and their causes, prevention, and treatment.

Lung Cancer

Lung cancer is the most common cause of cancer death in Canada; it is estimated that about 21 100 Canadians died from lung cancer in 2017 alone.

The chief risk factor for lung cancer is tobacco smoke, which accounts for 30% of all cancers.[7] When smoking is combined with exposure to other environmental carcinogens, such as asbestos particles, the risk of cancer can be multiplied by a factor of 10 or more. Quitting smoking substantially reduces risk, but ex-smokers remain at higher risk than those who never smoked. But the smoker is not the only one at risk. Long-term exposure to environmental tobacco smoke (ETS), or second-hand smoke, also increases risk for lung cancer. The risk for lung cancer is 20% greater for non-smokers exposed to second-hand smoke than for people who are unexposed.

Symptoms of lung cancer do not usually appear until the disease has advanced to the invasive stage. Signals such as a persistent cough, chest pain, or recurring bronchitis may be the first indication of a tumour's presence. Lung cancer is most often treated by some combination of surgery, radiation, and **chemotherapy**; if all the tumour cells can be removed or killed, a cure is possible. Unfortunately, lung cancer is usually detected only after it has begun to spread, and only about 17% of lung cancer patients are alive five years after diagnosis.[8]

chemotherapy   The treatment of cancer with chemicals that selectively destroy cancerous cells.

FIGURE 11.2

Estimated new cases and deaths for cancers by sex in Canada, 2013.

New Cases	Deaths	Male	Female	New Cases	Deaths
1650	1350	Brain	Brain	1342	1050
3196	860	Oral	Oral	1445	400
1753	1650	Esophagus	Esophagus	516	480
928	350	Larynx	Larynx	206	95
1650	95	Thyroid	Thyroid	5366	120
4021	790	Skin (melanoma)	Skin (melanoma)	3302	450
14 434	11 100	Lung	Lung	14 242	10 000
206	60	Breast	Breast	26 316	5000
2165	1250	Stomach	Stomach	1342	790
2784	2400	Pancreas	Pancreas	2683	2400
1856	950	Liver	Liver	619	270
4227	1200	Kidney	Kidney	2374	670
14 950	5100	Colon and rectum	Colon and rectum	11 868	4300
6702	1700	Bladder	Bladder	2167	680
21 342	4100	Prostate	Ovary	2786	1800
113	45	Testes	Uterus	7327	1150
			Cervix	1548	400
4640	1500	Non-Hodgkin's lymphoma	Non-Hodgkin's lymphoma	3715	1200
619	85	Hodgkin's lymphoma	Hodgkin's lymphoma	413	60
1650	810	Multiple myeloma	Multiple myeloma	1238	650
3609	1650	Leukemia	Leukemia	258	1250
9588	5500	Other	Other	991	4900
102 079	**42 545**	**Total**	**Total**	**92 065**	**38 115**

SOURCES: Canadian Cancer Society's Advisory Committee on Cancer Statistics. *Canadian Cancer Statistics 2013*. Toronto, ON: Canadian Cancer Society; 2013. Retrieved online at: https://www.cancer.ca/~/media/cancer.ca/CW/cancer%20information/cancer%20101/Canadian%20cancer%20statistics/canadian-cancer-statistics-2013-EN.pdf; Health Fact Sheets: The 10 leading causes of death, 2013. Table: 13-10-0394-01 (formerly CANSIM 102-0561). Contains information licensed under the Open Government Licence – Canada.

Wellness Tip

If you smoke, find a way to stop. There are many options for quitting smoking. See Chapter 14 for advice on giving up tobacco.

Colon and Rectal Cancer

Another common cancer in Canada is colorectal cancer. It is the second leading cause of cancer death, after lung cancer, in both men and women. Age is a key risk factor, with more than 90% of cases diagnosed in people age 50 and older.[9] This is likely the result of recommended colorectal examinations (i.e., colonoscopy) yearly in those with a higher than average risk of colorectal cancer, or those over 50 years of age. Many cancers arise from pre-existing polyps, which are small growths on the wall of the colon that may gradually develop into malignancies. Many colon cancers may be due to inherited gene mutations.

Lifestyle also affects colon cancer risk. Regular physical activity reduces risk, while obesity increases risk. Although the mechanisms are unclear, high intake of red meat, smoked meat and fish, and simple sugars appears to increase risk, as does excessive alcohol consumption and smoking. Protective lifestyle factors may include a diet rich in fruits, vegetables, and whole grains; adequate intake of folic acid, calcium, magnesium, and vitamin D; regular use of nonsteroidal anti-inflammatory drugs such as aspirin and ibuprofen; and, in women, the use of oral contraceptives.

Young polyps and early-stage cancers can be removed before they spread. Because polyps may bleed as they progress, the standard warning signs of colon cancer are bleeding from the rectum or a change in bowel habits. A stool blood test, performed during a routine physical exam, can detect small amounts of blood in the stool long before obvious bleeding would be noticed. The Canadian Cancer Society (CCS) recommends that this examination be performed annually after age 50 (earlier for people with a family history of the disease). Another test is the colonoscopy, in which a flexible fibre-optic device is inserted through the rectum, allowing the colon to be examined and polyps to be removed (Figure 11.3). Studies show that screening could reduce the occurrence of colorectal cancer by 90%, but only about 60% of adults age 50 and over undergo these tests.

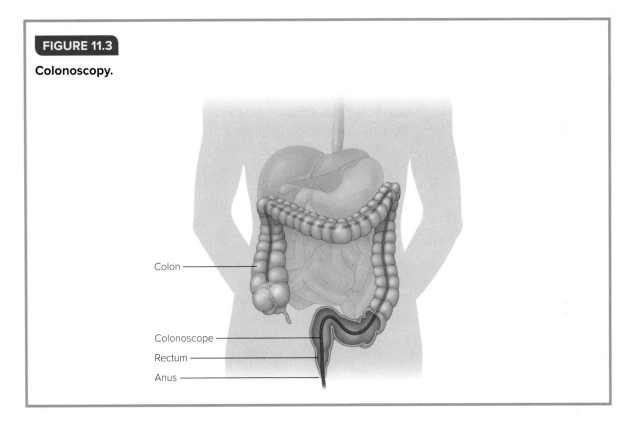

FIGURE 11.3

Colonoscopy.

Colon

Colonoscope

Rectum

Anus

Surgery is the primary method of treatment. The five-year survival rate is 95% for colon and rectal cancers detected early and 65% overall.

Breast Cancer

Breast cancer is the most common cancer in women and is second to lung cancer in the number of cancer deaths among women. In Canada, about one woman in nine will develop breast cancer in her lifetime. Breast cancer occurs only rarely in men.

Risk Factors

There is a strong genetic factor in breast cancer. A woman who has two close relatives with breast cancer is more than four times as likely to develop the disease than a woman who has no close relatives with breast cancer. However, only about 5–10% of cancers occur in women with a family history of it.

Other risk factors for breast cancer include the following:

- early onset menstruation or late-onset menopause
- having no children or having a first child after age 30
- current use of hormone replacement therapy
- obesity
- alcohol use
- smoking cigarettes

The female hormone estrogen may be a common element in some of these risk factors. Estrogen promotes cell growth in responsive tissues, such as the breast and uterus, so any factor that increases estrogen exposure may raise the risk of breast cancer. Fat cells also produce estrogen, and estrogen levels are higher in obese women. Alcohol can increase estrogen in the blood as well.

Prevention

Although some risk factors cannot be changed, important lifestyle risk factors can be controlled. Eating a low-fat, vegetable-rich diet, exercising regularly, limiting alcohol intake, and maintaining a healthy body weight can minimize the chance of developing breast cancer, even for women at risk from family history or other factors.

A dietary pattern rich in fruits, vegetables, and whole grains and lower in refined carbohydrates and animal products is associated with reduced risk of breast cancer. Some studies have found that people with higher vitamin D intakes or higher blood levels of vitamin D have a lower risk of breast and certain other cancers. (See Table 7.4 for key dietary sources of vitamin D.)

Detection

The early detection of breast cancer is promoted through a three-part approach:

1. **Mammography.** A **mammogram** is a low-dose breast X-ray that can spot abnormalities before physical symptoms arise. A newer type of mammography, called *digital mammography*, may provide more accurate results in some women, as may magnetic resonance imaging (MRI). The Canadian Cancer Society recommends that women over age 50 get a mammogram every two years.

> **mammogram**   A low-dose X-ray of the breasts used for the early detection of breast cancer.

2. **Breast self-awareness.** While the Canadian Cancer Society no longer recommends breast-self exams or clinical breast exams, a woman should be familiar with how her breasts look and feel, and alert her health-care provider to any changes right away. See the box Breast Awareness and Signs of Breast Cancer for more information.

If any of these methods detects a lump in the breast, it can be **biopsied** or scanned by **ultrasonography** to determine whether it is cancerous. Most lumps are benign.

> **biopsy**   The removal and examination of a small piece of body tissue for the purpose of diagnosis.
> **ultrasonography**   An imaging method in which inaudible high-pitched sound (ultrasound) is bounced off body structures to create an image on a monitor.

Fitness Tip

If you are a woman, staying physically active can reduce your risk of breast cancer. Strive to meet the recommended minimum of 150 minutes of moderate-intensity activity every week.

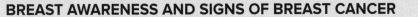

Take CHARGE

BREAST AWARENESS AND SIGNS OF BREAST CANCER

Women should be aware of how their breasts normally look and feel and report any symptoms or changes to their health-care provider. The following are warning signs of breast cancer, but keep in mind that these can also be caused by other conditions:

- a new lump in the breast or underarm
- thickening or swelling of part of the breast
- irritation or dimpling of breast skin
- redness or flaky skin in the nipple area or the breast
- pulling in of the nipple or pain in the nipple area
- nipple discharge other than breast milk, including blood
- any change in the size or the shape of the breast
- pain in any area of the breast

Remember, most breast lumps and changes are benign (not cancer).

Women can become familiar with their breast tissue by looking at and feeling their breasts. Experts used to suggest that women should do this in a certain way each month. Research shows that this isn't necessary. There really isn't a right or wrong way for women to examine their breasts. They just need to know their breasts well enough to notice changes. This includes the entire breast area up to the collarbone and under the armpits, as well as the nipples.

Being breast aware does not take the place of mammography, so be sure to keep up with the screening recommendations for your age and risk factors. And even if you've recently had mammography, see your health-care provider if you notice any changes to your breast.

For more information about breast cancer, visit cancer.ca/breast.

SOURCE: Canadian Cancer Society, cancer.ca/breast, "Screening for breast cancer" and "Signs and Symptoms," accessed 16 August 2018.

Treatment

If the lump is cancerous, one of several surgical treatments may be used, ranging from a lumpectomy (removal of the lump and surrounding tissue) to a mastectomy (removal of the breast). Chemotherapy or radiation may also be used to eradicate as many cancerous cells as possible.

Several drugs have been developed for preventing and treating breast cancer. These include selective estrogen-receptor modulators (SERMs), which act like estrogen in some tissues but block estrogen's effects in others. The two best-known SERMs are tamoxifen and raloxifene. Another category of drug, called trastuzumab (Herceptin), is a special type of antibody that binds to a specific cancer-related target in the body. Regardless of the treatments used, social support can also affect a patient's psychological and physical wellness.

If the tumour is discovered early, before it has spread to the adjacent lymph nodes, the patient with breast cancer has about a 98% chance of surviving more than five years. In Canada, the survival rate for all stages is 88% at five years.

Prostate Cancer

The prostate gland is situated at the base of the bladder in men; if enlarged, it can block the flow of urine. Prostate cancer is the most common cancer in men and the third leading cause of cancer death in men.

Age is the strongest predictor of the risk of prostate cancer, with about 75% of cases diagnosed in men over the age of 65. Inherited genetic predisposition may be responsible for 5–10% of cases; men with a family history of the disease should be vigilant about screening. Diets high in calories, dairy products, refined grains, and animal fats and low in plant foods (especially vegetable fibre) have been implicated as possible culprits, as have obesity, inactivity, and a history of sexually transmitted infections. Type 2 diabetes and insulin resistance are also associated with prostate cancer. Diet may be an important means of preventing prostate cancer. Soy foods, tomatoes, and cruciferous vegetables are being investigated for their possible protective effects.

Some cases are first detected by rectal examination during a routine physical exam. During this exam, a physician feels the prostate through the rectum to determine if the gland is enlarged or if lumps are present. Ultrasound and biopsy may also be used to detect and diagnose prostate cancer. A specialized test, called the **prostate-specific antigen (PSA) blood test**, is commonly used to detect prostate cancer and can be useful, but the test is controversial because it can yield false-positive results. The Canadian Cancer Society recommends that men over the age of 50 discuss the benefits of rectal exams and PSA testing with their physician. Men at high risk for the disease (such as African-Canadian men and men with a close relative who has been diagnosed with prostate cancer) should begin annual testing at age 40.

> **prostate-specific antigen (PSA) blood test**   A diagnostic test for prostate cancer that measures blood levels of prostate-specific antigen (PSA).

If the tumour is malignant, the prostate is usually removed surgically. However, a small, slow-growing tumour in an older man may be treated with watchful waiting because he is more likely to die from another cause before his cancer becomes life-threatening. A less invasive treatment involves radiation of the tumour by surgically implanting radioactive seeds in the prostate gland. Radiation from the seeds destroys the tumour and much of the normal prostate tissue, but leaves surrounding tissue relatively untouched. Alternative or additional treatments include external radiation, hormones that shrink tumours, cryotherapy, and chemotherapy. The five-year survival rate for all stages of prostate cancer is now nearly 100%.

Wellness Tip

Certain nutrients and over-the-counter (OTC) drugs have been promoted as reducing the risk of prostate cancer, but large-scale studies don't support such claims. Experts advise against taking supplements or OTC drugs to prevent prostate cancer.

Cancers of the Female Reproductive Tract

Several types of cancer can affect the female reproductive tract, and a few of these cancers are relatively common.

Cervical Cancer

Cancer of the cervix frequently occurs in women in their thirties and even twenties, and is at least in part a sexually transmitted disease. Most cases of cervical cancer stem from infection by the human papillomavirus (HPV), which causes genital warts and is transmitted during unprotected sex. Smoking and prior infection with the STIs herpes and chlamydia are other possible risk factors in cervical cancer.

Screening for the changes in cervical cells that precede cancer is done chiefly by means of the **Pap test**. During a pelvic exam, loose cells are scraped from the cervix and examined. If cells are abnormal, a condition commonly referred to as *cervical dysplasia*, the Pap test is repeated at intervals. In about one-third of cases, the cellular changes progress toward malignancy. If this happens, the abnormal cells must be removed, either surgically or by destroying them with an ultracold (cryoscopic) probe or localized laser treatment. In more advanced cases, treatment may involve chemotherapy, radiation, or hysterectomy (surgical removal of the uterus).

> **Pap test**   A scraping of cells from the cervix for examination under a microscope to detect cancer.

The Canadian Cancer Society recommends that women who are sexually active start having regular Pap tests by the age of 21 and have the tests every one to three years, depending on previous test results.

Cervical cancer can be prevented by avoiding infection with HPV. Sexual abstinence, mutually monogamous sex with an uninfected partner, or regular use of condoms can also reduce the risk of HPV infection. (See online Chapter 15 for more information on HPV and other STIs.)

Recently, some provinces began offering a vaccine (Gardasil) that protects against four types of HPV viruses. The vaccine can help prevent cervical cancer, as well as cancers of the vagina and vulva. The vaccine is recommended for all girls ages 11 to 12; the recommendation also allows vaccinations of girls as young as 9 and women up to age 26.

Uterine or Endometrial Cancer

Cancer of the lining of the uterus (endometrium), most often occurs after age 55. The risk factors are similar to those for breast cancer. Endometrial cancer is usually detectable by pelvic examination. It is treated surgically, as well as by radiation, hormones, and chemotherapy.

Ovarian Cancer

Although ovarian cancer is rare compared with uterine cancer, it causes more deaths. There are no approved screening tests to conclusively detect ovarian cancer so it is often diagnosed late in its development. The risk factors for ovarian cancer are similar to those for breast and endometrial cancer. Anything that lowers a woman's lifetime number of ovulation cycles—pregnancy, breast-feeding, or use of oral contraceptives—reduces the risk of ovarian cancer.

Early symptoms of ovarian cancer may include bloating, pelvic or abdominal pain, difficulty eating or feeling full quickly, and urinary problems (urgency or frequency). Women who experience these symptoms almost daily for a few weeks should see their physician. Some ovarian cancers are also detected through regular pelvic exams, sometimes with ultrasound imaging of the ovaries. Ovarian cancer is treated by surgical removal of one or both ovaries, the fallopian tubes, and the uterus.

Skin Cancer

Skin cancer is the most common cancer of all when cases of the highly curable forms are included in the count. Almost all cases of skin cancer can be traced to excessive exposure to **ultraviolet (UV) radiation** from the sun, including longer-wavelength ultraviolet A (UVA) and shorter-wavelength ultraviolet B (UVB) radiation. UVB radiation causes sunburns and can damage the eyes and immune system. UVA is less likely to cause a sunburn, but it damages connective tissue and leads to premature aging of the skin. Tanning lamps and tanning salon beds emit mostly UVA radiation. Both solar and artificial sources of UVA and UVB radiation are human carcinogens that cause skin cancer.

> **ultraviolet (UV) radiation**   Light rays of a specific wavelength, emitted by the sun; most UV rays are blocked by the ozone layer in the upper atmosphere.

Both severe, acute sun reactions (sunburns) and chronic low-level sun reactions (suntans) can lead to skin cancer. According to the American Academy of Dermatology, the risk of skin cancer doubles in people who have had five or more sunburns in their lifetime. People with fair skin have less natural protection against skin damage from the sun and a higher risk of developing skin cancer than people with naturally dark skin. Severe sunburns in childhood have been linked to a greatly increased risk of skin cancer in later life, so children in particular should be protected. Other risk factors include having many moles, particularly large ones, spending time at high altitudes, and a family history of the disease.

There are three main types of skin cancer, named for the types of skin cell from which they develop. **Basal cell** and **squamous cell carcinomas** together account for about 95% of the skin cancers diagnosed each year. They are usually found in chronically sun-exposed areas, such as the face, neck, hands, and arms. They usually appear as pale, wax-like, pearly nodules, or red, scaly, sharply outlined patches. These cancers are often painless, although they may bleed, crust, and form an open sore.

> **basal cell carcinoma**   Cancer of the deepest layers of the skin.
> **squamous cell carcinoma**   Cancer of the surface layers of the skin.

Melanoma is by far the most dangerous skin cancer because it spreads so rapidly. It can occur anywhere on the body, but the most common sites are the back, chest, abdomen, and lower legs. A melanoma usually appears at the site of a pre-existing mole. The mole may begin to enlarge, become mottled or varied in colour (colours can include blue, pink, and white), or develop an irregular surface or irregular borders. Tissue invaded by melanoma may also itch, burn, or bleed easily.

> **melanoma**   A malignant tumour of the skin that arises from pigmented cells, usually a mole.

You can help with early detection by making it a habit to examine your skin regularly. Most of the spots, freckles, moles, and blemishes on your body are normal. But if you notice an unusual growth, discolouration, or sore that does not heal, see your physician or a dermatologist immediately. The characteristics that may signal that a skin lesion is a melanoma are illustrated in Figure 11.4.

FIGURE 11.4

The ABCD test for melanoma. To see a variety of photos of melanoma and benign moles, visit the National Cancer Institute's Visual Online site (http://visualsonline.cancer.gov).

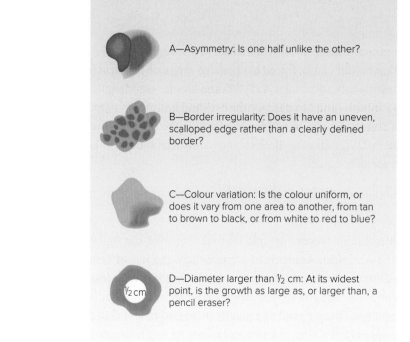

A—Asymmetry: Is one half unlike the other?

B—Border irregularity: Does it have an uneven, scalloped edge rather than a clearly defined border?

C—Colour variation: Is the colour uniform, or does it vary from one area to another, from tan to brown to black, or from white to red to blue?

D—Diameter larger than ½ cm: At its widest point, is the growth as large as, or larger than, a pencil eraser?

If you do have an unusual skin lesion, your physician will examine it and possibly perform a biopsy. If the lesion is cancerous, it is usually removed surgically, a procedure that can almost always be performed in the physician's office using a local anesthetic. Treatment is usually simple and successful when the cancer is caught early. Even for melanoma, the outlook after removal in the early stages is good, with a five-year survival rate of 98% if the tumour is localized but only 63% if the cancer has spread to adjacent lymph nodes. Most melanomas are detected in the early, localized stage.

To protect yourself against skin cancer, avoid overexposure to UV radiation. People of every age, including babies and children, need to be protected from the sun (see the box Sunscreen and Sun-Protective Clothing).

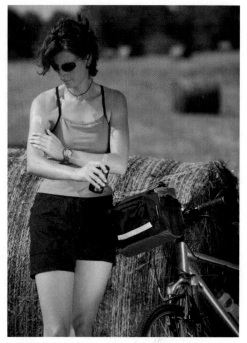

© Westend61 GmbH / Alamy Stock Photo

Sunscreen protects against skin cancer as well as sunburns.

Wellness Tip

The Skin Cancer Foundation recommends that everyone see their physician at least once a year for a head-to-toe skin evaluation. Depending on individual risk factors, some people may need to have their skin checked more frequently.

Critical CONSUMER

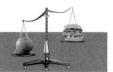

SUNSCREEN AND SUN-PROTECTIVE CLOTHING

With consistent use of the proper clothing, sunscreens, and common sense, you can lead an active outdoor life *and* protect your skin against most sun-induced damage.

Clothing

- **Wear long-sleeved shirts and long pants.** Dark-coloured, tightly woven fabrics provide reasonable protection from the sun. Another good choice is clothing made from special sun-protective fabrics; these garments have an Ultraviolet Protection Factor (UPF) rating, similar to the SPF for sunscreens.

continued

- **Wear a hat.** A good choice is a broad-brimmed hat or a legionnaire-style cap that covers the ears and neck. You still need to wear sunscreen on your face even if you are wearing a hat.
- **Wear sunglasses.** Health Canada suggests that if you spend a lot of time outdoors, you should wear sunglasses that block both UVA and UVB rays. Long-term exposure can damage the retina and can increase the risk for blindness in those over the age of 60.

Sunscreen

- **Use a sunscreen and lip balm with a sun protection factor (SPF) of 15 or higher.** An SPF rating refers to the amount of time you can stay out in the sun before you burn, compared with not using sunscreen; for example, a product with an SPF of 15 would allow you to remain in the sun without burning 15 times longer, on average, than if you didn't apply sunscreen. If you're fair-skinned, have a family history of skin cancer, are at high altitude, or will be outdoors for many hours, use a sunscreen with a high SPF (30+).
- **Choose a broad-spectrum sunscreen that protects against both UVA and UVB radiation.** The SPF rating of a sunscreen currently applies only to UVB, but a number of ingredients, especially titanium dioxide and zinc oxide, are effective at blocking most UVA radiation. In 2011, the Federal Drug Administration in the United States announced that sunscreens would be required to pass a new broad-spectrum test to determine how effectively they protect against both UVA and UVB radiation. Starting in summer 2012, products that have passed this test include the "broad spectrum" label. Canada has also adopted these labelling guidelines.
- **Use a water-resistant sunscreen if you swim or sweat quite a bit.** Under the new FDA regulations, sunscreens cannot be labelled as "waterproof" or "sweatproof" because these claims overstate the product's actual effectiveness. Labels for "water resistance" must now specify whether they are good for 40 or 80 minutes of swimming or sweating.
- **If you have acne, look for a sunscreen that is labelled "noncomedogenic."** This means that the sunscreen will not cause pimples.
- **Shake sunscreen before applying.** Apply it 30 minutes before exposure to allow it time to bond to the skin. Reapply sunscreen frequently and generously to all sun-exposed areas—many people overlook their temples, ears, and sides and backs of their necks. Most people use less than half as much as they need to attain the full SPF rating. One ounce of sunscreen is enough to cover an average-size adult in a swimsuit. Reapply sunscreen every two hours. Also be sure to reapply sunscreen after activities that could remove sunscreen, such as swimming.
- **If you're taking medications, ask your physician or pharmacist about possible reactions to sunlight or interactions with sunscreens.** Medications for acne, allergies, and diabetes are just a few of the products that can trigger reactions. If you're using sunscreen and an insect repellent containing DEET, use extra sunscreen since DEET may decrease sunscreen effectiveness.

Time of Day and Location

- **Avoid sun exposure between 10 a.m. and 2 p.m.** The sun's rays are most intense during this period. Clouds allow as much as 80% of UV rays to reach your skin. Stay in the shade when you can.
- **Consult the day's UV Index.** The index predicts UV levels on a scale from 0 to 10+, giving you a sense of the amount of sun protection you'll need. Take special care on days with a rating of 5 or above. UV Index ratings are available in local newspapers, from the television, or from certain websites.
- **Use water-resistant sunscreens if appropriate.** UV rays can penetrate at least 1 metre in water, so swimmers should wear water-resistant sunscreens. Snow, sand, water, concrete, and white-painted surfaces are also highly reflective.

Tanning Salons

- **Stay away from tanning salons!** Despite advertising claims to the contrary, the lights used in tanning parlours are damaging to your skin. Tanning beds and lamps emit mostly UVA radiation, increasing your risk of premature skin aging (such as wrinkles) and skin cancer.

Head and Neck Cancers

Head and neck cancers—cancers of the oral cavity, pharynx, larynx, and nasal cavity—can be traced principally to cigarette, cigar, or pipe smoking; the use of smokeless (spit) tobacco; and excessive consumption of alcohol. In addition, 50% of cancers of the tonsils and tongue base are related to HPV infection. Head and neck cancers occur twice as often in men as in women and most frequently in men over age 40.

Chemotherapy, radiation, and surgery are the primary methods of treatment for head and neck cancers. Patients often endure intense mouth and throat inflammation and some require disfiguring surgeries, but many can be cured. The five-year survival rate is about 62%.

Testicular Cancer

Testicular cancer is relatively rare, accounting for about 1% of cancers in men, but it is commonly found in men between the ages of 20 and 35. Testicular cancer is much more common among Caucasians than Latin, Asian, or African Canadians. Men with undescended testicles are at increased risk for testicular cancer, and for this reason the condition should be corrected in early childhood. Self-examination may help in the early detection of testicular cancer (see the box Testicle Self-Examination). Tumours are treated by surgical removal of the testicle and, if the tumour has spread, by chemotherapy. The five-year survival rate is 97%.

Take CHARGE

TESTICLE SELF-EXAMINATION

The best time to perform a testicular self-exam is after a warm shower or bath, when the scrotum is relaxed. First, stand in front of a mirror and look for any swelling of the scrotum. Then, examine each testicle with both hands. Place the index and middle fingers under the testicle and the thumbs on top; roll the testicle gently between the fingers and thumbs. Don't worry if one testicle seems slightly larger than the other—that's common. Also, expect to feel the epididymis, the soft, sperm-carrying tube at the rear of the testicle.

Perform the self-exam each month. If you find a lump, swelling, or nodule, consult a physician right away. The abnormality may not be cancer, but only a physician can make a diagnosis. Other possible signs of testicular cancer include a change in the way a testicle feels, a sudden collection of fluid in the scrotum, a dull ache in the lower abdomen or groin, a feeling of heaviness in the scrotum, or pain in a testicle or the scrotum.

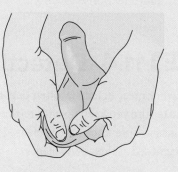

SOURCES: Testicular Cancer Resource Center. 2009. *How to Do a Testicular Self Examination* (http://www.acor.org/tcrc/tcexam.html, retrieved May 17, 2011); National Cancer Institute. 2009. *Testicular Cancer* (http://www.cancer.gov/cancertopics/types/testicular, retrieved May 17, 2011).

Other Cancers

Several other cancers affect thousands of people each year. Some have identifiable risk factors, but the causes of others are still under investigation.

- **Pancreatic cancer** is usually well advanced before symptoms become noticeable, and no effective cure is available. About three out of ten cases are linked to smoking. Other risk factors include being male, African-Canadian, or over age 60; having a family history of pancreatic cancer; having diabetes; being inactive and obese; and eating a diet high in fat and meat and low in vegetables.

- **Bladder cancer** is four times as common in men as in women, and almost two times higher in Caucasian men than in African-Canadian men. Smoking is the key risk factor. The first symptoms are likely to be blood in the urine and/or increased frequency of urination. These symptoms can also signal a urinary tract infection but should trigger a visit to a physician, who can evaluate the possibility of cancer. With early detection, 96% of bladder cancers are curable.

- **Kidney cancer** usually occurs in people over age 50; smoking and obesity are mild risk factors, as is a family history of the disease. Symptoms may include fatigue, pain in the side, and blood in the urine.

- **Brain cancer** commonly develops for no apparent reason and can arise from most of the cell types that are found in the brain. One of the few established risk factors for brain cancer is ionizing radiation, such as X-rays of the head. Symptoms are often nonspecific and include headaches, fatigue, behavioural changes, and sometimes seizures. Some brain tumours are curable by surgery or by radiation and chemotherapy, but most are not.

- **Leukemia**, cancer of the white blood cells, starts in the bone marrow but can then spread to the lymph nodes, spleen, liver, other organs, and central nervous system. Some possible risk factors include smoking, radiation, certain chemicals and infections. Most symptoms occur because leukemia cells crowd out the production of normal blood cells. The result can be fatigue, anemia, weight loss, and increased risk of infection.

- **Lymphoma** is a form of cancer that begins in the lymph nodes and then may spread to almost any part of the body. There are two types—Hodgkin's disease and non-Hodgkin's lymphoma (NHL). NHL is the more common and more deadly form of the disease; risk factors for NHL are not well understood but may include genetic factors, radiation, and certain chemicals and infections.

LO4 11.4 Detecting and Treating Cancer

Early cancer detection often depends on your willingness to be aware of changes in your own body and to make sure you keep up with recommended screening tests. Although treatment success varies with individual cancers, cure rates have increased—sometimes dramatically—in this century, especially for cancers that are diagnosed at their early stages.

Detecting Cancer

Unlike those of some other diseases, early signs of cancer are usually not apparent to anyone but the person who has them. Even pain is not a reliable guide to early detection because the initial stages of cancer may be painless. Self-monitoring is the first line of defence. By being aware of the risk factors in your own life, your immediate family's cancer history, and your own history, you may bring a problem to the attention of a doctor long before it would be detected at a routine physical (see the box Genetic Testing: Playing the Odds).

Take CHARGE

GENETIC TESTING: PLAYING THE ODDS

How far should we go to prevent potential cancers? Breast cancer genes *BRCA1* and *BRCA2* made the headlines in 2013 and again in 2015 when actor Angelina Jolie announced that she had had a preventive double mastectomy, followed by surgery to remove her ovaries and Fallopian tubes. After her mother struggled with ovarian and breast cancer for eight years until her death, Jolie learned that she harboured the same genetic minefield. Her 87% risk for breast cancer and 50% risk for ovarian cancer persuaded her to undergo surgery to remove her breasts, ovaries, and Fallopian tubes.

The reaction was mixed: some applauded Jolie's encouragement for women to be aware of genetic testing and their options for preventive, informed actions; others pointed out that worried women might pursue mastectomies that were medically unnecessary. Following Jolie's first announcement in *The New York Times*, cancer and genetic testing centres reported five times the number of calls they usually receive in a week related to genetic testing.

But having a mutation in the *BRCA1* or *BRCA2* gene is rare—only 5–10% of breast cancers and 10–15% of ovarian cancers result from this mutation among Caucasian women in the United States (data on other ethnicities are so far incomplete). Most women are advised not to opt for such extreme preventive surgery. Even if you have a mutation that suggests that you will ultimately get breast or ovarian cancer, other preventive measures are available, including several medications.

The Role of Drug and Diagnostic Companies

The so-called breast cancer genes were first discovered in the early 1990s, when Mary-Claire King, a geneticist at the University of California, Berkeley, isolated a single gene on chromosome 17. This later became known as *BRCA1*. King showed that as many as 5–10% of all cases of breast cancer may be hereditary. By 1994, Myriad Genetics had cloned *BRCA1* and filed a patent on the gene. The effect was to make screening extremely expensive. After 20 years of court battles, the US Supreme Court ruled that such a patent is not permitted because genes are a product of nature. As a result, the cost of testing for mutations on the *BRCA1* and *BRCA2* genes should decline from its current high of $4000. Many genetic tests used to detect other conditions cost in the $100 to $200 range.

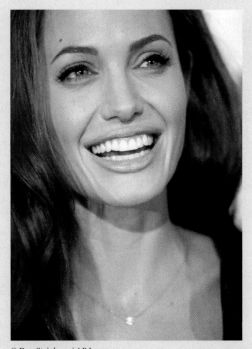

© Dan Steinberg / AP Images

The biotechnology industry and academics continue to look for better and cheaper ways to detect cancer and cancer risk. Molecular scientists can identify all of an individual's genes—at least 20 000 of them—for about $1000, which comes to about five cents per gene. One company, 23andMe, charges people $99 to see if they have gene variants that put them at higher risk for different diseases.

Identifying genes that make individuals or families susceptible to cancer play a major role in preventing the disease. Gene-based treatments can be devised to attack cancer at the molecular level, eliminating the need for surgery, radiation, or chemotherapy. Many biologists are engaged in gene therapy research focused on replacing a missing or defective gene with a healthy version. Further development in the fields of genetics and genomics will bring about

continued

more opportunities to diagnose and treat cancer. See For Further Exploration at the end of this chapter for links to reliable information about genetic testing.

SOURCES: Agus, D. B. 2013. The outrageous cost of a Gene Test. *New York Times,* May 20; Cook-Deegan, Robert. 2013. Are human genes patentable? *Annals of Internal Medicine,* June 11; Miller Tran, et al. 2013. Production of unique immunotoxin cancer therapeutics in algal chloroplasts. *Proceedings of the National Academy of Sciences* 110(1): E15–E22; M.D. Anderson Cancer Center. 2015. Gene therapy. http://www.mdanderson.org/patient-and-cancer-information/cancer-information/cancer-topics/cancer-treatment/chemotherapy/gene-therapy/index.html; Pitt, Angelina J. 2015. Diary of a surgery. *New York Times,* March 24, p. A23; Szabo, Liz. 2013. Angelina Jolie's news prompts women to call doctors. *USA Today,* May 15. (http://www.usatoday.com/story/news/nation/2013/05/15/jolie-genetics-counseling/2163783).

In addition to self-monitoring, specific screening tests for certain cancers are available. Consult the list and links in Table 11.2 for general screening guidelines from the Canadian Cancer Society (CCS). Discuss your personal risk factors, such as family history or cigarette use, with your health care provider to help determine the screening tests and schedule most appropriate for you. Digital reminders can be effective in increasing the likelihood that people follow through with cancer screening; see the box Cancer Screening Reminders (on page 484) for more information.

TABLE 11.2

Early detection of cancer in average-risk, asymptomatic people.

Site/Tests and Procedures	Description	CCS Links for more Information
BREAST		
Mammography	Yearly mammograms are the best way to find breast cancer early, when it is easier to treat. These imaging tests, which involve low-dose X-rays, are recommended for women between the ages of 50 and 69, or as long as they are in good health.	http://www.cancer.ca/en/prevention-and-screening/reduce-cancer-risk/find-cancer-early/get-screened-for-breast-cancer/when-should-i-be-screened-for-breast-cancer/?region=ab
Breast awareness	Routine examination of the breasts by health care providers or by women themselves starting in their 20s has not been shown to reduce deaths from breast cancer. However, any lump or other unusual change in the breast needs to be promptly reported to a doctor.	http://www.cancer.ca/en/about-us/a-future-without-breast-cancer/
CERVIX		
Pap and HPV cytology tests	Pap tests can find abnormal cells in the cervix that may turn into cancer, and they can find cervical cancer early, when the chance of a cure is high. Testing every 3 to 5 years should begin at age 21 and end at age 65, if results have been normal. Women who have been vaccinated against HPV still need HPV tests.	http://www.cancer.ca/en/prevention-and-screening/reduce-cancer-risk/find-cancer-early/get-screened-for-cervical-cancer/?region=ab

Site/Tests and Procedures	Description	CCS Links for more Information
COLON		
High-sensitivity fecal occult blood test (FOBT)	This yearly multiple-stool, take-home test reduces death from colorectal cancer and is recommended for people between the ages of 50 and 74. If a positive result is found, it is followed by a colonoscopy or sigmoidoscopy. If you are over age 74, consult your physician.	http://www.cancer.ca/en/cancer-information/cancer-type/colorectal/screening/?region=ab
Colonoscopy and sigmoidoscopy	Colonoscopy and sigmoidoscopy tests are typically completed if you have a high risk for colorectal cancer or if your stool test results were positive.	http://www.cancer.ca/en/cancer-information/diagnosis-and-treatment/tests-and-procedures/colonoscopy/?region=ab
LUNG		
Low-dose computed tomography (LDCT)	This imaging test has been shown to reduce lung cancer deaths among heavy smokers (30 pack-years*) between age 55 and 74 who still smoke or have quit within the last 15 years.	http://www.cancer.ca/en/cancer-information/cancer-type/lung/finding-cancer-early/?region=ab
OVARY AND UTERUS		
CA-125 blood test, transvaginal ultrasound	There is no evidence that any screening test reduces deaths from ovarian or uterine cancer. However, these tests can help in diagnosing ovarian (CA-125) and uterine (ultrasound) cancer. Women should report any unexpected bleeding or spotting to a health care provider.	http://www.cancer.ca/en/cancer-information/diagnosis-and-treatment/tests-and-procedures/cancer-antigen-125-ca-125/?region=ab and http://www.cancer.ca/en/cancer-information/cancer-type/uterine/diagnosis/?region=ab
PROSTATE		
Prostate specific antigen (PSA)	Although this blood test, which is often done with a digital rectal exam, can detect prostate cancer at an early stage, it is more likely to lead to overdiagnosis and overtreatment than to reduce deaths from prostate cancer. Starting at age 50, men should talk to a health care provider about the pros and cons of this test. African-Canadian men and men whose father or brother had prostate cancer before age 65 should talk to a health care provider about this test starting at age 45.	http://www.cancer.ca/en/cancer-information/diagnosis-and-treatment/tests-and-procedures/prostate-specific-antigen-psa/?region=ab

*A pack-year is calculated by multiplying the number of packs of cigarettes smoked per day by the number of years the person has smoked. For example, smoking two packs per day for 10 years is equal to 20 pack-years; smoking one-half pack per day for 10 years is equal to 5 pack-years.

SOURCE: Canadian Cancer Society.

Wellness *in the* DIGITAL AGE

CANCER SCREENING REMINDERS

Consider sending an e-card to help your mother, daughter, or female partner remember to get her next mammogram or Pap test. Many studies have shown that texts, emails, and e-cards are highly effective at prompting people to have regular health screenings. One study found that people who received an email reminder were significantly more likely than those who received only a verbal reminder from their physician to come to a medical office and pick up a fecal occult blood detection kit for colon cancer screening. Other studies have found that text messaging proved much more effective than telephone calls at prompting women to have mammograms.

If your physician or health care clinic doesn't offer a digital reminder service, it may fall on you to place those reminders in your calendar on your own.

To determine which screening tests are most appropriate for someone of your sex and age, discuss your individual risk factors and the risks and benefits of specific screening tests with your health care provider.

SOURCES: Kerrison, R.S., et al. 2015. Text-message reminders increase uptake of routine breast screening appointments: A randomised controlled trial in a hard-to-reach population. *Br J Cancer* 2015 Mar 17;112(6):1005–10. doi: 10.1038/bjc.2015.36; Muller, D., et al. 2009. The effectiveness of a secure email reminder system for colorectal cancer screening. *AMIA Annu Symp Proc. 2009.* Published online 2009 Nov 14. http://www.ncbi.nlm.nih.gov/pmc/articles/PMC2815450/.

Stages of Cancer

Physicians need to know the exact size and location of a tumour to treat it effectively. To confirm the type of tumour, a biopsy may be performed. Physicians can then classify the disease according to the extent of the cancer in a patient's body, whether the cancer has invaded nearby lymph nodes, and whether metastases are present. This is usually determined through imaging techniques such as MRI, computed tomography (CT) scanning, ultrasonography, or exploratory surgery. The classifying process is called *staging*, and the cancer is categorized in five stages, as shown in Table 11.3. By judging the extent of each criterion—size or extent, spread, metastases—physicians can determine the cancer's stage, establish how severe it is, and choose the most appropriate treatment based on the extent of the disease. Visit the Canadian Cancer Society's website to find more detailed information regarding staging.

TABLE 11.3

Cancer Stages

Stage	Description
0	Carcinoma in situ: abnormal cells are present only in the layer of cells in which they developed; not cancer but may become cancer
I, II, and III	Higher numbers indicate more extensive disease: larger tumour size and/or spread of the cancer beyond the organ in which it first developed to nearby lymph nodes or to tissues or organs adjacent to the primary tumour
IV	Cancer that has spread to distant tissues or organs

SOURCE: National Cancer Institute. 2015. Cancer staging (http://www.cancer.gov/about-cancer/diagnosis-staging/staging/).

Treating Cancer

The ideal cancer therapy would kill or remove all cancerous cells while leaving normal tissue untouched. Sometimes this is almost possible, as when a surgeon removes a small superficial tumour of the skin. Typically, however, the tumour is less accessible, so some combination of surgery, radiation therapy, and chemotherapy must be used. (See Common Questions Answered for information on new and emerging cancer treatments.)

Surgery

For most cancers, surgery is the most useful treatment. In many cases, the organ containing the tumour is not essential for life and can be partially or completely removed. Surgery is less effective when the tumour involves cells of the immune system, which are widely distributed throughout the body, or when the cancer has already metastasized.

Chemotherapy

Chemotherapy is the use of targeted drugs that destroy rapidly growing cancer cells. Many chemotherapy drugs work by interfering with DNA synthesis and replication in rapidly dividing cells. Normal cells, which usually grow slowly, are not destroyed by these drugs. However, some normal tissues such as intestinal, hair, and blood-forming cells are always growing, and damage to these tissues produces the unpleasant side effects of chemotherapy, including nausea, vomiting, diarrhea, and hair loss.

Radiation

In cancer radiation therapy, a beam of X-rays or gamma rays is directed at the tumour, killing the tumour cells. Occasionally, when an organ is small enough, radioactive seeds are surgically placed inside the cancerous organ to destroy the tumour; they are then removed later, if necessary. Radiation destroys both normal and cancerous cells, but because it can be precisely directed at the tumour, it is usually less toxic for the patient than either surgery or chemotherapy, and it can often be performed on an outpatient basis. Radiation may be used as an exclusive treatment or in combination with surgery and/or chemotherapy.

LO5 11.5 Preventing Cancer

Your lifestyle choices can radically lower your cancer risks, so take a practical approach to cancer prevention. Here are some guidelines:

- **Avoid tobacco.** Smoking is responsible for 80–90% of lung cancers and for about 30% of all cancer deaths. The carcinogenic chemicals in smoke are transported throughout the body in the bloodstream, making smoking a carcinogen for many forms of cancer other than lung cancer. The use of spit tobacco increases the risk of cancers of the mouth, larynx, throat, and esophagus. It's also important to avoid exposure to ETS.

- **Control diet and weight.** About one-third of all cancers are in some way linked to what we eat. Choose a low-fat, plant-based diet containing a wide variety of fruits, vegetables, and whole grains rich in phytochemicals. Drink alcohol only in moderation, if at all. Maintain a healthy weight.

- **Exercise.** Regular exercise is linked to lower rates of colon and other cancers. It also helps control weight.

- **Protect skin from the sun.** Almost all cases of skin cancer are sun-related. Wear protective clothing when you're out in the sun and use a sunscreen with an SPF rating of 15 or higher. Don't go to tanning salons.

- **Avoid environmental and occupational carcinogens.** Try to avoid occupational exposure to carcinogens and don't smoke; the cancer risks of many of these agents increase greatly when combined with smoking.

Your first line of defence against cancer involves the lifestyle changes described in this chapter. Your second line of defence against cancer is early detection. Stay alert for any of the seven major warning signs illustrated in Figure 11.5; you can remember these with the acronym CAUTION. The appearance of any of these warning signs, although not a sure indication of cancer, should send you to your physician.

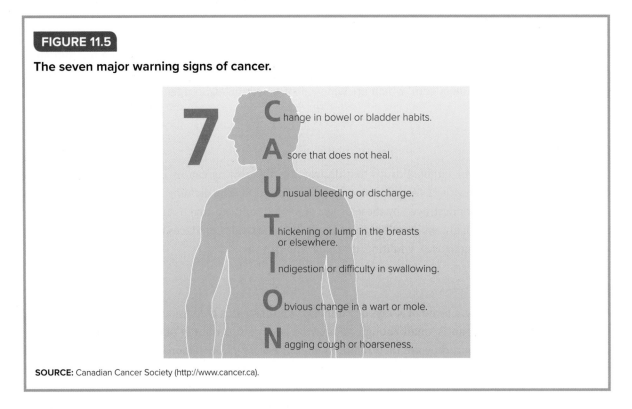

FIGURE 11.5

The seven major warning signs of cancer.

7 **CAUTION**

C hange in bowel or bladder habits.

A sore that does not heal.

U nusual bleeding or discharge.

T hickening or lump in the breasts or elsewhere.

I ndigestion or difficulty in swallowing.

O bvious change in a wart or mole.

N agging cough or hoarseness.

SOURCE: Canadian Cancer Society (http://www.cancer.ca).

Coping with Cancer

If you suffer from cancer or know someone who does, see For Further Exploration for tips on how to receive or provide support.

Tips for Today and the Future

A growing body of research suggests that you can take an active role in preventing many cancers by adopting a wellness lifestyle.

RIGHT NOW YOU CAN

- If you are a woman, do a breast self-exam; if you are a man, do a testicular self-exam.
- Buy multiple bottles of sunscreens and put them in places where you will most likely see them, such as your backpack, gym bag, or car.
- Check the cancer screening guidelines in this chapter and make sure you are up-to-date on your screenings.

IN THE FUTURE YOU CAN

- Learn where to find information about daily UV radiation levels in your area, and learn how to interpret the information. Many local newspapers and television stations (and their websites) report current UV levels every day.
- Gradually add foods with abundant phytochemicals to your diet, choosing from the list shown in Table 11.1.

Common Questions ANSWERED

Q **What is a biopsy?**

A A biopsy is the removal and examination of a small piece of body tissue. Biopsies enable cancer specialists to carefully examine cells that are suspected of having turned cancerous. Some biopsies are fairly simple to perform, such as those on tissue from moles or skin sores. Other biopsies may require the use of a needle or probe to remove tissue from inside the body, such as in the breast or stomach.

Q **Are other cancer treatments available beyond surgery, chemotherapy, and radiation?**

A Some experimental techniques that also show promise for some particular types of cancer include the following:

- **Bone marrow transplants.** Healthy bone marrow cells from a compatible donor are transplanted following the elimination of the patient's bone marrow by radiation or chemotherapy. Transplants of stem cells may provide a solution to the problem of donor incompatibility. These unique, unspecialized cells can divide and produce many specialized cell types, including bone marrow cells. Stem cells can be grown outside the body and then transplanted back into the cancer patient, allowing for safe repopulation of bone marrow. The Canadian Blood Services OneMatch Stem Cell and Marrow Network (https://www.blood.ca /en/stem-cells?utm_source=onematch&utm_edium=redirect&utm_campaign=onematch) is a database that attempts to match with a donor, those whose diseases inhibit their ability to produce these cells.

- **Vaccines and genetically modified immune cells.** These enhance the reaction of a patient's own immune system.

- **Anti-angiogenesis agents.** These starve tumours by blocking their blood supply.

- **Proteasome inhibitors.** Proteasomes help control the cell cycle—the process through which cells divide. If proteasomes malfunction, as is often the case in cancer cells, then cells may begin multiplying out of control. Proteasome inhibitors block the action of proteasomes, halting cell division and killing the cells. One proteasome inhibitor is now being used against certain cancers, and other such drugs are in development.

- **Enzyme activators/blockers.** Normal cells die after dividing a given number of times. Scientists believe that the enzyme caspase triggers the death of normally functioning cells. In cancer cells, caspase activity may be blocked. Conversely, if the enzyme telomerase becomes active in cancer cells, the life/death cycle stops and the cells duplicate indefinitely. In effect, inactive caspase or active telomerase may make cancer cells "immortal." Researchers are studying compounds that can either activate caspase or deactivate telomerase; either type of drug might lead cancer cells to self-destruct. No such drugs are now in clinical use.

- **Monoclonal antibodies.** The use of monoclonal antibodies to fight cancer mimics the way the immune system fights an infection. All cells in the body have markers on their surfaces, and the immune system develops antibodies, or special proteins, that can recognize these markers, bind to them, and trigger neutralization and destruction. Scientists carefully select cell-surface markers that are displayed on cancer cells and then administer antibodies to the patient. These monoclonal antibodies (the term *monoclonal* means they bind to only one particular cell-surface marker) target the cancer cells and enlist the help of the body's own immune system to selectively kill these cells. Rituximab (Rituxan) has been one of the most successful monoclonal antibodies, used effectively for patients with lymphoma. Many other monoclonal antibodies are currently in use, and the list of potential new agents in this category is growing rapidly.

In the future, gene sequencing techniques may allow treatments to be targeted at specific cancer subtypes, much as specific antibiotics are now used to treat specific bacterial diseases.

SUMMARY

- Cancer is an abnormal and uncontrollable growth of cells or tissue; cancer cells can metastasize.

- The genetic basis of some cancers appears to be mutational damage to suppressor genes, which normally limit cell division.

- Cancer-promoting dietary factors include meat, certain types of fat, and alcohol. Dietary elements that may protect against cancer include antioxidants and phytochemicals. An inactive lifestyle is associated with some cancers.

- Some carcinogens occur naturally in the environment; others are manufactured substances. Occupational exposure is a risk for some workers.

- All sources of radiation are potentially carcinogenic, including X-rays, the sun's UV rays, and radon gas.

- Lung cancer kills more people than any other type of cancer; tobacco smoke is the primary cause.

- Colon and rectal cancers are linked to age, heredity, obesity, and a diet rich in red meat and low in fruits and vegetables.

- Breast cancer has a genetic component, but lifestyle and hormones are also factors. Prostate cancer is chiefly a disease of aging; diet, heredity, and ethnicity are other risk factors.

- Cancers of the female reproductive tract include cervical, uterine, and ovarian cancer. Cervical cancer is linked to HPV infection; the Pap test is an effective screening test. Vaccination is recommended for girls and young women.

- Melanoma is the most serious form of skin cancer; excessive exposure to UV radiation in sunlight is the primary cause.

- Oral cancer is caused primarily by smoking, excess alcohol consumption, and use of spit tobacco. Some oral cancers have been recently linked to HPV.

- Testicular cancer can be detected early through self-examination.

- Self-monitoring and regular screening tests are essential to early cancer detection.

- Methods of cancer diagnosis include MRI, CT scanning, and ultrasound.

- Cancer treatment usually consists of some combination of surgery, chemotherapy, and radiation.

FOR FURTHER EXPLORATION

Organizations and Websites

Canadian Blood Services. Includes information about the OneMatch program and the various ways that blood can impact our lives.

    https://blood.ca

Canadian Cancer Society. Provides a wide range of free materials on the prevention and treatment of cancer.

http://www.cancer.ca

Canadian Cancer Society Research Institute. Offers information on treatment options, screening, clinical trials, and newly approved drugs.

https://www.cancerresearch.org/

EPA/Sunwise. Includes information about the UV Index and the effects of sun exposure, with links to sites with daily UV Index ratings for US and international cities.

https://www.epa.gov/sunsafety

MedlinePlus: Cancers. Provides links to reliable cancer information.

http://nlm.nih.gov/medlineplus/cancers.html

Skin Cancer Foundation. Offers information relating to skin cancer.

http://www.skincancer.org

Terry Fox Foundation. Advocates for cancer research, support, and development.

http://www.terryfox.org/

World Health Organization: Cancer. Home page of WHO's worldwide anti-cancer initiative.

http://www.who.int/cancer/en/

Laboratory Activities

Name _____ **Section** _____ **Date** _____

Lab 11.1 Cancer Prevention

connect

This lab looks at two areas of cancer prevention over which you have a great deal of individual control—diet and sun exposure. For a detailed personal risk profile for many specific types of cancer, complete the assessments at the Washington University School of Medicine's "Your Disease Risk" site (http://www .yourdiseaserisk.wustl.edu).

Part I Eating Cancer-Fighting Foods

Track your diet for three days, recording the number of servings from each of the following food groups that you consume.

Day 1	Day 2	Day 3	Potential Cancer Fighters
_____	_____	_____	Orange, deep yellow, pink, and red vegetables and some fruits (e.g., apricots, cantaloupe, carrots, corn, grapefruit, mangoes, nectarines, papayas, red and yellow bell peppers, sweet potatoes, pumpkin, tomatoes and tomato sauce, watermelon, winter squash such as acorn or butternut)
_____	_____	_____	Dark-green leafy vegetables (e.g., broccoli rabe, chard, kale, romaine and other dark lettuces, spinach; beet, collard, dandelion, mustard, and turnip greens)
_____	_____	_____	Cruciferous vegetables (e.g., bok choy, broccoli, Brussels sprouts, cabbage, cauliflower, kohlrabi, turnips)
_____	_____	_____	Citrus fruits (e.g., grapefruit, lemons, limes, oranges, tangerines)
_____	_____	_____	Whole grains (e.g., whole-grain bread, cereal, and pasta; brown rice; oatmeal; whole-grain corn; barley; popcorn; bulgur)
_____	_____	_____	Legumes (e.g., peas, lentils, and beans, including fava, navy, kidney, pinto, black, and lima beans)
_____	_____	_____	Berries (e.g., strawberries, raspberries, blackberries, blueberries)
_____	_____	_____	Garlic and other allium vegetables (e.g., onions, leeks, chives, scallions, shallots)
_____	_____	_____	Soy products (e.g., tofu, tempeh, soy milk, miso, soybeans)
_____	_____	_____	Other cancer-fighting fruits (e.g., apples, cherries, cranberries or juice, grapes, kiwifruit, pears, plums, prunes, raisins)
_____	_____	_____	Other cancer-fighting vegetables (e.g., asparagus, beets, chili peppers, eggplant, green peppers, radishes)
_____	_____	_____	**Daily Totals** **(Average for three days: _____)**

The goal is to eat at least 7 (for women) or 9 (for men) servings of cancer-fighting fruits and vegetables each day; the more servings, the better.

Note: Research is ongoing, and this list of cancer fighters is not comprehensive. Remember, nearly all fruits, vegetables, and grains are healthy, disease-fighting dietary choices.

Part II Skin Cancer Risk Assessment

Your risk of skin cancer from the ultraviolet radiation in sunlight depends on several factors. Take the quiz below to see how sensitive you are. The higher your UV-risk score, the greater your risk of skin cancer—and the greater your need to take precautions against too much sun. Score 1 point for each true statement.

_____ 1. I have blond or red hair.

_____ 2. I have light-coloured eyes (blue, grey, green).

_____ 3. I freckle easily.

_____ 4. I have many moles.

_____ 5. I had two or more blistering sunburns as a child.

_____ 6. I spent lots of time in a tropical climate as a child.

_____ 7. I have a family history of skin cancer.

_____ 8. I work outdoors.

_____ 9. I spend a lot of time in outdoor activities.

_____ 10. I like to spend as much time in the sun as I can.

_____ 11. I sometimes go to a tanning parlour or use a sunlamp.

_____ **Total Score**

Score	Risk of skin cancer from UV radiation
0	Low
1–3	Moderate
4–7	High
8–11	Very high

Using Your Results

How did you score?

(I) How close did you come to the goal of eating 7 to 9 or more servings of cancer fighters each day? Are you at all surprised by your results?

_____

_____

_____

Are you satisfied with your diet in terms of cancer prevention? If not, set a specific goal for a target number of servings of cancer-fighting fruits and vegetables:

_____

_____

_____

(II) What is your skin cancer risk assessment score? Are you at all surprised by the result? Does it indicate that you are at high or very high risk? Do you feel you need to take action because of your risk level?

_____

_____

_____

What should you do next? Enter the results of this lab in the Preprogram Assessment column in Appendix B.

If you've set a goal for the diet and cancer portion of the lab, select a target number of additional cancer fighters from the list to try over the next few days; list the foods below, along with your plan for incorporating them into your diet (as a side dish, as a snack, on a salad, as a substitute for another food, etc.).

Cancer fighter to try: *Plan for trying:*

_____   _____

_____   _____

_____   _____

_____   _____

You cannot control all of your risk factors for skin cancer, but you can control your behaviour with regard to sun exposure. Keep a journal to track your behaviour on days when you are outdoors in the sun for a significant period of time. Compare your behaviour with the recommendations for skin cancer prevention described in the chapter. Record such information as time of day, total duration of exposure, UV index for the day, clothing worn, type and amount of sunscreen used, frequency of sunscreen applications, and so on. From this record, identify ways to improve your behaviour to lower your risk of skin cancer. Put together a behaviour change plan.

Next, begin to put your strategies into action. After several weeks of a program to improve your diet or reduce your UV exposure, do this lab again and enter the results in the Postprogram Assessment column of Appendix B. How do the results compare?

_____

_____

_____

Stress

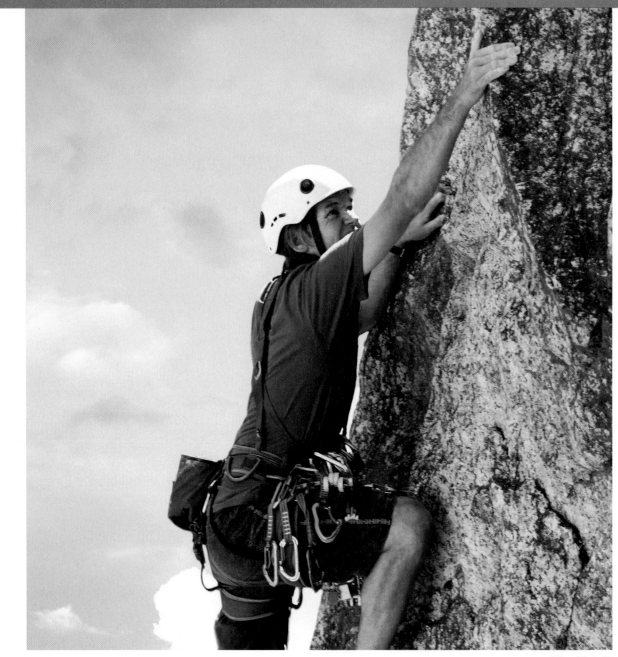

LEARNING OBJECTIVES

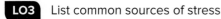

After reading this chapter, you should be able to

LO1 Explain what stress is and how people react to it—physically, emotionally, and behaviourally

LO2 Describe the relationship between stress and disease

LO3 List common sources of stress

LO4 Describe techniques for preventing and managing stress

LO5 Put together a plan for successfully managing the stress in your life

TEST YOUR KNOWLEDGE

1. **Which of the following events can cause stress?**
   a. taking out a loan
   b. failing a test
   c. graduating from university or college
   d. watching a hockey game

2. **Exercise stimulates which of the following?**
   a. analgesia (pain relief)
   b. birth of new brain cells
   c. relaxation

3. **Which of the following can be a result of chronic stress?**
   a. violence
   b. heart attack
   c. stroke

ANSWERS

1. **ALL FOUR.** Stress-producing factors can be pleasant or unpleasant and can include physical challenges and goal achievement as well as what are perceived as negative events.

2. **ALL THREE.** Regular exercise is linked to improvement in many dimensions of wellness.

3. **ALL THREE.** Chronic—or ongoing—stress can last for years. People who suffer from long-term stress may ultimately become violent toward themselves or others. They also run a greater than normal risk for certain ailments, especially cardiovascular disease.

Like the term *fitness*, stress is a word many people use without really understanding its precise meaning. Stress is popularly viewed as an uncomfortable response to a negative event, which probably describes *nervous tension* more than the cluster of physical and psychological responses that actually constitute stress. In fact, stress is not limited to negative situations; it is also a response to pleasurable physical challenges and the achievement of personal goals. Whether stress is experienced as pleasant or unpleasant depends largely on the situation and the individual. Because learning effective responses to whatever induces stress can enhance psychological health and help prevent a number of serious diseases, stress management is an important part of daily life.

This chapter explains the physiological and psychological reactions that make up the stress response and describes how these reactions can be risks to good health. The chapter also presents ways of managing stress.

LO1 12.1 What Is Stress?

In common usage, *stress* refers to two different things: situations that trigger physical *and* emotional reactions and the reactions themselves. In this text, we'll use the more precise term **stressor** for a situation that triggers physical and emotional reactions and the term **stress response** for those reactions. A first date and a final exam are examples of stressors; sweaty palms and a pounding heart are symptoms of the stress response. We'll use the term **stress** to describe the general physical and emotional state that accompanies the stress response. So, for example, a person taking a final exam experiences stress.

> **stressor**   Any physical or psychological event or condition that produces physical and emotional reactions.
> **stress response**   The physical and emotional reactions to a stressor.
> **stress**   The general physical and emotional state that accompanies the stress response.

Physical Responses to Stressors

Imagine a near miss: As you step off the curb, a car careens toward you. With just a fraction of a second to spare, you leap safely out of harm's way. In that split second of danger and in the moments following it, you experience a predictable series of physical reactions. Your body goes from a relaxed state to one prepared for physical action to cope with a threat to your life.

Two major control systems in your body are responsible for your physical response to stressors: the nervous system and the endocrine system. Through rapid chemical reactions affecting almost every part of your body, you are primed to act quickly and appropriately in time.

Actions of the Nervous System

The nervous system consists of the brain, spinal cord, and nerves. Part of the nervous system is under voluntary control, such as when you tell your arm to reach for a chocolate. The part that is not under conscious supervision—for example, the part that controls the digestion of the chocolate—is known as the **autonomic nervous system**. In addition to digestion, it controls your heart rate, breathing, blood pressure, and hundreds of other involuntary functions.

> **autonomic nervous system**   The branch of the nervous system that controls basic body processes; consists of the sympathetic and parasympathetic divisions.

The autonomic nervous system consists of two divisions:

- The **parasympathetic division** is in control when you are relaxed; it aids in digesting food, storing energy, and promoting growth.

- The **sympathetic division** is activated during times of arousal, including exercise, and when there is an emergency, such as severe pain, anger, or fear.

> **parasympathetic division** A division of the autonomic nervous system that moderates the excitatory effect of the sympathetic division, slowing metabolism and restoring energy supplies.
> **sympathetic division** A division of the autonomic nervous system that reacts to danger or other challenges by almost instantly accelerating body processes.

Sympathetic nerves use the neurotransmitter **norepinephrine** to exert their actions on nearly every organ, sweat gland, blood vessel, and muscle to enable your body to handle an emergency. In general, the sympathetic division commands your body to stop storing energy and instead to mobilize all energy resources to respond to the crisis.

> **norepinephrine** A neurotransmitter released by the sympathetic nervous system onto specific tissues to increase their function in the face of increased activity; when released by the brain, causes arousal (increased attention, awareness, and alertness); also called *noradrenaline*.

Actions of the Endocrine System

During stress, the sympathetic nervous system triggers the **endocrine system**. This system of glands, tissues, and cells helps control body functions by releasing **hormones** and other chemical messengers into the bloodstream to influence metabolism and other body processes. These chemicals act on a variety of targets throughout the body. Along with the nervous system, the endocrine system helps prepare the body to respond to a stressor.

> **endocrine system** The system of glands, tissues, and cells that secretes hormones into the bloodstream to influence metabolism and other body processes.
> **hormone** A chemical messenger produced in the body and transported in the bloodstream to target cells or organs for specific regulation of their activities.

The Two Systems Together

How do both systems work together in an emergency? Let's go back to your near collision with a car. Both reflexes and higher cognitive (thinking) areas in your brain quickly make the decision that you are facing a threat, and your body prepares to meet the danger. Chemical messages and actions of sympathetic nerves cause the release of key hormones, including **cortisol** and **epinephrine**. These hormones trigger a series of profound physiological changes (see Figure 12.1 on the next page), including the following:

> **cortisol** A steroid hormone secreted by the cortex (outer layer) of the adrenal gland; also called hydrocortisone.
> **epinephrine** A hormone secreted by the medulla (inner core) of the adrenal gland that affects the functioning of organs involved in responding to a stressor; also called *adrenaline*.

- Heart and respiration rates accelerate to speed oxygen through the body.

- Hearing and vision become more acute.

- The liver releases extra sugar into the bloodstream to boost energy.

- Perspiration increases to cool the skin.

- The brain releases **endorphins**—chemicals that can inhibit or block sensations of pain—in case you are injured.

endorphins   Brain secretions that have pain-inhibiting effects.

FIGURE 12.1

The fight-or-flight reaction. In response to a stressor, the autonomic nervous system and the endocrine system cause physical changes that prepare the body to deal with an emergency..

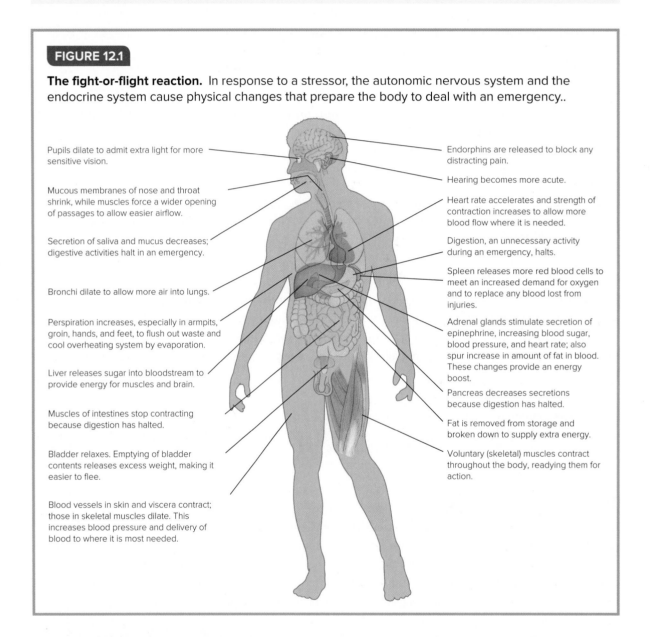

Pupils dilate to admit extra light for more sensitive vision.

Mucous membranes of nose and throat shrink, while muscles force a wider opening of passages to allow easier airflow.

Secretion of saliva and mucus decreases; digestive activities halt in an emergency.

Bronchi dilate to allow more air into lungs.

Perspiration increases, especially in armpits, groin, hands, and feet, to flush out waste and cool overheating system by evaporation.

Liver releases sugar into bloodstream to provide energy for muscles and brain.

Muscles of intestines stop contracting because digestion has halted.

Bladder relaxes. Emptying of bladder contents releases excess weight, making it easier to flee.

Blood vessels in skin and viscera contract; those in skeletal muscles dilate. This increases blood pressure and delivery of blood to where it is most needed.

Endorphins are released to block any distracting pain.

Hearing becomes more acute.

Heart rate accelerates and strength of contraction increases to allow more blood flow where it is needed.

Digestion, an unnecessary activity during an emergency, halts.

Spleen releases more red blood cells to meet an increased demand for oxygen and to replace any blood lost from injuries.

Adrenal glands stimulate secretion of epinephrine, increasing blood sugar, blood pressure, and heart rate; also spur increase in amount of fat in blood. These changes provide an energy boost.

Pancreas decreases secretions because digestion has halted.

Fat is removed from storage and broken down to supply extra energy.

Voluntary (skeletal) muscles contract throughout the body, readying them for action.

Taken together, these almost-instantaneous physical changes are called the **fight-or-flight reaction**. They give you the heightened reflexes and strength you need to dodge the car or deal with other stressors. Although these physical changes may vary in intensity, the same basic set of physical reactions occurs in response to any type of stressor—positive or negative, physical or psychological.

fight-or-flight reaction   A defence reaction that prepares a person for conflict or escape by triggering hormonal, cardiovascular, metabolic, and other changes.

The Return to Homeostasis

Once a stressful situation ends, the parasympathetic division of your autonomic nervous system takes command and halts the reaction. It restores **homeostasis**, a state in which blood pressure, heart rate, hormone levels, and other vital functions are maintained within a narrow range of normal. Your parasympathetic nervous system calms your body down, slowing a rapid heartbeat, drying sweaty palms, and returning breathing to normal. Gradually, your body resumes its normal "housekeeping" functions, such as digestion and temperature regulation. Damage that may have been sustained during the fight-or-flight reaction is repaired. The day after you narrowly dodge the car, you wake up feeling fine. In this way, your body can grow, repair itself, and acquire reserves of energy. When the next crisis comes, you'll be ready to respond again.

> **homeostasis**   A state of stability and consistency in a person's physiological functioning.

The Fight-or-Flight Reaction in Modern Life

The fight-or-flight reaction is a part of our biological heritage, and it's a survival mechanism that has served humans well. In modern life, however, it is often absurdly inappropriate. Many stressors we face in everyday life—such as an exam, a mess left by a roommate, or a stop light—do not require a physical response. The fight-or-flight reaction prepares the body for physical action regardless of whether such action is a necessary or appropriate response to a particular stressor.

Emotional and Behavioural Responses to Stressors

We all experience a similar set of physical responses to stressors, which make up the fight-or-flight reaction. These responses, however, vary from person to person and from one situation to another. People's perceptions of potential stressors—and their reactions to such stressors—also vary greatly. For example, you may feel confident about taking exams but may be nervous about talking to people you don't know, while your roommate may love challenging social situations but may be very nervous about taking tests. Many factors, some external and some internal, help explain these differences.

Your cognitive appraisal of a potential stressor will influence how it is viewed. Two factors that can reduce the magnitude of the stress response are successful prediction and the perception of control. For instance, obtaining course syllabi at the beginning of the term allows you to predict the timing of major deadlines and exams. Having this predictive knowledge also allows you to exert some control over your study and recreation plans and can help reduce the stress caused by exams.

The way we appraise potentially stressful situations is highly individual and strongly related to emotions. The facts of a situation—Who? What? Where? When?—are typically evaluated in the same way by each person involved. However, different people can evaluate the potential personal outcomes of a situation very differently: What does this mean for me? Can I do anything about it? Will it get better or worse? If you think you can't cope with a situation, you may respond negatively and with

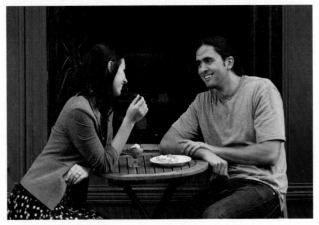
© Alan Bailey / Getty RF

Many people experience the set of almost-instantaneous physical changes that make up the stress response, such as increased heart rate and cold hands and feet, in reaction to positive stressors, such as a first date.

an inappropriate stress response. If, on the other hand, you think of a situation as a challenge you can manage, you are likely to have a more positive and appropriate response. A moderate level of stress, if coped with appropriately, can help promote optimal performance (Figure 12.2).

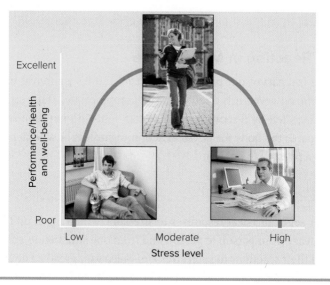

FIGURE 12.2

Stress level, performance, and well-being. A moderate level of stress challenges individuals in a way that promotes optimal performance and well-being. Too little stress, and people are not challenged enough to improve; too much stress, and the challenges become stressors that can impair physical and emotional health.

Wellness Tip

Chronic stress not only harms your health, it can also make you age faster. A study of women who were long-term caregivers to very sick children revealed that, over time, the women's bodies lost their ability to create new red blood cells. On average, these women were physically 10 years older than their actual chronological age. This is one reason it pays to learn to manage stress, especially when you're young!

Effective and Ineffective Responses

Common emotional responses to stressors include anxiety, depression, and fear. Although emotional responses are determined in part by inborn personality or temperament, you often can moderate or learn to control them. Coping techniques are discussed later in the chapter.

Behavioural responses to stressors—controlled by the **somatic nervous system**, which manages your conscious actions—are entirely under your control. Effective behavioural responses such as talking, laughing, exercising, meditating, learning time-management skills, and finding a more compatible roommate can promote wellness and enable you to function at your best. Ineffective behavioural responses to stressors include overeating, expressing hostility, and using tobacco, alcohol, or other drugs.

somatic nervous system The branch of the peripheral nervous system that governs motor functions and sensory information, largely under conscious control.

Personality and Stress

Some people seem to be nervous, irritable, and easily upset by minor annoyances; others are calm and composed even in difficult situations. Scientists remain unsure just why this is or how the brain's complex emotional mechanisms work. But **personality**, the sum of behavioural and emotional tendencies, clearly affects how people perceive and react to stressors. To investigate the links among personality, stress, and overall wellness, researchers have looked at different constellations of characteristics, or "personality types." Depending on the situation, most of us display some of the behaviours characteristic of one or more of the following types.

personality The sum of behavioural, cognitive, and emotional tendencies.

- **Type A.** People with Type A personality are often described as ultracompetitive, controlling, impatient, aggressive, and even hostile. Type A people have a higher perceived stress level and more problems coping with stress. They react explosively to stressors and are upset by events that others would consider only annoyances. Studies indicate that certain characteristics of the Type A pattern—anger, cynicism, and hostility—increase the risk of heart disease.

- **Type B.** The Type B personality is relaxed and contemplative. Type B people are less frustrated by daily events and more tolerant of the behaviour of others.

- **Type C.** The Type C personality is characterized by anger suppression, difficulties expressing emotions, feelings of hopelessness and despair, and an exaggerated stress response to minor stressors.

- **Type D.** The Type D personality tends toward negative emotional states such as anxiety, depression, and irritability. Type D people also avoid social interactions, worrying that others will react negatively toward them. Having this kind of personality predicts a number of poor health outcomes, including cardiovascular disease.

Researchers have also looked for personality traits that enable people to deal more successfully with stress. One such trait is hardiness, a particular form of optimism. People with a hardy personality view potential stressors as challenges and opportunities for growth and learning, rather than as burdens. Hardy people perceive fewer situations as stressful, and their reaction to stressors tends to be less intense. They are committed to their activities, have a sense of inner purpose and an inner locus of control, and feel at least partly in control of their lives.

The term *resilience* refers to personality traits associated with social and academic success in groups at risk for stress, such as people from low-income families and those with mental or physical disabilities. Resilient people tend to set goals and face adversity through individual effort. Resilience is also associated with emotional intelligence and violence prevention. There are three basic types of resilience, and each one determines how a person responds to stress.

- **Nonreactive resilience**, where a person does not react to a stressor
- **Homeostatic resilience**, where a person may react strongly but returns to baseline functioning quickly
- **Positive growth resilience**, where a person learns and grows from the stress experience

You probably can't change your basic personality, but you can change your typical behaviours and patterns of thinking and develop positive coping strategies. You can also use stress management techniques like those described later in the chapter.

Gender and Stress

Gender role—the activities, abilities, and behaviours that our culture expects of a person based on their sex—can affect an individual's experience of stress. Some behavioural responses to stressors, such as crying or openly expressing anger, may be deemed more appropriate for one gender than another. Strict adherence to gender roles can thus place limits on how a person responds to stress and can itself become a source of stress. Gender roles can also affect an individual's perception of a stressor. If a man derives most of his self-worth from his work, for example, retirement may be more stressful for him than for a woman whose self-image is based on several roles.

The Canadian Community Survey of 2014 reported that 23% of Canadians considered most days to be "quite a bit" or "extremely stressful," and that since 2003, more women than men are likely to report these feelings. In her book *Overwhelmed*, Brigid Schulte describes a continuing unequal gendered division of labour: families are working more hours than they used to (both parents combined worked an extra 13 hours per week in 2000 than they did in 1970), but American women spend even more time with their children than they did in the 1960s. How is this possible? Mothers tend to choose jobs that are flexible rather than very high-powered, they spend less time cleaning (either hiring someone else or leaving their houses dirtier), they sleep less, and they take less time for themselves.

Strengthening Mental Wellness

Think of the last time you faced a significant stressor. How did you respond? List the physical, emotional, and behavioural reactions you felt. Did these responses help you deal with the stress, or did they interfere with your efforts to handle it?

Experience

Past experiences can profoundly influence the evaluation of a potential stressor. Someone who has had a bad experience giving a speech in the past is much more likely to perceive an upcoming speech as stressful than someone who has had positive public speaking experiences. Effective behavioural responses, such as careful preparation and visualizing success, can help overcome the effects of negative past experiences.

The Stress Experience as a Whole

As Table 12.1 shows, the physical, emotional, and behavioural symptoms of excess negative stress are distinct—but they are also intimately interrelated. The more intense the emotional response, the stronger the physical response. Effective behavioural responses can lessen stress, while ineffective ones only worsen it. Sometimes people have such intense responses to stressors or such ineffective coping techniques that they need professional help to overcome the stress in their lives. More often, however, people can learn to handle stressors on their own.

TABLE 12.1

Symptoms of Excess Stress

Physical Symptoms	Emotional Symptoms	Behavioural Symptoms
Dry mouth	Anxiety or edginess	Crying
Excessive perspiration	Depression	Disrupted eating habits
Frequent illnesses	Edginess	Disrupted sleeping habits
Gastrointestinal problems	Fatigue	Harsh treatment of others
Grinding of teeth	Hypervigilance	Problems communicating
Headaches	Impulsiveness	Sexual problems
High blood pressure	Inability to concentrate	Social isolation
Pounding heart	Irritability	Increased use of tobacco, alcohol, or other drugs
Stiff neck or aching lower back	Trouble remembering things	

LO2 12.2 Stress and Wellness

The role of stress in health and disease is complex, but evidence suggests that stress can increase a person's vulnerability to numerous ailments. Several theories have been proposed to explain the relationship between stress and disease.

The General Adaptation Syndrome

Canadian biologist Hans Selye was one of the first scientists to develop a comprehensive theory of stress and disease. Based on his work in the 1930s and 1940s, Selye coined the term **general adaptation syndrome (GAS)** to describe what he believed is a universal and predictable response pattern to all stressors. Some stressors are pleasant, such as attending a party, while others are unpleasant, such as getting a bad grade. In the GAS theory, stress triggered by a pleasant stressor is called **eustress**; stress triggered by an unpleasant stressor is called **distress**. The sequence of physical responses associated with GAS (Figure 12.3) is the same for both eustress and distress and occurs in three stages:

> **general adaptation syndrome (GAS)**   A pattern of stress responses consisting of three stages: alarm, resistance, and exhaustion.
> **eustress**   Stress resulting from a pleasant stressor.
> **distress**   Stress resulting from an unpleasant stressor.

- **Alarm.** The alarm stage includes the complex sequence of events brought on by the fight-or-flight reaction. During this stage, the body is more susceptible to disease or injury because it is geared up to deal with a crisis. Someone in this phase may experience headaches, indigestion, anxiety, and disrupted sleeping and eating patterns.

- **Resistance.** With continued stress, the body develops a new level of homeostasis in which it is more resistant to disease and injury than normal. During this stage, a person can cope with normal life and added stress.

- **Exhaustion.** The first two stages of GAS require a great deal of energy. If a stressor persists, or if several stressors occur in succession, general exhaustion results. This is not the sort of exhaustion people complain of after a long, busy day. Rather it's a life-threatening type of physiological exhaustion.

FIGURE 12.3

The general adaptation syndrome. During the alarm phase, a lower resistance to injury is evident. With continued stress, resistance to injury is actually enhanced. With prolonged exposure to repeated stressors, exhaustion sets in, with a return of low resistance levels seen during acute stress.

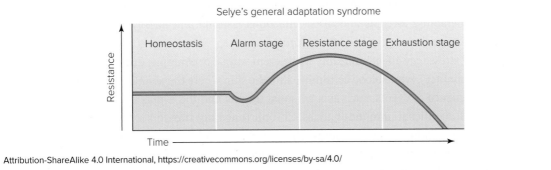

Attribution-ShareAlike 4.0 International, https://creativecommons.org/licenses/by-sa/4.0/

Allostatic Load

Although GAS is still viewed as a key contribution to the understanding of stress, some aspects of it are now outdated. For example, increased susceptibility to disease after repeated or prolonged stress is now thought to be due to the effects of the stress response itself rather than to a depletion of resources (exhaustion stage). In particular, long-term overexposure to such stress hormones as cortisol has been linked with health problems. Further, although physical stress reactions promote homeostasis (resistance stage), they also have negative effects on the body.

The long-term wear and tear of the stress response is called the **allostatic load**. An individual's allostatic load depends on many factors, including genetics, life experiences, and emotional and behavioural responses to stressors. A high allostatic load may be due to frequent stressors, poor adaptation to common stressors, an inability to shut down the stress response, or imbalances in the stress response of different body systems. High allostatic load has been linked with heart disease, high blood pressure, obesity, and reduced brain and immune system functioning. In other words, when your allostatic load exceeds your ability to cope, you are more likely to get sick.

allostatic load   The long-term negative impact of the stress response on the body.

Ask Yourself

QUESTIONS FOR CRITICAL THINKING AND REFLECTION

Have you ever felt so much stress that you felt ill in some way? If so, what were your symptoms? How did you handle them? Did the experience affect the way you reacted to other stressful events?

Stress and Specific Conditions

Although much remains to be learned, it is clear that people who have unresolved chronic stress in their lives or who handle stressors poorly are at risk for a wide range of health problems. In the short term, the problem might just be a cold, a stiff neck, or a stomachache. Over the long term, the problems can be more severe, such as cardiovascular disease or impairment of the immune system.

Stress and the Immune System

Study of the stress hormones cortisol and epinephrine has provided a physical link between emotions and immune function. In general, increased levels of stress hormones are linked to a decrease in the number or functioning of immune system cells. Some of the health problems linked to stress-related changes in immune function include vulnerability to colds and other infections, asthma and allergy attacks, and flare-ups of chronic diseases such as genital herpes and HIV infection.

Different types of stress may affect immunity in different ways. For example, during acute stress (typically lasting less than 100 minutes), white blood cells move into the skin where they enhance the immune response. During a stressful sequence of events, such as a personal trauma and the events that follow, however, there are typically no overall significant immune changes. Chronic (ongoing) stressors such as unemployment have negative effects on almost all functional measures of immunity. Chronic stress may cause prolonged secretion of cortisol and may accelerate the course of diseases that involve inflammation, including multiple sclerosis, heart disease, and type 2 diabetes.

Mood, personality, behaviour, and immune functioning are intertwined. For example, people who are generally pessimistic may neglect the basics of health care, become passive when ill, and fail to engage in health-promoting behaviours. People who are depressed may reduce physical activity and social interaction, which may in turn affect the immune system and the cognitive appraisal of a stressor. Optimism, successful coping, and positive problem solving, on the other hand, may positively influence immunity.

Cardiovascular Disease

The stress response profoundly affects the cardiovascular system. During the stress response, heart rate increases and blood vessels constrict, causing blood pressure to rise. Chronic high blood pressure is a major cause of atherosclerosis, a disease in which the lining of the blood vessels becomes damaged and caked with fatty deposits. These deposits can block arteries, causing heart attacks and strokes (see Chapter 10).

Certain types of emotional responses increase a person's risk of cardiovascular disease. People who exhibit extreme increases in heart rate and blood pressure in response to emotional stressors may face an increased risk of cardiovascular problems.[1]

Fitness Tip

Feeling too much stress? Then walk away—literally. Walking is a proven countermeasure against stress, and it contributes to your health in many other ways. A brisk, 10-minute walk may be enough to help you put things in perspective and get back to your normal routine. If not, just keep walking until you feel better. As you walk, try not to think too much about anything specific; the idea is to clear your head!

Other Health Problems

Many other health problems may be caused or worsened by excessive stress, including the following:

- digestive problems such as stomachaches, diarrhea, constipation, irritable bowel syndrome, and ulcers
- tension headaches and migraines
- insomnia and fatigue (see the box Overcoming Insomnia)
- injuries, including on-the-job injuries caused by repetitive strain
- menstrual irregularities, impotence, and pregnancy complications
- psychological problems, including depression, anxiety, panic attacks, eating disorders, and post-traumatic stress disorder (PTSD), which afflicts people who have suffered or witnessed severe trauma

Take CHARGE

OVERCOMING INSOMNIA

Most people can overcome insomnia by discovering the cause of poor sleep and taking steps to remedy it. Insomnia that lasts for more than six months and interferes with daytime functioning requires consultation with a physician. Sleeping pills are not recommended for chronic insomnia because they can be habit-forming; they also lose their effectiveness over time.

continued

If you're bothered by insomnia, try the following:

- Determine how much sleep you need to feel refreshed the next day, and don't sleep longer than that.
- Go to bed at the same time every night and, more important, get up at the same time every morning, seven days a week, regardless of how much sleep you got.
- Don't nap more than 30 minutes per day.
- Exercise regularly, but not too close to bedtime. Your metabolism needs at least six hours to slow down after exercise.
- Avoid tobacco and caffeine late in the day, and alcohol before bedtime (it causes disturbed, fragmented sleep).
- If you take any medications (prescription or not), ask your doctor or pharmacist if they interfere with sleep.
- Have a light snack before bedtime; you'll sleep better if you're not hungry.
- Use your bed only for sleep. Don't eat, read, study, or watch television in bed.
- Establish a relaxing bedtime routine that helps you unwind and lets your brain know it's time to go to sleep. Read, listen to music, or practise a relaxation technique. Don't lie down in bed until you're sleepy.
- If you don't fall asleep in 15 to 20 minutes, or if you wake up and can't fall asleep again, get out of bed, leave the room if possible, and do something monotonous until you feel sleepy. Try distracting yourself with imagery instead of counting sheep; imagine yourself on a pleasant vacation or enjoying some beautiful scenery.
- If sleep problems persist, ask your doctor for a referral to a sleep specialist in your area. You may be a candidate for a sleep study—an overnight evaluation of your sleep pattern that can uncover many sleep-related disorders.

LO3 12.3 Common Sources of Stress

Recognizing potential sources of stress is an important step in successfully managing the stress in your life.

Major Life Changes

Any major change in your life that requires adjustment and accommodation can be a source of stress. Early adulthood and the university/college years are typically associated with many significant changes, such as moving out of the family home. Even changes typically thought of as positive—graduation, job promotion, or marriage—can be stressful.

Clusters of life changes, particularly those that are perceived negatively, may be linked to health problems in some people. Personality and coping skills are important moderating influences, however. People with a strong support network and a stress-resistant personality are less likely to become ill in response to major life changes than people with fewer resources. Kelly McGonigal's book, *The Upside of Stress*, suggests that if you embrace stressful events as opportunities to learn and grow, your health will not be as negatively impacted as it is when you worry about them.

Daily Hassles

Although major life changes are undoubtedly stressful, they seldom occur regularly. Researchers have proposed that minor problems—life's daily hassles, such as losing your keys or wallet—can be an even greater source of stress because they occur much more often.

People who perceive hassles negatively are likely to experience a moderate stress response every time they are faced with one. Over time, this can take a significant toll on health. Studies indicate that for some people, daily hassles contribute to a general decrease in overall wellness.

University/College Stressors

University or college is a time of major life changes and abundant minor hassles. For many students, college means being away from home and family for the first time. Nearly all students share stresses like the following:

- **Academic stressors.** Exams, grades, and an endless workload await every university/college student but can be especially troublesome for young students just out of high school.

- **Interpersonal stressors.** Most students are more than just students; they are also friends, children, employees, partners, and so on. Managing relationships while juggling the rigours of university/college life can be daunting, especially if some friends or family are less than supportive.

- **Time pressures.** Class schedules, assignments, and deadlines are an inescapable part of university/college life. But these time pressures can be drastically compounded for students who also have a job and/or family responsibilities.

- **Financial concerns.** The majority of university/college students need financial aid not just to cover the cost of tuition, but also to survive from day to day while in school. For many, university/college life isn't possible without a job, and the pressure to stay afloat financially competes with academic and other stressors.

- **Worries about the future.** As university/college life comes to an end, students face the reality of life after school. This means thinking about a career, choosing a place to live, and leaving the friends and routines of school behind.

Job-Related Stressors

Surveys suggest that 30% of Canadians rate their jobs as the key source of stress in their lives. Tight schedules and overtime leave less time to exercise, socialize, and engage in other stress-proofing activities. Only a third of the Canadian workforce report working the standard 40-hour work week, while about a quarter spend 50 hours or more per week at their job.[2] Worries about job performance, salary, and job security and interactions with bosses, co-workers, and customers can contribute to stress. High levels of job stress are also common for people who are left out of important decisions relating to their jobs. When workers are given the opportunity to shape how their jobs are performed, job satisfaction goes up and stress levels go down.

If job-related (or education-related) stress is severe or chronic, the result can be *burnout*, a state of physical, mental, and emotional exhaustion. Burnout occurs most often in highly motivated and driven individuals who come to feel that their work is not recognized or that they are not accomplishing their goals. People in the helping professions—teachers, social workers, caregivers, police officers, and so on—are also prone to burnout. For some people who suffer from burnout, a vacation or leave of absence may be appropriate. For others, a reduced work schedule, better communication with superiors, or a change in job goals may be necessary. Improving time-management skills can also help.

Wellness Tip

If you worry about money, you definitely aren't alone. In 2007, Desjardins Financial Security reported that 44% of Canadians cited money as a key source of stress in their lives. If money is a constant cause of worry for you, see the advice on financial wellness in Chapter 1 and get help from a financial planner. It's never too early to have a solid financial plan in place.

Relationships and Stress

Human beings need social relationships; we cannot thrive as solitary creatures. Simply put, people need people. Even so, your interpersonal relationships—even your deepest, most intimate ones—can be some of the most significant sources of stress in your life.

The first relationships we form outside the family are friendships. Friendships give people the opportunity to share themselves and discover others, and are often more stable and longer lasting than intimate partnerships. Friends are often more accepting and less critical than lovers, probably because their expectations are different. Friendships also provide people with emotional support and buffer them from stress. During times of stress, in fact, many people initially turn to their friends for comfort, rather than family members or lovers.

Intimate love relationships are among the most profound human experiences. When two people fall in love, their relationship at first is likely to be characterized by high levels of passion and rapidly increasing intimacy. In time, passion decreases as the partners become familiar with each other. The diminishing of passionate love often creates stress between partners (usually affecting one partner more than the other) and can be experienced as a crisis in the relationship. If a quieter, more lasting love fails to emerge, the relationship will likely break up, and each person will search for another who will once again ignite their passion.

The key to developing and maintaining any type of friendship or intimate relationship is good communication. Miscommunication creates frustration and distances us from our friends and partners. (For more information, see the section Communication later in this chapter.)

Other Stressors

Environmental stressors—external conditions or events that cause stress—include loud noises, unpleasant smells, industrial accidents, violence, and natural disasters. In contrast, *internal stressors* are found not in your interactions with your environment, but rather within yourself. For example, people often put pressure on themselves to reach personal goals and then evaluate their progress and performance. Physical and emotional states such as illness and exhaustion are other examples of internal stressors.

LO4 12.4 Managing Stress

What can you do about all this stress? A great deal. By pursuing a wellness lifestyle—being physically active, eating well, getting enough sleep, and so on—and by learning simple ways to identify and moderate individual stressors, you can control the stress in your life.

Exercise

Researchers have found that people who exercise regularly react with milder physical stress responses before, during, and after exposure to stressors and their overall sense of well-being increases as well (see the box Does Exercise Improve Mental Health?). Although even light exercise can have a beneficial effect, an integrated fitness program can have a significant impact on stress.

For some people, however, exercise can become just one more stressor in a highly stressed life. People who exercise compulsively risk overtraining, a condition characterized by fatigue, irritability, depression, and diminished athletic performance. An overly strenuous exercise program can even make a person sick by compromising immune function. (For the details of a safe and effective exercise program, refer to Chapter 9.)

The Evidence *for* EXERCISE

DOES EXERCISE IMPROVE MENTAL HEALTH?

The overall conclusion from the many published studies is that exercise—even modest activity such as taking a daily walk—can help combat a variety of mental health problems. Overall, physically active people who exercise 2.5 to 7.5 hours per week are about 25–30% less likely to feel distressed than inactive people. Regardless of the number, age, or health status of the people being studied, those who were active managed stress better than their inactive counterparts. Among athletic teenagers, there is a correlation between exercise and improved social interaction, as well as between exercise and enhanced looks (e.g., better body structure), two factors that contribute to mental health. Physical activity has also been shown to improve conditions for people with anxiety; mood, eating, and substance use disorders; as well as schizophrenia and dementia. In some studies, therapeutic contact, social support, and distraction have been found to have some of the same positive effects of low-intensity exercise.

A simple walk can be very effective: One study found that taking a long walk can reduce anxiety and blood pressure. Another showed that a brisk walk for as little as 10 minutes can leave people feeling more relaxed and energetic for up to two hours. People who took three brisk 45-minute walks each week for three months reported that they perceived fewer daily hassles and had a greater sense of general wellness.

These findings are not surprising. The stress response mobilizes energy resources and readies the body for physical emergencies. If you experience stress and do not exert yourself physically, you are not completing the energy cycle. You may not be able to exercise while your daily stressors are occurring, but you can be active later in the day. Such activity allows you to expend the nervous energy you have built up and trains your body to return more readily to homeostasis after stressful situations.

Physical activity also helps you sleep better, and consistently sound sleep is critical to managing stress. According to the National Sleep Foundation, people who exercise vigorously are the most likely to report a good night's sleep. Of those who do not regularly exercise, about one-half report being wakeful during the night, every night. Quality sleep and regular exercise work in a cycle, so that a decrease in one can lead to a decrease in the other. There are about 70 known sleep disorders, and disordered sleep is associated with a variety of physical and neurological problems, including health problems relating to stress. Regular activity promotes better sleep and provides some protection against sleep interruptions such as insomnia and sleep apnea. Consistent, restful sleep is now regarded as a protective factor in disorders such as depression, anxiety, obesity, and heart disease.

SOURCES: Kim, Y.S., et al. 2012. Relationship between physical activity and general mental health. *Preventive Medicine* 55(5): 458–463; Monschouwer, Karin, et al. 2013. Possible mechanisms explaining the association between physical activity and mental health: findings from the 2001 Dutch health behaviour in school-aged children survey. *Clinical Psychological Science* January 1(1): 67–74; Zschucke, E., et al. January 2013. Exercise and physical activity in mental disorders: clinical and experimental evidence. *Journal of Preventive Medicine & Public Health* J46 (Suppl. 1): S12–S21; National Sleep Foundation. March 4, 2013. *National Sleep Foundation Poll Finds Exercise Key to Good Sleep.* Arlington, VA: National Sleep Foundation.

Nutrition

A healthy, balanced diet can help you cope with stress. In addition, eating wisely will enhance your feelings of self-control and self-esteem. Avoiding or limiting caffeine is also important in stress management. Although one or two cups of coffee a day probably won't hurt you, caffeine is a mildly addictive stimulant that leaves some people jittery, irritable, and unable to sleep. Consuming caffeine during stressful situations can raise blood pressure and increase levels of cortisol. (For more on sound nutrition and for advice on evaluating dietary supplements, many of which are marketed for stress, see Chapter 7.)

Sleep

Most adults need seven to nine hours of sleep every night to stay healthy and perform their best. Getting enough sleep isn't just good for you physically; adequate sleep also improves mood, fosters feelings of competence and self-worth, enhances mental functioning, and supports emotional functioning. See the box Apps for Improving and Tracking Sleep for suggestions to help you get enough sleep.

Wellness *in the* DIGITAL AGE

APPS FOR IMPROVING AND TRACKING SLEEP

Are you getting enough sleep? If you're like the average Canadian, you get less than the recommended 7 to 9 hours of sleep each night. Because chronic sleep disorders affect millions of people, sleep deprivation is often referred to as a national public epidemic.

Digital Devices and Sleep Before we look at sleep apps, it is important to consider how use of your digital devices can negatively impact your sleep. Tablets, Smartphones, and computers emit blue light that impedes the release of melatonin, a hormone that affects sleep and wake cycles. In one study, researchers compared the sleep of people who read an eBook on a digital device with people who read a print book in the hours before bedtime. Those who read the digital book took longer to fall asleep, had reduced melatonin release, and were less alert the next morning.

Could heavy texting affect sleep? Psychologist Karla Murdock reported that texting was a direct predictor of sleep problems among first-year students in a study that examined links among interpersonal stress, text-messaging behaviour, and three indicators of university/college students' health: burnout, sleep problems, and emotional well-being.

Murdock and other sleep experts suggest turning off your screens. Use them less during the day and also when preparing to sleep at night. If you have trouble relaxing and transitioning to sleep in the evenings, try shutting down all your devices an hour or more before you intend to sleep.

Now that you are resting in the dark, why would you consider using a sleep app or tracker on your digital device? Ironically, a Smartphone may help you get to sleep—if you tuck it into the corner of your bed.

Aids for Relaxation. There are many free and low-cost apps that help promote relaxation and improve sleep. Some include music, white noise, or sounds of nature (e.g., wind, rain, waves, or songbirds). Others offer specific techniques, such as guided meditation or breathing exercises, to promote relaxation to aid in falling asleep. Examples include Sleepmaker Rain, Nature Sounds Relax and Sleep, Sleep Soundly Hypnosis, Long Deep Breathing, and Relax & Sleep by Glenn Harrold.

Sleep Trackers. More complicated technologies attempt to track and analyze sleep. Many are based on movement detectors in Smartphones. These apps estimate the amount and type of sleep you get based on your movements during the night. They may generate detailed graphs of your sleep quality and then time your wake-up alarm to a specific sleep cycle. Some apps also include a sound recorder that detects sleep talking, snoring, and other night noises, providing further information. Sleep apps include Sleepbot, Sleep Cycle, Pillow, and Smart Alarm Clock.

In addition to Smartphone apps, specialized fitness wristbands such as Fitbit and Garmin include sleep trackers. Many of these are also based on movement detectors, but some incorporate heart-rate data as well; some preliminary research indicates that adding heart rate data to movement tracking may improve the accuracy of the results. Fitbit and other wearables, along with some apps, may combine sleep and fitness data into an overall picture of an individual's activity over the course of a day.

Apps and devices may be popular, but no consumer technology yet developed can equal the capability of a sleep lab at detecting sleep stages or diagnosing specific sleep disorders. If you enjoy the features of an app or wearable tracker, go ahead and use them; but don't rely on an app to diagnose the presence or absence of a serious sleep problem. One good effect of using a sleep tracker is simply the greater focus it places on sleep.

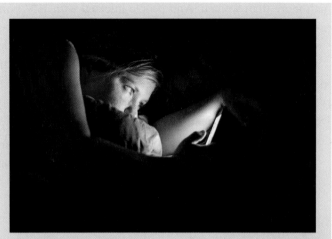

© Blend Images / Alamy Stock Photo

SOURCES: Chang, A. M., et al. 2015. Evening use of light-emitting eReaders negatively affects sleep, circadian timing, and next-morning alertness. *Proceedings of the National Academy of Sciences* 112(4): 1232–1237; Bhat, S., et al. 2015. Is there a clinical role for smartphone sleep apps? Comparison of sleep cycle detection by a smartphone application to polysomnography. *Journal of Clinical Sleep Medicine,* 3 Feb; Gradisar, M., et al. 2013. The sleep and technology use of Americans. *Journal of Clinical Sleep Medicine* 9(12): 1291–1299; Behar, J., et al. 2013. A review of current sleep screening applications for smartphones. *Physiological Measurement* 34(7): R29–46; Lewis, J. G. 2013. Sleep cycle app: precise, or placebo? Mind Read: Connecting Brain and Behavior (http://www.nature.com/scitable/blog/mind-read/sleep_cycle_app_precise_or); Murdock, K. K. Texting while stressed: Implications for students' burnout, sleep, and well-being. *Psychology of Popular Media Culture,* 2013; Burtchell, J. 2014. *The best sleep iPhone & Android apps of the year.* Medically reviewed by K. Hirsch. May 16, 2014. (http://www.healthline.com/health-slideshow/top-insomnia-iphone-android-apps#4).

Sleep and Stress

Stress hormone levels in the bloodstream vary throughout the day and are related to sleep patterns. Peak concentrations of these hormones occur in the early morning, followed by a slow decline during the day and evening. Concentrations return to peak levels during the final stages of sleep and in the early morning hours.

Even though stress hormones are released during sleep, it is the lack of sleep that has the greatest impact on stress. The Better Sleep Council of Canada reported that one-third of Canadians are unable to sleep at night at least once per week as a result of stress. In someone who is suffering from sleep deprivation (not getting enough sleep over time), mental and physical processes deteriorate steadily. A sleep-deprived person experiences headaches, feels irritable, is unable to concentrate, and is more prone to forgetfulness. Poor-quality sleep has long been associated with stress and depression. A small 2008 study of female university/college students further associated sleep deprivation with an increased risk of suicide.

Acute sleep deprivation slows the daytime decline in stress hormones, so evening levels are higher than normal. A decrease in total sleep time also causes an increase in the level of stress hormones. Together, these changes may cause an increase in stress hormone levels throughout the day and may contribute to physical and mental exhaustion. Extreme sleep deprivation can lead to hallucinations and other psychotic symptoms, as well as to a significant increase in heart attack risk.

Social Support

Meaningful connections with others can play a key role in stress management and overall wellness. Sharing fears, frustrations, and joys makes life richer and seems to contribute to the well-being of body and mind. One study of university/college students living in overcrowded apartments, for example, found that those with a strong social support system were less distressed by their cramped quarters than those who navigated life's challenges on their own. Other studies have shown that married people live longer than single people and have lower death rates from a wide range of conditions, although some studies suggest that marriage benefits men more than women. And people infected with HIV remain symptom-free longer if they have a strong social support network. A sense of isolation can lead to chronic stress, which in turn can increase a person's susceptibility to temporary illnesses, like colds, and to chronic illnesses, such as heart disease.

Although the mechanism isn't clear, social isolation can be as significant to mortality rates as factors like smoking, high blood pressure, and obesity. There is no single best pattern of social support that works for everyone. However, research suggests that having a variety of types of relationships may be important for wellness. Here are some tips for strengthening your social ties:

- **Foster friendships.** Keep in regular contact with your friends. Offer respect, trust, and acceptance, and provide help and support in times of need. Build your communication skills and express appreciation for your friends.

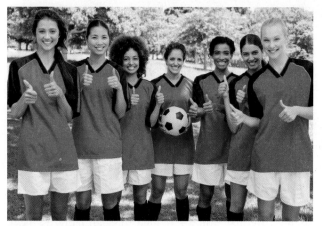
© Wavebreak Media ltd / Alamy

- **Keep your family ties strong.** Stay in touch with the family members you feel close to. If your family doesn't function well as a support system for its members, create a second "family" of people with whom you have built meaningful ties.

- **Get involved with a group.** Do volunteer work, take a class, attend a lecture series, or join a religious group. These types of activities can give you a sense of security, a place to talk about your feelings or concerns, and a way to build new friendships. Choose activities that are meaningful to you and that include direct involvement with other people.

Communication

Good communication skills can help everyone form and maintain healthy relationships. Communicating in an assertive way that respects the rights of others—as well as your own—can prevent potentially stressful situations from getting out of control. When friends or partners communicate effectively, they can reduce the stresses in their relationship and spend more time focusing on the positive aspects of being together.

Three keys to good communication in relationships are self-disclosure, listening, and feedback.

- **Self-disclosure** involves revealing personal information that you ordinarily wouldn't reveal because of the risk involved. It usually increases feelings of closeness and moves the relationship to a deeper level of intimacy.

- **Listening** is a rare skill. Good listening skills require that you spend more time and energy trying to fully understand another person's "story" and less time judging, evaluating, blaming, advising, analyzing, or trying to control. Empathy, warmth, respect, and genuineness are qualities of skillful listeners. Attentive listening encourages friends or partners to share more and, in turn, to be attentive listeners. In order to connect with other people and develop real emotional intimacy, listening is essential.

- **Feedback**, a constructive response to another's self-disclosure, is the third key to good communication. Giving positive feedback means acknowledging that the friend's or partner's feelings are valid—no matter how upsetting or troubling—and offering self-disclosure in response. Self-disclosure and feedback can open the door to change, whereas other responses block communication and change.

For tips on improving your skills, see the box Guidelines for Effective Communication.

Take CHARGE

GUIDELINES FOR EFFECTIVE COMMUNICATION

Getting Started

- When you want to have a serious discussion with your partner, choose an appropriate time and place. Find a private place and a time when you will not be interrupted.
- Face your partner and maintain eye contact. Use nonverbal feedback to show that you are interested and involved in the communication process.

Being an Effective Speaker

- State your concern or issue as clearly as you can.
- Use "I" statements—statements about how *you* feel—rather than statements beginning with "You," which tell another person how you think they feel. When you use "I" statements, you are taking responsibility for your feelings. "You" statements are often blaming or accusatory and will probably get a defensive or resentful response. The statement "I feel unloved," for example, sends a clearer, less blaming message than the statement "You don't love me."
- Focus on a specific behaviour rather than on the whole person. Be specific about the behaviour you like or don't like. Avoid generalizations beginning with "You always" or "You never." Such statements make people feel defensive.
- Make constructive requests. Opening your request with "I would like" keeps the focus on your needs rather than on your partner's supposed deficiencies.
- Avoid blaming, accusing, and belittling. Even if you are right, you have little to gain by putting your partner down. Studies have shown that when people feel criticized or attacked, they are less able to think rationally or solve problems constructively.
- Ask for action ahead of time. Tell your partner what you would like to have happen in the future; don't wait for them to blow it and then express anger or disappointment.

Being an Effective Listener

- Provide appropriate nonverbal feedback (nodding, smiling, and so on).
- Don't interrupt.
- Develop the skill of reflective listening. Don't judge, evaluate, analyze, or offer solutions (unless asked to do so). Your partner may just need to have you there in order to sort out feelings. By jumping in right away to "fix" the problem, you may be cutting off communication.
- Don't give unsolicited advice. Giving advice implies that you know more about what a person needs to do than they do; therefore, it often evokes anger or resentment.
- Clarify your understanding of what your partner is saying by restating it in your own words and asking if your understanding is correct.
- Be sure you are really listening, not off somewhere in your mind rehearsing your reply. Try to tune in to your partner's feelings as well as the words.
- Let your partner know that you value what they are saying and want to understand. Respect for the other person is the cornerstone of effective communication.

Some people have trouble either telling others what they need or saying no to the needs of others. They may suppress their feelings of anger, frustration, and resentment, and they may end up feeling taken advantage of or suffering in unhealthy relationships. At the other extreme are people who express anger openly and directly by being verbally or physically aggressive or indirectly by making critical, hurtful comments to others. Their abusive behaviour pushes other people away, so they also have problems with relationships.

If you typically suppress your feelings, you might want to take an assertiveness training course that can help you identify and change your patterns of communication. If you have trouble controlling your anger, you can benefit from learning anger management strategies; see the box Dealing with Anger.

Take CHARGE

DEALING WITH ANGER

Anger is a universal response to something perceived as a betrayal, injustice, threat, or some other wrong—whether real or imagined. You may respond physically with faster heart and breathing rates, increased muscle tension, a knot in the stomach, trembling, or a red face. When anger alerts you that something is wrong, it is a useful emotion that can lead to constructive change. When anger leads to loss of control and to aggression, it causes problems.

According to current popular wisdom, it's healthy to express your feelings, including anger. However, research has shown that people who are overtly hostile are at higher risk for heart disease and heart attacks than are calmer people. In addition, expressing anger in thoughtless or out-of-control ways can damage personal and professional relationships.

People who experience rage or explosive anger are particularly at risk for negative repercussions. Some of these people may have *intermittent explosive disorder*, characterized by aggressiveness that is impulsive and out of proportion to the stimulus. Explosive anger renders people temporarily unable to think straight or act in their own best interests. Counselling can help very angry people learn how to manage their anger.

In dealing with anger, it is important to distinguish between a reasonable degree of self-assertiveness and a gratuitous expression of aggression. When you are *assertive*, you stand up for your own rights at the same time that you respect the rights of others. When you are *aggressive*, you violate the rights of others.

Managing Your Own Anger

What are the best ways to handle anger? If you find yourself in a situation where you are getting angry, answer these questions:

- Is the situation important enough to get angry about?
- Are you truly justified in getting angry?
- Is expressing your anger going to make a positive difference?

If the answer to all these questions is yes, then calm, assertive communication may be appropriate. Use "I" statements to express your feelings ("I would like . . .," "I feel . . ."), and listen respectfully to the other person's point of view. Don't attack verbally or make demands; try to negotiate a constructive, mutually satisfying solution.

If you answer no to any of the questions, try to calm yourself. First, reframe the situation by thinking about it differently. Try these strategies:

- **Don't take it personally.** Maybe the driver who cut you off simply didn't see you.
- **Look for mitigating factors.** Maybe the classmate who didn't say hello was preoccupied with money concerns.
- **Practise empathy.** Try to see the situation from the other person's point of view.
- **Ask questions.** Clarify the situation by asking what the other person meant. Avoid defensiveness.
- **Focus on the present.** Don't let this situation trigger thoughts of past incidents that you perceive as similar.

Second, calm your body down by trying the following strategies:

- Use the old trick of counting to 10 before you respond.
- Concentrate on your breathing, and take long, slow breaths.

- Imagine yourself in a beautiful, peaceful place.
- If needed, take a longer cooling-off period by leaving the situation until your anger has subsided.

Dealing with Other People's Anger

If someone you are with becomes very angry, try these strategies:

- Respond asymmetrically—remain calm. Don't get angry in response.
- Apologize if you think you are to blame. Don't apologize if you don't think you are to blame.
- Validate the other person by acknowledging that they have some reason to be angry.
- Focus on the problem and ask what can be done to alleviate the situation.
- If the person cannot be calmed, disengage from the situation, at least temporarily. After a time-out, attempts at rational problem solving may be more successful.

Warning Signs of Violence

Violence is never acceptable. The following behaviours over a period of time suggest the potential for violence:

- a history of making threats and engaging in aggressive behaviour
- drug or alcohol abuse
- gang membership
- access to or fascination with weapons
- feelings of rejection or aloneness
- the feeling of constantly being disrespected
- victimization by bullies
- withdrawal from usual activities and friends; poor school performance
- failure to acknowledge the rights of others

The following are immediate warning signs of violence:

- daily loss of temper or frequent physical fighting
- significant vandalism or property damage
- increased risk-taking behaviour
- increased drug or alcohol abuse
- threats or detailed plans to commit acts of violence
- pleasure in hurting animals
- the presence of weapons

Don't spend time with someone who shows these warning signs of violence. Ask someone in authority or an experienced professional for help.

Conflict Resolution

Conflict is natural in any relationship, and it can become a key source of stress for friends, co-workers, family members, and intimate partners. No matter how close two people become, they still remain separate individuals with their own needs, desires, past experiences, and ways of seeing the world. Conflict itself isn't dangerous to a relationship; it may simply indicate that the relationship is growing. But if it isn't handled in a constructive way, conflict can damage—and ultimately destroy—a relationship.

Conflict is often accompanied by anger—a universal emotion, but one that can be difficult to handle. When angry, both parties should back off until they calm down and then come back to the issue later and try to resolve it rationally. Negotiation will help dissipate the anger so the conflict can be resolved. The following basic strategies are useful in successfully negotiating with a friend, family member, colleague, or intimate partner:

1. **Clarify the issue.** Take responsibility for thinking through your feelings and discovering what's really bothering you. Agree that one of you will speak first and have the chance to speak fully while the other

listens. Then reverse the roles. Try to understand the other person's position fully by repeating what you've heard and asking questions to clarify or elicit more information.

2. **Find out what each person wants.** Ask the other person to express their desires. Don't assume you already know what those desires are, and don't try to speak for the other person.

3. **Determine how you both can get what you want.** Brainstorm to generate a variety of options.

4. **Decide how to negotiate.** Work out a plan for change. For example, agree that one of you will do one task and the other will do another task, or that one of you will do a task in exchange for something they want.

5. **Solidify the agreements.** Go over the plan verbally and write it down, if necessary, to ensure that you both understand and agree to it.

6. **Review and renegotiate.** Decide on a time frame for trying out the new plan and set a time to discuss how it's working. Make adjustments as needed.

Wellness Tip

In a stressful situation, do you ever stop and count to 10? If not, you should. It works! In the few seconds it takes to count to 10, you can calm your mind, get your breathing under control, slow your heart rate, and lower your blood pressure. In effect, that quick 10-count can offset the stress reaction and help you avoid making things worse.

Striving for Spiritual Wellness

Spiritual wellness is associated with greater coping skills and higher levels of overall wellness. It is a very personal wellness component, and there are many ways to develop it. Researchers have linked spiritual wellness to longer life expectancy, reduced risk of disease and faster recovery, and improved emotional health. Although spirituality is difficult to study and researchers aren't sure how or why spirituality seems to improve health, several explanations have been offered. Lab 12.3 includes exercises designed to help you build spiritual wellness; choose activities that are most meaningful to you from among the ideas suggested in the lab.

Confiding in Yourself Through Writing

Keeping a diary is like confiding in someone else, except that you are confiding in yourself. This form of coping with severe stress may be especially helpful for those who are shy or introverted and find it difficult to open up to others. Although writing about traumatic and stressful events may have a short-term negative effect on mood, over the long term, stress is reduced and positive changes in health occur. A key to promoting health and well-being through journaling is to write about your emotional responses to stressful events. Set aside a special time each day or week to write down your feelings about stressful events in your life.

Time Management

Learning to manage your time successfully can be crucial to coping with everyday stressors. Overcommitment, procrastination, and even boredom are significant stressors for many people. Along with gaining control of nutrition and exercise to maintain a healthy energy balance, time management is an important element in a wellness program. Try these strategies for improving your time-management skills:

- **Set priorities.** Divide your tasks into three groups: essential, important, and trivial. Focus on the first two. Ignore the third.

- **Schedule tasks for peak efficiency.** You've undoubtedly noticed you're most productive at certain times of the day (or night). Schedule as many of your tasks for those hours as you can and stick to your schedule.

- **Set realistic goals and write them down.** Attainable goals spur you on. Impossible goals, by definition, cause frustration and failure. Fully commit yourself to achieving your goals by putting them in writing.

- **Budget enough time.** For each project you undertake, calculate how long it will take to complete. Then tack on another 10–15%, or even 25%, as a buffer.

- **Break up long-term goals into short-term ones.** Instead of waiting for or relying on large blocks of time, use short amounts of time to start a project or keep it moving.

- **Visualize achieving your goals.** By mentally rehearsing a task, you will be able to do it more smoothly.

- **Keep track of the tasks you put off.** Analyze the reasons why you procrastinate. If the task is difficult or unpleasant, look for ways to make it easier or more fun. For example, if you find the readings for one of your classes particularly difficult, choose an especially nice setting for your reading and then reward yourself each time you complete a section or chapter.

- **Consider doing your least-favourite tasks first.** Once you have the most unpleasant ones out of the way, you can work on the projects you enjoy more.

- **Consolidate tasks when possible.** For example, try walking to the store so that you run your errands and exercise in the same block of time.

- **Identify quick transitional tasks.** Keep a list of 5- to 10-minute tasks you can do while waiting or between other tasks, such as watering your plants, doing the dishes, or checking a homework assignment.

- **Delegate responsibility.** Asking for help when you have too much to do is no cop-out; it's good time management. Just don't delegate to others the jobs you know you should do yourself.

- **Say no when necessary.** If the demands made on you don't seem reasonable, say no—tactfully, but without guilt or apology.

- **Give yourself a break.** Allow time for play—free, unstructured time when you ignore the clock. Don't consider this a waste of time. Play renews you and enables you to work more efficiently.

- **Avoid your personal "time sinks."** You can probably identify your own time sinks, activities like watching television, surfing the Internet, or talking on the phone that consistently use up more time than you anticipate and put you behind schedule. Some days, it may be best to avoid problematic activities altogether; for example, if you have a big paper due, don't sit down for a five-minute TV break if it is likely to turn into a two-hour break. Try a five-minute walk if you need to clear your head.

- **Stop thinking or talking about what you're going to do, and just do it!** Sometimes the best solution for procrastination is to stop waiting for the right moment and just get started. You will probably find that things are not as bad as you feared, and your momentum will keep you going.

For more help with time management, complete Activity 10 in the Behaviour Change Workbook.

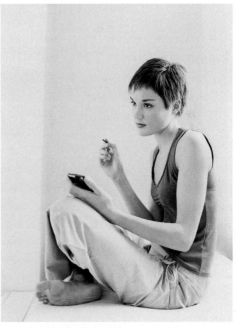

© Digital Vision / Getty RF

Managing the many commitments of adult life—including work, school, and relationships—can sometimes feel overwhelming and produce a great deal of stress. Time-management skills, including careful scheduling with a datebook or handheld computer, can help you cope with busy days.

Cognitive Techniques

Certain thought patterns and ways of thinking, including ideas, beliefs, and perceptions, can contribute to stress and have a negative impact on health. But other habits of mind, if practised with patience and consistency, can help break unhealthy thought patterns. An important skill is to distinguish between types of stressors: "eustress" or "challenge stressors" create positive experiences and opportunities for growth, while "distress" or "hindrance stressors" can impede growth and life satisfaction levels. The following suggestions can help you change destructive thinking:

- **Monitor your self-talk and try to minimize hostile, critical, suspicious, and self-deprecating thoughts.** Substituting positive self-talk for negative self-talk can help you build and maintain self-esteem and cope better with the challenges in your life (see Table 12.2).

- **Modify expectations.** They often restrict experience and lead to disappointment. Try to accept life as it comes.

- **Live in the present.** Clear your mind of old debris and fears so you can enjoy life as it is now.

- **"Go with the flow."** Accept what you can't change, forgive others for their faults, and be flexible.

TABLE 12.2

Avoiding Negative Self-Talk

Cognitive Distortion	Negative Self-Talk	Positive Self-Talk
Focusing on negatives	School is so discouraging—nothing but one hassle after another	School is pretty challenging and has its difficulties, but there certainly are rewards. It's really a mixture of good and bad.
Expecting the worst	Why would my boss want to meet with me this afternoon if not to fire me?	I wonder why my boss wants to meet with me. I guess I'll just have to wait and see.
Overgeneralizing	[*After getting a poor grade on a paper*] Just as I thought—I'm incompetent at everything.	I'll start working on the next paper earlier. That way, if I run into problems I'll have time to talk to the TA.
Minimizing	I won the speech contest, but none of the other speakers was very good. I wouldn't have done as well against stiffer competition.	It may not have been the best speech I'll ever give, but it was good enough to win the contest.
Blaming others	I wouldn't have eaten so much last night if my friends hadn't insisted on going to that restaurant.	I overdid it last night. Next time I'll make different choices.
Expecting perfection	I should have scored 100% on this test. I can't believe I missed that one problem through a careless mistake.	Too bad I missed one problem through carelessness, but overall I did very well on this test. Next time I'll be more careful.

SOURCE: Adapted from Scott, E. August 29, 2017. Reduce stress and improve your life with positive self talk: Develop the positive self talk habit! About. com: Stress Management. (https://www.verywellmind.com/how-to-use-positive-self-talk-for-stress-relief-3144816)

Cultivating your sense of humour is another key cognitive stress management technique. Even a fleeting smile produces changes in your autonomic nervous system that can lift your spirits. Hearty laughter triggers the release of endorphins, and after a good laugh, your muscles go slack and your pulse and blood pressure dip below normal; you are relaxed.

Relaxation Techniques

The **relaxation response** is a physiological state characterized by a feeling of warmth and quiet mental alertness. This response is the opposite of the fight-or-flight reaction. When you induce the relaxation response by using a relaxation technique, your heart rate, breathing, and metabolism slow down. Blood pressure and oxygen consumption decrease. At the same time, blood flow to the brain and skin increases, and brain waves shift from an alert beta rhythm to a relaxed alpha rhythm.

relaxation response A physiological state characterized by a feeling of warmth and quiet mental alertness.

The techniques described in this section are among the most popular techniques and the easiest to learn; also, see the box Relaxation Through Meditation. All these techniques take practice, so it may be several weeks before the benefits become noticeable in everyday life.

DIVERSITY Matters

RELAXATION THROUGH MEDITATION

Techniques for managing stress by inducing the relaxation response have been developed in many cultures over the centuries. Qigong, yoga, tai chi, and meditation can all complement or supplement other stress therapies.

At its most basic level, meditation, or self-reflective thought, involves quieting or emptying the mind to achieve deep relaxation. Some practitioners of meditation view it on a deeper level as a means of focusing concentration, increasing self-awareness, and bringing enlightenment to their lives. Meditation has been integrated into the practices of several religions—Buddhism, Hinduism, Confucianism, Taoism—but it is not a religion itself, nor does its practice require any special knowledge, belief, or background.

There are many styles of meditation, each based on different ways of quieting the mind. Here is a simple, practical technique for eliciting the relaxation response using one style:

1. Pick a word, a phrase, or an object to focus on. You can choose a word or phrase that has a deep meaning for you, but any word or phrase will work. Some meditators prefer to focus on their breathing.
2. Sit comfortably in a quiet place. Close your eyes if you're not focusing on an object.
3. Relax your muscles.
4. Breathe slowly and naturally. If you're using a focus word or phrase, silently repeat it each time you exhale. If you're using an object, focus on it as you breathe.
5. Keep your attitude passive. Disregard thoughts that drift in.
6. Continue for 10 to 20 minutes once or twice a day.
7. After you've finished, sit quietly for a few minutes with your eyes closed, then open. Then stand up.

Allow relaxation to occur at its own pace; don't force it. Don't be surprised if you can't tune your mind out for more than a few seconds at a time. It's nothing to get angry about. The more you ignore the intrusions, the easier it will become. If you want to time your session, peek at a watch or clock occasionally, but don't set a jarring alarm.

Although you'll feel refreshed even after the first session, it may take a month or more to get noticeable results. Be patient. Eventually, the relaxation response will become so natural that it will occur spontaneously or on demand when you sit quietly for a few moments.

Progressive Relaxation

In this simple relaxation technique, you tense then relax the muscles of the body one group at a time. Also known as deep muscle relaxation, this technique addresses the muscle tension that occurs when the body is experiencing stress. Consciously relaxing tensed muscles sends a message to other body systems to reduce the stress response.

To practise progressive relaxation, begin by inhaling as you contract your right fist. Then exhale as you release your fist. Repeat. Contract and relax your right bicep. Repeat. Do the same using your left arm. Then, working from forehead to feet, contract and relax other muscles. Repeat each contraction at least once, inhaling as you tense and exhaling as you relax. To speed up the process, tense and relax more muscles at one time—for example, both arms simultaneously. With practice you'll be able to relax quickly by simply clenching and releasing only your fists.

Visualization

Also known as using imagery, visualization is so effective in enhancing sports performance that it has become part of the curriculum at training camps for Canadian Olympic athletes. This same technique can be used to induce relaxation, to help change habits, or to improve performance on an exam, on stage, or on a playing field.

To practise visualization, imagine yourself floating on a cloud, sitting on a mountaintop, or lying in a meadow. Try to identify all the perceptible qualities of the environment—sight, sound, temperature, smell, and so on. Your body will respond as if your imagery were real.

An alternative is to close your eyes and imagine a deep purple light filling your body. Then change the colour into a soothing gold. As the colour lightens, so should your distress. Imagery can also enhance performance: Visualize yourself succeeding at a task that worries you.

Deep Breathing

Your breathing pattern is closely tied to your stress level. Deep, slow breathing is associated with relaxation. Rapid, shallow, often irregular breathing occurs during the stress response. With practice, you can learn to slow and quiet your breathing pattern, thereby also quieting your mind and relaxing your body. Try one of the breathing techniques described in the box Breathing for Relaxation for on-the-spot tension relief, as well as for long-term stress reduction.

Take CHARGE

BREATHING FOR RELAXATION

Controlled breathing can do more than just help you relax; it can also help control pain, anxiety, and other conditions that lead to or are related to stress. There are many methods of controlled breathing. Two of the most popular are belly breathing and tension-release breathing.

Belly Breathing

1. Lie on your back and relax.
2. Place one hand on your chest and one on your abdomen. Your hands will help you gauge your breathing.
3. Take in a slow, deep breath through your nose and into your belly. Your abdomen should rise significantly (check with your hand); your chest should rise only slightly. Focus on filling your abdomen with air.
4. Exhale through your mouth, gently pushing out the air from your abdomen.

Tension-Release Breathing

1. Lie down or sit in a chair and get comfortable.
2. Take a slow, deep breath into your abdomen. Inhale through your nose. Try to visualize the air moving to every part of your body. As you breathe in, say to yourself, "Breathe in relaxation."
3. Exhale through your mouth. Visualize tension leaving your body. Say to yourself, "Breathe out tension."

These techniques have many variations. For example, sit in a chair and raise your arms, shoulders, and chin as you inhale; lower them as you exhale. Or slowly count to four as you inhale, then again as you exhale.

Many yoga experts suggest breathing rhythmically, in time with your own heartbeat. Relax and listen closely for the sensation of your heart beating, or monitor your pulse while you breathe. As you inhale, count to four or eight in time with your heartbeat, then repeat the count as you exhale. Breathing in time with soothing music can work well, too.

Experts suggest inhaling through the nose and exhaling through the mouth. Breathe slowly, deeply, and gently. To focus on breathing gently, imagine a candle burning several centimetres in front of you. Try to exhale softly enough to make the candle's flame flicker, not hard enough to blow it out.

Practice is important, too. Perform your chosen breathing exercise two or more times daily, for 5 to 10 minutes per session.

Listening to Music

Music can relax you by influencing your pulse, blood pressure, and the electrical activity of your muscles. Listening to soothing, lyrical music can lessen depression, anxiety, and stress levels. To experience the stress-management benefits of music, set aside a period of at least 15 minutes to listen quietly. Choose music you enjoy and selections that make you feel relaxed.

Fitness Tip

Activities like yoga and tai chi are well known for their relaxing, meditative aspects—but they're also great workouts. If you're looking for a way to improve your flexibility and muscle tone while exercising in a quiet, pressure-free environment, check out a local yoga or tai chi class. Be sure the class is led by a qualified professional.

Other Stress-Management Techniques

Techniques such as biofeedback, hypnosis and self-hypnosis, and massage require a partner or professional training or assistance. As with the relaxation techniques presented, all take practice, and it may be several weeks before the benefits are noticeable.

Biofeedback helps people reduce their response to stress by enabling them to become more aware of their level of physiological arousal. In biofeedback, some measure of stress—perspiration, heart rate, skin temperature, or muscle tension—is mechanically monitored, and feedback is given using sound (a tone or music), light, or a meter or dial. With practice, people begin to exercise conscious control over their physiological stress responses. The point of biofeedback training is to develop the ability to transfer the skill to daily life without the use of electronic equipment.

Counterproductive Strategies for Coping with Stress

As we've seen, there are many effective coping techniques for dealing with stress. However, university/college students sometimes develop habits in response to stress that are ineffective and even unhealthy. Here are a few unhealthy coping techniques to avoid:

- **Alcohol**. A few drinks might make you feel at ease, and getting drunk may help you forget the stress in your life—but any relief alcohol provides is temporary. Binge drinking and excessive alcohol consumption are not effective ways to handle stress, and using alcohol to deal with stress puts you at risk for all the short- and long-term problems associated with alcohol abuse.

- **Tobacco**. The nicotine in cigarettes and other tobacco products can make you feel relaxed and may even increase your ability to concentrate. Tobacco, however, is highly addictive, and smoking causes cancer, heart disease, sexual problems, and many other health problems. Tobacco use is the leading preventable cause of death in Canada.

- **Other drugs.** Altering your body chemistry to cope with stress is a strategy with many pitfalls. Caffeine, for example, raises cortisol levels and blood pressure and can disrupt sleep. Repeated use of marijuana can elicit panic attacks.

- **Binge eating.** Eating can induce relaxation, which reduces stress. Eating as a means of coping with stress, however, may lead to weight gain and to binge eating, a risky behaviour associated with eating disorders.

There is one other problem with these methods of fighting stress: None of them addresses the actual cause of the stress in your life. To combat stress in a healthy way, learn some of the stress-management techniques described in this chapter.

LO5 12.5 Getting Help

You can use the principles of behavioural self-management described in Chapter 1 to create a stress-management program tailored specifically to your needs. The starting point of a successful program is to listen to your body. When you learn to recognize the stress response and the emotions and thoughts that accompany it, you'll be in a position to take charge of how you handle stress. Labs 12.1 and 12.2 can guide you in identifying and finding ways to cope with stress-inducing situations.

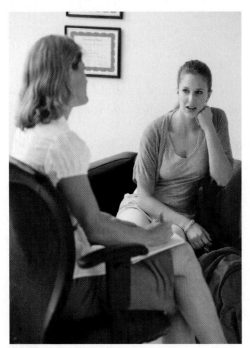

Tetra Images / Getty Images

Many people seek help from professional therapists when dealing with stress-related problems.

If you feel you need guidance beyond the information in this text, excellent self-help guides can be found in bookstores or the library; helpful websites are listed in For Further Exploration; and most university/college campuses have counselling services that assist students in dealing with stresses that may be specific to them.

Peer Counselling and Support Groups

If you still feel overwhelmed despite efforts to manage your stress, you may want to seek outside help. Peer counselling is often available through the student health centre or counselling centre, and is usually staffed by people with special training. This type of support emphasizes maintaining confidentiality. Peer counsellors can steer those seeking help to appropriate campus and community resources or just offer sympathetic listening.

Support groups are typically organized around a particular issue or problem: all group members might be entering a new school, re-entering school after an interruption, struggling with single parenting, experiencing eating disorders, or coping with particular kinds of trauma. Simply voicing concerns that others share can relieve stress.

Professional Help

Psychotherapy, especially a short-term course of sessions, can also be tremendously helpful in dealing with stress-related problems. Not all therapists are right for all people, so it's a good idea to shop around for a compatible psychotherapist with reasonable fees. (See the box Choosing and Evaluating Mental Health Professionals.)

Critical CONSUMER

CHOOSING AND EVALUATING MENTAL HEALTH PROFESSIONALS

University and college students are usually in a good position to find convenient, affordable mental health care. Larger schools typically have both health services that employ psychiatrists and psychologists and counselling centres staffed by professionals and peer counsellors. Resources in the community may include a school of medicine, a hospital, and a variety of professionals who work independently. It's a good idea to get recommendations from physicians, friends who have been in therapy, or community agencies, rather than picking a counsellor or therapist at random.

Financial considerations are also important. Find out the cost of different services and what your health insurance will cover. If you're not adequately covered by your provincial/territorial health plan, don't let that stop you from getting help; investigate low-cost alternatives on campus and in your community. The cost of treatment is linked to how many therapy sessions will be needed, which in turn depends on the type of therapy and the nature of the problem. Psychological therapies focusing on specific problems may require 8 or 10 sessions at weekly intervals. Therapies aiming for psychological awareness and personality change can last months or years.

Deciding whether a therapist is right for you will require meeting the therapist in person. Before or during your first meeting, find out about the therapist's background and training:

- Do they have a degree from an appropriate professional school and a license to practise in your province?
- Have they had experience treating people with problems similar to yours?
- How much will therapy cost? Or is it free?

You have a right to know the answers to these questions and should not hesitate to ask them. After your initial meeting, evaluate your impressions:

- Does the therapist seem like a warm, intelligent person who would be able to help you and is interested in doing so?
- Are you comfortable with the personality, values, and beliefs of the therapist?
- Is the therapist willing to talk about the techniques to be used? Do these techniques make sense to you?

If you answer yes to these questions, this therapist may be satisfactory for you. If you feel uncomfortable—and you're not in need of emergency care—it's worthwhile to set up one-time consultations with one or two others before you make up your mind. Take the time to find someone who feels right for you.

Later in your treatment, evaluate your progress:

- Are you being helped by the treatment?
- If you are displeased, is it because you aren't making progress or because therapy is raising difficult, painful issues you don't want to deal with?
- Can you express dissatisfaction to your therapist? Such feedback can improve your treatment.

If you're convinced your therapy isn't working or is harmful, thank your therapist for their efforts and find another.

Is It Stress or Something More Serious?

Most of us have had periods of feeling down when we become pessimistic, anxious, less energetic, and less able to enjoy life. Such feelings and thoughts can be normal responses to the ordinary challenges of life. Symptoms that may indicate a more serious problem that requires professional help include the following:

- Depression, anxiety, or other emotional problems begin to interfere seriously with school or work performance or in getting along with others.
- Suicide is attempted or is seriously considered.
- Symptoms such as hallucinations, delusions, incoherent speech, or loss of memory occur.
- Alcohol or drugs are used to the extent that they impair normal functioning; finding or taking drugs occupies much of the week; or reducing the dosage leads to psychological or physical withdrawal symptoms.

Depression is of particular concern because severe depression is linked to suicide, the second leading cause of death among Canadians between the ages of 15 to 25.[3] In some cases, depression, like severe stress, is a clear-cut reaction to a specific event, such as the loss of a loved one or failing in school or work. In other cases, no trigger event is obvious.

> depression   A mood disorder characterized by loss of interest, sadness, hopelessness, loss of appetite, disturbed sleep, and other physical symptoms.

Symptoms of depression include the following:

- negative self-concept
- pervasive feelings of sadness and hopelessness
- loss of pleasure in usual activities
- poor appetite and weight loss
- insomnia or disturbed sleep
- restlessness or fatigue
- thoughts of worthlessness and guilt
- trouble concentrating or making decisions
- thoughts of death or suicide

Not all of these symptoms are present in everyone who is depressed, but most do experience a loss of interest or pleasure in their usual activities. Warning signs of suicide include expressing the wish to be dead; revealing contemplated suicide methods; increasing social withdrawal and isolation; and a sudden, inexplicable lightening of mood (which can indicate the person has finally decided to commit suicide).

If you are severely depressed or know someone who is, expert help from a mental health professional is essential. Most communities have emergency help available, often in the form of a hotline telephone counselling service, and many universities and colleges have health services and counselling centres that can provide help. Treatments for depression and many other psychological disorders are highly effective.

The Canadian Association for Suicide Prevention website provides links to local crisis centres across Canada (https://suicideprevention.ca/need-help/). The Kids Help Phone, available at 1-800-668-6868, is a nationally recognized resource in Canada.

Ask Yourself

QUESTIONS FOR CRITICAL THINKING AND REFLECTION

What percentage of your daily stress is time-related? How effective are your time management skills? Identify one thing you can start doing right now to manage your time better, and describe how you can apply it to one aspect of your daily routine.

Tips for Today and the Future

For the stress you can't avoid, develop a range of stress-management techniques and strategies.

RIGHT NOW YOU CAN

- Practise deep breathing for 5 to 10 minutes.
- Visualize a relaxing, peaceful place and imagine yourself experiencing it as vividly as possible. Stay there as long as you can.
- Do some stretching exercises.
- Schedule what you'll be doing the rest of today and tomorrow on your calendar or Smartphone. Include a short walk and a conversation with a friend.

IN THE FUTURE YOU CAN

- Take a class or workshop that can help you overcome a source of stress, such as one in assertiveness training or time management.
- Find a way to build relaxing time into every day. Just 15 minutes of meditation, stretching, or massage can induce the relaxation response.

Common Questions ANSWERED

Q Are there any relaxation techniques I can use in response to an immediate stressor?

A Yes. Try the deep breathing techniques described in the chapter, and try some of the following to see which work best for you:

- **Do a full-body stretch while standing or sitting.** Stretch your arms out to the sides and then reach them as far as possible over your head. Rotate your body from the waist. Bend over as far as is comfortable for you.
- **Do a partial session of progressive muscle relaxation.** Tense and then relax some of the muscles in your body. Focus on the muscles that are stiff or tense. Shake out your arms and legs.
- **Take a short, brisk walk** (three to five minutes). Breathe deeply.
- **Engage in realistic self-talk about the stressor.** Mentally rehearse dealing successfully with the stressor. As an alternative, focus your mind on some other activity.
- **Briefly reflect on something personally meaningful.** In one study of college students, researchers found that self-reflection on important personal values prior to a stressful task reduces the hormonal response to the stressor.

continued

Q   Can stress cause headaches?

A   Stress is one possible cause of the most common type of headache, the tension headache. About 90% of headaches are tension headaches, characterized by a dull, steady pain, usually on both sides of the head. It may feel as though a band of pressure is tightening around the head, and the pain may extend to the neck and shoulders. Acute tension headaches may last from hours to days, while chronic tension headaches may occur almost every day for months or even years. Stress, poor posture, and immobility are leading causes of tension headaches. There is no cure, but the pain can be relieved with over-the-counter painkillers; many people also try such therapies as massage, relaxation, hot or cold showers, and rest. Stress is also one possible trigger of migraine headaches, which are typically characterized by throbbing pain (often on one side of the head), heightened sensitivity to light and noise, and visual disturbances such as flashing lights, nausea, and fatigue.

If your headaches are frequent, keep a journal with details about the events surrounding each one. Are your tension headaches associated with late nights, academic deadlines, or long periods spent sitting at a computer? Are migraines associated with certain foods, stress, fatigue, specific sounds or odours, or (in women) menstruation? If you can identify the stressors or other factors that are consistently associated with your headaches, you can begin to gain more control over the situation. If you suffer persistent tension or migraine headaches, consult your physician.

SUMMARY

- Stress is the collective physiological and emotional response to any stressor. Physiological responses to stressors are the same for everyone.

- The autonomic nervous system and the endocrine system are responsible for the body's physical response to stressors. The sympathetic nervous system mobilizes the body and activates key hormones of the endocrine system, causing the fight-or-flight reaction. The parasympathetic system returns the body to homeostasis.

- Behavioural responses to stress are controlled by the somatic nervous system and fall under a person's conscious control.

- The general adaptation syndrome model and research in psychoneuroimmunology contribute to our understanding of the links between stress and disease. People who have many stressors in their lives or who handle stress poorly are at risk for cardiovascular disease, impairment of the immune system, and many other problems.

- Potential sources of stress include major life changes, daily hassles, school- and job-related stressors, and interpersonal and social stressors.

- Positive ways of managing stress include regular exercise, good nutrition, support from other people, clear communication, spiritual wellness, effective time management, cognitive techniques, and other relaxation techniques.

- If a personal program for stress management doesn't work, peer counselling, support groups, and psychotherapy are available.

FOR FURTHER EXPLORATION

Organizations and Websites

American Psychiatric Association: Healthy Minds, Healthy Lives. Provides information on mental wellness, especially for college and university students.

http://apahealthyminds.blogspot.com/

Canadian Association for Suicide Prevention. Works to reduce suicide and its impact on Canadians.

http://www.suicideprevention.ca/

Canadian Headache Society. Includes information for consumers and clinicians about different types of headaches, their causes, and their treatment.

https://headachesociety.ca/

Canadian Institute of Stress. Offers a number of tools and educational programs for the workplace, home, and others.

http://www.stresscanada.org/

Canadian Mental Health Association. Promotes good mental health for all, including those experiencing mental illness.

http://www.cmha.ca

Canadian Sleep Society. Works to help the public understand sleep and sleep disorders through the support of sleep-related research, education, and advocacy.

https://css-scs.ca/

Harvard Mind-Body Medical Institute. Provides information about stress management and relaxation techniques.

http://www.mbmi.org

The Humor Project. Consists of a clearinghouse for information and practical ideas related to humour.

http://www.humorproject.com

The Financial Consumer Agency of Canada. Provides an interactive calculator designed to help you balance income and expenses.

http://itools-ioutils.fcac-acfc.gc.ca/yft-vof/eng/ieb-4-3.aspx

Laboratory Activities

Name _____ Section _____ Date _____

Lab 12.1 Identifying Your Stress Level and Key Stressors

connect

How Much Stress Do You Suffer From?

To help determine how much stress you experience on a daily basis, answer the following questions. How many of the symptoms of excess stress in the list below do you experience frequently? _____

Physical Symptoms	*Emotional Symptoms*	*Behavioural Symptoms*
Dry mouth	Anxiety or edginess	Crying
Excessive perspiration	Depression	Disrupted eating habits
Frequent illnesses	Fatigue	Disrupted sleeping habits
Gastrointestinal problems	Hypervigilance	Harsh treatment of others
Grinding of teeth	Impulsiveness	Problems communicating
Headaches	Inability to concentrate	Sexual problems
High blood pressure	Irritability	Social isolation
Pounding heart	Trouble remembering things	Increased use of tobacco, alcohol, or other drugs
Stiff neck or aching lower back		

Yes   No

_____ _____ 1. Are you easily startled or irritated?

_____ _____ 2. Are you increasingly forgetful?

_____ _____ 3. Do you have trouble falling or staying asleep?

_____ _____ 4. Do you continually worry about events in your future?

_____ _____ 5. Do you feel as if you are constantly under pressure to produce?

_____ _____ 6. Do you frequently use tobacco, alcohol, or other drugs to help you relax?

_____ _____ 7. Do you often feel as if you have less energy than you need to finish the day?

_____ _____ 8. Do you have recurrent stomachaches or headaches?

_____ _____ 9. Is it difficult for you to find satisfaction in simple life pleasures?

_____ _____ 10. Are you often disappointed in yourself and others?

_____ _____ 11. Are you overly concerned with being liked or accepted by others?

_____ _____ 12. Have you lost interest in intimacy or sex?

_____ _____ 13. Are you concerned that you do not have enough money?

Experiencing some of the stress-related symptoms or answering yes to a few questions is normal. However, if you experience a large number of stress symptoms or you answered yes to a majority of the questions, you are likely experiencing a high level of stress. Take time out to develop effective stress-management techniques. Many coping strategies that can help you deal with your university/college stressors are described in this chapter. Your school's counselling centre can also provide valuable support.

Weekly Stress Log

Now that you are familiar with the signals of stress, complete the weekly stress log to map patterns in your stress levels and identify sources of stress. Enter a score for each hour of each day according to the ratings listed below.

	A.M.							P.M.													Average
	6	7	8	9	10	11	12	1	2	3	4	5	6	7	8	9	10	11	12	Average
Monday																				
Tuesday																				
Wednesday																				
Thursday																				
Friday																				
Saturday																				
Sunday																				
Average																				

Ratings: 1 = No anxiety; general feeling of well-being

2 = Mild anxiety; no interference with activity

3 = Moderate anxiety; specific signal(s) of stress present

4 = High anxiety; interference with activity

5 = Very high anxiety and panic reactions; general inability to engage in activity

To identify daily or weekly patterns in your stress level, average your stress rating for each hour and each day. For example, if your scores for 6:00 a.m. are 3, 3, 4, 3, and 4, with blanks for Saturday and Sunday, your 6:00 a.m. rating would be 17 ÷ 5, or 3.4 (moderate to high anxiety). Finally, calculate an average weekly stress score by averaging your daily average stress scores. Your weekly average will give you a sense of your overall level of stress.

Using Your Results

How did you score? How high are your daily and weekly stress scores? Are you at all surprised by your score for average stress level?

_____

_____

_____

Are you satisfied with your stress rating? If not, set a specific goal:

_____

_____

_____

What should you do next? Enter the results of this lab in the Preprogram Assessment column in Appendix B. If you've set a goal for improvement, begin by using your log to look for patterns and significant time periods in order to identify key stressors in your life. Below, list any stressors that caused you a significant amount of discomfort this week; these can be people, places, events, or recurring thoughts or worries. For each, enter one strategy that would help you deal more successfully with the stressor; examples of strategies might include practising an oral presentation in front of a friend or engaging in positive self-talk.

_____

_____

_____

Next, begin to put your strategies into action. In addition, complete Lab 12.2 to help you incorporate lifestyle stress-management techniques into your daily routine.

Name _____ Section _____ Date _____

Lab 12.2 Stress Management Techniques

Mc Graw Hill Education **connect®**

Part I Lifestyle Stress Management

For each of the areas listed in the table below, describe your current lifestyle as it relates to stress management. For example, do you have enough social support? How are your exercise and nutrition habits? Is time management a problem for you? For each area, list two ways that you could change your current habits to help you manage your stress. Sample strategies might include calling a friend before a challenging class, taking a short walk before lunch, and buying and using a datebook to track your time.

	Current lifestyle	Lifestyle change #1	Lifestyle change #2
Social support system			
Exercise habits			
Nutrition habits			
Time management techniques			
Self-talk patterns			
Sleep habits			

Part II Relaxation Techniques

Try two relaxation techniques described in this chapter (progressive relaxation, visualization, deep breathing, meditation, yoga, tai chi, massage, listening to music). If a taped recording is available for progressive relaxation or visualization, these techniques can be performed by your entire class as a group.

List the techniques you tried.

1. _____

2. _____

How did you feel before you tried these techniques?

_____

_____

_____

What did you think or how did you feel during each of the techniques you tried?

1. _____

_____

_____

2. _____

_____

How did you feel after you tried these techniques?

_____

_____

_____

Name _____ **Section** _____ **Date** _____

Lab 12.3 Developing Spiritual Wellness

connect

To develop spiritual wellness, it is important to take time out to think about what gives meaning and purpose to your life and what actions you can take to support the spiritual dimension of your life.

Look Inward

This week, spend some quiet time alone with your thoughts and feelings. Slow the pace of your day, remove your watch, turn your phone off, and focus on your immediate experience. Try one of the following activities or develop another that is meaningful to you and that contributes to your sense of spiritual well-being.

- **Spend time in nature**. Experience continuity with the natural world by spending solitary time in a natural setting. Watch the sky (day or night), a sunrise, or a sunset; listen to waves on a shore or wind in the trees; feel the breeze on your face or raindrops on your skin; smell the grass, brush, trees, or flowers. Open all your senses to the beauty of nature.

- **Experience art, architecture, or music**. Spend time with a work of art or architecture or a piece of music. Choose one that will awaken your senses, engage your emotions, and challenge your understanding. Take a break and then repeat the experience to see how your responses change the second time.

- **Express your creativity**. Set aside time for a favourite activity, one that allows you to express your creative side. Sing, draw, paint, play a musical instrument, sculpt, build, dance, cook, garden—choose an activity in which you will be so engaged that you will lose track of time. Strive for feelings of joy and exhilaration.

- **Engage in a personal spiritual practice**. Pray, meditate, do yoga, or chant. Choose a spiritual practice that is familiar to you or try one that is new. Tune out the outside world and turn your attention inward, focusing on the experience.

Describe the personal spiritual activity you tried and how it made you feel—both during the activity and after.

_____

_____

_____

Reach Out

Spiritual wellness can be a bond among people and can promote values such as altruism, forgiveness, and compassion. Try one of the following spiritual activities that involve reaching out to others.

- **Share writings that inspire you**. Find two writings that inspire, guide, and comfort you, such as passages from sacred works, poems, quotations from literature, or songs. Share them with someone else by reading them aloud and explaining what they mean to you.

- **Practise kindness.** Spend a day practising small acts of personal kindness for people you know as well as for strangers. For example, compliment a friend, send a card, let someone go ahead of you in line, pick up litter, do someone else's chores, help someone with packages, say please and thank you, smile.

- **Perform community service**. Foster a sense of community by becoming a volunteer. Find a local nonprofit group and offer your time and talent. Mentor a youth, work at a food bank, support a literacy project, help build low-cost housing, or visit seniors in a nursing home. You can also work on national or international issues by writing letters to your elected representatives and other officials.

Describe the spiritual activity you performed and how it made you feel—during the activity and after. Include details about the writings you chose or the acts of kindness or community service you performed.

_____

_____

_____

Keep a Journal

One strategy for continuing on the path toward spiritual wellness is to keep a journal. Use a journal to record your thoughts, feelings, and experiences; to jot down quotes that engage you; or to sketch pictures and write poetry about what is meaningful to you. Begin your spiritual journal today.

Name _____ Section _____ Date _____

Lab 12.4 Time Management Skills

connect

One method of reducing stress may be to examine the ways that you spend your time. Effectively spending time means that you are able to prioritize your daily activities and accomplish those things that are most important to you. Meeting deadlines, due dates, and preparing for classes and exams are all things that many students consider important.

Log Your Time

- Log your daily activities for a span of three days.
- For each day, use a table similar to the one below to record your activities and the total time you spend on each activity (in half-hour units), and to indicate the priority level of each.
- Your priority levels are:
  - A—activities that MUST GET DONE that day
  - B—activities you would like to get done, but if you cannot complete them that day, they can wait until the next day
  - C—activities that NEVER should have been done on that day

Activity	Time Spent (in ½ hour blocks)	Priority level

Total the time you spent on each of A, B, and C activities for all three days and record below. Note that the total of all three days should add up to 72 hours.

"A" Activities = _____ hours

"B" Activities = _____ hours

"C" Activities = _____ hours

Next, begin to put your priorities and strategies into action. Complete Lab 12.2 to help you incorporate lifestyle stress-management techniques into your daily routine.

CHAPTER 13

Wellness for Life

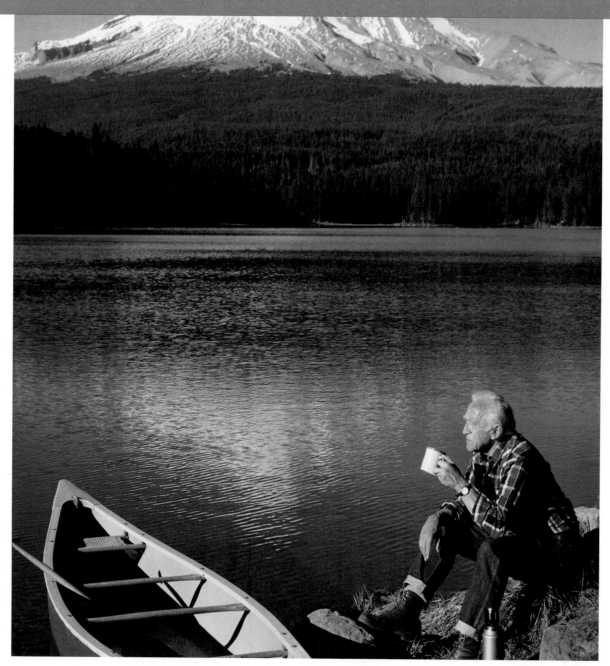

© Royalty-free / CORBIS

LEARNING OBJECTIVES

After reading this chapter, you should be able to

LO1 Explain what individuals can do to promote healthy aging

LO2 Discuss strategies for effective self-care and effective use of the health care system

LO3 Describe the role that the environment plays in personal wellness and the steps individuals can take to preserve and restore the environment

TEST YOUR KNOWLEDGE

1. **By the year 2031, Canada's population will include what percentage of adults over the age of 65?**
   a. 15%
   b. 25%
   c. 35%

2. **Most of the energy used by a standard incandescent light bulb is converted into light.**

   True or false?

3. **At what annual rate is the world's population increasing?**
   a. 0.76 million
   b. 7.6 million
   c. 76 million

ANSWERS

1. **B.** By the year 2031, it is estimated that Canada's population will include 9 million people over age 65, which is about 25% of the population. Healthy aging can potentially delay and/or minimize the effects of chronic disease and disability later in life. This has massive financial and social benefits to society.

2. **FALSE.** About 90% of the energy used by a standard bulb is wasted because it is given off as heat, not light. If each Canadian replaced one incandescent bulb with a compact fluorescent bulb, the yearly energy savings would equal the total production of four nuclear power plants. Fluorescent lights, however, contain higher levels of mercury, which can pose problems for landfills when these bulbs are thrown away.

3. **C.** The world's population currently stands at about 7.1 billion and is growing at a rate of about 76 million people per year—about 150 people per minute. The United Nations projects that the planet's population will reach 10 billion by the year 2200.

The goal of this book has been to introduce the concept of wellness and to provide the knowledge and skills you need to live a fit and well lifestyle. Knowing the facts about the effects of your actions on your health enables you to make informed choices. Using behavioural self-management allows you to make important lifestyle changes. This chapter briefly addresses some other skills that are important for a lifetime of wellness: meeting the challenges of aging, using the health care system intelligently, and understanding environmental health.

LO1 13.1 Meeting the Challenges of Aging

Aging is a normal process of development that occurs over the entire life span. Although youth is not entirely a state of mind, your attitude toward life and your attention to your health significantly influence the satisfaction you derive from life, especially when new physical and mental challenges occur in later years. If you take charge of your health during young adulthood, you can exert greater control over the physical and mental aspects of aging, and you can respond better to events that might be out of your control. With foresight and energy, you can shape a creative, graceful, and even triumphant old age.

Wellness Tip

Remember that modest changes in lifestyle maintained over the long term are more beneficial than dramatic changes that last only a few weeks. Long-term maintenance of behaviour change is challenging.

What Happens as You Age?

Aging results from biochemical processes that aren't yet fully understood. Physiological changes are caused by a combination of gradual aging and injury from disease. Because most organ systems have an excess capacity for performing their functions, the body's ability to function is not affected until damage is fairly extensive. Studies of healthy people indicate that general functioning remains essentially constant until after age 70. Even so, a fair number of older Canadians describe themselves as being in poor health (see Table 13.1).

TABLE 13.1

Canadian Self-Rated Health, by Age, 2012

Age	Excellent or Very Good Health	Fair or Poor Health
12–19 years	69.6%	4.2%
20–34 years	68.4%	5.8%
35–44 years	64.8%	7.6%
45–64 years	56.1%	12.7%
65+ years	44.2%	22.2%

SOURCE: Statistics Canada. Health indicator profile, annual estimates, by age group and sex, Canada, provinces, territories, health regions (2012 boundaries) and peer groups, occasional. Table 13100451; Formerly CANSIM Table 105-0501. Contains information licensed under the Open Government Licence – Canada.

The physical changes that accompany aging include the following:

- Skin becomes looser, drier, and less elastic.

- The ability to hear high-pitched and certain other sounds declines in most people.

- *Presbyopia*, the inability of the eyes to focus sharply on nearby objects, occurs gradually in most people beginning in their 40s. The eyes require more time to adapt to dark conditions, and depth perception may become distorted.

- The sensations of taste and smell diminish somewhat.

- Cells at the base of hair follicles produce progressively less pigment and eventually die. (Hair is thickest at age 20; individual hair shafts shrink after that.)

- Bone mass is lost and muscles become weaker, although both of these changes can be minimized significantly through regular exercise, a proper diet, and other measures.

- The heart pumps less blood with each beat, and maximum heart rate drops. Most of the other changes in the cardiovascular system that are associated with aging can be largely controlled through lifestyle.

- Sexual response slows, but an active and satisfying sex life can continue for both men and women throughout life.

The cumulative effects of these physical changes result in an increase in susceptibility to chronic health conditions such as those described in Chapter 10 and Chapter 11. In addition, the more we age, the more likely we are to suffer from more than just one chronic health condition (see Figure 13.1).

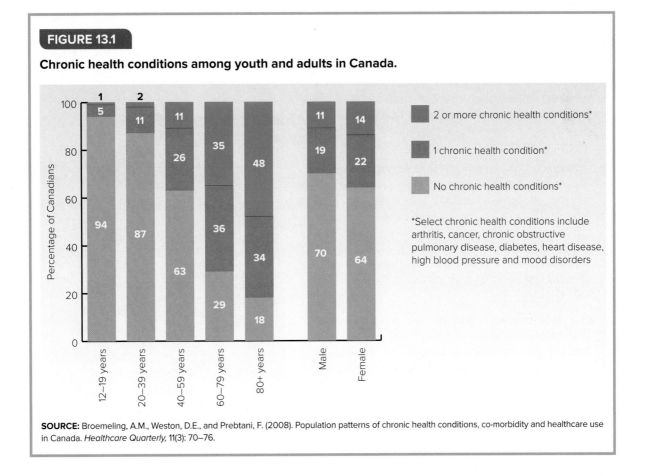

FIGURE 13.1

Chronic health conditions among youth and adults in Canada.

Legend:
- 2 or more chronic health conditions*
- 1 chronic health condition*
- No chronic health conditions*

*Select chronic health conditions include arthritis, cancer, chronic obstructive pulmonary disease, diabetes, heart disease, high blood pressure and mood disorders

SOURCE: Broemeling, A.M., Weston, D.E., and Prebtani, F. (2008). Population patterns of chronic health conditions, co-morbidity and healthcare use in Canada. *Healthcare Quarterly,* 11(3): 70–76.

Life-Enhancing Measures

Many of the characteristics associated with aging aren't due to aging at all, but instead are the result of neglect and abuse of our bodies and minds. These assaults lay the foundation for later mental health problems and chronic conditions. You can prevent, delay, lessen, or even reverse some of the changes associated with aging through good health habits. A few simple things you can do every day will make a vast difference to your health, your appearance, and your energy and vitality. For example:

- **Challenge your mind.** Creativity and intelligence remain stable in healthy individuals. Staying involved in learning as a lifelong process can help you stay sharp and retain all your mental abilities.
- **Plan for social changes.** Social roles change over time and require a period of adjustment. Retirement and an "empty nest" confer the advantage of increased leisure time, but many people do not know how to enjoy it. Throughout life, cultivate interests and hobbies you enjoy, both alone and with others, so you can continue to live an active and rewarding life in your later years. Volunteering in your community can enhance self-esteem and allow you to be a contributing member of society (see the box Help Yourself by Helping Others).

Take CHARGE

HELP YOURSELF BY HELPING OTHERS

Volunteering can enhance emotional, social, spiritual, and physical wellness. Surveys and studies indicate that the sense of purpose, service, and the feelings of generosity and kindness that go with helping others may be as important a consideration for wellness as good nutrition and regular exercise.

A 2006 study followed sedentary older people who joined a volunteer group called Experience Corps. The subjects' volunteer activities resulted in many of the same benefits as regular exercise, such as increased energy and vitality. Older adults who volunteer have higher levels of emotional and social wellness and lower rates of death.[*] In a national survey of volunteers from all fields, helpers reported the following benefits:

- "helper's high," or physical and emotional sensations such as sudden warmth, a surge of energy, and a feeling of euphoria that occur immediately after helping
- feelings of increased self-worth, calm, and relaxation
- a perception of greater physical health
- fewer colds and headaches, improved eating and sleeping habits, and some relief from the pain of chronic diseases such as asthma and arthritis

In helping others, you focus on things other than your own problems, and you get a special kind of attention from the people you help. Helping others can also expand your perspective and enhance your appreciation for your own life. Helping improves mood, banishes the blues, and may benefit physical health by providing a temporary boost to the immune system and by combating stress and hostile feelings linked to the development of chronic disease.

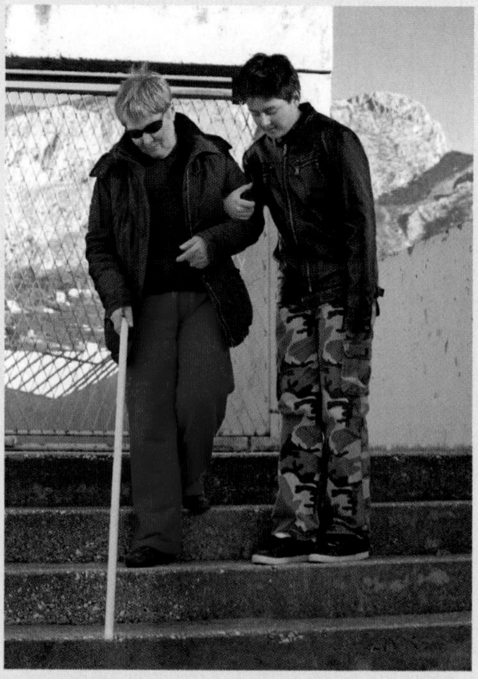

© Landd09 / Dreamstime.com / GetStock.com

No matter what your age, to get the most out of helping, keep the following guidelines in mind:

- Remember that helping others doesn't require a huge time commitment or a change of career.
- Choose an activity that involves personal contact. Work with a group to form bonds with other helpers who support your interests and efforts.
- Focus on the process, not the outcome. You can't always measure or know the results of your actions.
- Practise random acts of kindness. Smile, let people go ahead of you in line, pick up litter, and so on.
- Adopt a pet. Several studies suggest that pet owners enjoy better health, perhaps by feeling needed or by having a source of unconditional love.
- Avoid burnout. Recognize your own limits, pace yourself, and try not to feel guilty or discouraged.

In addition to benefiting you, volunteering has the added bonus of increasing the well-being of others. It fosters a sense of community and can provide some practical help for many of the problems facing our society today.

SOURCES: Adapted from Musick, M.A., A.R. Herzog, and J.S. House. 1999. Volunteering and mortality among older adults. *Journal of Gerontology: Social Sciences* 54B(3): 5173; Sobel, D.S., and R. Ornstein. 1996. *The Healthy Mind, Healthy Body Handbook.* Los Altos, CA: DRx Publishers; Morrow-Howell, N., McCrary, S., Hong, S-I., & Blinne, W. (2008). *Experience Corps: Benefits of Volunteering* (CSD Research Brief 08-23). St. Louis, MO: Washington University, Center for Social Development.

- **Develop physical fitness.** Exercise enhances both psychological and physical health. A 2010 study showed that elderly people who met the PHAC daily activity guidelines had a much lower mortality rate and longer healthy years than their peers who did not exercise. Even in people over age 80, endurance and strength training can improve balance, flexibility, and physical functioning and reduce the potential for dangerous falls (see the box Can Exercise Delay the Effects of Aging?).

The Evidence *for* EXERCISE

CAN EXERCISE DELAY THE EFFECTS OF AGING?

As people age, they often experience declines in functional health—the ability to perform the tasks of everyday life—and related declines in the quality of life. According to the Human Resources and Skills Development Canada, about 22% of Canadians over age 55 report their health as only "fair" or "poor." Similarly, according to a US Medicare survey, 31% of men and 42% of women ages 65 to 74 reported some sort of mobility limitation in 2003 (meaning they had difficulty walking one-quarter mile or 0.4 kilometre).

Can physical activity and exercise combat the degenerative effects of aging in middle-aged and older adults? The evidence indicates that they can. In reviewing the research, the US government's Physical Activity Guidelines Advisory Committee concluded that physical activity can prevent or delay the onset of limitations and declines in functional health in older adults, can maintain or improve functional health in those who already have limitations, and can reduce the incidence of falls and fall-related injuries.

One mechanism by which physical activity prevents declines in functional health is through maintenance or improvement of the physiological capacities of the body, such as aerobic power, muscular strength, and balance—in other words, through improvements in physical fitness. Declines in these physiological capacities occur with biological aging and are often compounded by disease-related disability. But evidence shows that older adults who participate in regular aerobic exercise are 30% less likely than inactive individuals to develop functional limitations (such as a limited ability to walk or climb stairs) or role limitations (such as a limited ability to be the family grocery shopper). Although studies found that both physical activity and aerobic fitness were associated with reduced risk of functional limitations, aerobic fitness was associated with a greater reduction of risk. Evidence also suggests that regular physical activity is safe and beneficial for older adults who already have functional limitations.

continued

An example is a 2006 study called the Lifestyle Interventions and Independence for Elders Pilot Trial, involving 424 men and women between the ages of 70 and 89. Participants were divided into a multimodal exercise group and a health education (control) group. Those in the exercise group participated in aerobic activity (primarily walking), strength training (focusing on the lower limbs), and flexibility exercises over the course of a year. The study found that the individuals in the exercise group significantly improved their physical performance and their walking speed compared with the control group. Also observed in the exercise group was an apparent trend toward reduced risk of major mobility disability. Another study, the 2005 Women's Health and Aging Study, found that older women who walked at least eight blocks per week had better health and functioning after one year than did nonwalkers.

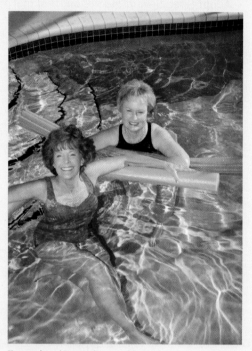

Katseyephoto / Dreamstime.com / GetStock.com

In addition, numerous studies have shown that regular exercise—particularly strength training, balance training, and flexibility exercises—can improve muscular strength, muscular endurance, and stability and provide some protection against falls. Falls are a leading cause of injury among people over age 65, affecting nearly 1.4 million older Canadians per year. In many cases, serious falls lead to long-term hospitalization or nursing home stays. Whether through direct injury or related complications, falls are a significant cause of death for older Canadians. Aerobic activity, especially walking, also helps reduce risk of falls, and some evidence indicates that tai chi exercise programs are beneficial as well. Regular exercise not only reduces the incidence of falls, but also greatly enhances mobility, allowing older people to live more independently and with greater confidence.

Of course, physical activity throughout life helps prevent such chronic conditions as cardiovascular disease, stroke, diabetes, and arthritis, all of which cause disability in older adults. Research also shows that regular physical activity can reduce anxiety and depression in older adults. Exercise stimulates blood flow to the brain and can even increase brain mass, helping the brain to function more efficiently and improving memory. Some evidence indicates that exercise may stave off mental decline and the occurrence of age-related dementia.

Current physical activity recommendations for older adults from the Public Health Agency of Canada include moderate- to vigorous-intensity aerobic activity, strength training, and flexibility exercises, as well as balance exercises for older adults at risk for falls. Unfortunately, a large percent of Canadians age 65 and older (63% of women and 51% of men) do not get the recommended amounts of physical activity, and many get no exercise at all beyond the activities of daily living. Older adults are the least active group of Canadians. Although it is important to exercise throughout life, the evidence indicates that older adults who become more active even late in life can experience improvements in physical fitness and functional health. It is never too late to start enjoying the benefits of regular physical activity.

SOURCES: Human Resources and Skills Development Canada. 2012 (http://www4.hrsdc.gc.ca/.3ndic.1t.4r@-eng.jsp?iid=10, retrieved January 30, 2012); Pahor, M., et al. 2006. Effects of a physical activity intervention on measures of physical performance: Results of the Lifestyle Interventions and Independence for Elders Pilot (LIFE-P) study. *Journal of Gerontology Biological Sciences and Medical Sciences* 61(11): 1157–1165; Paterson, D.H., et al. 2007. Aging and physical activity: Evidence to develop exercise recommendations for older adults. *Canadian Journal of Public Health* 98 (Suppl. 2): S69–S108; Physical Activity Guidelines Advisory Committee. 2008. *Physical Activity Guidelines Advisory Committee Report,* 2008. Washington, DC: Physical Activity Monitors, 2008. Available at http://www.cflri.ca/node/82, retrieved January 30, 2012, U.S. Department of Health and Human Services; Simonsick, E.M., et al. 2005. Just get out the door! Importance of walking outside the home for maintaining mobility: Findings from the Women's Health and Aging Study. *Journal of the American Geriatrics Society* 53(2): 198–203; U.S. Department of Health and Human Services, Centers for Medicare & Medicaid Services. 2006. *Medicare Current Beneficiary Survey* (http://www.cms.hhs.gov/MCBS, retrieved January 30, 2012).

- **Eat wisely.** A varied diet with special attention to calorie intake and nutrient density improves health at every age. (See Chapter 7 for detailed information on nutrition.)

- **Maintain a healthy body composition.** Sensible eating habits and an active lifestyle can help you maintain a healthy body composition throughout your life.

- **Control drinking and overdependence on medications.** Alcohol abuse ranks with depression as a common hidden mental health problem, affecting 10% of older adults. The problem is often not identified because the effects of alcohol or drug addiction can mimic disease, such as Alzheimer's disease. Don't use alcohol to relieve anxiety or emotional pain; don't take medications when safer forms of treatment are available.

- **Don't smoke.** The average pack-a-day smoker can expect to live about 12 years less than a nonsmoker and to be susceptible to disabilities that affect the quality of life. Premature balding, skin wrinkling, and osteoporosis are also associated with smoking.

- **Recognize and reduce stress.** Don't wear yourself out through lack of sleep, abuse of drugs, or overwork. Practise relaxation and stress management using the techniques described in Chapter 12.

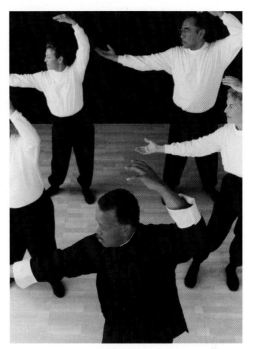

© Ryan McVay / Getty Images / PhotoDisc

Managing stress is one of the challenges of aging. These people practise stress management and relaxation through taijiquan, an activity that also helps them maintain physical fitness.

Other strategies for successful aging include getting regular physical examinations to detect treatable diseases, protecting your skin and eyes from the sun, and avoiding extremely loud noises to protect your hearing.

Strengthening Mental Wellness

How do you envision your old age? Do you want it to resemble the old age of older adults you know now, or do you want it to be different? What specific attributes and abilities will make your old age happy and productive? What are you doing now to ensure that you will be able to reach your goals?

LO2 13.2 Using the Health Care System Intelligently

Just as people can prevent many illnesses through healthy lifestyle choices, they can also avoid many visits to the medical clinic by managing their own health care—by gathering information, soliciting advice, making their own decisions, and taking responsibility for following through. People who manage their own health care are informed partners in medical care; they also practise safe, effective self-care.

How can you develop this self-care attitude and take a more active role in your own health care? First, you have to learn to identify and manage medical problems. Second, you have to learn how to make the health care system work for you. This section will help you become more competent in both of these areas.

Managing Medical Problems

The first step in managing medical problems is observing your body and assessing your symptoms. Symptoms—pain, fever, coughing, diarrhea, and so on—are signals that something isn't working right. Many self-tests are available to help you evaluate medical problems at home, such as blood pressure monitoring equipment, blood sugar tests for those with diabetes, pregnancy tests, self-tests for urinary tract infections, and more than a dozen other do-it-yourself kits and devices. Careful self-observation and the selective use of self-tests can help provide you with the type of information you need to make informed self-care decisions and participate more actively in your care.

Knowing When to See a Physician

In most cases, and with sufficient time and rest, the body heals itself. The decision to seek professional assistance for a symptom is generally guided by the nature of the symptom and by your own history of medical problems. If you're unsure about a symptom, call your physician.

Seek professional assistance for any symptom that is severe, unusual, persistent, or recurrent. Medical emergencies requiring a trip to the nearest hospital emergency room include broken bones, severe burns, deep wounds, uncontrollable bleeding, chest pain, loss of consciousness, poisoning or drug overdose, and difficulty breathing.

Self-Treatment

In most cases, your body can itself relieve your symptoms and heal a disorder. The prescriptions filled by your body's internal pharmacy are frequently the safest and most effective treatment. Patience and careful self-observation (watchful waiting) are often the best choices in self-treatment.

Nondrug options are often highly effective. For example, massage, ice packs, and neck exercises may be at times more helpful than drugs in relieving headaches and other pains. Adequate rest is just one of the many nondrug options for preventing or relieving many common health problems. For a variety of disorders either caused or aggravated by stress, the treatment of choice may be relaxation, visualization, humour, changing negative thoughts, and other stress-management strategies (see Chapter 12). Before reaching for medications, consider all of your nondrug options.

Nonprescription, or **over-the-counter (OTC) medications** play an important role in the health care system. Many OTC drugs are highly effective in relieving symptoms and sometimes curing illnesses. Common OTC drugs include antihistamines, expectorants, cough suppressants, pain relievers, and other products.

over-the-counter (OTC) medications Medications or medical products that a consumer can purchase without a prescription.

Any drug can have side effects. These simple guidelines will help you use medicines safely and effectively.

- Always read drug labels and follow directions.
- Do not exceed the recommended dosage or length of treatment unless your physician approves.
- Because OTC drugs, prescription drugs, and herbal remedies can interact, let your physician or pharmacist know before taking more than one type of drug or health remedy at the same time.
- Select medications with one active ingredient rather than combination products. Using single-ingredient products allows you to adjust the dosage of each medication separately for optimal symptom relief; you'll also avoid potential side effects from drugs you don't really need.

- Never take or give a drug from an unlabelled container or in the dark when you can't read the label.

- If you are pregnant, are nursing, or have a chronic medical condition, consult your physician before self-medicating.

- Store medications in a safe place out of the reach of children. Avoid locations where dampness or heat might ruin them. Dispose of all expired medications.

- Use special caution with aspirin. Because of an association with a rare but serious problem known as Reye's syndrome, aspirin should not be used for children or adolescents who may have the flu, chicken pox, or any other viral illness.

Getting the Most out of Medical Care

Although many health problems can be self-treated, many others require treatment by trained professionals. The key to using the health care system effectively is good communication with your physician and other members of the health care team.

The Canadian Health Care System

Canada has a government-funded, national health care system based on principles from the *Canada Health Act* that reinforce a health care system that is:

- universally available to permanent residents
- comprehensive in the services it covers
- accessible without income barriers
- portable within and outside the country
- publicly administered

Each province and territory is responsible for administering its own health care plan and for providing medically necessary services such as prescription drugs, dental care, and optometric services, to name a few. In an effort to provide efficient services, some provinces/territories have chosen to introduce their own supplemental plans (i.e., drug plan), while others have chosen to partner with private insurers such as Blue Cross.

The cost of health care in Canada is supplemented by federal and provincial/territorial taxes that all residents are required to pay. In addition, some provinces/territories, like Ontario, collect a health care premium from each of its residents. Recently, some provinces/territories have introduced P3s, or "private-public-partnerships," which represent a way for private companies to use public funds in serving patients who may be willing to pay for services. P3s have proven to be controversial and it remains to be seen whether a "tiered" system of health care will be created by these initiatives.

Communicating with Your Physician

When interacting with health care providers, you should be assertive in a firm but not aggressive manner. Feel free to ask questions, express your concerns, and be persistent. Strategies for good communication include the following:

- **Before the visit.** Make a written list of your questions and concerns and include notes about your symptoms. Bring a list of all medications (prescription and nonprescription) you are taking, or bring them with you to the office.

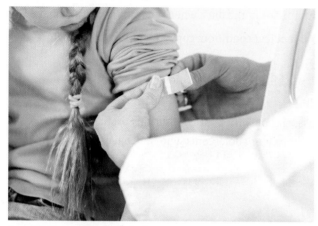

Arne9001 / Dreamstime.com / GetStock.com

Your health care provider is the best source of reliable information about any prescription or OTC medication you may need to take.

- **During the visit.** Present your major concerns at the beginning of the visit. Be specific and concise. Try to be as open and honest as you can in sharing your thoughts, feelings, and fears. It is particularly important to be truthful about your concerns so you receive the best possible advice from your physician. If you're not sure about something your physician has said, ask to go over it again. If appropriate, ask your physician to write down their instructions or to recommend reading material.

- **At the end of the visit.** In your own words, briefly state what you understood the physician to say about your problem and what you're supposed to do. Make sure you understand what the next steps are.

Obtaining Appropriate Screening Tests

Another important part of preventive health care is regular screening for various conditions and diseases. Be sure to follow the cholesterol and blood pressure testing recommendations provided in Chapter 10, the cancer screening guidelines given in Chapter 11, and the sexually transmitted infection (STI) screening and testing recommendations given in Chapter 15 (online). If you have symptoms, or if you are at risk for a particular disease, see your physician to discuss your needs.

Using Complementary and Alternative Medicine

Complementary and alternative medicine (CAM) is defined as those therapies or practices that do not form part of conventional, or mainstream, health care and medical practice as taught in most medical schools and offered in most hospitals. The inclusion of the term *complementary* indicates that most people use such approaches in addition to conventional medical treatments rather than in their place. Consumer surveys show that more and more people are using various forms of CAM. In Canada, the Fraser Institute reported that 73% of Canadians claim to have used at least one CAM in their lives. The most common forms of CAM used by Canadians are chiropractic (36%), relaxation techniques and massage (23% each), and prayer (21%). Despite their growing popularity, many CAM practices remain controversial, and you need to be critically aware of safety issues (see the box Avoiding Health Care Fraud and Quackery).

complementary and alternative medicine (CAM)   Therapies or practices that are not part of conventional or mainstream health care and medical practice as taught in most North American medical schools and available at most North American health care facilities.

Because there is less information available about CAM therapies, as well as less regulation of associated products and providers, it is important for consumers to take an active role. The National Centre for Complementary and Alternative Medicine (NCCAM), which is a part of the National Institutes of Health, advises consumers not to seek CAM therapies without first visiting a conventional health care provider for an evaluation and diagnosis of their symptoms. It's usually best to try conventional treatments that have been shown to be beneficial for your condition.

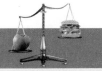

Critical CONSUMER

AVOIDING HEALTH CARE FRAUD AND QUACKERY

Consumers waste billions of dollars on unproven, fraudulently marketed, and sometimes useless or even harmful health care products and treatments. In addition, those with serious medical problems may waste valuable time before seeking proper treatment. Health care fraud is a business that sells false hope. It preys on people who are victims of diseases that have no medical cure and on people who want shortcuts to weight loss or improvements to personal appearance.

The first rule of thumb for evaluating any health claim is that if it sounds too good to be true, it probably is. Also, be on the lookout for the typical phrases and marketing techniques fraudulent promoters use to deceive consumers, such as the following:

- The product is advertised as a quick and effective cure-all for a wide range of ailments.
- The promoters use words like *scientific breakthrough, miraculous cure, secret ingredient*, or *ancient remedy*. Also remember that just because a product is described as "natural" or unprocessed does not necessarily mean it's safe.
- The promoter claims the government or the medical profession has conspired to suppress the product.
- The advertisement includes undocumented case histories claiming amazing results.
- The product is advertised as available from only one source, and payment is required in advance.
- The promoter promises a no-risk "money-back guarantee." Be aware that many fly-by-night operators are not around to respond to your request for a refund.

To check out a particular product, talk to a physician or another health care professional and to family members and friends. Be wary of treatments offered by people who tell you to avoid talking to others. Check with the Better Business Bureau to see whether other consumers have lodged complaints about the product or the product's marketer. You can also check with the appropriate health professional group. For example, check with the Canadian Diabetes Association or the National Arthritis Foundation if the products are promoted for diabetes or arthritis. Take special care with products and devices sold online; the broad reach of the Internet, combined with the ease of setting up and removing websites, makes online sellers particularly difficult to regulate.

SOURCES: Federal Trade Commission. 2001. "Miracle" Health Claims: Add a Dose of Skepticism (http://www.ftc.gov/bcp/conline/pubs /health/frdheal.htm, retrieved December 14, 2002); Kurtzweil, P. 1999. How to spot health fraud. *FDA Consumer,* November/December.

If you are thinking of trying any alternative therapies, it is critically important to talk with your physician or pharmacist to avoid any dangerous interactions. For example, some dietary supplements block or enhance the actions of prescription and over-the-counter drugs. Areas to discuss with your physician include the following:

- **Safety.** Is there anything unsafe about the treatment in general or for you specifically? Are there safety issues you should be aware of?

- **Effectiveness.** Is there any research about the use of the therapy for your condition?

- **Timing.** Is the immediate use of a conventional treatment indicated?

- **Cost.** Is the therapy likely to be very expensive, especially in light of the potential benefit?

You can also get information from individual CAM practitioners and from schools, professional organizations, and provincial licensing boards. Ask about education, training, licensing, and certification. When talking with a CAM practitioner, ask for a full description of the therapy and any potential side effects, how long the therapy should continue before it can be determined if it is beneficial, and how much it will cost. Tell the practitioner about any conventional treatments you are receiving. If anything a CAM practitioner recommends directly conflicts with advice from your physician, discuss it with your physician before making any major changes in any current treatment regimen or in your lifestyle.

You can investigate CAM therapies on your own by going to the library or doing research online, although caution is in order when using websites for the various forms of CAM. A good place to start are the websites of government agencies like Health Canada and of universities and hospitals that conduct government-sponsored research on CAM approaches.

Ask Yourself

QUESTIONS FOR CRITICAL THINKING AND REFLECTION

Drug manufacturers use television and magazine advertising to sell their products directly to consumers, telling them, "Ask your doctor about . . ." Has such an ad ever led you to believe you had a condition you didn't know you had or informed you about a treatment you didn't know existed? What do you think are the advantages and disadvantages of direct-to-consumer advertising?

LO3 13.3 Environmental Health

Because of the close relationship between human beings and the environment, even the healthiest lifestyle can't protect a person from the effects of polluted air, contaminated water, or a nuclear power plant mishap. Environmental health encompasses all the interactions between humans and the environment and the health consequences of these interactions.

Environmental health still focuses on such longstanding concerns as clean air and water, food inspection, and waste disposal, but in recent years its focus has expanded and become more complex. Many of the health challenges of the twenty-first century will involve protecting the environment from the by-products of human activity. Technological advances and rapid population growth have increased the ability of humans to affect and damage the environment. Water supplies are being depleted; landfills are filling up; toxic wastes threaten to contaminate both soil and water; and air pollution is altering the Earth's atmosphere and climate. Today there is a growing recognition that we hold the world in trust for future generations and for other forms of life. Our responsibility is to pass on an environment no worse—and preferably better—than the one we enjoy today.

Population Growth

The rapid expansion of the human population, particularly during the past 50 years, is generally believed to be responsible for most of the stress humans put on the environment. At the beginning of the first century CE, there were about 300 million people alive. By the seventeenth century, the world's population had gradually increased to 500 million. But then it started to rise exponentially, zooming to 1 billion by about 1800, to 2 billion by 1930, and then doubling again in just 40 years. The world's population, currently about 7.3 billion, is increasing at a rate of about 76 million per year—150 per minute. The United Nations now projects that world population will reach 9.6 billion by 2050.

The average number of children per woman fell from five in 1950 to half that (2.5) in 2017. This decline in fertility began in Western countries decades ago and is now also happening in poor countries. In sub-Saharan Africa, Asia, and Latin America, women with more education have fewer children; these regions nevertheless contribute the most to population size. Changes are also projected for the world's age distribution. For the first time in history, there are more older people than young children. During the second half of the twenty-first century, the number of older persons (aged 60 years or more) will increase to almost 3 billion, while the number of children will decrease to 1.94 billion.

Although population trends are difficult to influence, many countries recognize the importance of population management. A key goal of population management is to improve the conditions of people's lives so they feel less pressure to have large families. Research indicates that improved health, better education, and increased opportunities for women in the economic, political, and social realms work together with family planning and improved access to effective contraception to cut fertility rates and uncontrolled population growth (see the box Checking Your Environmental "Footprint").

Take CHARGE

CHECKING YOUR ENVIRONMENTAL "FOOTPRINT"

Environmental health may seem like a global challenge, but each person has a unique impact on our planet's health. In fact, there are ways to measure the environmental impact of your individual lifestyle.

For an estimate of how much land and water your lifestyle requires, take the Ecological Footprint quiz at http://myfootprint.org. You can also determine your carbon footprint at the Global Footprint Network website (http://www.footprintcalculator.org/) or at The Nature Conservancy website (https://www.nature.org/greenliving/carboncalculator/index.htm?intc=nature.tnav.getinvolved).

Go online to take one or all of these quizzes and compare your results with the results of your classmates. Then identify ways you can reduce the size of your ecological and carbon footprints, both as an individual and as a class.

Air Quality and Pollution

Air pollution is not a human invention or even a new problem. The air is polluted naturally with every forest fire, dust storm, and pollen bloom, as well as with countless other natural pollutants. In addition, humans contribute the by-products of their activities to these natural sources.

Air pollution is linked to a wide range of health problems, with the very young and the elderly being among the most susceptible to its effects. For people with chronic ailments such as diabetes or heart failure, even relatively brief exposure to particulate air pollution increases the risk of death by nearly 40%. Recent studies have linked exposure to air pollution to reduced birth weight in infants, reduced lung capacity in teens, and atherosclerosis (thickening of the arteries) in adults.

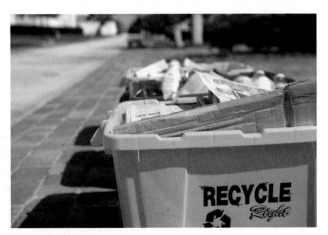

© Getty Images / Fuse

Recycling paper, cans, bottles, and plastics conserves resources, saves energy, and keeps large amounts of solid wastes out of landfills. Many communities have curbside recycling; others have drop-off sites.

Ask Yourself

QUESTIONS FOR CRITICAL THINKING AND REFLECTION

How often do you think about the environment's impact on your personal health? In what ways do your immediate surroundings (your home, neighbourhood, school, workplace) affect your well-being? In what ways do you influence the health of your personal environment?

Air Quality and Smog

Environment Canada uses a measure called the **Air Quality Health Index (AQHI)** to indicate whether air pollution levels pose a health concern. The AQHI is calculated based on the relative risk of the following three major air pollutants:

> **Air Quality Health Index (AQHI)**   A measure of local air quality and what it means for health.

- **Nitrogen dioxide (NO_2).** NO_2 is a reddish-brown, highly reactive gas formed when nitric oxide combines with oxygen in the atmosphere. Major sources include motor vehicles and power plants. In people with respiratory diseases such as asthma, NO_2 affects lung function and causes symptoms such as wheezing and shortness of breath. Exposure to NO_2 may also increase the risk of respiratory infections.

- **Particulate matter (PM).** Particles of different sizes are released into the atmosphere from a variety of sources, including combustion of **fossil fuels**, crushing or grinding operations, industrial processes, and dust from roadways. PM can accumulate in the respiratory system, aggravate cardiovascular and lung diseases, and increase the risk of respiratory infections.

> **fossil fuels**   Buried deposits of decayed animals and plants that are converted into carbon-rich fuels by exposure to heat and pressure over millions of years; oil, coal, and natural gas are fossil fuels.

- **Ground-level ozone (O_3).** At ground level, O_3 is a harmful pollutant. Where it occurs naturally in the upper atmosphere, it shields the Earth from the sun's harmful ultraviolet rays. (The health hazards from the thinning of this protective ozone layer are discussed later in the chapter.) O_3 is formed when pollutants emitted by cars, power plants, industrial plants, and other sources react chemically in the presence of sunlight (photochemical reactions). It can irritate the respiratory system, reduce lung function, aggravate asthma, increase susceptibility to respiratory infections, and damage the lining of the lungs. Short-term elevations of O_3 levels have also been linked to increased death rates.

AQHI is measured on a scale from 1 to 10+; the higher the AQHI, the greater the level of pollution and associated health danger. When the AQHI exceeds 10, air quality is considered to be a very high health risk—at first for certain sensitive groups of people and then for everyone as AQHI values get higher. Local AQHI information is often available in newspapers, on television and radio, and on the Internet (http://www.ec.gc.ca/cas-aqhi/).

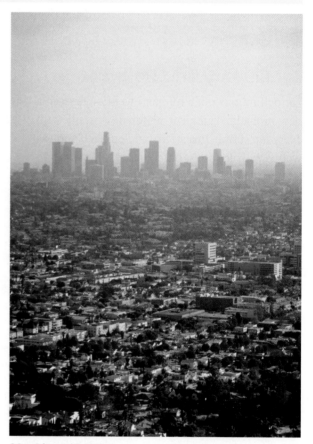

© Izzy Schwartz / Getty Images

Smog tends to form over cities because of geographical features and because of the tremendous amount of motor vehicle exhaust in the air.

The term **smog** was first used in the early 1900s in London to describe the combination of smoke and fog. What we typically call smog today is a mixture of pollutants, with ground-level ozone being the key ingredient. Major smog occurrences are linked to the combination of several factors: Heavy motor vehicle traffic, high temperatures, and sunny weather can increase the production of ozone. Pollutants are also more likely to build up in areas with little wind and/or where a topographic feature such as a mountain range or valley prevents the wind from pushing out stagnant air.

smog Hazy atmospheric conditions resulting from increased concentrations of ground-level ozone and other pollutants.

Fitness Tip

Exercising in polluted outdoor air can actually reduce lung function, at least temporarily. When the air quality outside is bad, exercise indoors.

The Greenhouse Effect and Global Warming

The temperature of the Earth's atmosphere depends on the balance between the amount of energy the planet absorbs from the sun (mainly as high-energy ultraviolet radiation) and the amount of energy radiated back into space as lower-energy infrared radiation. Key components of temperature regulation are carbon dioxide, water vapour, methane, and other **greenhouse gases**—so named because, like the glass panes in a greenhouse, they let through visible light from the sun but trap some of the resulting infrared radiation and re-radiate it back to the Earth's surface. This re-radiation causes a buildup of heat that raises the temperature of the lower atmosphere, a natural process known as the **greenhouse effect**. Without it, the atmosphere would be far cooler and much more hostile to life.

greenhouse gas A gas (such as carbon dioxide) or vapour that traps infrared radiation instead of allowing it to escape through the atmosphere, resulting in a warming of the Earth (the *greenhouse effect*).
greenhouse effect A warming of the Earth due to a buildup of greenhouse gases in the atmosphere.

There is scientific consensus that human activity is causing **global warming**, or *climate change*. The concentration of greenhouse gases is increasing because of human activity, especially the combustion of fossil fuels (see Table 13.2 on the next page). Carbon dioxide levels in the atmosphere have increased rapidly in recent decades. The use of fossil fuels worldwide pumps more than 20 billion tonnes of carbon dioxide into the atmosphere every year. Experts believe carbon dioxide may account for about 60% of the greenhouse effect. Analysis of ice core samples shows that carbon dioxide levels are now about 25% higher than at any other time in the past 650 000 years.

global warming An increase in the Earth's atmospheric temperature when averaged across seasons and geographical regions; also called *climate change*.

TABLE 13.2

Sources of Greenhouse Gases

Greenhouse Gas	Sources
Carbon dioxide	Fossil fuel and wood burning, factory emissions, car exhaust, deforestation
Chlorofluorocarbons (CFCs)	Refrigeration and air conditioning, aerosols, foam products, solvents
Methane	Cattle, wetlands, rice paddies, landfills, gas leaks, coal and gas industries
Nitrous oxide	Fertilizers, soil cultivation, deforestation, animal feedlots and wastes
Ozone and other trace gases	Photochemical reactions, car exhaust, power plant emissions, solvents

As consumers, we can all participate in the reduction of global warming and the greenhouse effect by doing the following:

- Reduce waste, recycle, and use reusable products instead of disposables.

- Drive less (e.g., walk or cycle) or drive smarter (e.g., use hybrid vehicles, properly inflate tires).

- Use the "off" switch on lights and electronics when they aren't in use.

- Use less (e.g., less heat, less air conditioning, less hot water) or buy energy-efficient products.

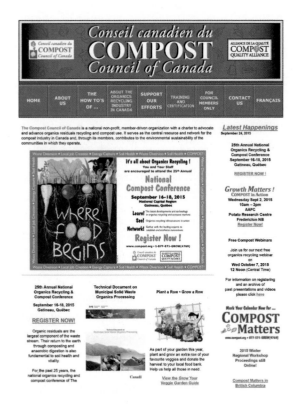

Composting is one simple but effective way to help protect the environment.

To date, 2016 was the warmest year on record since record-keeping began in 1880. The global temperature has risen more than 0.85°C (1.53°F) in the last century. There is agreement among scientists that temperatures will continue to rise, although estimates vary as to how much they will change. If global warming persists, experts say the impact may be devastating. Possible consequences include the following:

- Increased rainfall and flooding in some regions, and increased drought in others. Coastal zones, where half the world's people live, would be severely affected.

- Increased mortality from heat stress, urban air pollution, and tropical diseases. Deaths from weather events such as hurricanes, tornadoes, droughts, and floods might also increase.

- A poleward shift of about 80 to 560 kilometres (50–350 miles) in the location of vegetation zones, affecting crop yields, irrigation demands, and forest productivity.

- Alterations of ecosystems, resulting in possible species extinction.

- Increasingly rapid and drastic melting of the Earth's polar ice caps. Arctic ice melts to some extent during the summer each year, but melting has increased by 20% since 1979. Extensive melting could mean increased flooding in the Northern Hemisphere, further changes in weather patterns, and the elimination of habitats for species that live in the Arctic.

At the September 2014 United Nations Climate Summit, some groups endorsed the current scientific consensus that keeping the increase in global temperature below 2°C is necessary to stave off the worst effects of climate change. Although this conference did not end with a binding agreement among the world's nations, the parties did pledge to reduce greenhouse gas emissions.

Increasing research on climate change has revealed that significant amounts of greenhouse gases come from sources other than manufacturing industries. The United Nations has reported, for example, that raising cattle produces more greenhouse gases than driving cars.

Ask Yourself

QUESTIONS FOR CRITICAL THINKING AND REFLECTION

What are your views on the issue of climate change? Do you believe it is a real problem, or do you think it has been overly hyped by the media and some politicians and activist groups? How do you support your views?

Thinning of the Ozone Layer

Another air pollution problem is the thinning of the **ozone layer** of the atmosphere, a fragile, invisible layer about 16 to 50 kilometres above the Earth's surface that shields the planet from the sun's hazardous ultraviolet (UV) rays. Since the mid-1980s, scientists have observed the seasonal appearance and growth of a hole in the ozone layer over Antarctica. More recently, thinning over other areas has been noted.

ozone layer   A layer of ozone molecules (O_3) in the upper atmosphere that screens out UV rays from the sun.

The ozone layer is being destroyed primarily by **chlorofluorocarbons (CFCs)**, industrial chemicals used as coolants in refrigerators and air conditioners, as foaming agents in some rigid foam products, as propellants in some kinds of aerosol sprays (most of which were banned in 1978), and as solvents. When CFCs rise into the atmosphere, winds carry them toward the polar regions. During winter, circular winds form a vortex that keeps the air over Antarctica from mixing with air from elsewhere. CFCs react with airborne ice crystals, releasing chlorine atoms, which destroy ozone. When the polar vortex weakens in the summer, winds richer in ozone from the north replenish the lost Antarctic ozone.

chlorofluorocarbons (CFCs)   Chemicals used as spray-can propellants, refrigerants, and industrial solvents, implicated in the destruction of the ozone layer.

The largest and deepest ozone hole on record, measured at 29.9 million square kilometres, occurred on September 6, 2000. In 2014, the maximum size of the ozone hole was 24.1 million square kilometres, or the area of the United States, Canada, and Mexico combined. The Antarctic ozone layer likely will not return to its early 1980s state until about 2040 because of the long lifetimes of ozone-depleting substances in the atmosphere. As a result of an international agreement that regulates the production of ozone-depleting chemicals, overall atmospheric ozone is no longer decreasing. The gradual recovery is masked by annual variations caused by weather fluctuations over Antarctica.

Without the ozone layer to absorb the sun's UV radiation, life on Earth would be impossible. (UV radiation levels under the Antarctic ozone hole were high enough to cause sunburn within 7 minutes.) The potential effects of increased long-term exposure to UV light for humans include skin cancer, wrinkling and aging of the skin, cataracts and blindness, and reduced immune response. The United Nations Environment Programme predicts that a drop of 10% in overall ozone levels would cause a 26% rise in the incidence of nonmelanoma skin cancers. Some scientists blame ozone loss for many cases of melanoma.

UV light may interfere with photosynthesis and cause lower crop yields; it may also kill phytoplankton and krill, the basis of the ocean food chain. And because heat generated by the absorption of UV rays in the ozone layer helps create stratospheric winds, the driving force behind weather patterns, a drop in the concentration of ozone could potentially alter the earth's climate systems.

What Can You Do?

Faced with an array of complex and confusing environmental issues, you may feel overwhelmed and conclude that there isn't anything you can do. But in reality, you can take many actions to limit your negative impact on the environment and to promote environmentally sound practices in the social and political arenas. If everyone made even small changes in their life, the impact would be tremendous. Refer to the box What You Can Do for the Environment for actions you can take.

Assuming responsibility for your actions in relation to the environment isn't very different from assuming responsibility for your own health behaviours. It involves knowledge, awareness, insight, motivation, and commitment. You can use the same strategies that work to change personal health behaviours to change environment-related behaviours.

Take CHARGE

WHAT YOU CAN DO FOR THE ENVIRONMENT

- Ride your bike, walk, use public transportation, or carpool in a fuel-efficient vehicle instead of driving.
- Keep your car tuned up and well maintained.
- Make sure your residence is well-insulated.
- Use compact fluorescent light bulbs instead of incandescent bulbs to save energy.
- Buy energy-efficient appliances and use them only when necessary.
- Run the washing machine or dishwasher only when they have full loads.
- Buy products with the least amount of packaging you can, or buy products in bulk. Avoid disposable products. Buy recycled or recyclable products.
- Recycle newspapers, glass, cans, paper, and other recyclable items.
- Store food in glass jars and reusable plastic containers rather than plastic wrap.
- Take your own bags along when you go shopping.
- Dispose of household hazardous wastes according to instructions.
- Take showers rather than baths to save water.
- Install sink faucet aerators, water-efficient showerheads, and water-displacement devices in toilets.
- Don't let the water run when you're brushing your teeth, shaving, or hand-washing clothes or dishes.
- Buy products and services from environmentally responsible corporations. Don't buy products made from endangered species.
- Join or support organizations working on environmental causes.
- Vote for political candidates who support environmentally sound practices. Communicate with your elected representatives about environmental issues.

13.4 Fit and Well for Life

Adopting a wellness lifestyle is the most important thing you can do to ensure a high quality of life for yourself, now and in the future (see Lab 13.1 Looking to the Future: Your Values, Goals and Lifestyle for help in discovering what is important to you). The first chapter of this book described a behaviour change program that can be used to change problem behaviours and move toward wellness. Subsequent chapters have provided information on important areas of wellness—physical fitness, weight management, nutrition, stress management, cardiovascular health, and cancer. As you learned about these aspects of wellness and assessed your own status in relation to each of them, you probably identified personal behaviours that fell short of the ideal. Take the opportunity now (if you haven't already) to consider which of these behaviours you can begin to change. As you do so, let's review the basics of behaviour change, such as the following.

- Choose one behaviour to change at a time. Begin with something simple.

- Make sure your motivation and commitment are sufficient to carry you through to success. If they're not, review the health consequences of not changing this behaviour.

- Follow the five-step program outlined in Chapter 1: (1) monitor your behaviour and gather data; (2) analyze the data and identify patterns; (3) be "smart" about setting goals; (4) devise a plan of action; (5) make a personal contract.

- Build rewards into the plan.

- Make sure the new behaviour is enjoyable and fits into your routine.

- Get support from family and friends.

- Forgive yourself when you slip. Don't blame yourself or others or undermine yourself by feeling guilty.

- Expect to succeed. Use positive self-talk to create a new self-image—one that includes your new behaviour.

You live in a world in which your own choices and actions have a tremendous impact on your health. Don't let the broad scope of wellness be an excuse for apathy; instead, let it be a call to action. The time to start making changes in your lifestyle—to start becoming fit and well—is right now!

Tips for Today and the Future

On every level, from personal to planetary, we can all take an active role in shaping our environment and our level of wellness—now and in the future.

RIGHT NOW YOU CAN

- Determine which healthy aging behaviours you participate in and discover if you need to incorporate more.

- Research any alternative or complementary practice or product you are using to find out if it is considered safe.

- Turn the lights off in any unoccupied rooms. Turn the heat down a few degrees and put on a sweater, or turn the air conditioner off and change into shorts.

IN THE FUTURE YOU CAN

- Stay mentally challenged by taking up a new hobby (such as chess) or learning a new language.

- As your existing light bulbs burn out, replace them with compact fluorescent bulbs, which last longer and use much less electricity than standard incandescent bulbs.

- Have your car checked to make sure it runs efficiently and produces the least amount of emissions possible.

SUMMARY

- Many of the changes associated with aging are the result of an unhealthy lifestyle. There are many things you can do to prevent, delay, lessen, or reverse these changes.

- Managing your own health care involves identifying and managing medical problems and making the best use of the existing health care system.

- Self-care means knowing which symptoms need professional attention and understanding how to self-treat responsibly, with or without over-the-counter and prescription drugs.

- The best use of the health care system requires good communication with physicians and regular medical screenings. You need to use critical thinking skills when considering complementary and alternative therapies.

- Today's environmental health challenges include protecting the environment from the by-products of human activity. Overpopulation contributes to environmental problems, including pollution.

- Individual actions to minimize negative environmental effects can have a tremendous impact on air quality and smog, the greenhouse effect and global warming, and the thinning of the ozone layer.

FOR FURTHER EXPLORATION

Organizations and Websites

Active Aging Canada. Promotes a healthy lifestyle for older adults in Canada. Funded by Health Canada and the Public Health Agency of Canada.

> https://www.activeagingcanada.ca/

Alberta Centre for Active Living. Presents research and promotes a physically active lifestyle for all segments of the community.

> http://www.centre4activeliving.ca/

Canadian Centre for Activity and Aging. Focuses on enhancing the lives of Canadian adults from research to practice. Run through Western University.

> http://www.uwo.ca/ccaa/

Canadian Complementary Medical Association. Provides a network of Canadian physicians, residents, and medical students with an interest in complementary and alternative medical therapies.

> http://www.ccmadoctors.ca/

International Society for Complementary Medicine Research. Facilitates completion and promotion of research in the area.

> http://www.iscmr.org/content/incam/about-incam

Canadian Medical Association (CMA). Provides information about physicians, including their training, licensing, and board certification; also provides recent medical news, advice for consumers, and links to related sites.

> http://www.cma.ca

Many national and international organizations work on environmental health problems. A few of the largest and best known are listed below:

Greenpeace: http://www.greenpeace.org

National Wildlife Federation: http://www.nwf.org

The Nature Conservancy: http://www.tnc.org

Sierra Club: http://www.sierraclub.org

Laboratory Activities

Name _____ Section _____ Date _____

Lab 13.1 Looking to the Future: Your Values, Goals, and Lifestyle

connect

Your Values

1. List the personality traits or characteristics that you most value (e.g., friendly, patient, successful, outgoing, cooperative, loyal to family and friends, respectful of diversity). These can be characteristics of your own or of others.

   _____

   _____

   _____

2. List the activities and accomplishments that you most value(e.g., making lots of money, getting good grades, spending time with friends, making your own decisions). These can be accomplishments of your own or of others, or goals you have for the future.

   _____

   _____

   _____

Your Goals and Aspirations

1. Describe the person you want to become. What is the purpose of your life? What is its meaning? What are you trying to accomplish?

   _____

   _____

   _____

2. What significant goals have you yet to realize? These can be creating something or having a particular experience.

   _____

   _____

   _____

3. What can you do to help reach these goals and become the person you want to become? What would you most like to change about yourself?

   _____

   _____

   _____

4. What do you want your life to be like in 5 years? In 10 years? In 20 years?

   _____

   _____

   _____

Your Lifestyle

1. Keeping your values and goals in mind—along with what you've learned from this text about the effects of lifestyle on wellness—examine your current lifestyle. Are you doing everything you can now to enhance the quality of your life in the future? Does your current lifestyle reflect your values and goals? List 10 positive behaviours you engage in now that will help you maintain wellness throughout your life and achieve your goals (e.g., exercising regularly, taking a yoga class to manage stress, maintaining close relationships with family and friends, drinking alcohol moderately or not at all, not smoking, and always wearing a safety belt). Next to each behaviour, list how it helps you achieve wellness and your long-term goals.

_____

_____

_____

2. Next, list your current habits and behaviours that detract from wellness and may keep you from acting in accordance with your values and achieving your goals (e.g., if you smoke, you may not be able to participate in your favourite recreational activities as you get older; you may also find that smoking goes against your values because the habit has a significant amount of control over your daily routine—loss of control and freedom—and you negatively affect the health of those you care about by exposing them to environmental tobacco smoke).

_____

_____

_____

Lifestyle Management: Now and in the Future

1. Briefly describe the behaviour change plan(s) you worked on during this course. What behaviour(s) did you target? How successful was your program for behaviour change? Do you think you'll be able to maintain your healthier behaviour(s) in the future?

_____

_____

_____

2. How would you rate your wellness status now? Has it improved in recent weeks or months? Are you more aware of your behaviour and its effect on your level of wellness? Look back at the lab activities you completed for Chapter 1. Has your lifestyle improved? Have you moved up the wellness continuum? If you haven't already retaken some of the assessment lab activities, do so now to check your progress (see Appendix B).

_____

_____

_____

3. List several behaviours that could be targets for behaviour change in the future (see the list you prepared under item 2 in the previous section). Think about which of these behaviours you might want to try to change now. Begin working through the steps in Chapter 1 (and the Behaviour Change Workbook). Every positive change is a step toward wellness.

_____

_____

_____

Nutritional Content of Popular Food Items

If you are developing a behaviour change plan to improve your diet, or if you simply want to choose healthier foods, you may want to know more about the nutritional content of common food items.

Daily Food Items

You can track your daily food intake and calculate your nutrient intake from foods with Health Canada's Canadian Nutrient File (http://www.hc-sc.gc.ca/fn-an/nutrition/fiche-nutri-data/index-eng.php). This database lists foods by both description and nutrient content to give you as precise as possible a calculation of the types and quantities of nutrients you are consuming.

Apps such as eaTracker or MyFitnessPal provide mobile methods of keeping track of both your input and output on a daily basis. Check out these resources for efficient, fun ways to understand the foods you eat.

Fast-Food Items

Although most foods served at fast-food restaurants are high in calories, fat, saturated fat, cholesterol, sodium, and sugar, some items are healthier than others. If you eat at fast-food restaurants, knowing the nutritional content of various items can help you make better choices. Fast-food restaurants provide nutritional information both online and in print brochures available at most restaurant locations. To learn more about the items you order, visit the restaurants' websites. The following is a list of some common fast-food restaurants and URLs for accessing their nutrition guides:

- Arby's: http://cds.arbys.ca/pdfs/nutrition/Canada_Nutrition_July_2014.pdf
- Burger King: http://www.burgerking.ca/en/ca/menu-nutrition/lunch-and-dinner-menu-202/index.html
- Domino's Pizza: http://cache.dominos.com/ca021700/base/pdf/Canadian+Nutrition+Guide+Final+Secure.pdf
- KFC: http://www.kfc.ca/en/assets/pdf/KFC11834_NutritionalChart_Eng.pdf
- McDonald's: http://www.mcdonalds.ca/ca/en/food/nutrition_calculator.html
- Pizza Hut: http://www.pizzahut.ca/nutrition.aspx
- Subway: http://www.subway.com/en-ca/menunutrition/nutrition
- Taco Bell: https://www.tacobell.ca/assets/coupons/TB_REGULAR_MENU_NUTRITION_GUIDE_EN.pdf
- Tim Hortons: http://www.timhortons.com/ca/en/menu/menu-info.html
- Wendy's: https://www.wendys.com/en-us/nutrition-info

Monitoring Your Progress

Name _____ **Section** _____ **Date** _____

As you completed the 12 labs listed below, you entered the results in the Preprogram Assessment column of this lab. Now that you have been involved in a fitness and wellness program for some time, do the labs again and enter your new results in the Postprogram Assessment column. You will probably notice improvement in several areas. Congratulations! If you are not satisfied with your progress thus far, refer to the tips for successful behaviour change in Chapter 1 and throughout this book. Remember—fitness and wellness are forever. The time you invest now in developing a comprehensive, individualized program will pay off in a richer, more vital life in the years to come.

	Preprogram Assessment	**Postprogram Assessment**
LAB 2.2 Overcoming Barriers to Being Active	Key Barriers: _____	Key Barriers: _____
LAB 3.1 Cardiorespiratory Endurance		
1.6-km walk test	$\dot{V}O_{2max}$: _____ Rating: _____	$\dot{V}O_{2max}$: _____ Rating: _____
3-minute step test	$\dot{V}O_{2max}$: _____ Rating: _____	$\dot{V}O_{2max}$: _____ Rating: _____
2.4-km run-walk test	$\dot{V}O_{2max}$: _____ Rating: _____	$\dot{V}O_{2max}$: _____ Rating: _____
The beep test	$\dot{V}O_{2max}$: _____ Rating: _____	$\dot{V}O_{2max}$: _____ Rating: _____
12-minute swim test	$\dot{V}O_{2max}$: _____ Rating: _____	$\dot{V}O_{2max}$: _____ Rating: _____
LAB 4.1 Muscular Strength		
Maximum bench press test	Weight: _____ lb Rating: _____	Weight: _____ lb Rating: _____
Functional lower body strength tests	Weight: _____ lb Rating: _____	Weight: _____ lb Rating: _____
1. Chair squat	1. Rating: _____	1. Rating: _____
2. Single-leg step-up	2. Rating: _____	2. Rating: _____
3. Unweighted squat	3. Rating: _____	3. Rating: _____
4. Single-leg lunge squat with rear-foot support	4. Rating: _____	4. Rating: _____
5. Single-leg lunge squat from a bench preparation	5. Rating: _____	5. Rating: _____
Hand grip strength test	Weight: _____ lb Rating: _____	Weight: _____ lb Rating: _____

	Preprogram Assessment	Postprogram Assessment
LAB 4.2 Muscular Endurance		
Partial curl-up test	Number: _____ Rating: _____	Number: _____ Rating: _____
Push-up test	Number: _____ Rating: _____	Number: _____ Rating: _____
Squat endurance test	Number: _____ Rating: _____	Number: _____ Rating: _____
LAB 5.1 Flexibility		
Sit-and-reach test	Score: _____ cm Rating: _____	Score: _____ cm Rating: _____
Shoulder abduction	Right: _____ Left: _____	Right: _____ Left: _____
Shoulder adduction	Right: _____ Left: _____	Right: _____ Left: _____
Shoulder flexion	Right: _____ Left: _____	Right: _____ Left: _____
Shoulder extension	Right: _____ Left: _____	Right: _____ Left: _____
Trunk/low-back lateral flexion	Right: _____ Left: _____	Right: _____ Left: _____
Hip abduction	Right: _____ Left: _____	Right: _____ Left: _____
Hip flexion (bent knee)	Right: _____ Left: _____	Right: _____ Left: _____
Hip flexion (straight leg)	Right: _____ Left: _____	Right: _____ Left: _____
Ankle dorsiflexion and plantar flexion	Right: _____ Left: _____	Right: _____ Left: _____
LAB 5.3 Low-Back Muscular Endurance		
Side bridge endurance test	Right: _____ sec Rating: _____ Left: _____ sec Rating: _____	Right: _____ sec Rating: _____ Left: _____ sec Rating: _____
Trunk flexors endurance test	Trunk flexors: _____ sec Rating: _____	Trunk flexors: _____ sec Rating: _____
Back extensors endurance test	Back extensors: _____ sec Rating: _____	Back extensors: _____ sec Rating: _____
Front plank test	Plank: _____ sec Rating: _____	Plank: _____ sec Rating: _____
LAB 6.1 Body Composition		
Body Mass Index	BMI: _____ kg/m^2 Rating: _____	BMI: _____ kg/m^2 Rating: _____
Waist circumference	Circumf.: _____ Rating: _____	Circumf.: _____ Rating: _____
Skinfold measurements (or other method for determining percent body fat)	Sum of 3 skinfolds: _____ mm % body fat: _____ % Rating: _____	Sum of 3 skinfolds: _____ mm % body fat: _____ % Rating: _____
LAB 7.1 Daily Diet		
Number of servings	Milk products: _____	Milk products: _____
Number of servings	Meat and alternatives: _____	Meat and alternatives: _____
Number of servings	Fruits and vegetables: _____	Fruits and vegetables: _____
Number of servings	Grain products: _____	Grain products: _____

	Preprogram Assessment	**Postprogram Assessment**
LAB 7.2 Dietary Analysis Percentage of calories Percentage of calories Percentage of calories Percentage of calories	From protein: _____% From fat: _____% From saturated fat: _____% From carbohydrate: _____%	From protein: _____% From fat: _____% From saturated fat: _____% From carbohydrate: _____%
LAB 8.1 Daily Energy Needs	Daily energy needs: ___ cal/day	Daily energy needs: __ cal/day
LAB 10.1 Cardiovascular Health CVD risk assessment Hostility assessment	Score: _____ Estimated risk: _____ Score: _____ Rating: _____	Score: _____ Estimated risk: _____ Score: _____ Rating: _____
LAB 11.1 Cancer Prevention Diet: Number of servings Skin cancer	Fruits/vegetables: _____ Score: _____ Risk: _____	Fruits/vegetables: _____ Score: _____ Risk: _____
LAB 12.1 Identifying Stressors	Average weekly stress score: _____	Average weekly stress score: _____

Endnotes

Chapter 1

1. Statistics Canada. (2012). *Health-adjusted life expectancy, at birth and at age 65, by sex and income group, Canada and provinces, occasional (years)* (CANSIM Table 102–0122). Ottawa: Statistics Canada, 2012.
2. Canadian Institute for Health Information. (2013). Spending and health workforce. Available online at: http://www.cihi.ca/CIHI-ext -portal/internet/EN/SubTheme/spending+and+health+workforce /spending/cihi015954.
3. Colley, R.C., Garriguet, D., Janssen, I., Craig, C.I., Clarke, J., & Tremblay, M.S. (2011). Physical activity levels of Canadian adults: Accelerometer results from the 2007 to 2009 Canadian Health Measures Survey. *Health Reports, 22*(1).
4. Public Health Agency of Canada. 2013. Health Status of Canadians 2016: Report of the Chief Public Health Officer—What is influencing our health? - Physical activity. Available online at: https://www.canada .ca/en/public-health/corporate/publications/chief-public-health -officer-reports-state-public-health-canada/2016-health-status -canadians/page-13-what-influencing-health-physical-activity.html.
5. Public Health Agency of Canada (2003). Healthy Living Unit. Physical Activity for Health–The Evidence (online). Available online at: http://www.phac-aspc.gc.ca/pau-uap/fitness/evidence.html#1.
6. Twells, L.K., Gregory, D.M., Reddigan, J., & Midodzi, W.K. (2014). Current and predicted prevalence of obesity in Canada: A trend analysis. *Canadian Medical Association Journal*, 2 (1), E18–E26.
7. Canadian Centre on Substance Abuse. (2006). *The costs of substance abuse in Canada 2002: Highlights.* Ottawa, ON: Canadian Centre on Substance Abuse.
8. Physicians for a smoke-free Canada (2013). Tobacco use in Canada: Findings from the CCHS. Available online at: http://www.smoke -free.ca/factsheets/pdf/cchs/Canada-smokingratesbyprovince.pdf.
9. Health Canada. (2007). Reducing alcohol-related harm in Canada: Toward a culture of moderation. A report from the National Alcohol Strategy Working Group. Available online at: http://www .nationalframework-cadrenational.ca/uploads/files/FINAL_NAS _EN_April3_07.pdf.

Chapter 2

1. Canadian Fitness and Lifestyle Research Institute. (2008). Bulletin 09: Attitudes towards physical activity. *Physical Activity Monitor.* Available online at: http://www.cflri.ca.
2. Lee, C.D., Blair, S.N., & Jackson, A.S. (1999). Cardiorespiratory fitness, body composition, and all-cause and cardiovascular disease mortality in men. *American Journal of Clinical Nutrition,* 69(3): 373–380.
3. Thomas, D.Q., Kotecki, J.E., & McCormack Brown, K. (2006). *Physical activity and health: An interactive approach* (2nd ed.). Toronto: Jones & Bartlett.
4. McArdle, W.D., Katch, F.I., & Katch, V.L. (2007). *Exercise physiology: Energy, nutrition, & human performance* (6th ed.). New York: Lippincott Williams & Wilkins.

Chapter 3

1. Malina, R.M., Bouchard, C., & Bar-Or, O. (2004). *Growth, maturation, and physical activity.* Champaign, IL: Human Kinetics.
2. McTiernan, A., Yasui, Y., Sorensen, B., Irwin, M.L., Morgan, A., Rudolph, R.E., et al. (2006). Effect of a 12-month exercise intervention on patterns of cellular proliferation in colonic crypts: A randomized controlled trial. *Cancer Epidemiology Biomarkers and Prevention, 15,*1588–1597.
3. Bernstein, L., Patel, A., Ursin, G., Sullivan-Halley, J., Press, M.F., Deapen, D., et al. (2005). Lifetime recreational exercise activity and breast cancer risk among black women and white women. *Journal of the National Cancer Institute, 97*(22), 1–9.
4. Shang, M., Lee, A.H., & Binns, C.W. (2003). Physical activity and epithelial ovarian cancer risk: A case-control study in China. *International Journal of Cancer, 105*(6), 838–843; Fang, C.Y., Miller, S.M., Bovjerg, D. H., Bergman, C., Edelson, M.I., & Rosenblum, N.G. (2008). Perceived stress is associated with impaired T-cell response to HPV16 in women with cervical dysplasia. *Annals of Behavioral Medicine, 17*(1), 87–96.
5. Canadian Diabetes Association (2007). Think diabetes can't affect you because you're young? Available online at: http://www .diabetes.ca/getserious/facts.htm.
6. Persinger, R., Foster, C., Gibson, M., Fater, D.C.W., & Porcari, J.P. (2004). Consistency of the Talk Test for exercise prescription. *Medicine and Science in Sport and Exercise, 36,* 1632–1636.
7. Vetter, R.E. (2007). Effects of six warm-up protocols on sprint and jump performance. *Journal of Strength and Conditioning Research, 21*(3), 819–823.

Chapter 4

1. Heart and Stroke Foundation of Canada. (n.d.). Types and amounts of physical activities. Available online at: http://www.heartandstroke .com/site/c.ikIQLcMWJtE/b.3484261/.

Chapter 5

1. Kiblmer, W.B., Chandler, T.J., Uhl, T., & Maddus, R.E. (1989). A musculoskeletal approach to the preparticipation physical examination. *American Journal of Sports Medicine, 17:* 525–531.
2. Shrier, I. (2004). Does stretching improve performance? A systematic and critical review of the literature. *Clinical Journal of Sport Medicine, 14*(5): 267–273.
3. Gross, D.P., Ferrari, R., Russell, A.S., Battié, M.C., Schopflocher, D., Hu, R.W., et al. (2006). A population-based survey of back pain beliefs in Canada. *Spine, 31*(18): 2142–2145.
4. Shrier, I. (2004). Does stretching improve performance?: A systematic and critical review of the literature. *Clinical Journal of Sport Medicine, 14*(5): 267–273.
5. National Institute for Neurological Disorders and Stroke. (n.d.). Low back pain fact sheet. Available online at: http://www.ninds.nih.gov /disorders/backpain/detail_backpain.htm. Retrieved December 2011.
6. Church, J., Schneider, M., Shipka, P., Triska, O., Smith, D., Slater, L., et al. (2004). *Review of current knowledge on the effectiveness and cost effectiveness of treatments for low back conditions.* Edmonton, AB: Alberta Health Services Outcome Commission.
7. National Institute for Neurological Disorders and Stroke. (n.d.) Low back pain fact sheet. Available online at: http://www.ninds.nih.gov /disorders/backpain/detail_backpain.htm. Retrieved December 2011.

Chapter 6

1. Statistics Canada. (2014). Body mass index, overweight or obese, self-reported, adult, by sex, provinces and territories 2013. *Health Facts Sheets* (Statistics Canada, Catalogue 82-221-X). Available online at: http://www.statcan.gc.ca/tables-tableaux/sum-som/l01 /cst01/health82b-eng.htm.
2. Esmail, N., & Basham, P. (2014). *Obesity in Canada: Overstated problems, misguided policy solutions.* Available online at: http://www .fraserinstitute.org/uploadedFiles/fraser-ca/Content/research-news /research/publications/obesity-in-canada.pdf.

3. National Center for Health Statistics. (2006). 2003–2004 *National Health and Nutrition Examination Survey* (NHANES). Hyattsville, MD: National Center for Health Statistics.
4. Birmingham, C.L., Muller, J.L., Palepu, A., Spinelli, J.J., & Anis, A.H. (1999). The cost of obesity in Canada. *Canadian Medical Association Journal,* 160(4): 483–488.
5. Centers of Disease Control and Prevention. (2008). *Preventing Obesity and Chronic Diseases Through Good Nutrition and Physical Activity.* Available online at: http://www.cdc.gov/nccdphp/publications/factsheets/Prevention/obesity.htm.
6. Blackwell Publishing Ltd. (2007, March 12). Dialysis patients with metabolic syndrome show increased risk for heart disease. *ScienceDaily.* Available online at: http://www.sciencedaily.com/releases/2007/03/070307152542.htm.

Chapter 7

1. Garriguet, D. (2004). *Nutrition: Findings from the Canadian Community Health Survey.* Statistics Canada, Catalogue 82-620-MIE-No. 2.
2. Garriguet, D. (2004). *Nutrition: Findings from the Canadian Community Health Survey.* Statistics Canada, Catalogue 82-620-MIE-No. 2.
3. Health Canada. (2009). Food and nutrition: General questions and answers about trans fats. Available online at: http://www.hc-sc.gc.ca/fn-an/nutrition/gras-trans-fats/tfa-age_question-eng.php.
4. Health Canada. (2009). Food and nutrition: General questions and answers about trans fats. Available online at: http://www.hc-sc.gc.ca/fn-an/nutrition/gras-trans-fats/tfa-age_question-eng.php.
5. Health Canada. (2009). Food and nutrition: General questions and answers about trans fats. Available online at: http://www.hc-sc.gc.ca/fn-an/nutrition/gras-trans-fats/tfa-age_question-eng.php.
6. Health Canada. (2009). Food and nutrition: General questions and answers about trans fats. Available online at: http://www.hc-sc.gc.ca/fn-an/nutrition/gras-trans-fats/tfa-age_question-eng.php.

Chapter 8

1. Canadian community health survey: Adult obesity in Canada: Measured height and weight (2008, November 18). Statistics Canada. Available online at: http://www.statcan.ca/english/research/82-620-MIE/2005001/articles/adults/aobesity.htm.
2. National Center for Health Statistics. (2006). *Health, United States, with chartbook on trends in the health of Americans.* Hyattsville, MD: National Center for Health Statistics.
3. Roche Canada. (1997, December). Canadian national obesity survey. Toronto, ON: Pollara. Available online at: http://www.pollara.com/Library/News/news_1201.html.
4. King, S., & Hendricks, K. (2005, March). Addressing obesity and physical inactivity in Canadian children: National study shows it can be done. Available online at: http://www.activehealthykids.ca/Ophea/ActiveHealthyKids_v2/upload/Obesity-and-Physical-Inactivity.pdf.
5. Katzmarzyk, P.T., Gledhill, N, & Shephard, R.J. (2000). The economic burden of physical inactivity in Canada. *Canadian Medical Association Journal,* 163(11): 1435–1440.
6. Agras, W.S., Hammer, L.D., McNicholas, F., & Kraemer, H.C. (2004). Risk factors for childhood overweight: A prospective study from birth to 9.5 years. *Journal of Pediatrics,* 145: 19–24.
7. Gray-Donald, K., Jacobs Starkey, L., & Johnson-Down, L. (2000). Food habits of Canadians: Reduction in fat intake over a generation. *Canadian Journal of Public Health,* 91(5): 381–385.
8. Canadian community health survey: Adult obesity in Canada: Measured height and weight (2008, November 18). Statistics Canada. Available online at: www.statcan.ca/english/research/82-620-MIE/2005001/articles/adults/aobesity.htm.
9. Canadian community health survey: Adult obesity in Canada: Measured height and weight (2008, November 18). Statistics Canada. Available online at: www.statcan.ca/english/research/82-620-MIE/2005001/articles/adults/aobesity.htm.
10. Schwartz, J., & Byrd-Bredbenner, C. (2006). Portion distortion: Typical sizes selected by young adults. *Journal of the American Dietetic Association,* 106(9): 1494–1495.

11. Tjemkema, M. (2006). Adult obesity in Canada: Measured height and weight. Statistics Canada, Catalogue 82-620-MWE2005001.
12. Canadian Mental Health Association. (n.d.). About mental illness: Eating disorders. Available online at: http://www.cmha.ca/bins/content_page.asp?cid=3-98&lang=1.
13. Heweitt, P.L., Coren, S., & Steel, G.D. (2001). Death from anorexia nervosa: Age span and sex differences. *Aging and Mental Health,* 5(1): 41–46.
14. Canadian Mental Health Association. (n.d.). About mental illness: Eating disorders. Available online at: http://www.cmha.ca/bins/content_page.asp?cid=3-98&lang=1.
15. Hudson, J.I., Hiripi, E., Pope, H.G., Kessler, R.C. (2007). The prevalence and correlates of eating disorders in the National Comorbidity Survey replication. *Biological Psychiatry,* 61(3): 348–358.

Chapter 9

1. Conference Board of Canada. (2005). *Strengthening Canada: The Socio-economic Benefits of Sport Participation in Canada—Report August 2005.* Available online at: http://www.conferenceboard.ca/documents.aspx?did=1340.
2. Active Healthy Kids Canada. (2011). *Active Healthy Kids Report Card on Physical Activity for Children and Youth.* Available online at: http://www.activehealthykids.ca/ReportCard/2011ReportCardOverview.aspx.

Chapter 10

1. Heart and Stroke Foundation of Canada. (2015). Statistics. Available online at: http://www.heartandstroke.com/site/c.iklQLcMWJtE/b.3483991/k.34A8/Statistics.htm. Retrieved August 22, 2015.
2. Heart and Stroke Foundation of Canada. (2016). Stroke Report 2016. Available online at: http://www.strokebestpractices.ca/news-feature/stroke-report-2016-just-released/.
3. Linton, M. (2001). Healthy living a numbers game. Available online at: http://chealth.canoe.ca/columns.asp?columnsid=7&articleid=2387&relation_id=3224.
4. Canadian Stroke Network. (2007). Reducing salt intake would eliminate hypertension in one million Canadians. Available online at: http://ww2.heartandstroke.ca/Page.asp?PageID=33&ArticleID=6207&Src=news&From=Category.
5. Health Canada. (2007). Canadian Tobacco Use Monitoring Survey. Available online at: http://www.hc-sc.gc.ca/hl-vs/tobac-tabac/research-recherche/stat/ctums-esutc_2007-eng.php.
6. Statistics Canada. (2003). Community Health Survey (June 15, 2004). Available online at: http://www.statcan.ca/Daily/English/040615/d040615b.htm.
7. Physicians for a smoke-free Canada (n.d.). Tobacco and the health of Canadians. Available online at: http://www.smoke-free.ca/Health/pscissues_health.htm.
8. Hu, G., Sarti, C., Jousilahti, J., Silventoinen, K., Barengo, N.C., & Tuomilehto, J. (2005). Leisure time, occupational, and commuting physical activity and the risk of stroke. *Stroke,* 36: 1994–1999.
9. Grover, S.A., Coupal, L., Kaouache, M., & Lowensteyn, I. (2007). Preventing cardiovascular disease among Canadians: What are the potential benefits of treating hypertension or dyslipidemia? *The Canadian Journal of Cardiology,* 23(6): 467–473.
10. Public Health Agency of Canada. (1997). Heart disease and stroke in Canada. Available online at: http://www.phac-aspc.gc.ca/publicat/hdsc97/s06_e.html.
11. Grover, S.A., Coupal, L., Kaouache, M., & Lowensteyn, I. (2007). Preventing cardiovascular disease among Canadians: What are the potential benefits of treating hypertension or dyslipidemia? *The Canadian Journal of Cardiology,* 23(6): 467–473.
12. Public Health Agency of Canada. (1997). Heart disease and stroke in Canada. Available online at: http://www.phac-aspc.gc.ca/publicat/hdsc97/s06_e.html.
13. N.A. (2000). *First Nations and Inuit regional health survey: National report 1999.* St. Regis, PQ: First Nations and Inuit Regional Health Survey Steering Committee.
14. Sheth, T., Nair, C., Nargundkar, M., Anand, S., & Yusul, S. (1999). Cardiovascular and cancer mortality among Canadians of

European, south Asian, and Chinese origin from 1979 to 1993: An analysis of 1.2 million deaths. *Canadian Medical Association Journal*, 161(2): 132–138.

15. Heart and Stroke Foundation of Canada. (2003). *The growing burden of heart disease and stroke in Canada* 2003 (10896242 -30-8). Ottawa, ON: Author.

16. Heart and Stroke Foundation of Canada. (2003). *The growing burden of heart disease and stroke in Canada* 2003 (10896242 -30-8). Ottawa, ON: Author.

Chapter 11

1. Canadian Cancer Society. (2018). Available online at: http://www. cancer.ca/en/cancer-information/cancer-101/cancer-statistics-at-a -glance/?region=ab. Retrieved April 30, 2018.

2. Statistics Canada. (2008). Health Statistics Division, Leading Causes of Death, by sex, 2008 (Table 102-0561).

3. Prostate Cancer Canada. (2008). Statistics. Available online at: http://www.prostatecancer.ca/Prostate-Cancer/Prostate-Cancer /Statistics.aspx.

4. Enger, S.M., Geif, J.M., Polokoff, J., & Press, M. (2004). Body weight correlates with mortality in early-stage breast cancer. *Archives of surgery*, 139(9): 954–960; Bianchini, F., Kaaks, R., & Vainio, H. (2002). Overweight, obesity, and cancer risk. *The Lancet Oncology*, 3(9): 565–574.

5. Bianchini, F., Kaaks, R., & Vainio, H. (2002). Overweight, obesity, and cancer risk. *The Lancet Oncology*, 3(9): 565–574.

6. Canadian Cancer Society. (2018). Available online at: http://www .cancer.ca/~/media/cancer.ca/CW/cancer%20information/cancer%20 101/Canadian%20cancer%20statistics/Canadian-Cancer-Statistics -2017-EN.pdf?la=en

7. Statistics Canada. (2005). *Canadian Community Health Survey* (CCHS)–Cycle 3.1.

8. Statistics Canada. (2005). *Canadian Community Health Survey* (CCHS)–Cycle 3.1.

9. Canadian Cancer Society. (2011). *Canadian Cancer Statistics, 2011.* Available online at: http://www.cancer.ca/Canada-wide/Publications /Alphabetical%20list%20of%20publications/Canadian%20Cancer %20Statistics.aspx?sc_lang=en.

Chapter 12

1. Morrow-Howell, N., McCrary, S., Hong, S-I., & Blinne, W. (2008). *Experience Corps: Benefits of Volunteering* (CSD Research Brief 08-23). St. Louis, MO: Washington University, Center for Social Development.

Chapter 13

1. Eliot, R.S. (1995). From stress to strength. *Stress Medicine*, 11(1): 139–140.

2. Duxbury, L., Higgins, C., & Coghill, D. (2003). *Voices of Canadians: Seeking work-life balance* (Cat. No. RH54-12/2003). Hull, PQ: Human Resources Development Canada.

3. Crisis Intervention and Suicide Prevention Centre. Key suicide statistics. Available online at: http://www.crisiscentre.bc.ca/learn/stats.php.

Chapter 14

1. Martins, S.S., Tavares, H., Sabbatini da Silva Lobo, D., Galetti, A.M., & Gentil, V. (2004). Pathological gambling, gender, and risk-taking behaviours. *Addictive Behaviours*, 29(6): 1231–1235.

2. Responsible Gaming Council (2015). Canadian Gambling Digest: 2013-2014. Available online at: http://www.responsiblegambling

.org/docs/default-source/default-document-library/cprg_canadian -gambling-digest_2013-14.pdf.

3. Canadian Centre on Substance Abuse. 2018. *Canadian Drug Summary: Alcohol.* Available online at: http://www.ccsa.ca/Resource%20Library /CCSA-Canadian-Drug-Summary-Alcohol-2017-en.pdf.

4. Mann, R. (2008). Reducing alcohol-related deaths on Canada's roads. Presentation to the Standing Committee on Justice and Human Rights. Available online at: http://www.camh.net/Public _policy/Standing%20CommitteeImpaired%20Driving08.pdf.

5. Public Health Agency of Canada (2006). It's your health: Fetal alcohol spectrum disorder. Available online at: http://www.hc-sc .gc.ca/hl-vs/iyh-vsv/diseases-maladies/fasd-etcaf-eng.php.

6. Boffetta, P., Pershagen, G., Jockel, K-H., Forastiere, F., Gaborieau, V., Henirich, J., et. al. (1999). Cigar, pipe smoking and lung cancer risk: A multicenter study from Europe. *Journal of the National Cancer Institute*, 91(8): 607–701.

7. Boffetta, P., Hecht, S., Gray, N., Gupta, P., & Staif, K. (2008). Smokeless tobacco and cancer. *The Lancet Oncology*, 9(7): 667–675.

8. Physicians for a smoke-free Canada (n.d.). Tobacco and the health of Canadians. Available online at: http://www.smoke-free.ca/Health /pscissues_health.htm.

9. Health Canada (2007). Canadian tobacco use monitoring survey (CTUMS). Available online at: http://www.hc-sc.gc.ca/hl-vs/tobac -tabac/research-recherche/stat/index-eng.php.

10. Health Canada (2007). Canadian tobacco use monitoring survey (CTUMS). Available online at: http://www.hc-sc.gc.ca/hl-vs/tobac -tabac/research-recherche/stat/index-eng.php.

11. Crawford, J.T., Tolosa, J.E., Goldenberg, R. L. (2008). Smoking cessation in pregnancy: Why, how, and what next. *Clinical Obstetrics & Gynecology*. 51(2): 419–435.

12. Health Canada (2010). Canadian tobacco use monitoring survey (CTUMS). Available online at: http://www.hc-sc.gc.ca/hc-ps/tobac -tabac/research-recherche/stat/_ctums-esutc_2010/ann-eng.php#t6.

13. Health Canada (2010). Canadian tobacco use monitoring survey (CTUMS). Available online at: http://www.hc-sc.gc.ca/hc-ps/tobac -tabac/research-recherche/stat/_ctums-esutc_2010/ann-eng.php#t6.

Chapter 15

1. UNAIDS: Joint United Nations Programme on HIV/AIDS (2008). 2007 AIDS epidemic update. Available online at: http://www.unaids .org/en/KnowledgeCentre/HIVData/EpiUpdate/EpiUpdArchive/2007 /default.asp.

2. Public Health Agency of Canada Summary (2015) Estimates of HIV Incidence, Prevalence and Proportion Undiagnosed in Canada, 2014. Surveillance and Epidemiology Division, Professional Guidelines and Public Health Practice Division, Centre for Communicable Diseases and Infection Control. Available online at: http://www.catie.ca/sites/ default/files/2014-HIV-Estimates-in-Canada-EN.pdf

3. Rotermann, M. (2005). Sex, condoms, and STDs among young people. *Statistics Canada: Health Reports*, 16(3): 39–45.

4. Rotermann, M. (2005). Sex, condoms, and STDs among young people. *Statistics Canada: Health Reports*, 16(3): 39–45.

5. Rotermann, M. (2005). Sex, condoms, and STDs among young people. *Statistics Canada: Health Reports*, 16(3): 39–45.

6. Rotermann, M. (2005). Sex, condoms, and STDs among young people.*Statistics Canada: Health Reports*, 16(3): 39–45.

7. Public Health Agency of Canada (2017) Report on Sexually Transmitted Infections in Canada: 2013-2014. Available online at: https://www.canada.ca/en/public-health/services/publications /diseases-conditions/report-sexually-transmitted-infections-canada -2013-14.html.

Fit for Life: Index